£4.95

369 0276120

KU-407-175

Foundations of Clinical Nurse Specialist Practice

Janet S. Fulton, PhD, RN, ACNS-BC, Associate Professor, Indiana University School of Nursing, is the program coordinator for the Adult Clinical Nurse Specialist (CNS) major. She has many years of experience as both a CNS and CNS educator in the area of adult health with a focus in oncology. She is actively engaged in promoting the CNS role and practice nationally and internationally, having served as a member of the executive committee for the American Nurses Association Council of Clinical Nurse Specialists, president of the National Association of Clinical Nurse Specialists and coordinator of the CNS Specialist Interest Group for the Oncology Nursing Society. Dr. Fulton is currently the Editor of *Clinical Nurse Specialist: The Journal for Advanced Nursing Practice.*

Brenda L. Lyon, DNS, RN, FAAN, is a professor in the Adult Health Department at Indiana University (IU) School of Nursing and is a Fellow in both the American Academy of Nursing and the National Academies of Practice. Dr. Lyon has taught in the Adult Health CNS program at IU since 1971. She had a private practice as an adult health clinical nurse specialist in treating stress-related physical illnesses for over 25 years. In addition to serving in leadership roles in state, regional, and national nursing organizations, she is a founder and past president of the National Association of Clinical Nurse Specialists. She has authored over 45 articles and book chapters on the topics of stress, CNS practice, and regulation of CNS practice.

Kelly A. Goudreau, DSN, RN, ACNS-BC, is the director of education/designated learning officer at the Portland VA Medical Center. Dr. Goudreau oversees staff development at all levels in the organization, patient education, and academic affiliations that bring multidisciplinary students into the VA health care environment. She is involved in nursing initiatives at the local, state, and national level and is a past president of the National Association of Clinical Nurse Specialists and an associate editor of *Clinical Nurse Specialist: The Journal for Advanced Nursing Practice.*

Foundations of Clinical Nurse Specialist Practice

EDITORS Janet S. Fulton, PhD, RN, ACNS-BC
Brenda L. Lyon, DNS, RN, FAAN
Kelly A. Goudreau, DSN, RN, ACNS-BC

SPRINGER PUBLISHING COMPANY

New York

NATIONAL ASSOCIATION OF
CLINICAL NURSE SPECIALISTS

Springer Publishing Company, LLC
11 West 42nd Street
New York, NY 10036
www.springerpub.com

Acquisitions Editor: Margaret Zuccarini
Project Manager: Mark Frazier
Cover design: Steve Pisano
Composition: Apex CoVantage, LLC

Ebook ISBN: 978-0-8261-1068-8

09 10 11 12 / 5 4 3 2 1

The author and the publisher of this Work have made every effort to use sources believed to be reliable to provide information that is accurate and compatible with the standards generally accepted at the time of publication. Because medical science is continually advancing, our knowledge base continues to expand. Therefore, as new information becomes available, changes in procedures become necessary. We recommend that the reader always consult current research and specific institutional policies before performing any clinical procedure. The author and publisher shall not be liable for any special, consequential, or exemplary damages resulting, in whole or in part, from the readers' use of, or reliance on, the information contained in this book. The publisher has no responsibility for the persistence or accuracy of URLs for external or third-party Internet Web sites referred to in this publication and does not guarantee that any content on such Web sites is, or will remain, accurate or appropriate.

Library of Congress Cataloging-in-Publication Data

Foundations of clinical nurse specialist practice / editors, Janet S. Fulton, Brenda L. Lyon, Kelly Goudreau.
   p.; cm.
  Includes bibliographical references and index.
   ISBN 978-0-8261-1067-1 (alk. paper)
  1. Nurse practitioners. I. Fulton, Janet S. II. Lyon, Brenda L. III. Goudreau, Kelly.
   [DNLM: 1. Nurse Clinicians—organization & administration.
2. Nursing Process—organization & administration.
WY 128 F771 2009]
   RT82.8.F68   2009
   610.7306'92—dc22   2009029259

Printed in the United States of America by Bang Printing

Dedication

This book is dedicated to clinical nurse specialists everywhere. To those who preceded this work, we thank you for showing us the way. For our contemporary colleagues, we celebrate your dedication to creativity, leadership, and innovation. To future generations, we wish you success. May you grow in wisdom while carrying on a proud tradition of advancing the practice of nursing. We are proud to introduce this work in the year commemorating the 100-year anniversary of Hildegard Peplau's birth; Dr. Peplau being the creator of the first CNS program in 1954.

Contents

U N I T   I

THE NATURE OF CNS PRACTICE

U N I T   I I

DESIGNING AND EVALUATING NURSING INTERVENTIONS

U N I T   I I I

PROMOTING INNOVATION, CHANGE, AND DIFFUSION IN PRACTICE

U N I T   I V

DELIVERING CARE TO CLIENTS

U N I T   V

THE BUSINESS OF CLINICAL NURSE SPECIALIST PRACTICE

U N I T   V I

EXEMPLARS OF THE CLINICAL NURSE SPECIALIST ROLE IN A VARIETY OF SETTINGS

U N I T V I I

EXEMPLARS OF CLINICAL NURSE SPECIALIST PRACTICE IN A VARIETY OF SPECIALTY AREAS

Contributors

Carol Baird, DNS, RN
Associate Professor, Indiana University
School of Nursing
Indianapolis, IN

Nancy Benton, PhD, RN, CNS, CPHQ
Quality Management Officer, Department of
Veterans Affairs, Northwest Network VISN20
Portland, OR

Diane Billay, MN, RN
Doctoral Student, University of Alberta
Alberta, Edmonton, Canada

Janet M. Bingle, MS, RN
Chief Nursing Officer, Community Health Network
Indianapolis, IN

Leeann Blue, MSN, RN
Chief Nursing Officer, Wishard Health Services
Indianapolis, IN

Jane L. Bromund, MSN, RN
Clinical Research Scientist
Eli Lilly and Company, Indianapolis, IN

**Kathryn Ann "Katie" Brush, MS, RN, CCRN,
CCNS, FCCM (Deceased)**
Massachusetts General Hospital
Boston, MA

Garrett Chan, PhD, APRN-BC, CEN
Lead Advanced Practice Nurse, Emergency
Department, Stanford Hospital & Clinics and
Assistant Clinical Professor, University of California
Schools of Nursing and Medicine
San Francisco, CA

Kathleen M. Chapman, MSN, RN, NEA-BC, FACHE
Deputy Director/Chief Nurse Executive,
Portland Veterans Affairs Medical Center
Portland, OR

Victoria Church, MS, RN, CNS
Medical Surgical & Telemetry Program Manager,
Patient Safety Center for Inquiry,
Portland Veterans Affairs Medical Center, Portland, OR

Ann L. Cupp Curley, PhD, RN
University of Medicine and Dentistry of
New Jersey—School of Nursing
Newark, NJ

Sue B. Davidson, PhD, RN, CNS
Assistant Executive Director Nursing Practice
Education & Research
Oregon Nurses Association, Tualatin, OR

Tammie DiPietro, MN, RN
Doctoral Student, Lawrence S. Bloomberg Faculty
of Nursing, University of Toronto
Toronto, Ontario, Canada

Diane M. Doran, PhD, RN, FCAHS
Lawrence S. Bloomberg Professor in
Patient Safety, Lawrence S. Bloomberg Faculty
of Nursing, University of Toronto
Toronto, Ontario, Canada

Susan Dresser, MSN, RN, CCRN, CNS, APRN
Cardiovascular Clinical Nurse Specialist,
Deaconess Hospital
Oklahoma City, OK

Kathleen L. Dunn, MS, RN, CRRN, CNS
Clinical Nurse Specialist & Rehabilitation
Case Manager,
Spinal Cord Injury Center,
VA San Diego Healthcare System
San Diego, CA

Patricia R. Ebright, DNS, RN
Associate Professor, Indiana University
School of Nursing
Indianapolis, IN

Naomi E. Ervin, PhD, RN, APRN-BC, FAAN
Professor, Eastern Michigan University
School of Nursing, Ypsilanti, MI

Ginette G. Ferszt, PhD, RN, CNS-BC
Associate Professor, University of Rhode Island
College of Nursing
Kingston, RI

Mary L. Fisher, PhD, RN, NEA, BC
Associate Vice Chancellor for Academic Affairs,
Indiana University—Purdue University Indianapolis
and Professor, Indiana University School of Nursing
Indianapolis, IN

Frank D. Hicks, PhD, RN
Associate Professor, Rush University
College of Nursing Chicago, IL

Barbara Holmes Gobel, MS, RN, AOCN
Oncology Clinical Nurse Specialist,
Northwestern Memorial Hospital
Chicago, IL

Lisa Hopp, PhD, RN
Director, Indiana Center for Evidence Based Nursing
Practice: A Joanna Briggs Collaboration Center
Hammond, IN

Mary Pat Johnston, MS, RN, AOCN
Oncology Clinical Nurse Specialist, ProHealth Care
Regional Cancer Center,
Waukesha Memorial Hospital
Waukesha, WI

Diana Jones, MSN, RN
Clinical Nurse Specialist
St. Vincent Hospital, Indianapolis, IN

Jeffrey S. Jones, DNP, CNS, BC
Psychiatric Clinical Nurse Specialist,
Pinnacle Mental Health Associates, Inc.
Mansfield, OH

Robert Loo, PhD, CPsych
Professor of Management
The University of Lethbridge
Alberta, Canada

Pamela A. Minarik, PhD, RN, PMHCNS-BC, FAAN
Professor, Interim, Samuel Merritt College
School of Nursing
San Francisco, CA

Ann F. Minnick, PhD, RN, FAAN
Senior Associate Dean for Research and Julia Eleanor
Chenault Professor of Nursing,
Vanderbilt University
School of Nursing, Nashville, TN

Patricia S. Moore, MSN, RN, CNS, CDE
Director of Diabetes Education & Resource Center and
Diabetes CNS, Columbus Regional Hospital
Columbus, IN

Theresa Murray, MSN, RN, CCRN, CCNS
Critical Care Clinical Nurse Specialist,
Community Health Network, Indianapolis, IN

Florence Myrick, PhD, RN
Professor, University of Alberta
Alberta, Edmonton, Canada

Barbara S. O'Brien, PhD, RN
Assistant Professor, University of
Rhode Island College of Nursing
Kingston, RI

Patricia O'Malley, PhD, RN, CNS
Nurse Researcher, Miami Valley Hospital
Dayton, OH

Christine M. Pacini, PhD, RN
Director, Professional Development,
Research and Innovation,
University of Pennsylvania Health System
Philadelphia, PA

Geraldine S. Pearson, PhD, PMHCNS-BC, FAAN
Director, HomeCare Program,
University of Connecticut Health Center
Farmington, CT

Jeannette Richardson, MS, RN, CNS, CNRN
Critical Care Clinical Nurse Specialist
Portland Veterans Affairs Medical Center
Portland, OR

Jo Ellen Rust, MSN, RN, CNS
Clinical Nurse Specialist, Riley Hospital for Children
Indianapolis, IN

Maria R. Shirey, PhD, MBA, RN, CNAA, BC, FACHE
Principal Consultant, Shirey & Associates
Evansville, IN

Mary A. Short, MSN, RN
Clinical Research Scientist
Eli Lilly and Company, Indianapolis, IN

Souraya Sidani, PhD
Professor and Canada Research Chair,
Ryerson University School of Nursing
Toronto, Ontario, Canada

Kathleen C. Solotkin, MSN, RN
Medical Information Consultant
Eli Lilly and Company, Indianapolis, IN

Michelle Treon, MSN, RN, OCN
Oncology Clinical Nurse Specialist,
Indiana University Hospital, Indianapolis, IN

Kathleen M. Vollman, MSN, RN, CCNS, FCCM
Clinical Nurse Specialist/Educator/Consultant,
Advanced Nursing, LLC, Northville, MI

Kathy Wright, MSN, RN, CWOCN, AHRN, APRN
Regional Director of Clinical Services,
National Healing Corporation
Boca Raton, FL

Reviewers

Barbara Habermann, PhD, RN
Associate Professor,
Indiana University School of Nursing
Indianapolis, IN

Jan Powers, PhD, RN
Critical Care Clinical Nurse Specialist,
St. Vincent Hospital
Indianapolis, IN

Mary Beth Riner, DNS, RN
Associate Professor,
Indiana University School of Nursing
Indianapolis, IN

Mary Sitterding, MSN, RN, CNRN
Director, Nursing Practice Research & Innovation,
Columbus Regional Hospital
Columbus, IN

Diane Von Ah, PhD, RN
Assistant Professor,
Indiana University School of Nursing
Indianapolis, IN

The National Association of Clinical Nurse Specialists (NACNS) represents all clinical nurse specialists (CNSs) regardless of specialty or practice setting. Drs. Fulton, Lyon, and Goudreau have included information in this book that is applicable to the various specialties and settings in which the CNS practices and reflects the work of the CNS in today's health care environment. *Foundations of Clinical Nurse Specialist Practice* explains the basis for CNS practice from inception and Hildegard Peplau's concept of the CNS to the world of today, with a focus on quality, safety, technology, reimbursement issues, and financial constraints. Evidence-based practice, transformational leadership, and regulatory issues affecting CNS practice are other areas of focus of the book. The exemplars in Unit VI cite specific examples of the work the CNS does on a daily basis. Each project may have appeared to be a monumental task, but the CNS proceeded step by step until the final, quality outcome was achieved. NACNS is honored to support a comprehensive work of this magnitude that addresses the multiple facets of CNS practice.

Melanie Duffy, MSN, RN, CCRN, CCNS
President, NACNS

Preface

Clinical nurse specialists (CNSs) make unique contributions to the health and safety of the public by working directly and indirectly with patients, families, groups, and communities. These contributions often occur through clinical intervention and leadership at the point of nursing care delivery or by influencing factors that impact the point of delivery. CNSs are clinical experts in a delimited specialty area of practice, while also diffusing expert knowledge about phenomena central to nursing practice—such as pain, mobility, and skin integrity—that cut across specialties. CNSs help to shape specialty-focused practice innovations by identifying new or changing nursing care needs and by bringing new advanced nursing knowledge to well-established specialty practice areas.

Across diverse specialties, CNSs exhibit core practice competencies that cluster into three domains. The domains, also referred to as spheres of influence, are client, nursing practice/nurses, and system/organization. CNSs bridge the gap between what is known and what is practiced and collaborate in the removal of system barriers that impede the delivery of safe and cost-effective care. A wide range of knowledge is required to practice effectively in all three domains.

The inception of the National Association of Clinical Nurse Specialists (NACNS) in 1995 was a milestone in the continuing evolution of the CNS role and education. NACNS's mission includes making visible the unique contributions of CNSs to health care. Today, perhaps more than ever, the contributions of CNSs to quality, cost-effective patient care are vital. NACNS's curricular recommendations represented the first ever comprehensive overview of CNS educational program content. Prior to the recommendations, CNS educational programs varied based on specialty focus, local needs, and university/school considerations. The trend in textbooks was toward generic advanced practice, resulting in a lack of educational materials for CNS educators and students.

The book is written as a textbook to be used in the education of CNSs and the continuing development of practicing CNSs and is consistent with NACNS curricular recommendations. No one book can ever include the expanse of knowledge needed by CNSs. As editors, we included content believed to be core foundational knowledge for CNS practice, knowledge that will help CNS students and practicing CNSs achieve the core competencies. Unit I begins with an overview of the evolution of CNSs from the 1940s to present, setting the stage for understanding contemporary CNS practice. Also included are chapters describing the professional attributes of CNSs, the philosophical underpinnings of CNS practice, and nursing-sensitive outcomes. Units II, III, and IV include content supporting the *how* of CNS practice. For example, there are chapters devoted to clinical reasoning, designing and evaluating interventions, working in complex systems, influencing quality, and promoting patient safety. Unit V addresses the business of CNS practice, such as interviewing, entrepreneurship, billing and reimbursement, and understanding regulation. Unit VI includes exemplars demonstrating CNS practice in different settings—hospital, private practice, business and industry, and entrepreneurship ventures. The last unit, Unit VII, offers 10 short vignettes describing CNS practice in various specialties.

It is our fervent belief that the future of CNSs and CNS practice is bright and that the need for the unique contributions of CNSs will be increasingly in demand as hospitals and other health care settings are moved to performance-based reimbursement. We hope that faculty teaching in programs preparing CNSs, CNS students, and practicing CNSs will find this book to be a helpful resource.

Janet S. Fulton
Brenda L. Lyon
Kelly A. Goudreau

Acknowledgments

Many thanks are in order for making this book a reality. We are particularly grateful to Laura Parker, administrative assistant, for her steadfast support in coordinating the logistical, contractual, and structural elements necessary to move the work forward. Thanks to the staff at Springer Publishing, especially Margaret Zuccarini, acquisitions editor, for her guidance and support. Developing a book is, as we learned, a challenging and time-consuming process. We thank our colleagues in the nursing community for generously sharing their expertise as chapter editors and reviewers.

We would also like to thank our family, friends, and colleagues for their support in the long journey that is this book.

"Thanks to my family, husband, Morgan, and sons, Alexander and David, for their spirit, humor, and patience. You're the best. And to colleagues, faculty and staff."

Jan Fulton

"Thanks to my close CNS colleagues (Jan Bingle, Sue Davidson, Nancy Dayhoff, Lois Meier, and Kathleen Vollman) and to hundreds of CNS students who over the years have challenged me to both grow in the role and to help shape the evolution of CNS practice in the educational and regulatory arena."

Brenda Lyon

"Thanks to my husband, Serge, and my daughters, Kelsey and Christianne Goudreau, who had to wait as Mum went to 'go write and edit chapters' just one more day. Thanks also to all the CNSs whose thought provoking ideas have challenged and shaped my skills. You all have helped me to learn and grow in ways I would never have imagined."

Kelly Goudreau

The Nature of CNS Practice

Evolution of Clinical Nurse Specialist Role and Practice in the United States

Janet S. Fulton

Much has been written about the clinical nurse specialist (CNS) role beginning in the 1950s, yet CNS curricula are often void of content about the evolution of the role. The two most commonly used curricular recommendations for CNS programs—the *Statement on Clinical Nurse Specialist Practice and Education* (National Association of Clinical Nurse Specialists [NACNS], 2004) and *Essentials of Master's Education for Advanced Practice Nursing* (American Association of Colleges of Nursing [AACN], 1996)—are silent on the topic of history pertaining to the role. An electronic search of the Cumulative Index to Nursing and Allied Health Literature (CINAHL) database from 1981 (earliest date available for e-search) to 2008 found about 3,800 articles under the search term *clinical nurse specialist*. Earlier articles have been reproduced in books, and some significant works are available in JSTOR, a digital archive for scholarship. In exploring the evolution of the CNS's role and practice, it is important to consider the context of nursing in society as a major influence shaping the CNS role. For an expanded understanding, readers are encouraged to explore the historical references cited in this chapter and other related historical works.

EARLY HISTORICAL ROOTS

Evidence suggests that the idea for a clinical expert in nursing emerged in the 1940s and '50s. In the first textbook written for CNSs, *The Clinical Nurse*

Specialist: Interpretations by Riehl and McVay (1973), the editors suggested that the 1923 Winslow-Goldmark Committee report on nursing education, sponsored by the Rockefeller Foundation, set in motion events creating a need for clinical experts in nursing practice. Also called *The Study of Nursing and Nursing Education in the United States,* the report noted inadequacies in hospital nursing education and identified as a central problem the extended hours of service worked by students in the apprenticeship hospital training programs. A poor educational option, hospital training was made worse by lack of curricular standards, insufficient pedagogical knowledge among faculty, and inadequate instruction in the application of science and theory to practice (Bullough & Bullough, 1979; Ellis & Hartley, 2004; McHenry, 1983). As a result of these findings, nursing placed great emphasis on roles of teaching and administration in an effort to improve nursing education and clinical education experiences. Evidence of this focus can be seen in the preface to Wolf's 1947 textbook for nurses:

> The never-ending task of improving the quality of nursing practice falls squarely upon the shoulders of the teaching personnel in school of nursing and in public health nursing agencies. Those who are responsible for planning and providing the classroom and field practice experiences for nurse students are constantly striving to enrich these learning experiences and keep them in line with newer developments in the broad field of public health and preventative medicine. (p. v)

The 1948 release of Esther Lucile Brown's *The Future of Nursing* further reinforced the need to improve nursing education. Called the *Brown Report,* it also criticized hospital training programs and strongly advocated collegiate education for nursing. Less well identified with the report was Brown's observation about the overemphasis on teaching and administration at the expense of patient care. She called for increasing efforts to help students develop clinical knowledge and skill supporting direct care of patients; to better prepare nurses for care of persons both sick and well; and to teach scientific knowledge and create opportunities for students to apply knowledge in the care of patients. Nurses, Brown argued, needed to possess discriminative judgment and be able to exert leadership. Under leadership she included: (1) making a unique contribution to the prevention and treatment of illness; (2) improving nursing skills and developing new nursing skills; (3) teaching and supervising other nurses and ancillary workers; and (4) cooperating with other professions in planning for health at community, state, national, and international levels (Allen, Koos, Bradley, & Wolf, 1948).

In 1956, the National League for Nursing (NLN) sponsored the National Working Conference in Williamsburg, Virginia, to discuss the need for a psychiatric clinical expert (NLN, 1958). Against a backdrop of programs to train teachers and administrators, conference participants affirmed the need and determined that a new role should be created. The purpose of this new role, labeled *clinical specialist,* was "to bring about advances in the art and science of psychiatric nursing and to promote the application of new knowledge and methods in the care of patients" (NLN, 1958/1973, p.8). The final conference report included a description of clinical competencies for the new role and basic elements of a graduate-level curriculum to prepare nurses for the role.

Concerns about the lack of attention to developing clinical nursing experts continued. Appointed the first dean of the Graduate School of Nursing at New York Medical College, Frances Reiter became a leading voice for developing educational programs to prepare advanced clinical experts in many different specialty areas (Hiestand, 2006). Reiter's 1961 essay *Improvement in Nursing Practice* criticized hospital nursing service departments for devaluing direct patient care provided by the graduate nurses (*graduate nurse* being the term used for now registered nurses). She asserted that hospital nursing services were controlled by nurses who were not clinically skilled, but highly influenced by policies of hospital administration (Reiter, 1961). In addressing the American Nurses Association (ANA), she forecast a preferred future:

> I believe that some day an Academy of Nursing will be established. Membership in this academy will be an honorable one. The members will be selected from those practitioners who are clinical nursing specialists. Because of their values in practice, their clinical knowledge and their judgment, this corps of practitioners will give us professional leadership in advancing the excellence of our practice. (p. 18)

Reiter's goal as dean was to prepare a new kind of expert clinical nurse. In 1948, she had chaired the second of five studies funded by the W. K. Kellogg Foundation to develop teaching and learning experiences for nurses, the *Study of Advanced Clinical Nursing Education* (Hiestand, 2006). In 1966, she again called for a renewed emphasis on clinical practice and described an expert nurse-clinician. Reiter's expert nurse-clinician was a master practitioner for all dimensions of nursing practice—able to provide both basic and technical care while using discriminative judgment in assessing problems (diagnosis), determining care priorities, and selecting nursing measures (interventions) to achieve therapeutic objectives (outcomes). The expert nurse-clinician would possess sound knowledge of basic sciences and principles underlying care and would use this knowledge to promote quality of care and remove system-level barriers to care delivery. As she expressed it, the expert nurse-clinician would be "committed to 'hacking' her way down through the personnel pyramid so that her professional knowledge and judgment are exerted on behalf of every patient" (Reiter, 1966, p. 9). Further, the expert nurse-clinician's motivation, judgment, and expert nursing skills were envisioned to benefit patients both directly and indirectly because the visible expertise of this clinician was expected to provide leadership for the nursing staff in the delivery of patient care.

In summary, the early history of the CNS included a vision of a clinical role in nursing in response to a growing need for knowledgeable and skilled experts in the delivery of nursing care. An expert clinical nurse should be grounded in theory and scientific evidence, possess clinical skill, and be able to advance nursing care techniques, mentor nursing staff, assure excellence and quality, collaborate with other care providers, and remove system barriers to care delivery. This vision of the clinical expert created the CNS role.

THE CNS ROLE TAKES SHAPE

Although the psychiatric CNS is recognized as the first CNS specialty, the role of the CNS as a clinical expert was conceived before being linked to a specialty. *Role* is defined as expected functions of a person and is characterized by a pattern of behavior in a given social context. CNS is a functional role in nursing. The functional role is actualized through a set of professional practice competencies.

Not until 1998 were the common functional role competencies of CNS practice enunciated (NACNS, 1998). However, the establishment of the first-ever CNS core practice competencies relied heavily on a review of the literature (Baldwin et al., 2007). Multiple articles, beginning in the 1960s, helped to define and establish the core practice competences of the CNS role. Table 1.1 summarizes the role description and core competencies identified in the literature of the 1960s and early 1970s.

ADVANCED SPECIALTY PRACTICE

At the same time the CNS role was being conceptualized, specialization in health care was evolving and creeping into nursing practice. In 1949, the idea of specialization was introduced at a conference of graduate program directors convened at the University of Minnesota (Sills, 1983). In 1967, Little noted that specialization in nursing had moved well beyond the usual fields of practice (public health and hospital nursing) and the usual functions of teaching, supervision, and administration. Specialization was emerging in clinical areas based on body systems, age, type of illness, and scientific content areas. She conceded that specialization in nursing had indeed arrived.

The idea of specialty-focused practice for nurses was discussed in the very first issue of the *American Journal of Nursing* in an article by Katherine DeWitt (1900). In "Specialties in Nursing," DeWitt noted that nurses should be trained as generalists, and while she

 Summary of Selected Early Publications About CNS Role and Competencies Descriptions

DESCRIPTIONS OF CNS ROLE	DESCRIPTIONS OF CNS COMPETENCIES	YEAR	REFERENCE
Independent provider for continuity of care; clinical leader for nursing staff.	Explore and study (research) ways to improve patient care; understand patient needs; apply theory to practice; observe and report results objectively.	1964	Crawford
Independent clinician; model of expertness representing advanced or newly developing practices.	Clinical expert; develop innovations in practice based on emerging knowledge; interdisciplinary collaboration.	1965	Peplau
Expert nurse in direct care of patients; working with other nurses to improve performance.	Work with difficult patients; analyze needs; problem solve; interpret nursing care principles to nursing personnel.	1966	Anderson
Expert professional practitioner; assumes direct and continuing responsibility for nursing care of patients.	High levels of knowledge and cognitive ability demonstrated in practice; skilled decision maker; high level of ability in identifying patient problems and selecting intervention.	1967	Johnson, Wilcox, & Moidel
Professional nurse with advanced knowledge and competence in nursing.	Activities include many things: teaching, providing leadership in planning patient care, or exclusively practicing direct nursing care.	1968	Towner
A nurse who practices nursing by applying specific, relevant theories and knowledge from nursing and allied disciplines to person requiring specialized nursing services.	Deliver expert care; guide allied nursing personnel as teacher and model; innovate or initiate change; contribute to nursing knowledge through research and practice; coordinate activities with persons in allied disciplines; consult with those requiring clinical nursing judgment and knowledge.	1969	Berlinger
Expert nurse with definite responsibility for influencing patient care.	Uses a theoretical framework for change—one that allows for description and analysis of problems for organizing and interpreting what she perceives; brings about through conscious, deliberate, and collaborative effort the improvement of patient care.	1969	Gorden
Nurse with special preparation through education and experience to serve as expert practitioner and consultant.	Practitioner providing direct care; consultant directing, guiding, and assisting nursing staff to provide nursing care to patients; educator providing staff development to improve clinical competence; collaborates in initiating and facilitating patient care programs with health team members.	1973	Kurihara

saw no immediate need for specialists, she conceded that nurses could pursue specialty practice out of personal interest. DeWitt's comments were prompted by the turn-of-the-century emergence of specialties in medicine. Physicians were becoming more focused on medical practice; dentistry and pharmacology were becoming autonomous specialty practices and no longer services provided by the physician. DeWitt stated that when a nurse chooses a specialty, she (all nurses were referred to using the feminine pronoun in most early nursing literature) should engage in additional and continued studies in the specialty area and likewise should keep abreast of advances in science in the specialty. Her remarks indicate a belief that generalist education should precede specialty education.

Specialization is the mark of advancement of a profession (ANA, 1980; Snyder, 1990). In a landmark paper, Peplau (1965) discussed the nature of specialties in clinical nursing practice. She noted three social trends that gave rise to specialty practice: (1) increasing knowledge about a phenomenon, (2) new technology emerging from new knowledge, and (3) emerging areas of public need. The areas for specialty practice suggested by Peplau are summarized in Table 1.2. The suggested categories and examples were not intended to be either exhaustive or static, only suggestions based on Peplau's observation about nursing practice at the time.

Specialization is a division or partitioning of a more general area of practice along some logical lines. It involves a narrowing and deepening of focus or a recombination of aspects of different areas of knowledge and practice competencies with a simultaneous narrowing and deepening of focus (Peplau, 1965). Specialties are the inevitable result of new knowledge and demands of the public for new services (Smoyak, 1976). As such, specialties are adaptations arising in response to scientific and technological discoveries and continuously evolving to meet health concerns in a society. Specialties evolve and are refined, promoted, and molded. Specialties become outdated and are discarded. Most importantly, specialties are determined by society. Specialization gives nursing the ability to address the public's need for health services by expanding and contracting focus.

In discussing specialty practice, Peplau (1965) offered two cautions. The first caution addressed the growing complexity of health care delivery, particularly in post–World War II hospitals, which saw the emergence of multiple types of care providers. Peplau noted that "nurses must pinpoint intersecting, overlapping, and identical functions and activities which they share with other professional disciplines. *And nurses must identify their unique nursing functions*" (Peplau, 1965, p. 276, emphasis added). This caution echoes Brown's recommendation that nursing identify its unique contribution to patient care. Peplau was concerned that nurses not gravitate into practice areas and specialties where they would merely be duplicating the services offered by others. Peplau's second caution addressed keeping specialization efforts focused on developing *clinical experts* in patient care. Experts in the delivery

1.2 | Areas of Specialization Suggested by Peplau

AREAS OF SPECIALIZATION	EXAMPLES
Areas of practice	General hospitals, psychiatric hospitals, tuberculosis hospitals, mental retardation centers, industry
Organs and body systems	Cardiac, renal, and cardiac surgery
Age of client	Infant, premature infant, child, juvenile, adolescent, adult, and geriatric
Degree of illness	Progressive care, acute illness, convalescent care, and chronic illness services
Length of illness	Short-term (ambulatory), intermediate, and long-term
Fields of knowledge	Knowledge gives rise to new terminology, for example, nuclear nursing, interpersonal nursing, electronics nursing, and space nursing
Subroles of the work role of staff nurse	Mother-surrogate nurse, expert technical nurse, health teacher, nurse counselor
Professional goal	Rehabilitation nursing, prevention nursing, curative nursing, ameliorative nursing
Clinical services	Medical, surgical, maternal, pediatric, psychiatric-mental health

From "Specialization in Professional Nursing," by H. Peplau, 1965, *Nursing Science, 3,* pp. 268–287.

of patient care services, such as care coordinators or others with responsibilities for supervisory or administrative duties, were different from and should not be substituted for clinical experts in patient care.

Specialties ebb and flow, adapting to the availability of knowledge, advances in technology, and public health demands. Today, due to advances in antibiotic therapies, we don't need nurses specializing in tuberculosis hospital care as Peplau (1965) suggested. Similarly, Peplau could not have foreseen a need for clinical specialists in acquired immune deficiency syndrome (AIDS), a disease that was only described in the 1980s. It has been and remains the responsibility of CNSs, grounded in nursing theory, science, and use of evidence in practice, to interpret needs and bring nursing expertise to new and emerging specialties for the public good.

Defining Specialty Practice

In 1980, ANA defined specialization in nursing as "a narrowed focus on a part of the whole field of nursing. It entails application of broad range of theories to selected phenomena within the domain of nursing, in order to secure depth of understanding as a basis for advances in nursing practice" (p. 21). Currently, specialty is defined by the NACNS (2004) and the ANA (2004) as a delimited or concentrated area of expert clinical practice with focused knowledge and competencies. NACNS stated that specialties could be identified as population, type of problem, setting, type of care, or disease. The American Board of Nurse Specialties (ABNS) defined a specialty as: (1) a distinct and well-defined field of nursing that subscribes to the overall purpose and function of nursing and is national in scope, and (2) possessing a tested body of research or data-based knowledge related to the nursing specialty (Burns & Welk, 1997). ABNS criteria for a specialty fit a mature specialty, one that is linked to a professional association that sets standards and promotes activities to contribute to the conduct, review, and dissemination of knowledge in the specialty.

Styles (1990) pointed out that a single, central authority should be designated to recognize specialties and specialty standards to give nursing a source of authority for its specialties. Without a central authority in nursing, Style argued, specialties are self-declared and self-ordained, susceptible to internal fluctuations and disorganization, and vulnerable to outside forces competing for power and resources. In contrast, Snyder (1990) noted that because nursing is continuously developing its body of knowledge and is also part of a dynamic health care system and society, any organizing framework for specialization in nursing would be, of necessity, continuously evolving. At present, CNSs practice in small, emerging specialties and in well-established specialties attached to large professional organizations. Several specialty organizations have established scope and standards for CNS practice, such as the *Scope of Practice and Standards of Professional Performance for Acute and Critical-Care Clinical Nurse Specialist* (American Association of Critical Care Nurses, 2002) and the *Oncology Clinical Nurse Specialist Competencies* (Oncology Nursing Society, 2008).

A Model for Evolving CNS Specialty Practice

A three-stage model has been proposed to describe the evolution of advanced practice roles (Hanson & Hamric, 2003). According to Hanson and Hamric's model, in Stage I, a specialty develops in a practice setting. The specialty emerges in response to unmet needs in the health care system, particularly unmet patient needs, often involving activities not valued by physicians and not seen as a nursing role. Nurses in this stage attain on-the-job skills and expand practice to encompass these new skills. Clinical research coordinator is cited as an example of an emerging specialty currently in Stage I (Hanson & Hamric, 2003). In Stage II, organized training develops for the specialty. Training may be institution or agency specific and characterized as an apprentice model. Anesthesia, midwifery, and nurse practitioner are examples of specialties that began with training programs (Hanson & Hamric, 2003). In Stage III, graduate education with standardized curriculum emerges for the specialty. Salyer and Hamric (2008) add a fourth stage to the model; in Stage IV, the specialty is well-articulated and recognized by other providers, and certification exams are developed.

CNS role evolution does not fit well into Hanson and Hamric's model (2003). The CNS role emerged before specialty practice, conceived by nursing to address a void in clinical practice expertise in nursing and initiated with an expectation of graduate education. The emphasis on graduate education has been consistent since the earliest descriptions of the role and reinforced across the years. Nonacademic/nonuniversity–based training programs never existed for the CNS role. Certification options exist for some CNS specialties, but not all. A modified model of evolution for CNS role and practice would be as follows. Stage I, scientific discovery, knowledge, and technology create a public need for nursing services in a new area. CNSs practicing in related specialties pursue specialty knowledge from many sources; no one owns knowledge. Stage II, CNSs combine new scientific knowledge with existing clinical expertise and identify the level and type of nursing care necessary to meet the public need. Stage III, CNSs provide leadership to nursing services in the area by disseminating knowledge, role modeling, mentoring, and other activities.

CNSs develop norms and standards of care for nursing practice in the newly emerging specialty. Depending on the scope of the newly emerging specialty, CNSs may engage in developing and promoting specialty certification or other mechanisms to advance quality care for the patient population. For example, as patients were appearing with a yet undefined disease in the early 1980s, CNSs and other nurses with specialties in infection control, oncology, and palliative care began providing care for this group. AIDS was eventually described, a scientific literature amassed, professional organizations developed, and care standards established. A new specialty emerged based on public need.

The CNS role has a unique and rich history contributing texture and dimension in an ongoing evolutionary journey. For the CNS role, specialty practice represents an interpretation of nursing services into a discrete area of public need.

CNS EDUCATION

In 1943, the NLN appointed a committee to identify guiding assumptions and basic principles for developing clinical post-graduate courses (Mayo, 1944). One assumption set forth by the committee stated: "The fundamental purpose of all advanced clinical nursing courses is the further preparation of qualified graduate nurses as clinical nursing specialists in order to ensure a constantly improving quality of nursing practice" (Mayo, 1944, p. 581). As graduate education became available, very few nurses held bachelor degrees, and it was difficult to establish cohorts of baccalaureate-prepared nurses for master's level classes. Throughout the 1940s and '50s, diploma and bachelor prepared nurses often enrolled in the same courses; the only determinant of the degree granted was the degree held upon enrollment. Course content varied widely, and classes did not always contain theory and science. During this same time, specialty education was largely controlled by hospitals and used by administration to recruit nurses and manipulate the nursing workforce for hospital goals (Smoyak, 1976). Not until specialty knowledge (science and theory) was embedded in academic curricula did the reality of a graduate-prepared specialist as expert clinician emerge. The first graduate specialty program to prepare only CNSs as expert clinicians was the graduate program in advanced psychiatric nursing at Rutgers University in New Jersey. The design and delivery of the program as a specialty-focused graduate program was important because up to this point graduate courses included students seeking options in administration or teaching and were not necessarily always taught by faculty in the specialty or with an advanced degree (Smoyak, 1976).

Curriculum recommendations were developed for CNS educational programs but not formally organized as a standardized curriculum. The 1969 NLN report *Extending the Boundaries of Nursing Education* noted that the role should be flexible, but no single definition of the clinical specialist could be reached. A cluster of role components were identified and set forth: therapist/practitioner, teacher, consultant, researcher, and change agent. The therapist/practitioner component was a direct care provider in a specialty area of expertise and included assessment, interpreting cues (diagnosis), and intervention. The teacher component included one-on-one bedside work with staff nurses, formal (classes) and informal (in-service) staff development programs, assessment of staff competencies, interpreting the nursing literature, and building staff nurses' skills. The consultant component was linked to the ability to move about in the system—"unit to unit"—offering expertise and knowledge as needed and responding to calls by staff nurses for assistance in solving problems. For the researcher component, no description was included in the report. The change agent component is described as effecting changes in the system of delivering health care. The report emphasized placing a CNS in the clinical setting so she would be able to move about without interference while being an integral part of the staff because she would be able to identify staff needs and help then develop professionally. To prepare a graduate student to perform competently in the role components, four educational requirements were recommended. These requirements are listed in Table 1.3. In the same 1969 NLN report, Berlinger advocated four educational strands for all CNS education: the process of nursing, the process of clinical nursing specialization, the process of scientific investigation, and the process of communication. Further, she recommended that each student evolve a philosophy of nursing practice congruent with her philosophy of nursing and adopt or develop a conceptual framework for nursing practice. Clinical experiences in the specialty area were recommended for the purpose of knowledge of scientific investigation, critical analysis of current research, and the conduct of independent research as well as the care of patients in the specific specialty.

Descriptions of CNS curricula were published. For example, McIntyre (1970) listed five essential content areas underpinning the CNS program at the University of California—San Francisco: (1) intense study and experience with complex, specialized health problems; (2) opportunity to use advanced technology; (3) deliberative and continuous exchange with members of other health professions; (4) participation with members of the community in the improvement of nursing care; and (5) opportunity to identify the unknowns in care, including participation in research. Rhein (1973) outlined

1.3 | Early CNS Educational Requirements

EDUCATIONAL REQUIREMENTS

1. A broad base in the psychopathology and pathophysiology related to the clinical specialty. Even though the nurse planned to specialize in the nursing care of patient with neurological conditions, for example, her preparation should include a sound foundation in the whole medical-surgical nursing.

2. Knowledge and skills in the clinical practice of the specialty and in teaching and research.

3. The behavioral sciences essential to the leadership role and to prepare the person to be a change agent.

4. Knowledge and understanding of the social framework in which health care is given. Some participants felt that public health nursing concepts would be sufficient; others suggested a breadth of knowledge of social agencies and societal influences.

From (NLN, 1969, pp. 78–79).

the curriculum at University of California—Los Angeles, noting a strong emphasis on the care of patients and families with one academic quarter of introduction to clinical practice and two quarters of actual clinical practice. The focus of clinical was assessment, diagnosis, and planning interventions for patients within a philosophy-conceptual framework. Rubin (1969) reported implementing a specialty-focused PhD degree for maternity and pediatric nursing at the University of Pittsburgh.

The number of CNS programs began to expand after the Nurse Training Act of 1964 (PL 88–581), Title II of the 1968 Health Manpower Act (PL 92–158), and the Nurse Training Act of 1975 (PL 94–63; Hawkins & Thibodeau, 1993). In 1974–1975, the NLN reported 65 universities were offering master's programs in nursing. Of these, 90% offered some type of clinical focus. Program titles varied, making it difficult to distinguish the specialty focus and depth of clinical experiences (Smoyak, 1976). By 1984, the NLN reported 129 accredited programs preparing CNSs (NLN, 1984). In 2003, Walker and colleagues identified 157 separate CNS programs/majors offered by 139 different schools (Walker et al., 2003). In a national survey conducted several years later, Spross and colleagues reported a total of 215 schools self-reporting CNS programs/majors (Spross, Gerard, & France, 2006).

In the practice setting, the title of CNS was not always protected, and nurses not prepared in CNS graduate programs often assumed or were given the title *clinical specialist.* In 1980, the ANA published the first edition of its *Social Policy Statement,* recognizing the CNS as an expert clinician with a specialty focus and a graduate degree. This document helped further to entrench the criteria for CNS education.

The specialist in nursing practice is a nurse who, through study and supervised practice at the graduate level (master's or doctorate) has become an expert in a defined area of knowledge and practice in a selected clinical area of nursing. (ANA, 1980, p. 23)

While CNS education was available at the graduate level, CNS curricula varied by school and specialty. Throughout the 1980s and most of the 1990s, publications appeared discussing CNS education, but no organized effort existed to create national standards for CNS education. Schools relied on the NLN recommendations to guide curricula. Sills (1983) reported CNS graduate programs varying in length from 9 to 28 months with most programs taking 2 full academic years to complete. Some CNS programs were designated "clinical" options to distinguish them from administration and teaching options. Other CNS programs were linked to a specialty and had separate curricular tracks for each specialty. For example, at some point between mid-1970 and mid-1990, the University of Cincinnati College of Nursing offered distinct CNS specialty tracks for pulmonary, medical-surgical, burn-trauma, occupational health, gerontology, oncology, adult mental health, and child/adolescent mental health.

In 1996, the AACN published *The Essentials of Master's Education for Advanced Practice Nursing.* The *Essentials* recommended content to be included in advanced practice nursing curricula preparing clinical specialists, nurse midwives, nurse anesthetists, and nurse practitioners. In 1999, the National Advisory Council on Nurse Education and Practice (NACNEP), established by Title VIII of the Public Health Service Act to advise the Secretary on nursing workforce issues, completed a comprehensive report addressing federal support for the preparation of the CNS workforce. Among the recommendations, the report called for the federal government to support and encourage the profession's efforts to standardize requirements for educational preparation for core competencies of the CNS role. In 1998, NACNS published the first edition of *The Statement on Clinical Nurse Specialist Practice and Education*, which included both core practice competencies for the CNS role and recommendations for educational preparation of the CNS. In 2003, Walker and colleagues found that 56% of schools preparing CNSs used the NACNS recommendations to guide curricula. The second edition of the *Statement* was published in 2004 and again included core practice competencies and curricular recommendations. At this writing, NACNS has a national effort under way to move the recommendations to the level of curricular standards. Curricular standards are anticipated to help with more consistent competencies among graduates; however, a more prescriptive standardized curriculum is not envisioned because it could be constraining and may hamper CNS programs in respond to public needs for nursing care.

SUB-ROLES MODEL OF CNS PRACTICE

The CNS role components identified in the 1969 NLN report—therapist/practitioner, teacher, consultant, researcher, and change agent—continued to be cited in the literature in the 1970s. With slight variations, these role components became the unifying description of the CNS role. Throughout the 1980s, greater emphasis was placed on understanding the CNS role. Hamric (1983) noted that the change agent component involved a variety of indirect activities to improve care quality and suggested that the CNS role included both direct and indirect functions. Direct care functions included expert practitioner, role model, and patient advocate. Indirect care functions included change agent, consultant/resource person, clinical teacher, supervisor, researcher, liaison, and innovator. Hamric's 1983 observation was consistent with Reiter's 1966 vision of the CNS as engaged in both directly and indirectly contributing to patient outcomes. Further, Hamric (1983) described the CNS role as a constellation of sub-roles.

Well over 1,000 articles were published in the 1980s describing CNS practice in many different specialties and focusing on one or more of the role components. In 1986, the ANA Council of Clinical Nurse Specialists published *The Role of the Clinical Nurse Specialist*, which listed the dimensions of the CNS role as specialist in clinical practice, educator, consultant, researcher, and administrator. The administrator dimension was controversial; many authors argued against administrative functions, citing a move to a supervisory function over staff negated the clinical focus of the role. The ANA considered the administrator component optional and provided examples of the CNS assuming responsibility for direct care programs in the area of specialization and in situations for maintaining a direct client-based practice.

In further describing the CNS role, Hamric (1989) identified three foundational elements—primary criteria, skills and competencies, and sub-roles. Primary criteria were those conditions required for the role, such as an earned graduate degree in nursing with a focus on clinical practice, eligibility for certification by a professional society, and a practice focus on patient/client/family. Sub-roles were identified as expert practice, consultation, education, and research. Skills and competencies were identified as change agent, collaborator, clinical leader, role model, and patient advocate. The rationale for deciding to classify an item under competencies or sub-roles was not addressed. Nonetheless, by the end of the 1980s, the role components of expert clinician, educator, and researcher were solidified. Other role components frequently associated with the CNS role were consultant, collaborator, role model, and change agent.

The sub-roles description became a de facto organizing framework for the CNS role. Textbooks began to appear emphasizing the sub-roles. Hamric and Spross's 1989 book included chapters on the sub-roles, one each discussing direct patient care provider, consultant, educator, researcher, collaborator, and clinical leader. Sparacino, Cooper, and Minarik's (1990) book included a chapter on the role components—clinician, consultant, educator, researcher, administrator, and clinical leader. Gawlinski and Kern's (1994) text for CNSs in the critical care specialty was organized according to sub-roles and included sections on practitioner, educator, consultant, researcher, and leader/manager. Additional publications, articles, and books used the sub-roles framework.

At the same time, research about the CNS role was appearing in the literature. The methods and methodologies used for these studies helped codify the sub-roles by assuming a sub-role framework and designing instruments to collect data fitting each sub-role. Surveys often asked CNSs to identify the percentage of time spent in sub-role activities. An often expressed critique of this research was the conceptualization of role components as discrete entities when, in practice, the role was highly integrated.

Additionally, the distinction between sub-roles and clinical competencies is not clear. Practitioner, educator, researcher, consultant, collaborator, change agent, patient advocate, and leader are all expected professional competencies associated with nursing practice. These competencies exist on a continuum; the level of performance in the competency varies based on academic preparation and job role. All nurses provide clinical care, teach patients, collaborate, act as patient advocates, and so forth. For example, bachelor-prepared nurses engage in research activities, as do masters and doctorally prepared CNSs, albeit not at the same level. The sub-roles framework did little to distinguish the CNS from other nursing roles. What were not articulated in the sub-roles framework were the performance expectations—clinical competencies unique to the CNS role.

INTEGRATED MODEL OF CNS PRACTICE

Core CNS Practice Competencies

Finally, after many years of waiting, core competencies for CNS practice were identified in the 1998 publication of the NACNS *Statement on Clinical Nurse Specialist Practice and Education*. The development of the core practice competencies represented a rigorous process, including an extensive review of the literature, interviews of practicing CNSs and administrators, and a national external review (Baldwin et al., 2007). The final list of core competencies reflected CNS practice regardless of specialty. Following the release of the 2004 revisions of the *Statement*, a national validation study was conducted further demonstrating the validity of the core competencies for CNSs regardless of specialty (Baldwin, Clark, Fulton, & Mayo, 2009). At this writing, a third revision of CNS core practice competencies is undergoing review.

Domains of Practice

The core competencies represented a more integrated description of CNS practice. However, the competencies did cluster into domains representing consumers and stakeholders of CNS services. The domains were patient/client, nurses and nursing practice, and organizations and systems (NACNS, 1998). The domains were labeled s*pheres of influence* to denote the scope or breadth of practice activities and the target outcomes associated with a particular sphere. The patient/client sphere was identified as central, reinforcing the long-standing view of CNSs as clinical experts. The nurses and nursing practice sphere recognized the CNS practice involved in working one-on-one with nurses to deliver care and improving norms of care and standards that direct the actions of nurses and nursing personnel. The organizations/system sphere reflects the practice of CNSs in articulating the value of nursing care at the organizational level and influencing decision making at the system level to remove barriers and facilitate quality care and improved patient outcomes (NACNS, 2004). CNS role core competencies are actualized in specialty knowledge, standards, and skills, as demonstrated in Figure 1.1. Outcomes of CNS practice were also identified for each domain, demonstrating the link between CNS practice consistent with the core competencies and anticipated clinical outcomes.

This more integrated model of CNS practice, commonly referred to as the *spheres of influence* model, is

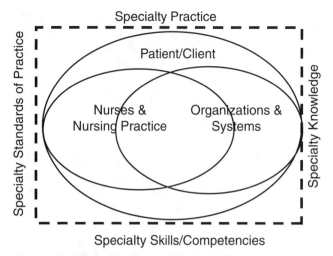

Figure 1.1   Clinical nurse specialist practice conceptualized as core competencies in three interacting spheres actualized in specialty practice and guided by specialty knowledge and specialty standards.
© J. S. Fulton 2004. Used with permission.

more descriptive of CNS practice than the previous sub-roles model. The addition of core competencies adds greater clarity to curriculum content because educators know the performance expectations of graduates. Identifying core competencies and expected outcomes also informs employers, the public, and other providers what to expect from CNS practice.

OPPORTUNITIES FOR THE FUTURE

The CNS is an expanded nursing role prepared at the graduate level, either master's or doctorate. CNSs acquire and apply scientific knowledge and skills for the purpose of meeting the public need for clinically expert nursing services with both newly emerging and established specialty populations. CNSs are leaders in providing innovative nurse-initiated interventions resulting in improved health outcomes for specialty populations. Through hundreds of articles about the CNS role and practice available in the professional literature, this consistent core representation of the CNS role and practice has emerged. It is curious, however, that so many publications include commentary noting CNS role ambiguity and a poor understanding of the CNS role by nurses, administrators, and other health care providers. Continued assertion about CNS role ambiguity is a curiosity given the many CNSs successfully practicing in the role and the many administrators supporting the role. With the focus of the CNS role on interpreting and advancing nursing practice, it seems likely that ambiguity about the CNS role is a reflection of a lack of clarity about nursing, nursing practice, and the unique contributions nursing makes to the public good. Understanding the CNS role and practice is tied inextricably to the ability to articulate the value of nursing. Lacking the ability to articulate nursing clearly, it becomes even more challenging to describe nursing practiced at an advanced level.

This is the dual challenge for CNSs in the future to continue moving forward with the advice offered by Brown (1948)—to clearly articulate the unique contributions of nursing to patient care, while describing, implementing, and evaluating nursing practice at an advanced level. It's difficult to manage what is not measured. CNS core competencies have been developed, and CNS practice outcomes described. The next decade should be dedicated to intense efforts to measure the outcomes of CNS practice, which will, in turn, demonstrate the value of nursing practiced at the advanced level. If CNSs successfully address the opportunity, much will be achieved for the benefit of our patients, their families, and general public welfare.

DISCUSSION QUESTIONS

1. Discuss the significance of collegiate education on the emergence of the CNS role. What social and/or professional influences surrounded moving nursing education from the hospital training program to university academic programs? How have these influences changed over time; are they similar or nonexistent today?
2. Discuss the development of a framework for the CNS role and practice. Identify themes in early descriptions of the CNS role that are present in the current integrated spheres of influence framework.

ANALYSIS AND SYNTHESIS EXERCISES

1. Clinical expertise in nursing practice is central to the CNS role and practice. Trace the development of a selected specialty practice. Explore the relationships among the specialty and scientific knowledge development, technological influences, and public need for nursing services.
2. Analyze trends in nursing that influenced development of nursing and the CNS role. The *American Journal of Nursing* is electronically archived in JSTOR and available through Google Scholar; explore this historical literature for influences on today's CNS role.

CLINICAL APPLICATION

Review the NACNS core practice competencies and outcomes. Identify methods for measuring outcomes related to CNS practice. Compare and contrast variations in methods and data needed to measure the same outcome in different specialties.

REFERENCES

Allen, R. B., Koos, E. L., Bradley, F. R., & Wolf, L. K. (1948). The Brown report. *American Journal of Nursing, 48*(12), 736–742.

American Association of Colleges of Nursing. (1996). *The essentials of master's education for advanced practice nursing.* Washington, DC: Author.

American Association of Critical-Care Nurses. (2002). *Scope of practice and standards of professional performance for the acute and critical care Clinical Nurse Specialist.* Aliso Viejo, CA: Author.

American Nurses Association. (1980). *Social policy statement.* Kansas City, MO: Author.

American Nurses Association. (2004). *Nursing scope and standards of practice.* Washington, DC: Author.

American Nurses Association, Council of Clinical Nurse Specialists. (1986). *The role of the Clinical Nurse Specialist.* Kansas City, MO: Author.

Anderson, L. C. (1966). The clinical nursing expert. *Nursing Outlook, 14,* 62–64.

Baldwin, K. M., Clark, A. P., Fulton, J. S., & Mayo, A. (2009). Validation of the NACNS Clinical Nurse Specialist core competencies through a national survey. *The Journal of Nursing Scholarship, 41*(2), 193–201.

Baldwin, K. M., Lyon, B. L., Clark, A. P., Fulton, J., Davidson, S., & Dayhoff, N. (2007). Developing clinical nurse specialist practice competencies. *Clinical Nurse Specialist, 21*(6), 297–302.

Berlinger, M. R. (1969). The preparation and roles of the clinical specialist at the master's level. In *Extending the boundaries of nursing education* (pp. 15–21). New York: National League for Nursing.

Brown, E. L. (1948). *Nursing for the future.* New York: Russell Sage Foundation.

Bullough, V. L., & Bullough, B. (1979). *Care of the sick: The emergence of modern nursing.* London: C. Helm.

Burns, K., & Welk, D. (1997). American Board of Nursing Specialties: Past, present and future. *Nursing Outlook, 45,* 114–117.

Crawford, M. I. (1964). Use of the clinical specialist. In *Blueprint for action in hospital nursing* (pp. 87–90). New York: National League for Nursing.

DeWitt, K. (1900). Specialties in nursing. *American Journal of Nursing, 1*(1), 14–17.

Ellis, J. R., & Hartley, C. L. (2004). *Nursing in today's world: Trends, issues and management* (8th ed.). Philadelphia: Lippincott Williams Wilkins.

Gawlinski, A., & Kern, L. S. (1994). *The clinical nurse specialist role in critical care.* Philadelphia: W.B. Saunders.

Gorden, M. (1969). The clinical nurse specialist as change agent. *Nursing Outlook, 17,* 37–39.

Hamric, A. B. (1983). Role development and functions. In A. B. Hamric & J. Spross (Eds.), *The clinical nurse specialist in theory and practice* (pp. 39–56). New York: Grune & Stratton.

Hamric, A. B. (1989). History and overview of CNS role. In A. B. Hamric & J. A. Spross (Eds.), *The clinical nurse specialist in theory and practice* (pp. 1–18). Philadelphia, PA: Saunders.

Hanson, C. M., & Hamric, A. B. (2003). Reflections on the continuing evolution of advanced practice nursing. *Nursing Outlook, 51*(5), 203–211.

Hawkins, J. W., & Thibodeau, J. A. (1993). *The advanced practitioner: Current practice issues.* New York: Tiresias Press.

Hiestand, W. C. (2006). Frances U. Reiter and the Graduate School of Nursing at the New York Medical College, 1960–1973. *Nursing History Review, 14,* 213–226.

Johnson, D. E., Wilcox, J. A., & Moidel, H. C. (1967). The clinical specialist as a practitioner. *American Journal of Nursing, 67*(11), 2298–2303.

Kurihara, M. (1973). A nursing care specialist in cardiopulmonary disease and medical intensive care unit. In J. P. Riehl & J. W. McVay (Eds.), *The clinical nurse specialist: Interpretations* (pp. 258–267). New York: Appleton-Century-Crofts.

Little, D. (1967). The nurse specialist. *American Journal of Nursing, 67,* 552–556.

Mayo, A. A. (1944). Advanced courses in clinical nursing: A discussion of basic assumptions and guiding principles. *American Journal of Nursing, 44*(6), 579–585.

McHenry, R. (1983). *Famous American women: A biographical dictionary from colonial times to present.* New York: Dover Publications.

McIntyre, H. M. (1970). The nurse-clinician—One point of view. *Nursing Outlook, 18*(9), 26–29.

National Advisory Council on Nurse Education and Practice. (1999). *Federal support for the preparation of the clinical nurse specialist workforce through Title VIII.* Department of Health and Human Services, Health Resources and Services Administration, Bureau of Health Professions, Division of Nursing. HRSA 99–40. Retrieved March 25, 2009, from: http://www.eric.ed.gov/ERICDocs/data/ericdocs2sql/content_storage_01/0000019b/80/16/36/30.pdf

National Association of Clinical Nurse Specialists. (1998). *Statement on clinical nurse specialist practice and education.* Harrisburg, PA: Author.

National Association of Clinical Nurse Specialists. (2004). *Statement on clinical nurse specialist practice and education* (2nd ed.). Harrisburg, PA: Author.

National League for Nursing. (1958). *Report of the National Working Conference: Education of the clinical specialist in psychiatric nursing.* New York: Author.

National League for Nursing. (1969). *Extending the boundaries of nursing education.* New York: Author.

National League for Nursing. (1958/1973). Report of the National Working Conference: Education of the clinical specialist in psychiatric nursing. In J. P. Riehl & J. W. McVay (Eds.), *The clinical nurse specialist: Interpretations* (p. 8). New York: Appleton-Century-Crofts.

National League for Nursing. (1984). *Master's education in nursing: Route to opportunities in contemporary nursing.* New York: Author.

Oncology Nursing Society. (2008). *Oncology clinical nurse specialists competencies.* Pittsburgh, PA: Author.

Peplau, H. (1965). Specialization in professional nursing. *Nursing Science, 3,* 268–287.

Riehl, J. P., & McVay, J. W. (1973). *The clinical nurse specialist: Interpretations.* New York: Appleton-Century-Crofts.

Reiter, F. (1961/1973). Improvement in nursing practice. In J. P. Riehl & J. W. McVay (Eds.), *The clinical nurse specialist: Interpretations* (pp. 9–18). New York: Appleton-Century-Crofts.

Reiter, F. (1966). The nurse-clinician. *American Journal of Nursing, 66,* 274–280.

Rhein, M. (1973). The education of the clinical specialist. In J. P. Riehl & J. W. McVay (Eds.), *The clinical nurse specialist: Interpretations* (pp. 131–144). New York: Appleton-Century-Crofts.

Rubin, R. (1969). Graduate programs in maternity and pediatric nursing leading to the degree of doctor of philosophy at the University of Pittsburgh. In *Extending the boundaries of nursing education* (pp. 22–27). New York: National League for Nursing.

Salyer, J., & Hamric, A. B. (2008). Evolving and innovative opportunities for advanced practice nursing. In A. B. Hamric, J. A. Spross, & C. M. Hanson (Eds.), *Advanced practice nursing: An integrative approach* (pp. 520–540). St. Louis: Saunders.

Sills, G. M. (1983). The role and function of the clinical nurse specialist. In N. L. Chaska (Ed.), *The nursing profession: A time to speak* (pp. 563–579). New York: McGraw-Hill.

Smoyak, S. A. (1976). Specialization in nursing: From then to now. *Nursing Outlook, 24*(11), 565–681.

Snyder, M. (1990). Specialization in nursing: Logic or chaos. In N. L. Chaska (Ed.), *The nursing profession: Turning points.* St. Louis: C. V. Mosby.

Spross, J. A., Gerard, P. S., & France, N. (2006). Directory of clinical nurse specialist programs in the United States, 2005. *Clinical Nurse Specialist, 20*(1), 34–48.

Sparacino, P. A. S., Cooper, D. M., & Minark, P. A. (1990). *The clinical nurse specialist: Implementation and impact.* Norwalk, CT: Appleton & Lange.

Styles, M. M. (1990). Clinical nurse specialists and the future of nursing. In P. S. A. Sparacino, D. M. Cooper, & P. A. Minarik (Eds.), *The clinical nurse specialist: Implementation and impact* (pp. 279–298). Norwalk, CT: Appleton-Century-Crofts.

Towner, A. M. (1968). No more supervisors? *Nursing Outlook, 16,* 56–58.

Walker, J., Gerard, P. S., Bayley, E., Coeling, H., Clark, A. P., Dayhoff, N., et al. (2003). A description of clinical nurse specialist programs in the United States. *Clinical Nurse Specialist, 17*(1), 50–57.

Wolf, L. K. (1947). *Nursing.* New York: Appleton-Century-Crofts.

Professional Attributes in the Context of Emotional Intelligence, Ethical Conduct, and Citizenship of the Clinical Nurse Specialist

Janet M. Bingle
Sue Davidson

Note to reader. The content of this chapter has provided the professional opportunity for reflection on our rich and extensive careers over a 45-year period in a continually changing context of nursing, health care, and society. In this reflection, we realize that there are different ways that the professional attributes discussed in this chapter have been acquired/developed or enhanced. A good part of this development did not occur in our various academic and professional practice experiences as CNSs, but rather, the development has occurred through interactions in life experiences that we regard as our personhood. There were times in this reflection that we were joyful and other times that we became sad or angry. This reflection has, however, made conscious our thoughts for your consideration, and our hope is that learning and growth will occur.

The context of the current health care system in the United States is one in which there is a level of conflict, a need for influence, and the requirement to deliver care. The student clinical nurse specialist (CNS) or practicing CNS stands at the intersection of practice and outcomes and in the initiatives shifting from process to outcomes. This is true not only in acute care but in every place in which health care and nursing care are provided. The essential characteristics of the student or practicing CNS that are described in the second CNS scope statement (National Association of Clinical Nurse Specialists, 2004) are: clinical expertise in the specialty; collaboration skills; leadership skills; consultation skills; *professional attributes,* including but not limited to honesty, integrity, emotional competence, a willingness for self review, and a value for diversity; *ethical conduct*; and *professional citizenship.* The professional attributes are embodied in the concept of emotional intelligence.

These seven essential characteristics are critical to the CNS's ability to influence in the absence of position or line authority. *Influence* is the power to produce desired effects or outcomes by moving others to action (*Webster's Dictionary of the American Language,* 1962; see also chapter 11). For a CNS to be effective in today's health care system, development of the essential characteristics is not a luxury but a requisite.

The characteristics taken together reflect a gestalt that is partly innate, partly developed, and continuously refined in the practice so that the CNS is growing and expanding his/her practice in these areas.

This chapter begins with an overview of the development of essential characteristics of the CNS. Then the professional attributes of the CNS are discussed in the context of emotional intelligence, followed by an overview of ethical conduct, including ethical principles and dealing with ethical dilemmas. The chapter concludes with an overview of professional citizenship including organizational citizenship. The three characteristics discussed in this chapter form the basis for other essential characteristics of the CNS, such as clinical expertise, leadership, consultation, and collaboration, which are addressed in other chapters.

DEVELOPMENT OF THE ESSENTIAL CHARACTERISTICS OF A CNS

The professional attributes, ethical conduct, and citizenship attributes are critical elements of CNS practice. Knowing where you stand with reference to them is critical in choosing to become a CNS, in learning to be a CNS, and in practicing as a CNS. (See Table 2.1.) The curriculum in a CNS program hones the intellectual abilities in mastery of the discipline of nursing and within a nursing specialty and assumes that these attributes are present. These attributes, however, require attention and development across the career because they are significant predictors of the success of the CNS in practice.

Undergraduate nursing education is designed to ensure that the graduate has competency and skill in the *caring* delivery of safe patient care as a generalist. Clinical practice experiences following completion of the program are assumed to enable the nurse to become competent in the delivery of specialized nursing care in a variety of settings to a specific population of patients, for example, oncology, critical care, mother/baby, and so on.

There is an assumption that intellectual development in courses combined with clinical experiences in the nursing program and the student's *intention to care for others* will be sufficient. Two factors suggest that this assumption is questionable. First, research has shown that emotional competency is critical to provision of caring assessment and intervention—the basis for nursing practice (McQueen, 2004; Porter O'Grady & Malloch, 2002). Such competency should be taught and can be learned. Secondly, evidence related to the presence of high turnover, burnout, de-energizing and/or reduced overall productivity of teams/units, reduced patient satisfaction, ineffective communication resulting in error and/or workplace injury, as well as horizontal violence in the workplace (nurse to nurse; Bartholomew, 2005, 2006; Robert, 1983) are problems that plague the nursing component in the health care system. Many of these situations are directly or indirectly linked to emotional intelligence, effective communication, and positive workplaces. The findings suggest that preparation of nurses in content related to emotional competency is needed (Cosby & Croskerry, 2004; Kerfoot, 1999, 2005; Lynch & Cole, 2006).

2.1 | Definitions of Selected Essential Characteristics and Professional Attributes of a CNS

ESSENTIAL CHARACTERISTICS OF CNS	DEFINITION
Professional attributes	Personal characteristics such as honesty, integrity, mastery in managing thoughts and emotions, positive self-regard and confidence, willingness to take risks, knowledge of one's own strengths and weaknesses coupled with openness to continued learning and development, self-review, willingness to solicit and accept peer review, ability to value and support diversity. Self-awareness Self-management Social awareness Relationship management (communication, negotiation, and team building)
Ethical conduct	Application of ethical principles to the identification and analysis of ethical dilemmas, and demonstration of decision making characterized by thoughtful consideration of multiple competing values in an ethical dilemma.
Professional citizenship	Awareness and action that is based on membership in the community of all CNSs, with rights and obligations to shape and influence the destiny of all CNSs.

If there is not an equivalent focus in the undergraduate and graduate nursing programs on the development of emotional competency as well as intellectual competency, the nurse may lack self-awareness, have self-doubt, and be unskilled or undeveloped in controlling their emotions, understanding patterns of behavior, and having organizational and political savvy (Arena & Page, 1992). A lack of emotional competency can have a significant impact on the nurse's ability to thrive and grow in the clinical practice of nursing. As an example, practice competencies of an experienced registered nurse (RN) and those of an experienced CNS with full role development are depicted in Table 2.2.

The preparation of the CNS must include content, experience, and self-assessment of emotional intelligence/competency, including understanding and dealing with stress emotions, relationship building, and citizenship in organizations and external entities. The CNS role includes expectations of emotional intelligence and emotional competency because the role is built on role modeling and persuasion and not line authority.

PROFESSIONAL ATTRIBUTES IN THE CONTEXT OF EMOTIONAL INTELLIGENCE

Why is there a need to describe professional attributes of the CNS? First, because these professional attributes link to competencies for effectiveness of the CNS in organizations (Goleman, 1998; National Association of Clinical Nurse Specialists [NACNS], 2004). Individuals who provide leadership in health care are judged by a different yardstick, not just by clinical expertise, but by how well they manage themselves and each other. New leaders are not predicted based solely on academic learning, but who has attributes and the personal qualities of initiative, empathy, adaptability, and persuasiveness (Skinner & Spurgeon, 2005). For example, in a national survey of employers, the skills, competencies, and attributes that were highly valued were not technical skills

 | Description of the Developmental Differences Between an Experienced RN and the CNS

DEVELOPMENTAL DIFFERENCE	REGISTERED NURSE	CNS
Focus	Within a specialty unit	Within specialty populations and organization/system
Clinical expertise	Competency and excellence with patients and families	Excellence with patient, families, and related system-level initiatives
System skills	Some	Role models skills to other nurses; coaches development of skills; collaborates with and provides consultation to other members of the health care team
Emotional competence	Varies from novice to expert given the variability in expectations for emotional competence in the practice	Expectation is for expert competence in self-awareness, resilience, handles difficult information, openness in thinking and feeling, open to differing viewpoints, active coaching and mentoring, well-developed impulse control (Porter O'Grady, 2002, p. 210).
Ethical conduct	Uses Code of Ethics for Nurses to guide practice; delivers care that preserves and protects patient autonomy, dignity, and rights; maintains patient confidentiality within legal/regulatory parameters; maintains therapeutic/professional patient–nurse relationship; contributes to resolution of ethical issues of patients, colleagues, and unit of work. Source: ANA, 2004	Involved in bioethics (patient, family) as well as organizational and business ethical dilemmas; educates others and has knowledge competency within the organization around ethical issues; informs patient of risks, benefits, and outcomes of health care regimens; participates in interdisciplinary teams addressing ethical risks and outcomes; leads ethics consultation and complete causal analysis of ethical dilemmas.
Professional citizenship	Varies from novice to expert, given the organization and the practice.	Meets expectations for strong stewardship/citizen of professional practice in an organization, within the specialty, and at the state and national level.

but competence in reading and writing, communication, interpersonal skills, and initiative (Goleman, 1998). Additionally, the general and specialty-based scope and standards of nursing practice presuppose these professional attributes (American Association of Critical Care Nurses [AACN], 2005; ANA, 2004, 2005; ANA Council of Clinical Nurse Specialists, 1986).

Professional attributes as described by NACNS (2004, p. 16) include "honesty and integrity, personal mastery in managing thoughts and emotions; positive self regard and confidence; willingness to take risks and be wrong, knowledge of one's own strengths and weaknesses coupled with openness to continued learning goals for development; self review and willingness to solicit and accept peer review, and ability to value and support diversity." These attributes collectively have been described in the literature in relation to emotional competence and emotional intelligence (EI) of the leader, in particular, the transformational leader (Beauman, 2006; Davidhizer, 1992; Gurka, 1995). Emotional intelligence is measured as emotional intelligence quotient (EQ). The emotional competency of the CNS is critical to personal and professional success and fulfillment. Although traditionalists in health care have often looked at this competency and EQ as the soft side of work, research evidence has emerged over the past decade to demonstrate the stunning interdependence between IQ and EQ (McKinnon, 2005). In fact, the attributes most coveted in many types of professionals and businesses are those of emotional intelligence (Goleman, 1998). Porter O'Grady (2003) points out that emotional intelligence is like other intelligences in that it provides the potential to learn, in this case, how to be emotionally competent.

Social intelligence, in which emotional intelligence has its roots, was first described by Thorndyke in the 1920s (McQueen, 2004). In the 1990s, this intelligence was further elucidated by Gardner, who spoke of *intra-* and *inter*personal intelligence, with *intra*personal intelligence being the knowledge of self and *inter*personal intelligence being the knowledge of self and others. Building on that work, the research and work of Goleman (1995, 1998) gave substance and definition to EQ so that its requisite skills and competencies could be elucidated and studied (Goleman, Boyatzis, & McKee, 2002). Goleman outlined four leadership competencies associated with EQ: self-awareness, self-management, social awareness, and relationship management. Each competency has subcompetencies that resonate with the professional attributes identified in the NACNS *Statement on Practice and Education* (2004).

Self-Awareness

CNSs must recognize their moods, emotions, and drives. They need to understand how these emotions affect others and their performance. This self-awareness requires disciplined inquiry into their personal thoughts and experiences. It requires deliberate analysis of their feelings and how these emotions drive thoughts and behaviors. Humans often have automatic reactions to certain interpersonal stimuli. These reactions may result from deep-seated assumptions that have taken root over time. Probably the best example of an automatic reaction can be seen when watching a group of cows head out to pasture. For whatever reasons, the cows always follow the same path. Day in and day out, they create the "cow path" for their route. Humans also create symbolic "cow paths" in their responses to certain situations (e.g., responses to failure or interpersonal conflict), thoughts, and emotions. The CNS needs to understand his/her "cow paths" in order to raise their self-knowledge and to have confidence in situations fraught with the various emotional triggers found in health care.

Self-Management

Self-management or self-control is critical to a professional who is immersed in daily conflict. The CNS, regardless of what sphere of influence they are functioning within, must remain clear-headed, exhibit composure, and find ways to steer the emotions to positive outcomes. Professionals with a high degree of self-regulation are transparent to others. Through personal disclosure, humor, and optimism, they are open to discussing their feelings and behaviors, receiving feedback, and experiencing personal learning. This transparency allows the individual to suspend judgment, assume accountability, and take the initiative to be solution-oriented. Self-management is critical to the CNS, who is expected to be the expert in situations that are loaded with intense emotions, a steep authority gradient, and unclearly defined outcomes. The self-confidence that comes with personal awareness and control gives the CNS the courage to navigate these critical dilemmas and create a model for how difficult situations are managed (Arena & Page, 1992; Kerfoot, 1999).

Social Awareness

The CNS is the role model for emotional competence. His/her EQ provides for social awareness, organizational savvy, and agility. Given high levels of empathy, CNSs are sensitive to a wide range of emotions from individuals, groups, and the organization as a whole. As they move through the organization, they cultivate relationships with diverse groups of professionals and clients. They can read the political climate at the time and accurately describe the emotional reality of the situation (Goleman et al., 2002). Social awareness implies engagement, availability, and service competence.

In this competence, there's a level of approachability that keeps the communication lines open, relationships intact, and social networks functioning.

Relationship Management

Relationship management is the fourth leadership competency associated with emotional intelligence, and it builds on the previous three competencies (Goleman et al., 2002). As Goleman describes the leader with relationship competency, he draws a clear picture of the transformational leader, in general, and the CNS, in particular (Institute of Medicine [IOM], 2004; see also chapter 5). This leader is inspirational, has power derived from his/her ability to influence, and is committed to the development of others. Because of these attributes, the leader is a trusted change agent skilled in conflict management and collaboration. Being able to effectively manage relationships to ensure desired outcomes is fundamental to the core competencies outlined in the *Statement on CNS Practice and Education* (NACNS, 2004). The CNS is expected to serve as a leader, consultant, mentor, and change agent among nurses and across systems. The role is also required to lead multidisciplinary groups and to establish and enhance collaboration with other disciplines to attain mutually agreed upon outcomes. These core competencies are essential for establishing and maintaining a highly reliable care delivery system and healthy work environment. Fundamental to these functions and outcomes, however, are effective communication and team building skills.

The communication skills of the CNS must be as proficient as the clinical skills. One's ability to effectively communicate creates the pathway to successful organizational change through influence and inspiration. The ability to articulate ideas, opportunities for improvement, and the mission, vision, and values inherent in those concepts and improvements requires a command of the language, knowledge of the power of linguistics, the ability to find the right appeal to a diverse audience, and the knowledge of how to build buy-in from key stakeholders. To be able to communicate a controversial, conflict-laden issue so that all participants can hear and become engaged in solution building is critical to CNS credibility and organizational success. As CNSs today become immersed in error management, root cause analysis, and sentinel event disclosure to professional as well as public audiences, skilled communication will be a required competency (Frankel, Leonard, & Denham, 2006). Through active listening, respectful interaction, and compassionate dialogue, trust is built so that crucial conversations can be had that result in learning and a safe, high-quality health care environment (Patterson, Grenny, McMillan, & Switzler, 2002). Conflicts and confrontations need to be managed effectively, keeping

them as part of a solution and not the focus of the problem or an issue to be avoided. Knowing how to language one's way through the confrontation is essential and often needs to be role-played or rehearsed so that all individuals emerge from the conversation intact and able to grow from the experience.

Another critical skill in managing relationships is the art of negotiation. Because the CNS brings together multiple disciplines to weigh in on a system issue or care improvement opportunity, there can be many lines drawn in the sand, none of which are connecting to a solution. These lines may be discipline-specific and compartmentalized, not system-focused and in alignment. Don Berwick, CEO for the Institute for Health Care Improvement, stated: "System-mindedness means cooperation. It means skills such as conflict resolution. It means asking yourself . . . not what are the parts of me, not what do I do, but what am I part of?" (IOM, 2003).

Berwick is talking about high levels of cooperation, coordination, and collaboration. The CNS, in leading multidisciplinary teams, is the catalyst for collaboration by helping members negotiate their differences and establish concessions without damaging relationships. The CNS needs to establish rapport and know how to find a common ground or platform on which all can agree. Storytelling, humor, self-disclosure, and a patient focus often allow the members to become grounded in the overall system and venture out of their specific paradigms. Successful negotiation can be thrilling for a CNS as long as he/she remains open to all possibilities and to the influence from others. Emotional intelligence and the competencies of self-awareness, self-management, and social awareness are critical to this process because the success of negotiating is more about the relationships than management of the deal itself. Many can relate to situations in which one has much time, energy, and emotional investment in an idea, policy and procedure, or plan for improvement. There is often fear and trepidation when bringing them forward for external or team review. One's emotional competency can wane as the critique becomes negative, and the desire to defend one's position inhibits the ability to listen, understand, and learn from the input. This is when the CNS needs to be at the top of his/her game in relationship management.

The ability to self-correct and take in the collective wisdom of the team is essential. To stop oneself from personalizing the feedback and focus on maintaining friendly collegiality is necessary for strong team building and collaboration. Keeping in mind there is no "I" in the word "TEAM," the CNS uses the words "we," "us," and "the team" when referring to results and outcomes of a particular initiative. Creating a collective identity drives cohesion in the group, which, in turn, facilitates high performance. Other characteristics of high-performing teams are they have a common vision, the members trust each other and will cover for each other, the members collectively have the talent to get the work done, and the team has the group skills to work effectively and efficiently. The CNS can create a spirit of innovation and experimentation in the team by communicating a learning attitude toward mistakes or failures. This type of team culture has fun while being highly productive. An atmosphere of learning, trust, and fun helps members develop into leaders. It also allows the CNS leader to coach and mentor through timely and effective feedback because the members feel safe and genuinely cared about.

The emotional competency of the CNS is critical to his/her success in the role. Both as a student and a practitioner, the CNS must conduct periodic self-reflection and seek structured feedback regarding one's emotional competence. Role-playing, improvisational theater, or simulation can provide great insight into one's self-awareness, social awareness, and self-management. Soliciting feedback from peers, coaches, mentors, and customers can facilitate this personal inquiry into how others perceive these competencies. Conducting a 360-degree feedback (Garmen, Tyler, & Darnall, 2004) and similar approaches give the CNS a well-rounded view from multiple, varied customers and lenses. Working on transparency through storytelling can help others to see the attributes that the CNS is working on and brings to each situation.

ETHICAL CONDUCT

Ethical conduct, an essential characteristic of the CNS, is embedded in beliefs and values. It involves application of knowledge related to ethical principles, analysis of situations that contain ethical dilemmas, and decision making in responding to these situations. Ethical conduct is based on the presence of emotional competency (self-awareness, self-management, social awareness, relationship competency) and knowledge of health care ethics and moral reasoning. It is also based on the foundational principles that the profession has articulated in two documents: the *Code of Ethics with Interpretive Statements* (ANA, 2005) and the *Scope and Standards of Nursing Practice* (ANA, 2004).

Code of Ethics

Nursing's ethical conduct is derived from universal principles of ethics (Edge & Groves, 1999; see Table 2.3). These principles include autonomy, truth telling, beneficence, nonmaleficence, confidentiality, justice, and role fidelity. The universal principles were the source for, and are woven into, the Code of Ethics for nursing.

Of the nine provisions of the Code of Ethics for nursing, three provisions address basic values and commitments of the nurse, three address duty and loyalty, and three address the health care environment and the nursing profession and its relationship to other health care professionals. For example, in the Code of Ethics, the nurse is expected to practice with compassion and respect for the dignity and worth of every individual unrestricted by status and personal attributes. This provision is linked to the ethical principles of dignity of all, respect for persons, and primacy of the interests of the patient. In the Code of Ethics provisions having to do with the boundaries of duty and loyalty, the nurse is expected to be responsible for his/her individual nursing practice and appropriately delegate consistent with the provision of optimum patient care. The associated ethical principles for these provisions are accountability and responsibility for nursing judgment, professional growth and maintenance of competency, and exercise of moral virtue and values. Finally, the Code of Ethics provisions having to do with duties beyond patient encounters are associated with advancement of the profession of nursing, responsibility to the public, conduct consistent with the profession, and intraprofessional integrity.

Conduct consistent with the Code is part of what it means to be a nurse, and such conduct is expected of all nurses regardless of level, role, or setting. The nurse commits to being reflective about his/her ethical conduct in practice situations. The Code of Ethics for Nursing is prescriptive and should be predictive of a nurse's ethical conduct.

The *Scope and Standards of Nursing Practice* "reflect the values of the nursing profession" (ANA, 2004, p. 1). One of the standards of professional performance of a nurse is to provide ethically sensitive care as described in this document.

These foundational documents of the profession of nursing lay the groundwork for ethical professional practice. Integration of these statements into practice behavior ensures ethical conduct at the level of the RN, an RN practicing in a specialty, and the CNS.

The setting of the practice of a CNS may be an office in which the CNS provides care independently or with other health care providers, in a business or the health care industry, within a health care organization, on a unit, a group of units, or all units where a particular population of patients exist, or less commonly, in a nonprofit organization related to health care or nursing. Regardless of setting, the CNS may recognize conflicts in care delivery that give rise to moral distress in nurses and present ethical dilemmas that may have implications for ethical conduct.

Various examples of ethical issues and dilemmas that may arise within components of the health care delivery and its associated management processes are illustrated here:

Universal Principles of Ethics and the Linkage to the Components of the Code of Ethics for Nurses

UNIVERSAL ETHICAL PRINCIPLES (EDGE & GROVES, 1999)		CODE OF ETHICS FOR NURSES (ANA, 2005)
Autonomy	Individual is free to choose and implement their own decisions. Includes the ability to decide, the power to act on the decision, and respect for the autonomy of others.	Respect for human dignity. Delivery of nursing with respect for human needs and value and without prejudice and irrespective of disease, disability, functional status, or proximity to death. Right of self-determination. Respect for all persons with whom nurse interacts.
Veracity (truth telling)	Applies to both patient and health care giver; patient must tell the truth so that appropriate care is given; provider discloses information so that patient can exercise personal autonomy.	Nurse's primary commitment is to patient (individual, family, group, community). Evaluate conflict. Collaboration. Maintain professional boundaries.
Beneficence	Action that benefits another, obligation to help, to promote health and welfare above other considerations. Means one ought to prevent harm or evil, ought to remove evil or harm, out to do or promote good.	Act on questionable practice(s). Accept accountability/responsibility. Be accountable in nursing judgments. Responsibility for nursing actions. Delegation of nursing activities.
Nonmaleficence	Ought not to inflict evil or harm.	Address impaired practice.
Confidentiality	Patient has the right to privacy regarding his own care program, treatments are conducted discreetly and confidentially, those not involved in the care must have permission to be present.	Privacy. Confidentiality. Protection of those in research projects. Standards and review mechanisms.
Justice	Equal distribution of scarce resources.	
Role fidelity	Individual must practice within the constraints of the role.	Moral self-respect. Professional growth and maintenance of competency. Wholeness of character. Preservation of integrity. Advance the profession through assertion of values, intra- and interprofessional integrity, social reform.

1. Conflicts over ownership and/or authorship of intellectual property and/or new products, or patient care process innovations; *Potential ethical issue/dilemma:* Justice, conflict of interest
2. Preeminence of personal versus institutional self-interest (Swidler, Seastrum, & Shelton, 2007); *Potential ethical issue/dilemma:* Justice, autonomy
3. Insufficient or underestimated resources to support care delivery that result in limitation or no access to care; *Potential ethical issue/dilemma:* Justice
4. Emergence of unintended consequences to redesign efforts; *Potential ethical issue/dilemma:* Beneficence, nonmaleficence
5. Practice outside of scope of practice; *Potential ethical issue/dilemma:* Role fidelity
6. Dishonest or deceptive interactions with patients, families, nurses, or others (Mohr & Mahon, 1996);

Potential ethical issue/dilemma: Role fidelity, truth telling, autonomy
7. Inability or unwillingness to provide the best-practice standard of care even though national guidelines for its use have been disseminated (Golomb, McGraw, Evans, & Dimsdale, 2007); *Potential ethical issue/dilemma:* Justice, beneficence/nonmaleficence, fidelity, autonomy
8. Presence of policies that deliberatively use the least experienced rather than appropriately experienced staff for nursing care delivery (Mohr & Mahon, 1996; Robert, 1983); *Potential ethical issue/dilemma:* Beneficence/nonmaleficence
9. Work environments where patients and the nurse are not treated with dignity and respect (AACN, 2005; Bartholomew, 2005); *Potential ethical issue/dilemma:* Respect, autonomy

10. Insufficient safeguards in clinical research projects with some patient populations (psychiatry, trauma) and in some clinical situations such as end of life (Curtin, 2007; Mohr & Mahon, 1996); *Potential ethical issue/dilemma:* Confidentiality, truth telling, beneficence/nonmaleficence
11. Conflicts in care management, such as futility of care, refusal of treatment, issue of second opinions; *Potential ethical issue/dilemma:* Justice, autonomy, truth telling, fidelity

Some researchers suggest that agreement over ethical issues and dilemmas varies between nurses who lead and nurses who deliver nursing care. A survey of nurse executives identified the failure to provide service of the highest quality in the eyes of the consumer, health care providers not employed by the organization, and by the purchasers of care (insurance companies) as being the most significant ethical issue they face, whereas staff nurses identified economic constraints and quality as the top issues (Cooper, Frank, Hansen, & Gouty, 2004).

DeWolf (1989) found in a study of medical surgical nurses that five precipitating factors were present before ethical issues arose to the unit-level discourse: (a) nurses experienced an emotional reaction and felt uncomfortable with a patient situation; (b) there was a sense of urgency with little time left to address the issue; (c) nurses personalized the situation and wondered how they would want to be treated if they were the patient, thus using the personal to act on the professional domain; (d) nurses recognized that a communication failure had occurred and information with which to make a decision was lacking; and (e) there was disagreement among the health care team regarding what should happen. These studies suggest that there was a lag between awareness of ethical dilemmas and action related to these dilemmas among staff nurses, or that there are varying skills/ability to articulate ethical dilemmas (Nelson, 2006). Alternatively, others suggest that, due to the demands of today's care environment, "fully capable health care professionals feel powerless and voiceless," even though they have awareness of ethical dilemmas and concerns (Austin, 2007).

Ethical problems, dilemmas, and issues arise when an individual perceives there is a conflict regarding the right thing to do (Bozek & Savage, 2007). The CNS may be among the first to recognize an ethical dilemma that is causing moral distress to him/herself, to staff nurses, and/or to other health care providers. Early recognition by the CNS of moral distress requires sensitivity, the ability to listen without judgment or premature closure, and maintenance of confidentiality of parties. Ethical conduct, demonstrated in any and all of the domains of CNS practice, includes direct and indirect actions based on the presence of "power, trust, inclusion, role

flexibility, and inquiry" (Wlody, 2007, p. S30). It means that the CNS thinks and acts, rather than retreats, in situations where there is moral distress and an ethical dilemma.

Examples illustrative of direct and indirect CNS ethical conduct include fostering truth telling in nursing staff in clinical situations with patients, families, and others; advocating for the rights of patients, families, and others, directly or indirectly; and participation in development and creation of protocols, policies, and/or practice guidelines that are consistent with ethical principles. It means the CNS supports identification, analysis, and response to ethical dilemmas that arise in the practice, rather than avoiding the issue. The CNS skilled in ethics and values clarification will demonstrate adherence to an appropriate and effective set of core values and beliefs during good and bad times, will act in line with those values, will provide constructive guidance to others in values clarification, and will seek alignment between ethical practices and the organization/setting and practice (Lombardo & Eichinger, 2006).

Roles of the CNS in Ethical Analysis and Reasoning

The CNS may be a catalyst for early identification of ethical problems through assisting nursing staff to address issues in rounds, report, in care conferences, and in dialogue with each other and other disciplines. The CNS may also act as an educator by ensuring that staff and patients and/or their families understand the issues, the language, and the options being discussed; this may occur by the CNSs leading or participating in an ethics consultation or conference. The CNS may lead or assist in clarifying assumptions that are impacting the ethical decision making of staff nurses and others. For example, the nursing staff may assume that there is limited time in which to consider the ethical dilemma, that ethical reasoning is relatively easy, that exploration of the ethical problem is unnecessary, and lastly, that the business of health care "trumps" the ethics of health care. The role the CNS plays in ethical analysis and reasoning will also depend on whether the ethical issue relates to the CNS's professional values, the patient's values, or the organization's (Bozek & Savage, 2007).

Ethical dilemmas are one type of conflict in care management. Conflicts in care management can arise from many sources, and confusion may exist about the root cause(s). For issues arising from questionable medical management, gaps in communication, legal issues, perceived harassment, and other conflicts, the resolution of conflict takes different paths, depending on the cause(s). If an issue is confirmed to be an ethical dilemma, it may be resolved through bedside consultation with members of the Ethics Committee, or, if the ethical dilemma is an issue of sufficient complexity and scope, resolution may take place in the Ethics Committee. The point is that conflicts in practice may have different root causes, some of which are ethical in nature. The CNS can be a valuable resource in clarifying the root causes in care management, thus enabling the organization to direct its resources toward the appropriate resolution of the dilemma (Community Hospitals Indianapolis, 1995).

Just as the root causes of conflicts in care management vary, so do frameworks for ethical reasoning. It is important that the CNS understand these various ethical frameworks because the individuals with whom they are practicing may see the dilemma and its solution from a unique, individual framework.

One framework for ethical reasoning comes from Kohlberg (1981) who studied decision making of adult males. He found that, in adults, abstract concepts such as justice, respect for the rights and dignity of others, equality, and one's own conscience became the framework by which ethical dilemmas were analyzed and resolved. The focus is on rights and has been referred to a justice-based ethical framework. This model, however, has come under criticism for several reasons: (a) rules apply, no matter who is involved; (b) this approach may lead to a focus on some aspects of an ethical dilemma and ignore others; (c) the individual using this approach to an ethical dilemma is stepping outside of the situation, and the unintended outcome may be to objectify the patient; (d) some ethical principles, for example, autonomy, may lead to ethical uncertainty because they are not universally applicable and because they apply in one situation but not in another situation. Other have criticized the justice-based approach because it is markedly different than the ethical reasoning of women.

A second model, inductive in style, focuses on "concern for individual cases" and is called care-based reasoning. This approach has been associated with ethical reasoning in women (Gilligan, 1982) and is characterized by full knowledge of the particularities of the case through knowledge of the relationships between the principals in the situation. It is called the "ethics of attachment" because it focuses on the responsibility to give care to the patient, and less on people as carriers of rights. Care-based approaches are criticized because: (a) the ethical dilemma/situation is "rule-less" but contains the possibility of the good, the moral thing to do; (b) this approach damages the patient–provider relationship, which, although unequal, is not necessarily bad; (c) this approach does not result in generalizable knowledge to be used in the other/all patient–provider relationships.

The patient, family, CNS, relevant nursing staff, ethics team, and other providers such as physicians, chaplains, and social workers are part of ethical decision making. This multidisciplinary team approach avoids the situation in which biased or unilateral decision making takes place, and it fosters and sustains the environment of open discussion around ethical dilemmas. The common processes used, regardless of ethical framework, include identification of the ethical problem, identification and consideration of alternatives, implementation of a choice and the associated ethical rationale, and evaluation of the decision-making process and it's outcome (Bozek & Savage, 2007).

Ethical decision making occurs in a context and may involve substantial distress. A variety of other process approaches to ethical decision making have also been suggested, such as concerned argumentation, consensus formation, clarification, ranking, reassurances, review of cases, and rehearsal of arguments, as ways to uncover the various layers and nuances that may exist in ethical dilemmas (Häyry, 2005).

CITIZENSHIP

Citizenship is defined as "membership in a community with rights to political participation," for example, political rights of an individual within a society. This citizenship is similar to the *polis citizenship* of ancient Greece, when citizenship was not seen as a public matter separate from a person's life. The obligations of citizenship were deeply connected to everyone's life in the *polis* (Leydet, 2006). A core concept of the *polis citizenship* was that the destiny of an individual was strongly linked to the destiny of the community. Applied to nursing, this would suggest that the destiny of an individual nurse or CNS is tied to the destiny of the community of all nurses and all CNSs. This viewpoint suggests that being a good citizen or steward of the profession enables the CNS to influence an organization as well as to influence the profession at the local, state, and national levels. Professional citizenship is presented in the context of the CNS as an employee in terms of organizational citizenship and as a member of the nursing profession as a professional citizen of nursing.

Organizational Citizenship

An organizational citizen refers to someone who exhibits behaviors that exceed formal job requirements but that contribute indirectly to the organization's effectiveness. These behaviors include helping behaviors (helping others, volunteering, orienting others), keeping up with matters that affect the organization (civic virtue), sportsmanship (not complaining about trivial matters), organizational loyalty, organizational compliance, individual initiative, and self-development (Joireman, Kamdar, Daniels, & Duell, 2006). These behaviors are different from tasks; rather, they are directed at supporting the organizational environment in which tasks take place. Other facets of organizational citizenship are demonstrating concern for the well-being of others, concern with future consequences of one's actions, expectations that individual work will be identified as well as linked to groups, and the belief that contributions have a meaningful impact on the group outcome. These behaviors have been studied and, after meta-analysis across many studies, are now considered to be reflective of organizational citizenship (LePine, Erez, & Johnson, 2002).

The CNS moves through and across many layers of an organization as they conduct their clinical practice. Clinical expertise in a specialty serves as one kind of "passport" to traverse the organization; organizational citizenship is another kind of passport that creates visible fidelity of the CNS with the organization and its mission, vision, and goals. For example, the CNS who is tremendously gifted in the clinical practice but is at odds with his/her organization will be hampered until the issues attached to the "war" are resolved.

Organizational citizenship behaviors are similar, overlap, and, potentially, have synergy with emotional competency within an organization. Thus, both as an advanced practice nurse and as an employee in an organization, the CNS who demonstrates competency in self- and social awareness, self-management, and relationships is also likely to demonstrate behaviors associated with organizational citizenship.

Organizational citizenship behaviors can create dilemmas, or, as these theorists call it, a social delayed fence. This refers to a situation that requires immediate effort ("hurdling the fence") to obtain a long-term collective goal (Joireman, Kamdar, Daniels, & Duell, 2006). For example, a CNS is working on nursing care with staff and the family of a very complex patient; the CNS is asked to leave that work and refocus on participation in a failure mode effect analysis (FMEA) or another equally complicated project that has equal or higher priority over the current work. The new priority moves the CNS from direct care with a patient family situation to another issue of equal importance to the organization. This scenario is an accurate description of the practice of the CNS who is interacting with multiple customers who have differing priorities.

The CNS can resolve conflicts such as this between equally meaningful projects and activities by considering the short-term and long-term outcomes of the priorities, and through alignment of the new priority with other projects so that one project advances the other, and, finally, by assessing the resources needed to respond to both priorities. These responses to competing priorities require the CNS to step around the either/or dilemma and use the both/and response. It may be that to accomplish this, the CNS will ask the organization to bring its resources to bear on their work so that their expertise can be given to both priorities. This discussion highlights the dilemmas and the solutions that can be used by the CNS as an organizational citizen while fulfilling the unique characteristics of his/her clinical practice.

Organizational citizenship can be influenced by organizational politics. For example, when the organizational environment supports high levels of informal leader and coworker feedback, the perceptions of organizational politics (in this research defined as intrusive and negative) will be low, and higher morale is present. Recent research has shown that when there is a high-quality feedback environment, employees are more likely to know the standards of good performance, to believe that performing well leads to desired rewards, and to use the feedback to improve their performance, resulting in low perceptions of organizational politics (Rosen, Levy, & Hall, 2006).

Professional Citizenship

If a person's choices and activities indicate their values, needs, and beliefs, then it would be predicted that future behavior in conceptually similar situations would be consistent with those values, needs, and beliefs. Thus, if a CNS valued and demonstrated organizational citizenship, it could be predicted that the CNS would also value and demonstrate professional citizenship. Professional citizenship behaviors are conceptually similar to those of organizational citizenship; the difference is that organizational citizenship occurs within the context of an organization, and professional citizenship behavior occurs beyond the CNS's organization and in the nursing profession, the community, and in the civic arena.

Professional citizenship may be reflected in many differing ways. For example, a CNS may be a member or a leader/officer of a state nursing association and the ANA, a nursing specialty organization such as the Oncology Nurses Society, or a national organization related to his/her role, such as the NACNS. Professional citizenship may also be reflected by the CNS's use and integration of various products and services from national organizations into their practice, for example, the use of national standards in the CNS's specialty or of the ANA, or through use of the Code of Ethics (ANA, 2005).

A CNS may demonstrate professional citizenship through leadership or participating in a project in his/her community. For example, recently, scholarship awardees of the national association for CNSs were selected because of their involvement in issues facing a particular patient population in their community (e.g., institutionalized teens, high-risk mothers, etc.; see http://www.nacns.org).

CNSs may determine that an issue affecting their practice requires resolution in the state legislature or with a regulatory board. An example of this occurred when CNSs in the state of Oregon sought changes in statute and participated in writing the language of administrative rules related to CNS practice (Davidson et al., 2001; Ponto, Sabo, Fitzgerald, & Wilson, 2002). Other CNSs have sought expansion of regulations to include prescriptive privilege for all advanced practice nurses, including CNSs (Carson & Minarik, 2007).

It may be that the CNS, through his/her professional organization(s), joins others at the national level in addressing issues such as health care reform, tobacco control, or end-of-life care (Long, 2005). Each and all of these levels of involvement add dimension and give meaning to professional citizenship of the CNS.

There are indications that nurses in particular have been reluctant to engage in professional citizenship. The reasons are complex and include the following factors: (1) perception of ethical conflict between professional values and political involvement (Gordon & Nelson, 2006), (2) lack of awareness or comfort with the political process (Buresh & Gordon, 2000), (3) sense of powerlessness and apathy (Des Jardin, 2001a, 2001b), (4) inability to frame and defend issues and present them so the public can understand (Mason, 2006), and (5) fear of retribution from peers and others.

The impact of these factors and the reluctance that nurses may have at the national level has limited but not extinguished the efforts of nursing to extend its reach beyond the clinical setting. Rather, nursing has achieved through professional citizenship in national nursing organizations and a small increase in the numbers of nurses elected to political office. These elected nurses have helped secure intermittent increases in federal budgets that support nursing education and practice, have secured funds supporting recruitment into nursing, and have obtained the passage of some laws addressing health care reform (Twedell & Webb, 2007).

Many baccalaureate programs now include curriculum content related to professional citizenship so that as graduates enter practice and then seek to become a CNS, they have received preparation in professional citizenship (Brown, 1996; Byrd, Costello, Shelton, Thomas, & Petrarca, 2004; Des Jardin, 2001a, 2001b; Rains & Barton-Kriese, 2001; Williams, 1993). Most, if not all, graduate programs include course work on health policy in the graduate core courses (Ennen, 2001). The NACNS has extensive influence on issues related to CNS practice at the national level (Baldwin, Clark, Fulton, & Mayo, 2009; Baldwin et al., 2007).

Professional citizenship by the CNS may take many forms. It is, however, dependent on the voice of CNSs in various arenas outside of the CNS's primary practice unit and organization. Full development of professional citizenship competency is not only an expectation of the CNS, but a requisite for the role.

SUMMARY

This chapter has presented three of the essential characteristics of CNSs, including the professional attributes of a CNS with an emphasis on emotional intelligence, ethical conduct, and professional citizenship, incorporating theoretical tenets and relevant research. The ability of CNSs to understand emotions as drivers to thoughts and behaviors, including how these emotions affect relationships, allows CNSs to interact ethically and as good citizens in the communities in which they live and work.

CNSs are often evaluated on their intellectual capacity, knowledge competence, and clinical acumen. While these are essential characteristics, the abilities of the CNS within an organization will be incompletely realized should the professional characteristics, including emotional competence, ethical conduct, and professional citizenship, be underdeveloped. Conversely, when emotional competence, ethical conduct, and professional citizenship are highly tuned, the effectiveness of the CNS is ensured and will be recognized by staff, peers, the organization, and by society. It is essential that curricula, work experiences, and lifelong learning be dedicated, in part, to the continual refinement of these attributes and characteristics. As a recognized clinical leader, the role modeling of these behaviors creates understanding and potential cultural transformation within the organization. This transformation supports the growth and development of all members of the team and, subsequently, results in more effective teamwork, reduced conflict, and better outcomes.

DISCUSSION QUESTIONS

I. Self-awareness/self-management

Scenario: With your class, identify a professional situation in which you experienced the emotion of anger or frustration.

a. *Discussion, analysis, synthesis*: Describe the incident and disclose your responses to the incident, both behavioral as well as your thoughts. Does a symbolic "cow path" emerge? What would you do differently next time as you experience these emotions to realize a healthier outcome for you and others in this scenario?
   Caution: Honesty and transparency are essential to one's growth in this exercise.
b. *Clinical application:* Establish a journal in which you narrate your emotional responses to professional situations, focusing on self-awareness and

self-management. Has the self-management of your emotions over time reflected a change?

II. Social awareness

Scenario: A multidisciplinary group is assigned to refine and implement a clinical practice guideline. This guideline impacts pharmacy, medicine, social work, nursing, and the dietitian. Members of the class assume the roles of the different disciplines.

  a. *Discussion, analysis, synthesis*: From the lens of the discipline to which you have been assigned, discuss barriers and facilitators to implementation. Reflect on your thoughts and emotions as you view this situation from a totally different perspective. Discuss how that experience increases your organizational savvy and political acumen.
  Caution: Reverse role-playing can uncover deep-seated mental models regarding other disciplines or individuals with whom you have previously worked.

  b. *Clinical application*: The next time a conflict arises between yourself and another discipline, practice reverse role-playing, step into the shoes of the other discipline, and now look at the situation. Is your response to the conflict different? Make journal entries as to whether your view of the situation has been enhanced to result in a win/win for both parties.

III. Relationships

Scenario: An accrediting agency is at the doorstep. You need to implement a policy rapidly in order to fulfill the requirements of the standards. The policy will require a substantive change in practice (e.g., national patient safety goals). You have been assigned to outline the implementation process for the policy. You bring together a group of stakeholders. Everybody is grumbling: "it's the other person's work" and "I'm not changing my practice" are the mantras.

  a. *Discussion, analysis, synthesis*: How you would move the group to a win/win situation for all, moving from "you/they" to "I/we"? A collective identity for the group is essential to negotiating this conflict.
  Caution: This exercise focuses on accelerated group process, appropriate linguistics, and effective communication. Avoid getting stuck in silos.

  b. *Clinical application*: In a group in which you currently participate, reflect on how your interaction patterns and style either accelerate or inhibit group productivity. Reflect on whether the group productivity is different when you are absent as compared to when you are present. Make journal entries related to this.

IV. Ethical conduct

Scenario: You have been approached by three staff nurses that there is a serious ethical dilemma in one of the units. The nurses express extreme frustration over the physician's lack of engagement, the family's veiled threats of suit, and the lack of agreement among the caregivers as to what is appropriate care for this patient. The patient wants to refuse treatment for a very treatable condition.

  a. *Discussion, analysis, synthesis:* Discuss the root causes involved in this care conflict, for example, is this a legal matter, or poor communication and understanding, or truly an ethical dilemma? How would you, as a CNS, proceed to analyze which of the root causes is driving the conflict? Talk this through with your group, focusing on the values that are in conflict for you personally, the members of the team involved, the patient, and the family.
  Caution: Be clear with the members involved in the conflict as to what their expectations are of you and the process that you will use to clarify the drivers involved in the conflict.

  b. *Clinical application:* Have conversations with nurses in your work unit regarding their perception of conflicts in care management. Is moral distress among the nurses evident? Think about your role in working through these conflicts? How would you know if moral distress was reduced?

V. Professional citizenship

Scenario: You are the CNS within a specific specialty. This specialty has a national professional organization and a national certification examination. You work on a unit where only two of the nurses belong to the professional organization, and no one has their certification. It is the organization's intent to receive magnet status within the next 3 years. The unit leadership wants you to get the majority of the RNs on the unit certified and actively engaged in their professional organization. There is a local chapter of the national specialty organization in the city in which you work. In fact, you are the vice president of that local chapter and an author of questions that are in the certification examination.

  a. *Discussion analysis synthesis*: Discuss how to move the nurses from employee to organizational citizen to reach the goals established by the system.
  Caution: Are the nurses with whom you are working connected to the magnet vision? Do they see themselves as professionals within an organization, or employees to do a job?

  b. *Clinical application*: Assess the level of professional citizenship in the work unit in which you currently are employed. What variables would you use to assess professional citizenship?

REFERENCES

American Association of Critical Care Nurses. (2005). *AACN standards for establishing and sustaining healthy work environments: A journey to excellence.* Aliso Viejo, CA: Author.

American Nurses Association. (2004). *Nursing: Scope and standards of practice.* Washington, DC: Author.

American Nurses Association. (2005). *Code of ethics for nurses with interpretive statements.* Washington, DC: Author.

American Nurses Association Council of Clinical Nurse Specialists. (1986). *The role of the clinical nurse specialist.* Washington, DC: American Nurses Association.

Arena, D. M., & Page, N. E. (1992). The imposter phenomenon in the clinical nurse specialist role. *Image: Journal of Nursing Scholarship, 24,* 121–125.

Austin, W. (2007). The ethics of every day practice: Health care environments as moral communities. *Advances in Nursing Sciences, 30,* 81–88.

Baldwin, K. M., Clark, A. P., Fulton, J., & Mayo, A. (2009). National validation of the NACNS clinical nurse specialist core competencies. *Journal of Nursing Scholarship, 41,* 193–201.

Baldwin, K. M., Lyon, B. L., Clark, A. P., Fulton, J., Davidson, S., & Dayhoff, N. (2007). Developing clinical nurse specialist practice competencies. *Clinical Nurse Specialist, 9,* 297–301.

Bartholomew, K. (2005). *Speak your truth: Proven strategies for effective nurse-physician communication.* Marblehead, MA: HCPro, Inc.

Bartholomew, K. (2006). *Ending nurse to nurse hostility: Why nurses eat their young and each other.* Marblehead, MA: HC Pro, Inc.

Beauman, S. S. (2006). Leadership and the clinical nurse specialist: From traditional to contemporary. *Newborn and Infant Nursing Reviews, 6,* 22–24.

Bozek, M. S., & Savage, T. A. (2007). *The ethical component of nursing education: Integrating ethics into clinical experience.* Philadelphia: Lippincott, Williams & Wilkins.

Brown, S. G. (1996). Incorporating political socialization theory into baccalaureate nursing education. *Nursing Outlook, 4,* 120–123.

Buresh, B., & Gordon S. (2000). *From silence to voice: What nurses know and must communicate to the public.* Ottawa: Canadian Nurses Association.

Byrd, M. E., Costello, J., Shelton, C. R., Thomas, P. A., & Petrarca, D. (2004). An active learning experience in health policy of baccalaureate nursing students. *Public Health Nursing, 21,* 501–506.

Carson, W. Y., & Minarik, P. A. (2007). Advanced practice nurses: A new skirmish in the continuing battle over scope of practice. *Clinical Nurse Specialist, 21,* 52–54.

Community Hospitals Indianapolis. (1995). *Patients rights & responsibilities: The partnership.* Indianapolis: Author.

Cooper, R. W., Frank, G. L., Hansen, M. M., & Gouty, C. A. (2004). Key ethical issues encountered in healthcare organizations: The perceptions of staff nurses and nurse leaders. *Journal of Nursing Administration, 34,* 149–156.

Cosby, K. S., & Croskerry, P. (2004). Profiles in patient safety: Authority gradients in medical error. *Academy of Emergency Medicine, 11,* 1341–1345.

Curtin, L. L. (2007). Facing up to fallibility: A manager's guide to ethical decision-making. *Nurse Leader, 5,* 23–27.

Davidhizer, R. (1993). Clinical nurse specialist leading with charisma. *Journal of Advanced Nursing, 18,* 675–679.

Davidson, S., Beardsley, K., Busch, A. H., Garner, A., Heresa, S., Hodges, N. D., et al. (2001). Statutory and regulatory recognition of clinical nurse specialists in Oregon. *Clinical Nurse Specialist, 15,* 276–283.

Des Jardin, K. E. (2001a). Political involvement in nursing—Education and empowerment, Part I. *Association of periOperative Registered Nurses Journal, 74,* 468–477.

Des Jardin, K. E. (2001b). Political involvement in nursing—Politics, ethics, and strategic action, Part II. *Association of periOperative Registered Nurses Journal, 74,* 614–622.

DeWolf, M. S. (1989) Clinical ethical decision-making; A grounded theory method. *Dissertation Abstracts International, 50*(11), 4980.

Edge, R. S., & Groves, J. R. (1999). *Ethics of health care: A guide for clinical practice.* Albany: Delmar Publishers.

Ennen, K. A. (2001). Shaping the future of practice through political activity. *American Association of Occupational Health Nurses Journal, 49,* 557–569.

Frankel, A. S., Leonard, M. W., & Denham, C. R. (2006). Fair and just culture, team behavior and leadership engagement. *Health Services Research, 41,* 1690–1709.

Garmen, A. N., Tyler, J. L., & Darnall, J. S. (2004). Development and validation of a 360 degree feedback instrument for health care administrators. *Journal of Health Care Management, 49,* 307–322.

Gilligan, C. (1982). *In a different voice.* Cambridge, MA: Harvard University Press.

Goleman, D. (1995). *Emotional intelligence: Why it can matter more than IQ* (10th ed.). New York: Bantam Books.

Goleman, D. (1998). *Working with emotional intelligence.* New York: Bantam Books.

Goleman, D., Boyatzis, L., & McKee, A. (2002). *Primal leadership: Learning to lead with emotional intelligence.* Boston: Harvard Business School Press.

Golomb, B. A., McGaw, J. J., Evans, M. A., & Dimsdale, J. E. (2007). Physician response to patient reports of adverse drug effects: Implications for patient-targeted adverse effect surveillance. *Drug Safety, 30,* 669–675.

Gordon, S., & Nelson, S. (2006). *The complexities of care: Nursing reconsidered.* New York: ILR Press.

Guralnik, D. (1962). *Webster's Dictionary of the American Language.* Cleveland: The Word Publishing Company.

Gurka, A. (1995). Transformational leadership: Qualities and strategies for the CNS. *Clinical Nurse Specialist Journal, 9,* 169–174.

Häyry, M. (2005). Can arguments address concerns? *Journal of Medical Ethics, 31,* 598–600.

Institute of Medicine. (2003). *Health professions education: A bridge to quality.* Washington, DC: National Academies Press.

Institute of Medicine. (2004). *Keeping patients safe: Transforming the work environment of nurses.* Washington, DC: National Academies Press.

Joireman, J., Kamdar, D., Daniels, D., & Duell, B. (2006). Good citizens to the end? Empathy and concern with future consequences moderate the impact of a short-term time horizon on organizational citizenship behaviors. *Journal of Applied Psychology, 91,* 1307–1320.

Kerfoot, K. (1999). The culture of courage. *Pediatric Nursing, 25,* 558–559.

Kerfoot, K. (2005). Healthy work environments: En route to excellence. *Critical Care Nurse, 25,* 71–72.

Kohlberg, L. (1981). *Philosophy of moral development.* San Francisco: Harper and Rose.

LePine, J. A., Erez, A., & Johnson, D. E. (2002). The nature and dimensionality of organizational citizenship behaviors: A critical review and meta-analysis. *Journal of Applied Psychology, 87,* 52–65.

Leydet, D. (2006). *Citizenship.* Retrieved June 21, 2009, from http://plato.stanford.edu/entries/citizenship

Lombardo, M. M., & Eichinger, R. W. (2006). *For your improvement: A guide for development and coaching* (4th ed.). Minneapolis: Lominger International.

Long, R. E. (2005). From revelation to revolution: Critical care nurses' emerging roles in public policy. *Critical Care Nursing Clinics of North America, 17,* 191–199.

Lynch, A. E., & Cole, E. (2006). Human factors in emergency care: The need for team resource management. *Emergency Nurse, 14,* 32–35.

Mason, D. (2006). Pride and prejudice: Nurse's struggle with reasoned debate. In S. Nelson & S. Gordon (Eds.), *The complexities of care: Nursing reconsidered* (pp. 40–49). Ithaca, NY: ILR Press.

McKinnon, J. (2005). Feeling and knowing: Neural scientific perspectives on intuitive practice. *Nursing Standard, 20,* 41–46.

McQueen, A. C. H. (2004). Emotional intelligence in nursing work. *Journal of Advanced Nursing, 47,* 101–108.

Mohr, W. K., & Mahon, M. M. (1996). Dirty hands: The underside of marketplace health care. *Advances in Nursing Science, 19,* 28–37.

National Association of Clinical Nurse Specialists. (2004). *Statement on clinical nurse specialist practice and education* (2nd ed.). Harrisburg: Author.

Nelson, S. (2006). Ethical expertise and the problem of the good nurse. In S. Nelson & S. Gordon (Eds.), *The complexities of care: Nursing reconsidered* (pp. 69–87). Ithaca, NY: ILR Press.

Patterson, K., Grenny, J., McMillan, R., & Switzler, A. (2002). *Crucial conversations: Tools for talking when stakes are high.* Provo, UT: Vital Smarts.

Ponto, J., Sabo, J., Fitzgerald, M. A., & Wilson, D. E. (2002). Operationalizing advanced practice registered nurse legislation. *Clinical Nurse Specialist, 16,* 263–269.

Porter O'Grady, T. P. (2003). New age for leadership: New rules, new roles. *Journal of Nursing Administration, 33,* 173–178.

Porter O'Grady, T. P., & Malloch, K. (2002). *Quantum leadership: A textbook for new leadership.* Gaithersburg, MD: Aspen Publications.

Rains, J. W., & Barton-Kriese, P. (2001). Developing political competence: A comparative study across disciplines. *Public Health Nursing, 18,* 219–224.

Robert, S. J. (1983). Oppressed group behavior: Implication for nursing. *Advances in Nursing Science, 5,* 21–30.

Rosen, C. C., Levy, P. E., & Hall, R. J. (2006). Placing perceptions of politics in the context of feedback environment, employee attitudes, and job performance. *Journal of Applied Psychology, 91,* 211–220.

Skinner, C., & Spurgeon, P. (2005). Empathy: 4 distinct dispositions: Empathetic concern, perspective taking, personal distress and empathetic matching. 3 empathy scales related to transformational behaviors. *Health Services Management Research, 18,* 1–12.

Swidler, R. N., Seastrum, T., & Shelton, W. (2007). Difficult hospital inpatient discharge decisions: Ethical, legal and clinical practice issues. *American Journal of Bioethics, 7,* 23–28.

Twedell, D. M., & Webb, J. A. (2007). The value of the political action committee: Dollars and influence for nurse leaders. *Nursing Administration Quarterly, 31,* 279–283.

Webster's Dictionary of the American Language. (1962). Cleveland: The Word Publishing Company.

Williams, A. (1993). Community health learning experiences and political activism: A model for baccalaureate curriculum revolution content. *Journal of Nursing Education, 32,* 352–356.

Wlody, G. S. (2007). Nursing management and organizational ethics in the intensive care unit. *Critical Care Medicine, 35,* S29–S35.

Philosophical Underpinnings of Advanced Nursing Practice: A Synthesizing Framework for Clinical Nurse Specialist Practice

Frank D. Hicks

Professional nursing has made significant progress since its inception 150 years ago. Moving from a skills-based vocation to a profession and discipline, nursing has produced talented practitioners, scientists, entrepreneurs, and executives. Despite its increasingly recognized contribution to health care, nursing continues to justify its unique place among other health care professions. The need for this justification arose, in my opinion, as a response to two factors. First, as nursing matured and moved into academe, it became increasingly important to establish and justify a unique identity and body of knowledge to be acceptable to the other scholarly and scientific disciplines. Second, as nurses began to take on more sophisticated roles, it became necessary to establish nurses' efficacy and cost-effectiveness. At the heart of this justification was and continues to be the need to clearly articulate what it is about nursing that is so crucial and necessary to the health and well-being of humankind. Thus, the search to uncover, describe, and categorize nursing's body of knowledge continues.

The generation of nursing science, a body of knowledge unique to nursing with direct applicability to nursing practice, has lead to numerous philosophical and theoretical formulations that attempt to give voice to a fundamental and seemingly implicit understanding of the nature of nursing. Importantly, these theoretical formulations have led to philosophical considerations that have helped to elucidate nursing's nature and the structure of its knowledge.

As a clinical nurse specialist (CNS), I have often grappled with questions of the nature of nursing (nursing's ontology) and the structure of its knowledge (nursing's epistemology). I believe that it is important for the CNS to have an understanding of these concepts for several reasons. First, understanding nursing's ontology and epistemology helps us to understand that our practice emerges from a particular worldview. As nurses, each of us has a view about the nature of health, people, the environment, and the discipline and practice of nursing. This worldview comes from our education and experience and most certainly influences the way in which we deliver nursing care, and this ultimately influences client outcomes. Second, as CNSs, we are in a remarkable position to influence the generation of theory that is grounded in practice, something that has long been advocated by several theorists and philosophers of science (Ellis, 1969). As championed by Reed (2006), the time has come to end the dichotomy between theory and practice and place the development of theory where it should be, in a practice-oriented discipline such as nursing, with the nurse engaged in the practice of nursing. Given the varied roles and responsibilities of the CNS and the breadth of CNS influence, there is no one better to engage in the generation and application of theory. To that end, this chapter has three goals:

1. Describe nursing's metatheoretical space as it helps define nursing's autonomous domain of practice.
2. Discuss nursing's ontological perspective as it informs nursing processes for CNS practice.
3. Discuss nursing's epistemological perspective related to phenomena of concern for CNS practice and nursing's unique contribution to health care outcomes.

Exploration of these topics will address concerns generated by the growing emphasis on pathology, pharmacology, and the diagnosis and treatment of disease, readily apparent in current advanced practice nursing (APN) education and practice. This emphasis may be obfuscating the essential core of nursing knowledge (Arslanean-Engorin, Hicks, Whall, & Algase, 2005; Whall & Hicks, 2002). CNSs, and indeed all APNs, need to be able to clearly articulate the unique role of nursing in health care.

METATHEORY AND AUTONOMOUS CLINICAL NURSE SPECIALIST PRACTICE

Metatheory deals with the broad conceptual issues concerning how theory is situated, discussed, and developed within a particular discipline. As such, metatheory proffers an overarching framework (the metaparadigm) for understanding important concepts within a field of study. The metaparadigm of nursing—considered to be the concepts of person, environment, health, and nursing—has gained acceptance as the essential concepts that underlie nursing's view of reality. A majority of scholarly work undertaken in the past four decades can be seen to address, to some degree, the four concepts. Virtually all theories of nursing deal with these four concepts to one degree or another, though the definitions of these concepts vary greatly, depending upon the theorist's paradigm. The essential message implied by the metaparadigm, however, is that disciplinary focus of nursing is concerned with the person–environment–health interface. The metaparadigm provided the framework for nursing scholars to begin to think about the relationships among the

essential concepts of person, environment, health, and nursing. Accordingly, the metaparadigm has given rise to several paradigms.

A *paradigm* is a worldview that frames the assumptions, methods, and theories scientists use to engage in the work of discovery and understanding (Kuhn, 1972). Logical positivism and phenomenology are two such examples of paradigms that have influenced science over the last 100 years, including nurse scientists (Whall & Hicks, 2002). Parse (1981) posited that nursing's scientific endeavors arose from two predominate worldviews: totality and simultaneity. Essential differences in these paradigms arise from how each one defines the nature of person, environment, and health.

In the totality paradigm, the person is viewed as a holistic being comprised of biological, psychological, sociological, and spiritual components that are in constant interaction with the environment. The person and environment are believed to influence one another, as well as to determine health. Health is often seen as well-being or wholeness that results from the human-environment interaction. The simultaneity paradigm, based in the science of unitary human beings (Rogers, 1970), sees person and environment as inseparable energy fields that are in continuous and mutual exchange with one another. Health is viewed as a social construction (Rogers, 1970), thus it has no inherent value in itself. Newman (1986), who was influenced by Rogers, sees health as a transcendental process resulting in expanding consciousness. Both of these paradigms have assisted nurses in constructing unique ways of viewing nursing and of delineating the focus and work of nursing. From these paradigms arose the grand theories of nursing, such as Orem (1971), King (1971), Roy (1984), Parse (1981), and Newman (1986).

The argument could be made that none of the concepts contained in the metaparadigm are unique to nursing. Certainly, physicians, occupational and physical therapists, social workers, and other health care workers would say they were concerned with aspects of person, environment, and health. The unique view of nursing, however, comes from the belief that these realities are viewed as holistic and inseparable, in mutual process, and ever-evolving. The particularities and specifics of each of these concepts, as defined by the various theorists, may differ, but the unifying theme found in these various theories and worldviews is that nurses deal with humans in their totality and unity and are concerned with the continual and mutual interactions and reactions that occur as a result of the human–environment–health interface. The uniqueness of the discipline, science, and practice of nursing lies at the heart of this interaction and emerges from both trying to understand its results and dealing with its consequences.

To summarize, I suggest that the theories of nursing, though diverse, have some strong underlying, unified themes that speak to essential truths and that can be used to help construct a framework for CNS practice:

A. Nursing is relational by nature. Effective nursing cannot occur if the nurse cannot establish a therapeutic relationship with the patient/client.
B. Nursing does not occur in a vacuum. There must always be consideration of the context in which the person, environment, and the resulting patterns of health occur.
C. Nursing focuses on health, wholeness, and well-being rather than disease, dysfunction, and disability.
D. Nursing always strives not only to maintain but to enhance the unique and indivisible wholeness inherent in the human being and their environment.

NURSING'S ONTOLOGICAL PERSPECTIVE: NURSING PROCESSES

Ontology is the branch of philosophy that deals with understanding being, existence, or reality. Thus, as applied to nursing (and nursing science), ontology explores the nature of nursing and essential elements defining that nature. For nearly 40 years, nursing scholars attempted to define the nature of nursing with several unique ontological formulations coming to the fore. As previously noted, Rogers (1970) asserted that humans and their environment could best be understood as energy fields in mutual exchange. The science of nursing, therefore, emerged from the study of patterns generated of the mutual processes of human and environmental energy fields. Roy (1995) posited nursing's purpose as understanding human adaptive processes for attaining or maintaining health, while Orem (1971) focused on understanding self-care needs of nursing's clients. Alternatively, Parse (1981) saw nursing as understanding the process of *human becoming* (an evolving self-knowledge) and quality of life. More recently, Reed (1997) offered another ontological view of nursing that has much potential. Reed's unique view of the discipline of nursing is a synthesis of the work of several philosophers and theorists, including Nightingale (1859/1969), Henderson (1964) and Rogers (1970), among others (Kauffman, 1995; Lerner, 1986; von Bertalanffy, 1981; Waldrop, 1992; Werner, 1957).

In Reed's view (1997), nursing's focus of concern is the innate processes of well-being possessed by all human systems, which are manifested by their complexity and integration. The idea that human beings (and their systems) possess innate characteristics that foster well-being is not new in nursing. Similar ideas can be found in the writings of Nightingale (1859/1969), who

maintained that the work of nursing was to put the patient in the right state so the body could heal itself. Similarly, Henderson (1964) asserted that nursing was the work of supporting those activities and processes already possessed by the individual, while Watson (1985) referred to self-healing processes. Similarly, Schlotfeldt (1994) believed humans were able and disposed to seek and attain their health. Reed takes these ideas a step further. She asserts that inherent nursing processes are not necessarily an attempt to reverse disease; rather, nursing processes are intent on moving the human system (individual, group, community) forward toward a sense of well-being (Reed, 1997). Thus, nursing processes are not external mechanistic devices imposed by nurses, but are essentially relational, contextual, and transformational conceptions of the world perceived and employed by human systems. Reed believes that nursing is a participatory process transcending the boundary between patient and nurse and deriving value from the human systems' inherent propensity for innovation and change. Human systems emanate and participate in these nursing processes. For example, nursing processes can be seen in an individual experiencing fear and anxiety over a diagnosis of cancer (e.g., the physiological and psychosocial responses that result from the attempt to understand and integrate this event), or in the rituals and activities that emerge from the healing practices of a culture, which attempt to aid the individual as well as the community. The patterns emerging from these processes are potentially limitless, thus providing fodder for research and application to practice. Thus, for Reed (1997), the quest of the nursing discipline is to "understand the nature of and to facilitate nursing processes in diverse contexts of health experiences" (p. 77). The unique characteristic of the discipline of nursing is found in the intersection of three important concepts: complexity, integration, and well-being.

Complexity refers to the number of variables, factors, or events influencing an individual or group. Variables can be psychological, social, cultural, or physiological; the greater the number of variables, the greater the complexity. For example, consider the variables introduced into the life of a patient who sustains a spinal cord injury (SCI). Not only are there functional and physiological limitations for the individual to overcome, but there are many psychosocial and emotional challenges to meet that influence not only the patient, but the family and health care system, as well. Complexity results in quantitative change, not qualitative change of the whole (Reed, 1997).

Integration occurs when variables are synthesized and organized. Synthesis implies a change in form, not simply the number of events (Reed, 1997, p. 78). Change occurs through integration of an event's meaning and symbolism into one's life. Thus, integration is transformative and results in qualitative change

(Reed, 1997). Integration is more than adaptation, however. Integration involves constructing meaning of or identifying a pattern (or patterns) among variables experienced and incorporating these new meanings and patterns into a new understanding of the human-health experience. Elaborating on the example of a patient with SCI, integration occurs when the multiple variables confronting the patient and family become understood, interpreted, and incorporated into a new way of being for both the patient and those with whom the patient interacts and relates. Thus, out of this integration comes a new way of being, a synthesized reality that attempts to regain a sense of well-being.

Well-being emerges from the interaction of complexity and integration. As Reed (1997) stated, "Complexity provides life with the diversity, specialization, and depth in experiences, whereas integration provides organization, coherence, and breadth" (p. 78). The rhythm between complexity and integration determines well-being. The inability to achieve harmony between complexity and integration may result in a feeling of dis-harmony or dis-ease.

Reed's ontology provides the CNS with a unique view of nursing that holds great promise for helping to redefine and refine practice. By synthesizing views commonly expressed in nursing's theoretical history, Reed's ontology provides a flexible way of telescoping from the patient to the system. The concepts of complexity, integration, and well-being can be readily applied to a plethora of human experiences and systems. The idea that well-being evolves out of the way in which the system, whether that be the cardiovascular system or a nursing unit, integrates the complexity of its patterns and experiences provides a unique view to understand various phenomena at any level of abstraction.

PHENOMENA OF CONCERN FOR CLINICAL NURSE SPECIALIST PRACTICE

Having explicated a new ontological view of nursing, let us turn to a discussion of epistemology, or the structure of nursing knowledge. Until recently, the only valid form of scientific knowledge was empirical (Whall & Hicks, 2002), an idea championed by logical positivists who believed that only observable and verifiable knowledge was worthy of consideration for scientists. With the advent of postmodernism, philosophers of science have entertained the possibility that there may be multiple ways of knowing that may arise out of personal experience and knowledge, as well as from observables. This view has been embraced in nursing, as well.

One of the best known treatises on the structure of nursing knowledge is Carper's (1978) "Fundamental patterns of knowing in nursing." This work is significant because it went beyond empirical methods of knowledge development. Indeed, Carper argued that the complexities in the nature of nursing and in nursing practice required more than mere observation and confirmation of phenomena. Nurses require knowledge that not only builds their science, but that can also inform their art, morality, and self-knowledge.

Carper (1978) identified four patterns by which nursing knowledge can be understood. *Empirical* knowledge is knowledge acquired through the scientific process. *Ethical* knowledge arises out of the moral imperatives related to the right thing to do in patient/client encounters and is grounded in fundamental ethical principles. *Personal* knowledge refers to the understanding of self and how self influences interactions with others. Finally, *aesthetic* knowledge addresses the creative and original interpretation and application of other forms of knowledge. Each of these patterns helps structure observations and experiences encountered on a daily basis by nurses in practice. The complexity of nursing practice requires depth and breadth of empirical knowledge, a sound understanding of knowing the right thing to do (ethics), and understanding how self-knowledge "promotes wholeness and integrity in the personal encounter" (personal knowledge; Carper, as cited in Reed, Shearer, & Nicoll, 2004, p. 226). These ways of knowing culminate in the application of knowledge in a given context. Repeated application in similar contexts gives rise to knowledge based in experience. Although others have analyzed and expanded upon Carper's initial epistemological conceptualization (Munhall, 1993; Schultz & Meleis, 1988; White, 1995), these fundamental patterns still provide a solid foundation for exploring knowledge generation and categorization, and these ways of knowing can be used in conjunction with Reed's (1997) ontology to develop an organizing framework that helps to delineate the phenomena of concern for CNS practice.

If we accept the assumption that human systems generate patterns of innate nursing processes that compel the system toward integration and well-being, then it is possible to begin to examine nursing situations for these emerging patterns. Further, if we accept that there are four fundamental forms of nursing knowledge (empirical, aesthetic, personal, and ethical), then each pattern emerging from the human system should lend itself to examination within one of these four forms. By relating the patterns of innate processes to patterns of knowing, then a framework develops that assists in the generation and categorization of patterns that arise out of practice. Because the CNS has the theoretical and empirical knowledge of a specialist and engages regularly in the advanced practice of nursing, there is no individual better suited to generate and test nursing knowledge.

The development of knowledge from CNS practice may seem, at first, a daunting task. But, in fact, we all generate thoughts about the experiences we encounter in life, and we analyze them in an attempt to describe and categorize these thoughts and impressions. This description and categorization is the foundation of theory development. Theory is merely a set of hypotheses that create a framework to understand phenomena (Ellis, 1969). The works of Reed (1997) and Carper (1978) provide the CNS with a unique nursing lens through which the observations of phenomena encountered in practice can be described, categorized, and interpreted. As knowledge of these practice-related phenomena accumulates and multiplies, the CNS has a rich and varied resource upon which to design, implement, and evaluate nursing care. Furthermore, a synthesis of these two works provides a unique way of examining nursing phenomenon. Given the multiple roles in which most CNSs must engage today, it is increasingly important that they have the ability to see the wide-ranging connections and ramifications that phenomena have for the patient and the system within which they all interact.

A Pragmatic Application

The difficulty in reading a chapter such as this is that it often leaves the reader asking questions such as, "So, what can I do with this?" and "How can I apply this to my practice?" The application of philosophy finds its voice in the way in which it is embraced and the resulting influence it has in shaping how one looks at the world. Philosophy is not directly applicable to practice, but it can profoundly influence the values and beliefs of the practitioner. The beliefs and values of the practitioner, in turn, influence the theories chosen to direct nursing interventions. Thus, if a CNS were to accept the ontological perspective forwarded by Reed (1997), then the resulting worldview of nursing practice may be very different. For example, instead of concerning oneself with a low hemoglobin level, the CNS looking at nursing with a grounding in Reed's ontology would consider the nursing systems that are being influenced by the reduction in oxygen-carrying capacity of the blood and how that ultimately influences the client's well-being.

SUMMARY AND CONCLUSION

In this chapter, I have tried to provide a philosophical basis for CNS practice by positing a new way to look at nursing practice based on Reed's (1997) and Carper's (1978) work. This ontological and epistemological synthesis is not meant to replace ontological and epistemological perspectives from which previous nursing theories have evolved. Rather, it is meant to provide the CNS with

another way to examine and understand nursing phenomena. To recapitulate the beginning of the chapter, the need to establish nursing as a discipline and profession that brings a unique and clearly articulated perspective to health care cannot be overemphasized. This articulation is not only important to ensure that nursing has a role on the health care team, but it is also important to keep this unique perspective before the eyes of educators of advanced practice nurses to ensure that nursing is not lost in advanced practice nursing programs. Finally, nursing scientists need a perspective from which to develop a science that serves the needs of not only nurses, but also the patients for whom they care.

DISCUSSION QUESTIONS

1. What beliefs and values most influence your views of nursing and nursing care?
2. Examine the theories you use in your practice. What are the predominate paradigmatic views from which these theories are derived, and how do these views influence the development and implementation of nursing interventions?

ANALYSIS AND SYNTHESIS

1. Take two nursing theories and analyze them in terms of what the theorist says about each of the metaparadigm concepts (i.e., person, environment, nursing, health). How have the theorist's underlying assumptions (i.e., philosophy) driven the interpretation/ definition of these concepts?
2. Observe a CNS in his/her practice. In the course of their interactions with clients and other health care workers, what philosophical beliefs influence their practice?

CLINICAL APPLICATION

1. Take a recent client/family for whom you cared and evaluate the case from Reed's ontological perspective. Can you identify where and how the complexity and integration in the various nursing systems occurred?

REFERENCES

Arslanean-Engorin, C., Hicks, F. D., Whall, A. L., & Algase, D. L. (2005). An ontological view of advanced nursing practice. *Research and Theory for Nursing Practice: An International Journal, 19*(4), 315–322.

Carper, B. A. (1978). Fundamental patterns of knowing in nursing. *Advances in Nursing Science, 1*(1), 13–23.

Ellis, R. (1969). The practitioner as theorist. *American Journal of Nursing, 69*(7), 428–435.

Henderson, V. (1964). The nature of nursing. *American Journal of Nursing, 64*(8), 62–68.

Kauffman, S. (1995). *At home in the universe: The search for the laws of self-organization and complexity.* New York: Oxford University Press.

King, I. (1971). *Toward a theory of nursing: General concepts of human behavior.* New York: Wiley.

Kuhn, T. S. (1972). *The structure of scientific revolutions* (2nd ed.). Chicago: University of Chicago Press.

Lerner, R. M. (1986). *Concepts and theories of human development* (2nd ed.). New York: Random House.

Munhall, P. L. (1993). "Unknowing": Toward another pattern of knowing in nursing. *Nursing Outlook, 41,* 125–128.

Newman, M. (1986). *Health as expanding consciousness.* St. Louis: C. V. Mosby.

Nightingale, F. (1969). *Nursing: What it is and what it is not.* New York: Dover. (Original work published in 1859.)

Orem, D. E. (1971). *Nursing: Concepts of practice.* New York: McGraw-Hill.

Parse, R. R. (1981). *Man-living-health: A theory of nursing.* New York: Wiley.

Reed, P. G. (1997). Nursing: The ontology of the discipline. *Nursing Science Quarterly, 10,* 76–79.

Reed, P. G. (2006). The practice turn in nursing epistemology. *Nursing Science Quarterly, 19*(1), 36–38.

Reed, P. G., Shearer, N. C., & Nicoll, L. H. (2004). *Perspectives on nursing theory* (4th ed.). Philadelphia, PA: Lippincott, Williams & Wilkins.

Rogers, M. E. (1970). *Introduction to the theoretical basis of nursing.* Philadelphia: F. A. Davis.

Roy, C. (1984). *Introduction to nursing: An adaptation model* (2nd ed.). Englewood Cliffs, NJ: Prentice Hall.

Roy, C. L. (1995). Developing nursing knowledge: Practice issues raised from four philosophical perspectives. *Nursing Science Quarterly, 8,* 79–85.

Schlotfeldt, R. (1994). Resolving opposing viewpoints: Is this desirable? Is it practicable? In J. E. Kikuchi & H. Simmons (Eds.), *Developing a philosophy of nursing* (pp. 67–74). Thousand Oaks, CA: Sage.

Schultz, P. R., & Meleis, A. I. (1988). Nursing epistemology: Traditions, insights, and questions. *Image: Journal of Nursing Scholarship, 20*(4), 217–221.

von Bertalanffy, L. (1981). *A systems view of man* (Ed. P. A. LaViolette). Boulder, CO: Westview Press.

Waldrop, M. M. (1992). *Complexity: The emerging science at the edge of order and chaos.* New York: Simon and Schuster.

Watson, J. (1985). *Nursing: Human science and human care.* Norwalk, CT: Appleton-Century-Crofts.

Werner, H. (1957). The concept of development from a comparative and organismic point of view. In D. B. Harris (Ed.), *The concept of development* (pp. 125–148). Minneapolis: University of Minnesota Press.

Whall, A. L., & Hicks, F. D. (2002). The unrecognized paradigm shift in nursing: Implications, problems, and possibilities. *Nursing Outlook, 50,* 72–76.

White, J. (1995). Patterns of knowing: Review, critique, and update. *Advances in Nursing Science, 17*(4), 73–86.

Nurse Sensitive Outcomes

Diane M. Doran
Souraya Sidani
Tammie DiPietro

Outcomes measurement has become a primary focus as health care organizations tackle the major challenges of today and tomorrow, namely, cost and quality, effectiveness of care, and organizational performance. All practitioners in the health care field are being challenged to find ways to demonstrate that the care they provide leads to improvement in outcomes for patients. To accomplish that, practitioners are attempting to identify the relevant outcomes that can be linked in a meaningful way to their own practices. In this chapter, we review the most recent accumulated evidence related to patient and system outcomes that are associated with the role of the clinical nurse specialist (CNS). We review both the theoretical and empirical literature about patient outcomes that are sensitive to the CNS role, with the goal of providing sound evidence to clinicians, health care leaders, and researchers for evaluating the impact of CNSs in our health care system.

The three objectives of this chapter are:

1. To identify the essential characteristics or attributes defining CNS practice. This first objective is critical to developing a clear conceptual definition of their scope of practice, which will lay the foundation for identifying outcomes relevant for measuring the impact of their role. In particular, the framework for CNS practice described in the National Association of Clinical Nurse Specialists (NACNS) *Statement on Clinical Nurse Specialist Practice and Education* (http://www.nacns.org/) will be reviewed as a foundation

for identifying specific outcomes associated with the CNS role.
2. To identify outcomes associated with the CNS role.
3. To determine the extent to which each outcome has demonstrated sensitivity to the CNS role. This will be accomplished by examining relationships between CNS role variables and patient/team/system outcomes.

METHODOLOGY FOR LITERATURE REVIEW ON CNS PRACTICE

Step 1: Literature Search

The first step of the literature review/analysis consisted of identifying conceptual and empirical references that discuss or investigate advanced nursing practice, excluding nurse practitioners. The search involved four strategies:

1. Generating a comprehensive list of relevant articles, book chapters, books, or other documents that we have accumulated through our involvement in previous work.
2. Completing a computerized literature search to identify relevant literature about the outcomes of the CNS role. The computerized literature bases included in this step were the Cumulative Index to Nursing and Allied Health Literature (CINAHL), Health Planning,

MEDLINE, CANCERLIT, SocioFile, and PsychLit. This search strategy used the following key words to identify relevant articles:

a. Advanced practice nursing/ nurses *and or*
b. Clinical nurse specialist *and*
c. Nursing sensitive patient outcomes, role impact, role effectiveness, CNS interventions, quality of nursing care, patient outcomes, nursing organization
d. Patient satisfaction with nursing care, patient satisfaction, patient and quality of care, system outcomes

3. The references reported within the articles, in particular those reporting the results of meta-analytic studies or integrative literature review/synthesis, were traced to identify additional references.

Step 2: Literature Selection

The references identified were included in the literature review if they met the following criteria:

1. For theoretical/conceptual references:
   a. They discussed the definition and the domains/dimensions of advanced nursing practice.
   b. They presented the findings of a concept analysis or literature review performed to identify the essential characteristics, domains, and dimensions, as well as the empirical indicators or manifestations of the outcome concepts of interest.
   c. They reported the results of a qualitative study conducted to explore the understanding of role implementation or perception of outcomes related to advanced nursing practice.
2. For empirical references:
   a. They reported the results of studies that examined the relationships among the structure, process, and outcome variables for clinical nurse specialist practice.
   b. Studies with descriptive, experimental, or quasi-experimental designs were included. The inclusion of quasi-experimental studies was important for two reasons:
      i. It increased the number of references for a comprehensive literature review, particularly if the studies were conducted in the context of actual/everyday practice where randomization may not have been feasible or possible; and
      ii. It provided evidence for determining the extent to which the outcomes are responsive to change.

Differences in research designs across studies were accounted for when synthesizing the findings to address the objectives set for this literature review.

Step 3: Literature Compilation

1. A list of references was generated for each outcome variable.
2. Standardized tables for extracting the relevant data were used to review the literature.
3. Word files were generated for anecdotal observations and synthesis of the literature.
4. Two of the coauthors independently reviewed all of the empirical studies.

CONCEPTUALIZING CNS PRACTICE

In this section, we present a conceptualization of the CNS *role*, derived from a synthesis of essential characteristics developed by the NACNS (2004) and pertinent theoretical and empirical literature. The literature consisted of:

1. Reviews about the CNS role components done either as independent initiatives (Conger & Craig, 1998; Harrington & Smith, 2005; McAlpine, 1997; Raja-Jones, 2002) or in preparation for a research study (Barnason, Merboth, Pozehl, & Tietjen, 1998; Carroll, Robinson, Buselli, Berry, & Rankin, 2001; Mick & Ackerman, 2000; Wojner & Kite-Powell, 1997); or
2. Quantitative or qualitative studies that investigated the CNS role implementation in various settings (Bousfield, 1997; Dickerson, Wu, & Kennedy, 2006; Froggatt & Hoult, 2002; Linck & Phillips, 2005; McCreaddie, 2001; Scott, 1999).

A clear and sound understanding of the CNS role is required to appreciate its contribution to outcomes. Knowledge of the CNS domains of practice and role functions and activities is critical for delineating the mechanisms underlying the impact of CNSs' care on patient, nurse, and system outcomes (Sidani, Doran, & Mitchell, 2004).

CNSs are "licensed registered professional nurses with graduate preparation" demonstrated in an earned master's or doctorate degree (NACNS, 2004, p. 12). Through graduate preparation, CNSs acquire advanced knowledge and clinical expertise that enables them to function independently and in collaboration with other health care professionals for the purpose of achieving high-quality, cost-effective outcomes. Although CNSs develop expertise in particular specialty areas (Darmody, 2005), they exert their influence in three spheres: patients or clients and patient care; nurses and nursing practice; and organization and system (NACNS, 2004).

Patient and Patient Care

Within this sphere or domain of practice, CNSs follow the nursing process of assessment, diagnosis, intervention, and evaluation in order to maintain or improve health.

CNSs focus on identifying the needs of patients, selecting and implementing theory and evidence-based interventions to remedy or alleviate symptoms, enhancing physical and psychosocial functioning, and modifying risk behaviors and promoting healthy lifestyles (NACNS, 2004). In addition, CNSs manage patients' care through consultation and collaboration with health care professionals (Brooten, Youngblut, Deatrick, Naylor, & York, 2003; Harrington & Smith, 2005; Naylor, Bowles, & Brooten, 2000). Consultation and collaboration are directed toward clarifying complex patient problems, finding appropriate solutions to those problems, and providing and coordinating services to achieve the collaboratively identified goals or outcomes (NACNS, 2004).

The role functions and activities comprising the patient and patient care practice domain are specified in the conceptual and empirical literature included in this review. The specific activities are consistent with the NACNS's (2004) statement but are categorized into direct and indirect patient-care activities. Direct patient-care activities reflect the basic elements of the nursing process (assessment, diagnosis, intervention, and evaluation) and encompass surveillance, provision of care, and facilitation of support groups for patients and families. Indirect patient-care activities include case management and the provision of consultation regarding patient care (Brooten et al., 2003; Conger & Craig, 1998; Fowler Byers & Brunnell, 1998; Linck & Phillips, 2005; Naylor

et al., 2000; Scott, 1999; Wojner & Kite-Powell, 1997). Table 4.1 presents a list of specific activities illustrating direct and indirect patient-care functions of the CNS role.

Nurse and Nursing Care

This domain of CNS practice focuses on supporting nursing personnel in the delivery of high-quality, safe, and evidence-based care. CNSs engage in role-modeling, consultation, and education to improve nursing practice (NACNS, 2004). The specific activities representing this domain are classified into formal and informal education. Formal education consists of the organization of and participation in staff orientation to the specialty area and the design and provision of programs concerned with the continuous professional development of nurses (Barnason et al., 1998; Carroll et al., 2001; Fowler Byers & Brunnell, 1998; Martin, 1999; McCreaddie, 2001; Phillips, 2005; Scott, 1999). Informal education entails the role-modeling and consultation activities mentioned in the NACNS (2004) statement. For a list of specific activities related to formal and informal education provided by CNSs, refer to Table 4.2.

Organization and System

CNSs are leaders who advocate for patient care and professional nursing within the organization and the health care

4.1 | Specific Activities Illustrating Direct and Indirect Patient Care Functions

PATIENT CARE FUNCTIONS	SPECIFIC ACTIVITIES
Direct care	
Surveillance	1. Assessing patients' physical and psychosocial conditions, health behaviors, and environmental situations 2. Diagnosing patients' and family needs 3. Monitoring patients' condition and progress toward achieving outcomes
Provision of care	1. Planning comprehensive care for patients and family 2. Providing extended education and counseling 3. Troubleshooting complex patient care problems 4. Assessing effectiveness of interventions
Facilitation of support groups for patients and family	1. Planning support groups for patients and family 2. Organizing logistics of support groups
Indirect care	
Case management	1. Overseeing delivery of patient care 2. Facilitating interdisciplinary patient care conference 3. Coordinating interdisciplinary services 4. Discharge planning, including arrangement for required community services
Provision of consultation regarding patients' care	1. Applying advanced knowledge in crisis intervention 2. Providing support for front-line problem solving, including equipment problems

4.2 | Specific Activities Illustrating Formal and Informal Education Functions

EDUCATION FUNCTIONS	SPECIFIC ACTIVITIES
Formal	1. Participating in development, organization, and coordination of nursing staff orientation to specialty unit 2. Participating in initial and continuous assessment of nursing staff competencies 3. Designing and implementing ongoing educational programs to nursing staff based on identified learning needs/competencies 4. Providing certification review courses to nursing staff 5. Participating in and/or providing courses to undergraduate and/or graduate nursing students 6. Serving as clinical preceptor to nursing staff and students
Informal	1. Providing mentorship to nursing staff at bedside 2. Serving as role model in problem solving and case management 3. Serving as information resource to nursing staff (e.g., responding to questions related to unfamiliar policies, procedures, clinical problems; discussing evidence base for nursing interventions)

system. They initiate, implement, and coordinate innovative programs that address the needs of patients, nurses, and organizations and aim at achieving high-quality and cost-efficient health care across the full continuum of care (NACNS, 2004). The specific activities pertaining to this organizational domain of CNS practice and mentioned in the literature are grouped into those associated with: continuous quality improvement initiatives (Arbour, 2003; Conger & Craig, 1998; Wojner & Kite-Powell, 1997); policies, procedures, and best practice guidelines development (Froggatt & Hoult, 2002; Harrington & Smith, 2005; McCreaddie, 2001); program development and evaluation (Scott, 1999); evidence-based practice (Harrington & Smith, 2005; McCreaddie, 2001; Scott, 1999); and committee work. These activities operationalize the CNS role within the organizational domain, as described by the NACNS (2004) and presented in Table 4.3.

Only one study was found that investigated CNSs' implementation of role functions and activities related to the three domains of practice as identified by the NACNS (2004). Darmody (2005) conducted a pilot study to explore CNS ($n = 5$) engagement in patient care, nursing practice, and organization-related activities. CNS performance of these activities was assessed with direct observation and time study. The results provided a useful overview indicating that the CNSs spent 30% of their time in patient care, 44% in activities associated with improvement of nursing practice, 10% in organization activities, and 16% in other activities, such as personal time and managing e-mail communication.

CONCEPTUALIZING OUTCOMES OF CNS PRACTICE

In this section, we present a conceptualization of outcomes expected of CNS *practice*. The conceptualization was derived from a synthesis of the NACNS's (2004) statement, which identified specific outcomes for the three domains of CNS practice, and the available conceptual literature reflecting nursing scholars' propositions of outcomes sensitive to CNS care. We define *CNS-sensitive outcomes* as those that can be theoretically linked to the activities of CNSs and observed in the three domains of CNS practice: patient and patient care, nurse and nursing practice, and organization and system.

Patient-Related Outcomes

CNSs have an impact on patient outcomes through the accurate diagnosis of patients' needs and problems and the provision of appropriate interventions to remedy the problems, promote health, and prevent error. CNSs' practice in this domain is expected to achieve four categories of desired patient-focused outcomes: clinical, functional, perception, and cost of care (Fowler Byers & Brunnell, 1998; NACNS, 2004).

The *clinical* outcomes are subdivided into: (1) the successful management of disease-specific signs and of physical and psychosocial symptoms experienced as a result of disease, illness, or treatment, manifested by normal test values (e.g., blood glucose level, FEV1) and reduced symptom frequency and severity; and (2) the early identification and prevention of complications (e.g., nosocomial infections and deep vein thrombosis) and side effects of medications (Arbour, 2003; Barnason et al., 1998; Darmody, 2005).

Functional outcomes encompass: physical, psychological, and social functioning; ability to participate in activities of daily living and to meet role expectations; overall well-being; quality of life; and self-management knowledge and skills related to current condition and modification of risky health behaviors

Specific Activities Pertaining to Organization-System Domain of Practice

ORGANIZATION/SYSTEM FUNCTIONS	SPECIFIC ACTIVITIES
Continuous quality improvement initiatives	1. Designing methods and tools for continuous data (related to process and outcome of care) collection 2. Analyzing and synthesizing data obtained from multiple sources 3. Identifying care-related issues requiring remediation 4. Collaborating with members of interdisciplinary team in formulation of remedial strategies and change of practice 5. Overseeing implementation of remedial strategies and practice change 6. Facilitating ongoing outcome monitoring
Policies, procedures, and best practice guidelines development	1. Developing organization policies and procedures related to care delivery 2. Developing best practice guidelines based on available evidence 3. Providing leadership in dissemination and implementation of policies, procedures, and practice guidelines
Program development and evaluation	1. Collaborating with administrators and professionals (nursing and others) to identify clinical issues requiring intervention 2. Designing programs to address identified clinical issues 3. Coordinating implementation of programs and evaluation of their effects
Evidence-based practice	1. Leading or participating in research related to area of specialty 2. Assisting professionals (nursing and others) in conduct of clinical research 3. Participating in dissemination of research findings within organization and at conferences 4. Supporting nursing staff in change of practice or research utilization
Committee work	1. Participating in committees within organization, community, and profession

(Barnason et al., 1998; Carroll et al., 2001; Conger & Graig, 1998; Darmody, 2005).

Perception of care outcomes relate to the patient and family rating of the quality of services and satisfaction with the care received (Harrington & Smith, 2005).

Cost outcomes are associated with utilization of resources across the health care continuum operationalized in indices such as length of hospital stay, readmission, return visit to clinic, and visit to the emergency department (Harrington & Smith, 2005; Linck & Phillips, 2005; McAlpine, 1997; Scott, 1999). CNSs' engagement in indirect patient-care activities promotes coordination of patient care, which is reflected in prompt services required for patients (Harrington & Smith, 2005).

Nurse-Related Outcomes

CNSs' involvement in formal and informal education is anticipated to contribute to improving nursing staff's knowledge, skills, and practice that is theory- and evidence-based, enhancing nurse participation in continuing professional development, increasing nurse job satisfaction, and retaining competent nursing personnel (Arbour, 2003; Barnason et al., 1998; Darmody, 2005; NACNS, 2004).

Organization-Related Outcomes

The implementation of activities within this domain of CNS practice is expected to result in improved organizational performance in terms of innovative evidence-based models of care and cost savings associated with the purchase and use of equipment, supplies, and services (Fowler Byers & Brunnell, 1998; NACNS, 2004).

CNSs' achievement of these specific outcomes will contribute to the attainment of the ultimate goal summarized by the NACNS (2004) as "quality, cost-effective, patient-focused outcomes" (p. 6). The empirical evidence supporting the impact of CNS role on patient, nurse, and organization outcomes is presented next.

CATEGORIZING NURSING-SENSITIVE PATIENT OUTCOMES

In this section, we provide an overview of the historical work in classifying nursing-sensitive patient outcomes as a foundation for situating our discussion of outcomes sensitive to CNS practice. Nursing-sensitive outcomes are outcomes that can be empirically or theoretically linked to the actions of registered nurses

(RNs) or registered practical nurses (RPNs; Doran et al., 2003). There have been several attempts to generate a taxonomy of patient outcomes that can be expected to occur from the provision of nursing care (Hegyvary, 1991; Jennings, Staggers, & Brosch, 1999; Lohr, 1985).

Early categorizations of nursing-sensitive outcomes focused on the adverse aspects of treatment and have included mortality, morbidity (iatrogenic complications), unscheduled readmission, unscheduled repeat surgery, and unnecessary hospital procedures (e.g., cesarean section rates). Lohr (1985) proposed a list of six categories based on the continuum of care: mortality, adverse events and complications during hospitalization, inadequate recovery, prolongation of the medical problem, decline in health status, and decline in quality of life. Using a different approach, Hegyvary (1991) suggested four categories of outcome assessment from the perspectives of patients, providers, and purchasers: (a) clinical (patients' responses to interventions), (b) functional (improvement or decline in physical functioning), (c) financial (cost and length of stay), and (d) perceptual (patient satisfaction with care received and persons providing the care).

Jennings et al. (1999) reviewed the nursing, medical, and health services research literature from 1974 and on to locate all indicators of outcomes. These were classified as patient-focused, provider-focused, or organization-focused. Although not specific to the CNS role, this classification has potential applicability because of its broad conceptualization of outcomes and its recognition that nurses do impact system-level outcomes. Within the patient-focused category, a further subdivision into diagnosis-focused and holistically focused was proposed. Examples of the diagnosis-specific outcomes are laboratory values, Apgar scores, and vital signs. The holistically oriented outcomes include health status, health-related quality of life, patient satisfaction ratings, assessments of patient knowledge, and symptom management. Care provider–focused outcomes included complication rates, appropriate use of medications, and, when a family caregiver is involved, a measure of caregiver burden. Adverse events such as falls, deaths, and unplanned readmission were categorized as organization-focused outcomes.

In the Quality Health Outcomes Model developed by the American Academy of Nursing Expert Panel on Quality Health Care, five outcome categories expected to be sensitive to nursing care inputs were delineated: achievement of appropriate self-care, demonstration of health-promoting behaviors, health-related quality of life, perception of being well cared for, and symptom management to criterion (Mitchell, Armstrong, Simpson, & Lentz, 1989; Mitchell & Lang, 2004). In the Nursing Role Effectiveness Model, proposed by Irvine, Sidani, and McGillis Hall (1998), the following patient outcomes were hypothesized as sensitive to nursing:

patient satisfaction, functional status, self-care, symptom control, and safety/adverse occurrences.

These different frameworks for categorizing nursing-sensitive outcomes are quite consistent with the conceptualization of outcomes of CNS practice that were derived from the NACNS's (2004) statement on CNS practice and education. Most frameworks recognize that nurses have an impact on a broad set of patient outcomes, reflecting improvement in clinical, functional, and psychosocial outcomes, and that nurses minimize or mitigate the effect of adverse outcomes. The conceptualization of outcomes of CNS practice that was synthesized from the NACNS's statement has been used to organize our discussion of the evidence from the empirical literature presented in the next section.

EVIDENCE CONCERNING OUTCOMES SENSITIVE TO CNS PRACTICE

In identifying outcomes relevant for evaluating the impact of the CNS role within the health care system, we considered both the empirical evidence concerning the influence of CNS practice on patient outcomes and the empirical evidence concerning the influence of CNS practice on unit or system outcomes, recognizing that the processes by which CNSs impact outcomes is often mediated through other system variables, such as changes in the quality of nursing care. The studies that were identified through our search of the literature are summarized in the Appendix. Each study was reviewed using the following framework: research design, setting for practice, sample, method of accounting for confounding/control variables that could influence the results, CNS role activities, intervention tested, and research results. This information was helpful in determining the level of consistency in the evidence across studies with regard to outcomes sensitive to CNS practice.

Patient-Related Outcomes

As previously noted, patient-related or patient-focused outcomes include clinical, functional, perception, and cost of care (Fowler Byers & Brunnell, 1998; NACNS, 2004). The *clinical* outcomes have been subdivided into: (a) successful management of disease-specific signs and symptoms, and (b) early identification and prevention of complications.

Under subdivision (a), there are a number of *disease/condition–specific outcomes* that were identified from the empirical literature on CNS practice. These include: arthritis disease activity for a rheumatoid arthritis population (Ryan, Hassell, Lewis, & Farrell, 2006; Tijhuis, Zwinderman, Hazes, Breedveld, & Vliet, 2003), wound healing (Capasso, 1998), glycemic control for a diabetic population (Vrijhoef, Diederiks, Spreeuwenberg, &

Wolffenbuttel, 2001), mobility for patients with Parkinson disease (Hurwitz, Jarman, Cook, & Bajekal, 2005), physiological indicators (Graveley & Littlefield, 1992), and full-term delivery for high-risk women (Brooten et al., 2001). The types of CNS role activities that were investigated in these studies were case management (Ryan et al.; Vrijhoef et al.), patient education (Brooten et al.; Tijhuis et al.), multidisciplinary collaborative practice (Hurwitz et al., 2005), assessment, patient monitoring, counseling, and referrals (Brooten et al.; Graveley & Littlefield). With the exception of the research by Vrijhoef et al. and by Gravely and Littlefield, these studies employed a randomized controlled trial (RCT) design and focused on the expanded role of the CNS in outpatient settings. When this research was reviewed, we found that there was mixed evidence concerning the relationship between CNS practice and disease/condition–specific outcomes. Three studies found a significant positive relationship between CNS practice and the disease/condition–specific outcomes, whereas three studies did not. Two of the studies that did not find a significant relationship might have lacked power to detect significant effects because of small sample size (Graveley & Littlefield; Tijhuis et al.). However, the third study had a large sample size, included a 2-year follow-up, and utilized objective approaches to outcomes measurement (Hurwitz et al., 2005). Therefore, the empirical evidence suggests that CNSs can have a significant positive influence on patients' disease/condition–specific outcomes, however, this evidence is mixed and requires further validation in future research.

The second type of outcome reviewed under subdivision (a), "successful management of disease specific signs and symptoms," was *physical and psychosocial symptoms*. Under this grouping, researchers have investigated pain outcomes (Gaston-Johansson et al., 2000; Tranmer & Parry, 2004; White, 1999), perceived stress (Tsay, Lee, & Lee, 2005), depression (Gaston-Johansson et al., 2000; Naylor et al., 1999; Tsay et al., 2005), symptom distress (McCorckle et al., 1989; Tranmer & Parry, 2004), nausea, and fatigue (Gaston-Johansson et al., 2000). These studies have investigated the full scope of CNS practice from case management (McCorckle et al., Tranmer & Parry, Tsay et al.), to direct clinical practice (White), to group intervention (Gaston-Johansson et al.), and to discharge follow-up (Naylor et al.). The empirical evidence suggests that CNSs have a significant positive effect on physical and psychosocial outcomes through practice in inpatient settings (Gaston-Johansson et al.; White) and outpatient settings (McCorckle et al.; Tsay et al.).

The third category of outcome we consider in the *clinical* category is under subdivision (b), *early identification and prevention of complications*. Two types of outcomes are considered in this category: unanticipated mortality (Brooten et al., 2001) and hospital-acquired

complications, such as respiratory infection, foot drop, surgical wound infection, urinary tract infection, drug overdose, fever (Forster et al., 2005; Gurka, 1991; Jacavone, Daniels, & Tyner, 1999; Wheeler, 2000), and endotracheal reintubation (Crimlisky et al., 1997). The majority of studies demonstrated a positive impact of CNS practice on early identification and prevention of complications, although it is important to note that many of these studies employed weaker study designs than an RCT. The one RCT study found no significant difference in hospital-acquired complications between general medical inpatients who received care from a CNS-supported multidisciplinary team and those who received care on general medical units (Forster et al.). However, that RCT study had a relatively small sample size (175 patients in the intervention arm) and thus might have been too underpowered to detect significant differences.

Functional health outcomes encompass physical, psychological, and social functioning; self-management knowledge and skills; and modification of risky health behaviors. Under this category of outcome, we included studies that investigated the impact of CNS practice on functional health outcomes, quality of life, and self-management or adherence to treatment. Of the seven studies that investigated functional health outcomes, only two found a significant relationship between CNS practice and medical patients' self-reported functional health outcomes (Ryan et al., 2006; Tsay et al., 2005). This lack of evidence concerning the impact of CNS practice on functional health outcomes is somewhat puzzling; however, it could be a function of the way in which functional health was conceptualized and measured in those studies (Hurwitz et al., 2005; Naylor et al., 1999; Tijhuis et al., 2003; Vrijhoef et al., 2001; York et al., 1997). In our previous research, we observed that nurses have a significant influence on patients' functional health outcomes but for a specific subcategory only, namely, activities of daily living and instrumental activities of daily living (Doran, 2003). The studies investigating functional status outcomes of CNS practice have typically employed broad measures of patients' physical, social, and emotional role functioning, which might be less sensitive to CNS influence, especially within the context of a short hospital stay. Therefore, we suggest that further research is needed to investigate functional status as an outcome of CNS practice, with a particular focus on the conceptualization of appropriate indicators that will be amenable to change over relatively short periods of time. Functional health indicators that could be appropriately based on evidence from previous research include activities of daily living and instrumental activities of daily living.

Quality of life outcome is the most broadly conceptualized outcome under the functional health outcome category. Once again, the evidence in Table 4.4 indicates mixed findings, with one study reporting a significant relationship between CNS practice and quality of life outcome (Tijhuis et al., 2003) and one study reporting no significant relationship (Tranmer & Parry, 2004). Quality-of-life instruments typically combine into one measure the three dimensions of functioning: physical functioning, emotional functioning, and social functioning. That measure yields an assessment of general health status or health-related quality of life (McDowell & Newell, 1996). Such quality-of-life instruments have two characteristics that might make them insensitive to detecting the contribution of CNSs' practice to patient outcome. First, they often have a long-term time horizon, and thus, it is difficult to detect the influence of any particular direct-care activities from the influence of all the other events and circumstances that contribute to health and well-being. Second, because quality-of-life measures typically generate a global score, it is possible to miss the contribution of a clinicians' practice if, for instance, the effect of that practice is only on a particular subdimension of the patients' quality of life. Based on these observations and the aforementioned evidence, we suggest that quality of life may be sensitive to CNS practice but that its relationship can be difficult to detect.

The third type of functional health outcomes identified in the empirical literature was *self-management* or *adherence to treatment*. Three studies were found that investigated self-management or compliance with treatment as an outcome of CNS practice (Capasso, 1998; De Jong & Veltman, 2004; Hall, Callow, Evans, & Johnston, 1994). In each of these studies, CNS practice was positively associated with patients' self-management and risk modification behavior.

Patient satisfaction with care is another category of outcome identified in Table 4.4. Four studies were identified that included patient satisfaction as an outcome of CNS practice (Charles, Le Vasseur, & Castle, 1999; Forster et al., 2005; Graveley & Littlefield, 1992; Naylor et al., 1999). Two of these found a significant relationship between the care provided by CNSs and patient satisfaction outcome (Charles et al., 1999; Forster et al., 2005). Charles et al. randomly assigned patients presenting to the emergency department (ED) who required suturing for minor lacerations to the services of a CNS or to a physician. Patients in the CNS arm reported higher satisfaction with their care than patients in the physician arm. In another RCT, Forster et al. reported higher satisfaction for patients admitted to the services of a CNS-supported medical team than for patients admitted to routine hospital services. In contrast, neither Naylor et al. nor Gravely and Littlefield found significantly higher satisfaction for obstetrical patients assigned to CNS care than for patients assigned to routine care. Because these latter two studies involved women

in an obstetrical setting, it is possible that the women were already predisposed to feel positive about their care, and that could have resulted in high satisfaction scores for women in both the intervention group and the control group. Previous research in the context of general nursing practice offers strong evidence of the sensitivity of patient satisfaction outcome to nursing care (Laschinger & Almost, 2003). It, therefore, seems reasonable to expect a similar sensitivity to CNS practice. However, it will be important to carefully assess the process mechanisms that explain how CNS practice affects patient satisfaction, something we say more about in the discussion that follows.

Organizational outcomes identified from the empirical literature investigating CNS practice were: *unit length of stay, hospital length of stay,* and *total costs* for patient care. With only a couple of exceptions (Forster et al., 2005; Hurwitz et al., 2005), the research evidence suggests that CNS services can have a significant positive influence on cost outcomes (Ahrens, Yancey, & Kollef, 2003; Brooten et al., 2001; Graveley & Littlefield, 1992; Naylor et al., 1999; York et al., 1997). These findings were consistent across practice settings, including inpatient hospital settings (Ahrens et al., Naylor et al.), ambulatory care (Graveley & Littlefield), and home care (Brooten et al., York et al.). The CNS role activities in these studies included comprehensive discharge planning, case management, and home follow-up. These role activities had a significant impact on health care utilization and overall health care costs, demonstrating the CNSs' achievement of quality, cost-effective, patient-focused outcomes.

In summary, the following patient and organizational outcomes were found to be sensitive to CNS practice and are recommended as appropriate indicators for assessing the impact of clinical nurse specialists within the health care system:

1. Patient-Focused
   a. Disease/condition–specific outcomes
   b. Physical and psychosocial symptom outcomes
   c. Early identification and prevention of complications
   d. Self-management and adherence to treatment
   e. Patient satisfaction
2. Organization-Focused
   a. Unit/hospital length of stay
   b. Total health care charges

In addition, functional status was identified as potentially sensitive to CNS practice, however, further research is needed to determine the most appropriate indicators for its measurement. These will likely be indicators that are amenable to change over a relatively short period of time, such as activities of daily living and instrumental activities of daily living.

4.4 | Studies Investigating Clinical Nurse Specialist Practice and Patient Outcomes

AUTHOR(S)	DESIGN	SETTING/ SUBJECTS	CONTROL VARIABLES	OUTCOME	CNS ROLE COMPONENTS/ DOMAINS	INTERVENTION	RESULTS
Ahrens et al. (2003)	Quasi-experiment	Medical ICU patients at high risk of dying (N = 43 intervention, N = 108 control)	Patient demographics (chart review)	Clinical (chart review); Severity of Illness "Apache II scoring system"; Resource consumption (ICU and hospital length of stay, mortality and fixed cost per case, hospital variable indirect charge per case, hospital variable direct charge per case)	Physician and CNS collaborative ICU managed care vs. rotating physician managed care. Education, physical functioning, psychosocial functioning, administration, case management	Daily information to families, clarify issues and develop care plan	Patients receiving collaborative physician/CNS care had > improvements in severity of illness (32.1–28.6); length of stay in ICU (6.1–9.5 days); costs ($5320–$8484); and mortality (74%–93%) than physician managed care only.
Brooten et al. (2001)	RCT	173 women and 194 infants		Fetal/infant mortality; full-term deliveries; Re-hospitalization; Maternal affect "Multiple Affect Adjective State Form Checklist" (Zuckerman et al., 1983), α 0.73; Satisfaction with care "LaMonica-Oberst Patient Satisfaction Scale" (LaMonica-Oberst, 1986), α 0.92	Assessment, monitoring, environmental supports, individual teaching and counseling, referrals	Home visits by APNs	Experimental group had lower fetal/ infant mortality (2 vs. 9), fewer preterm infants, more twin pregnancies carried to term (77% vs. 33%), fewer prenatal hosp. (41 vs. 49), fewer infant rehosp. (18 vs. 24), and lower costs.
Charles et al. (1999)	Descriptive, comparative,	80 patients from emergency		Patient wait times; patient perceptions	Low acuity patients requiring simple	Nursing educational sessions related to	More patients were satisfied with CNS

(Continued)

4.4 | Studies Investigating Clinical Nurse Specialist Practice and Patient Outcomes (*Continued*)

AUTHOR(S)	DESIGN	SETTING/ SUBJECTS	CONTROL VARIABLES	OUTCOME	CNS ROLE COMPONENTS/ DOMAINS	INTERVENTION	RESULTS
	randomly assigned	department in Melbourne, Australia		of wait time; patient satisfaction; wound complications	suture receiving CNS managed care vs. physician managed care. Physical functioning, administration, psychosocial functioning, role functioning	suturing of minor lacerations	than physician care (mean rank 47.65 & 33.35, 2 tailed $P = 0.0016$). No other significant findings
Crimlisk et al. (1997)	Prospective	Adult patients requiring endotracheal intubation in a trauma center during a 3-month period. Phase 1 $N = 862$ Phase 2 $N = 808$		Reintubation rate (the # of reintubations per total hospital intubations) Duration of intubation (# patient ventilated days)	Reintubation events documented for 3 months. Interventions instituted and evaluated for reintubation (3-month period). Similar data collected at 2 years	Continuous quality screening of high-risk patients. Staff nurses provided with inservices, education and posted signs	Multiple reintubation events decreased from 45% to 18.8% of all intubations
De Jong (2004)	Descriptive, convenience sampling. Baseline, 8, 12 weeks after initial questionnaire	Community-based COPD screening clinic $N = 243$	Questionnaire: demographics, symptoms, treatments, smoking history	Spirometry "GOLD"; Stage of Smoking (author prepared questionnaire)	CNS-managed COPD clinic to identify at-risk adults. Physical functioning, psychosocial functioning, counseling, self care	COPD screening questionnaire, spirometry testing, counseling and follow-up survey.	86% participants identified as current or past smokers. Of these, 23% had evidence of obstruction. 78% had never had spirometry testing. Post screening 40% stated they were contemplating quitting smoking and 5 had.

Author (year)	Design	Sample	Data/Measures	Outcomes (Instruments)	Comparison	Intervention	Results
Forster et al. (2005)	RCT	General medical in-hospital patients $N = 307$ CNS care $N = 313$ regular hospital care. Post discharge $N = 175$ CNS care $N = 186$ regular hospital care	Medical information demographics (chart review, patient interviews)	In-hospital: mortality, length of stay. Post discharge: time to ED visit, readmission or death; Patient satisfaction (Cleary et al., 1991); Risk of adverse events	Regular hospital care vs. CNS care	CNS arranged in-hospital consultations and investigations, organized follow-up visits and telephone calls post discharge	Addition of CNS to a medical team improved patient satisfaction but did not impact hospital efficiency or patient safety
Gaston-Johansson et al. (2000)	RCT	Patients with breast cancer with autologous bone marrow/peripheral blood stem cell transplantation $N = 58$ control; $N = 52$ treatment group	Socio-demographic questionnaire	Pain "(POM)-Gaston-Johansson Painometer" (Gaston-Johansson, 1996); Nausea "Nausea VAS" (Gift, 1989); Fatigue "Fatigue VAS" (Piper, 1989); Anxiety "State Trait Anxiety Inventory" (Spielberger et al., 1971); Depression "Beck Depression Inventory" (Beck & Steer, 1993)	Treatment group given CCSP vs. regular care. Pain, fatigue, psychological distress, nausea	CNS developed Comprehensive Coping Strategy Program (CCSP); Conducted baseline questionnaires (Social worker taught CCSP)	CCSP effective in reducing nausea/fatigue. Treatment group experienced mild anxiety; control group experienced moderate anxiety
Graveley & Littlefield (1992)	Descriptive/cost comparative analysis	3 prenatal clinics: Study period = 3 months $N = 156$	Demographics	Physiological—"Kessner Index" (Kessner et al., 1973); Patient satisfaction tool "PST" (Reed et al., 1978), α 0.83; Costs (personal costs/number of kept appointments)	CNS managed prenatal clinic compared to physician/NP managed and physician care. Maternal and infant physical function, psychosocial function, role function, administration, case management, research	CNS delivered total prenatal care & referrals to community agencies	CNS care was significantly lower costs per visit over physician and physician/NP managed care ($7.81, $11.18 & $9.23 respectively). No other differences noted.

(Continued)

4.4 | Studies Investigating Clinical Nurse Specialist Practice and Patient Outcomes (*Continued*)

AUTHOR(S)	DESIGN	SETTING/ SUBJECTS	CONTROL VARIABLES	OUTCOME	CNS ROLE COMPONENTS/ DOMAINS	INTERVENTION	RESULTS
Hall et al. (1994)	Retrospective 3, 6-month reviews	N = 70 referrals		Patient compliance (diary cards); Mean peak expiratory flow (PEF); Nursing consultation time (diary)	Home nebulizer CNS managed care	Patient assessment and nebulizer trial therapy. Referral assessment for appropriateness	19% CNS time spent on patient/nebulizer assessment. 24% CNS time spent on clerical duties. 54% of patients used nebulizer as prescribed. 18% used not at all/very little. 4 referrals inappropriate. PEF not reported.
Hurwitz et al. (2004)	RCT over 2 years	Total participants with Parkinson's disease in general practice N = 1859 N = 1028 CNS group N = 808 control group		Function & well-being "PDQ-39" (Jenkinson et al., 1995); Health-related quality of life "Euroqol" (Williams, 1995); Health care costs "Personal Social Services Research Unit" (Netten & Denett, 1996); Medicine use "Monthly index of Medical Specialists 1996 net ingredients costs" (MIMS, 1996); Mortality "National Health Services Central Registry" Visuomotor coordination (Gersten–brand et al., 1973); Ability to rise from sitting "Columbian Rating Scale" (Wade, 1994)	Attended by CNS vs. standard care with GP	CNS worked in collaboration with GP providing counseling, education and monitoring of patients	CNS had little effect on clinical conditions, but did improve patients' sense of well-being. No additional costs to care

Author (Year)	Design	Sample	Data Collection	Variables/Instruments	Intervention	APN Role	Findings
Jacavone et al. (1999)	Retrospective chart review Pre/post clinical pathway implement	N = 602 preimplement (control), N = 598 postimplement (intervention), Cardiac surgery patients		Surgical complications Prolonged ventilation (mechanical vent > 24 hours); Pneumonia (+ve sputum cultures or chest x-ray); Complications "Summit Medical Systems Inc database"; Length of stay "Information Technology Systems Department"; Costs "Information Technology Systems Department"	CNS facilitated cardiac surgery clinical pathway program. Role development, physical function, Administration, Practice development, health policy.	CNS facilitated interdisciplinary development/implementation of a clinical pathways for post cardiac surgery patients	Intervention group had decreased prolonged ventilation (10.3%–9.03%), pneumonia (2.49%–1.67%) and GI (0.66%–0.33%). Intervention group had shorter length of stay (8–7 days) and total cost savings of $201,000.
Lacko et al. (2000)	Quasi-experimental	Medical patients aged 65+ in community hospital N = 34 experimental N = 11 control	Demographics (chart review)	Mental Status "Memory Concentration Test (OMC)," Delirium "Confusion Assessment Method (CAM)" α 0.87, IRR = 1.0 Algorithm for both tests based on guidelines developed by the Task Force on Aging, American College of Physicians, 1995	Experimental group nurses educated to utilize a delirium screening tool vs. control nurses.	CNS/NP developed algorithm that identified tools to be used by staff nurses for screening delirium and defining physician vs. nurse responsibilities	Experimental nurses were able to identify all cases of delirium (100%). Control nurses identified none
McCorkle et al. (1989)	Longitudinal, RCT	N = 166 lung cancer patients Nursing home 3 groups: specialized oncology home care (OHC)-APN care; standard home care—interdisciplinary care (SHC); and office care—physician only (OC)	Baseline interview	Symptom distress "The Symptom Distress Scale"; Pain "McGill-Melzack Pain Questionnaire"; Concern "Inventory of Current Concerns" (Weisman & Worden, 1976); Mood state "Profile of Mood States" (Moinpour et al., 1992); Functional status "Enforced Social Dependency Scale"; Health perceptions "General Health Rating Index"; Utilization of services "Medical Record Review"	CNS home care managed personalized care for persons diagnosed with advanced cancer and their family members vs. interdisciplinary home care vs. physician managed care. Pain management, communication, Self care, psychosocial function.	5 interviews—1 within 8–10 days of diagnosis, 4 at 6-week intervals following. CNS conducted in-depth interviews re: physical and psychosocial health condition, hospitalization	OC experienced symptom distress and social dependency 6 weeks sooner than SHC and OHC. OHC and SHC reported worse health perceptions over time. OHC had fewer hospitalizations, but higher mean LOS in hospital. No difference in post-discharge acute care visits, functional status, depression, or patient satisfaction.

(Continued)

4.4 | Studies Investigating Clinical Nurse Specialist Practice and Patient Outcomes (*Continued*)

AUTHOR(S)	DESIGN	SETTING/ SUBJECTS	CONTROL VARIABLES	OUTCOME	CNS ROLE COMPONENTS/ DOMAINS	INTERVENTION	RESULTS
Naylor et al. (1999)	RCT 2, 6, 12, and 24 weeks follow-up	At-risk elders, 65+ for hospital readmission $N = 138$ control $N = 124$ experimental		Acute/hospital readmission Function "Enforced Social Dependency Scale" (Moinpour et al., 1992); Depression "Centre for Epidemiological Studies Depression Scale" (Radloff, 1997); Patient satisfaction (Author prepared); Costs "Standardized Medicare reimbursements"	CNS Transitional care vs. routine acute care discharge planning. Physical function, psychological function	APN visit within 48 hours of hospital admission, comprehensive discharge planning, 2 home follow-up visits and weekly telephone calls	Control group had more hospital readmissions (14.5% & 6.2% respectively); Greater length of stay (760 vs. 270, $p < 0.001$); and two times greater health care costs ($1,238,928 vs. $642,595, $p < 0.001$).
Rankin et al. (2005)	RCT	Unpartnered elders, 65+ post cardiac event, medically stable $N = 40$		Number of contacts with nurse (nursing log); Number of minutes spent talking to patients (nursing log); Nurse dose "FAMISHED"	Collaborative CNS/peer advisor intervention to improve social networks and enhance social efficacy by promoting social integration	2 CNSs contacted recovering patients 16 times with home visits and telephone calls. CNSs provided social support, emotional-informative-instrumental aid.	Nurse dose calculated as amount of time, intensity of nursing time and percentage of proposed intervention strategies completed = 270 minutes per 12-week period. Most important CNS role identified = emotional support

Author (Year)	Design	Sample	Measures	Setting/Role	Intervention	Findings
Ryan et al. (2006)	RCT Baseline, 2, 7, 12 months follow-up	Rheumatology clinic (hospital based) $N = 36$ intervention $N = 35$ control	Ability to control arthritis "Arthritis Impact Measure Scale" (Meenan et al., 1980); "Rheumatology Attitude Index" (Nicassio et al., 1985); Disease activity "Disease Activity Score" (Prevoo et al., 1995); Medications (Nursing records/notes)	Rheumatology clinic vs. outpatient clinic care. Management, role function	CNSs reviewed and monitored patients' conditions once per week for 4 weeks and then once monthly x year for drug reactions, changes in disease.	Intervention group: improved scores in perception of ability to control arthritis, control group scores declined at 12 months (1.8 & 0.3 respectively) and had greater improvements in disease activity (0.9 & 0.1, $p = 0.048$ respectively).
Savage & Grap (1999)	Descriptive	Convenience sample of open-heart surgery patients $N = 342$	Questionnaire related to post surgery recovery: areas investigated— healing of wounds/ incisions, Physical signs/symptoms, Appetite Activity (Author prepared)	Cardiovascular CNS role described in relation to facilitative recovery. Problems patients encounter post hospital discharge defined.	CNS conducted telephone interviews 7–14 days post discharge asking patients about certain aspects of care. Provided patients with written material on symptoms of infection, incision care and use of incentive spirometer	Implications noted for CNS postoperative management, Recommended scheduled telephone follow-up interviews post discharge, particularly within first 2 weeks of discharge
Tijhuis et al. (2003)	RCT Study period = 2 years Follow-up at 12, 52, and 104 weeks	Rheumatoid arthritis patients $N = 210$	Quality of Life "RAND 36 Health Survey" (Hays et al., 1993); Rheumatoid Arthritis Quality of Life "RAQoL" (De Jong et al., 1997); Function "Health Assessment questionnaire" "HAQ" (Siegert et al., 1984); "McMaster Toronto arthritis" "MACT AR" (Tugwell et al., 1987); Disease Activity "DAS" "Disease Activity Scale" (Prevoo et al., 1995); Uptake of Paramedical services and Practical Aids and adaptations	Clinical and socio-demographic	CNS provided care in outpatient clinic vs. inpatient care	CNS provided information about RA, medications prescribed, equipment, home adaptations, and additional referrals at 1-hour educational sessions and 9-day clinic treatment days. Patients also received 1.5 hours of bedrest per clinic visit	Care provided by CNS had similar long-term clinical outcomes to inpatient and day patient care in RA patients

(Continued)

AUTHOR(S)	DESIGN	SETTING/ SUBJECTS	CONTROL VARIABLES	OUTCOME	CNS ROLE COMPONENTS/ DOMAINS	INTERVENTION	RESULTS
Tranmer et al. (2004)	RCT	Cardiac surgery patients $N = 200$ Followed during first 5 weeks post hospital discharge		Health-related quality of life "Medical Outcomes Study Short Form 36" (Ware et al., 1994); Symptom distress "Memorial Symptom Assessment Scale" (Portenoy et al., 1994); Satisfaction with care recovery; Rate of unexpected health care contacts (ED/hospital admissions)	APN managed care vs. usual care	APN familiar with patient clinical condition/care needs conducted telephone calls twice in first week and then weekly x 4 weeks	No significant effects on selected outcomes noted
Tsay et al. (2005)	RCT, convenience sampling, pre/post intervention	End-stage renal disease patients from Taiwan $N = 33$ control $N = 33$ intervention		Perceived stress "Hemodialysis Stressor Scale" (Baldree et al., 1982), α 0.85; Depression "Beck Depression Scale" (Beck et al., 1961), α 0.89; Quality of Life "Medical Outcome Short Form 36" (Ware et al., 1994).	CNS managed care vs. usual care (pamphlet and routine treatment), Psychosocial function, mental health, self-care management, role function, counseling	Coping and cognitive behavioral group sessions x 8 weeks	Intervention group improved in perception of stress ($t = 3.39$, $p = 0.002$), depression ($t = 3.54$, $p = 0.001$) and quality of life ($t = 4.35$, $p = 0.001$) Control group worsened in perception of stress ($t = 0.05$, $p = 0.96$), depression ($t = 3.69$, $p = 0.001$) and quality of life ($t = 2.68$, $p = 0.01$).
Vrijhoef et al. (2001)	Quasi-experimental, nonequivalent control group, baseline, 2-, 6-, 9-, and 12-month follow-up	Type 2 diabetics from hospital in Netherlands $N = 47$ control $N = 74$ intervention		Clinical status: hemoglobin A1C, fasting total cholesterol, triglycerides, BMI, BP; Health Status "Dutch Version of COOP/	CNS substituted diabetes managed care vs. internist led diabetes managed care. Physical function, self-care management,	3 quarterly CNS consultations & annual internist follow-up.	Intervention group improved while control declined for: Hemoglobin A1C (8.6–8.3% vs. 8.6–8.8%, respectively); Self-care behaviors (3.2–3.5 & 3.6–3.5,

			WONCA charts" (Nelson et al., 1987); Quality of Life "Visual Analogue Scale" (Maxwell et al., 1978); Self care "Self care behaviour checklist" (Pennings-van der Eerden, 1992); Disease knowledge "Dutch Diabetes Specific Instrument" (Ripken et al., 1990) α 0.80; Patient satisfaction "Industrial Marketing Management"; Number of consults (chart review)	patient satisfaction, education, role function	respectively); and Number of consultations (4–24 & 21-9, respectively). At baseline 96% intervention group preferred internist care, but at 24 weeks, 89% preferred CNS managed care.
Wheeler (2000)	Comparative, correlational, retrospective, random chart review	4 hospital orthopedic units (2 with CNS, 2 without) 32 patients undergoing total knee replacement	Demographics; Quality of care "Acute Pain Process Instrument, APRI" "High Risks for Disuse Syndrome Process Instrument, HRDSPI" (Author prepared). APRI IRR 90.4%, HRDSPI 91%; Length of stay (date of discharge–date of admission); Number of preventable complications (physician notes, x-rays, laboratory tests)	Orthopedic unit based CNS vs. non-CNS care to delineate CNS processes and patient outcomes. Role function, physical function, role performance; Nursing processes within first 24 hours post surgery	CNS units had fewer complications than non-CNS (6 & 17 respectively), shorter length of stay (4.87 days vs. 6.84 days, $p = 0.001$), and better quality of care (140.44 & 102.16, $p = 0.0001$, respectively).

(Continued)

AUTHOR(S)	DESIGN	SETTING/ SUBJECTS	CONTROL VARIABLES	OUTCOME	CNS ROLE COMPONENTS/ DOMAINS	INTERVENTION	RESULTS
White (1999)	Descriptive, prospective chart audits on nursing documentation at 3 months and 2 years	Acute care patients undergoing spinal surgery N = 35		Present Pain "Present Pain Index of McGill Pain Questionnaire" (Melzack et al., 1975); Analgesia administration "Agency for home care policy guidelines for acute pain management equivalency table" (Acute Pain Management Guideline Panel, 1992); Nursing Documentation "Pain Management Audit Tool" (Ferrell et al., 1991); Education program	Baseline: 1) Assess patient pain intensity and nursing documentation of pain assessment/analgesia administration; 2) Assess nursing documentation of pain assessment/ management Evaluate 1 & 2 with chart audit for changes in patient intensity and nursing documentation (with same population). Pain management, physical function, role function, education	4-week pain assessment and management focused educational program & new routes for post-op analgesia.	Assessment: PPI = 3.4 mean, 40% charts documented pain assessment, 50% received analgesia as ordered. Evaluation: PPI <3.0 mean 3 months 90% charts documented pain assessment and 85% received analgesia as ordered.
Willoughby et al. (2001)	Descriptive, random selection	N = 48 Outpatient foot care clinic, N = 15 Did not attend clinic	Demographics	Questionnaire re: Foot pathology & foot care behaviors (Author prepared)	CNS managed foot care clinic vs. inpatient or outpatient care with no clinic visits	CNS foot assessment, education re: foot care, referrals, lesion treatment	69% attendees reported calluses/ corns vs. 40% nonattendees. 8% attendees vs. 0% nonattendees reported ulcers. 60% nonattendees vs. 25% attendees walk barefoot. 20% nonattendees vs. 2% attendees would treat own lesions.

Study	Design	Sample	Variables/Instruments	Comparison	Intervention	Results
York et al. (1997)	RCT, baseline, 2, 4, 8 weeks postpartum	High-risk pregnant woman with diabetes or hypertension (N = 52 control, N = 44 intervention) and their infants (N = 51 control, N = 42 intervention)	Function "Enforced social dependent scale" (Benoliel et al., 1980), α 0.65; Patient satisfaction "La Monica Oberst Patient Satisfaction Scale" (LaMonica et al., 1986), α 0.98; Maternal/infant length of stay; # hospital/ acute care visits; cost of care	Perinatal CNS care vs. routine care. Physical functioning, social functioning, administration	Transitional care with 3 weekly telephone & 5 (minimum) home visits Patient education & counseling	Maternal: intervention group<antepartum rehospitalizations (p = 0.048) Infant: intervention group< birth weight babies (2 vs. 9, p = 0.56) and 378 g heavier

RCT = randomized controlled trial;
N = sample size;
CNS = clinical nurse specialist;
α = alpha coefficients;
IRR = interrater reliability.

From "Outcomes of Clinical Nurse Specialist Practice," by D. M. Doran, S. Sidani, & T. Di Pietro (in press), in J. Fulton (Ed.), Essentials of Clinical Nurse Specialist Practice. Lippincott Williams & Wilkins: New York, New York.

DISCUSSION OF THE EVIDENCE

A systematic review of the theoretical and empirical literature was undertaken in order to describe the scope of CNS practice and to identify its impact on patient and organizational outcomes. The systematic review of the literature showed that the contribution of the CNS role to patient outcomes is variable and of a rather small magnitude. Most of the studies were not explicitly guided by a framework that clearly delineated the nature of the relationships between the CNS role functions or components and anticipated outcomes. The conceptualization of CNS practice, based on the NACNS (2004) statement and described earlier in this chapter, offers a potentially useful explanation of the observed variable and small effects of the CNS role on patient outcomes. As articulated in that statement, the CNS's contribution to patient outcomes encompasses both direct and indirect effects. While the direct effect may be small, the indirect effect, mediated by enhancements in the nurses and nursing care sphere of practice, may be more substantial. Such conceptualization could provide a comprehensive framework to guide future investigation and a more accurate understanding of the mechanisms underlying the impact of the CNS role.

The results of the review have implications for practice, quality monitoring, quality improvement, and future research. Each of these is discussed in turn.

With regard to practice, examples were found in the literature of CNSs engaged in the full range of practice roles described in the NACNS (2004) statement. The examples included direct-care activities, such as advanced nursing assessment, intervention, and follow-up care. They also involved several examples of CNSs engaged in collaborative practice with the multidisciplinary team and in case management for patients in hospital and community settings. It was also noted that CNSs practice in a wide range of settings, including hospital-based, ambulatory care, and community-based settings. Such diversity of practice and demonstrated scope of practice provides strong evidence of the depth and breadth of the CNS role in our health care system today.

Roberts-Davis and Read (2001) conducted a Delphi study to establish similarities and differences between nurse practitioners (NPs) and CNSs and found that the skills required for both roles are primarily nursing skills. Their research demonstrated differences between NPs and CNSs in the area of systematic physical examination, systematic patient history taking, making diagnostic decisions, and prescribing treatment. However, Roberts-Davis and Read also concluded that both roles may evolve within the changing care context and may become more alike in some contexts. We found examples of this in the literature, such as CNSs assuming primary care management for patients admitted to the ED

for suturing of minor lacerations (Charles et al., 1999) and of ambulatory care for patients with rheumatoid arthritis (Ryan et al., 2006).

The findings from our review have implications for selecting indicators for quality monitoring and quality improvement. Patient outcomes for quality monitoring and quality improvement are essentially the same types of outcomes that one would select for assessing the impact of any nursing role within our health care system. They are the types of outcomes that were identified in the American Academy of Nursing Expert Panel on Quality Health Care (Mitchell et al., 1989) and in the Nursing Role Effectiveness Model (Irvine et al., 1998). They include nurses' contribution to achievement of appropriate self-care, demonstration of health-promoting behaviors, functional status, perception of being well cared for, and symptom management to criterion (Irvine et al., Mitchell et al.). In addition, CNSs contribute to quality outcomes at the organizational level, as articulated in the NACNS (2004) framework. This contribution is demonstrated in reduced health care costs, reduced rehospitalizations, and reduced length of hospital stay.

Future research is needed both to confirm some of the outcome indicators for which there is mixed evidence of sensitivity to CNS practice and to establish appropriate indicators for assessing the impact of CNS practice on patients' functional health outcomes. Furthermore, future studies need to utilize research designs that both enable determination of causal inference and clarify the mechanisms by which CNS practice impacts patient and system outcomes. In doing so, we recommend a theory-driven approach to evaluating the quality of CNS practice (Sidani et al., 2004).

The world of practice is a complex system of multiple factors, multiple effects, and mutual causation (Hegyvary, 1993). Factors related to patients receiving care, to nurses providing care, to the setting or context in which care is provided, and to the nature of care provided interact and affect the outcomes expected as a result of care (Sidani & Braden, 1998). As a result Sidani and colleagues (2004) recommended a theory-driven approach to evaluating the impact of nursing care by theorizing about the relationships among all the factors that affect outcomes. In adopting this approach to theorize about the contribution of CNSs to outcomes, it is important to identify the expected outcomes of CNS practice, to explain the processes responsible for producing the expected patient and organizational outcomes, and to identify the factors that influence the occurrence of these processes and, subsequently, the effectiveness of nursing care in achieving the outcomes (Sidani et al.). In an evaluation study, the researcher will need to carefully identify and define the factors that influence the processes and outcomes. Sidani and Braden (1998) suggest there are five categories of factors. The first includes the personal, sociocultural, and health-related characteristics of the patients seeking and receiving care. The second category is the personal and professional characteristics of the nurse giving care. The third consists of the physical and social features of the setting in which care is delivered. The fourth is the type and dose of the interventions received by patients. The last category is related to the nature and timing of occurrence of outcomes expected as a result of the care provided. These five categories provide a comprehensive way of evaluating the impact of CNS practice within the health care system. We suggest that it is only through such careful theorizing that it will be possible to effectively demonstrate the impact of CNSs on patient and organizational outcomes.

DISCUSSION QUESTIONS

1. Consider your own practice as a CNS and identify which nurse-sensitive outcomes are appropriate for assessing the impact of your role in health care.
2. Why do we often observe only small effects of the CNS practice on patient outcomes?
3. Describe the different role mechanisms by which CNSs influence patient and organizational outcomes.
4. Identify four key strategies for planning an evaluation of the CNS role in health care delivery.

REFERENCES

Ahrens, T., Yancey, V., & Kollef, M. (2003). Improving family communications at the end of life: Implications for length of stay in the intensive care unit and resource use. *American Journal of Critical Care, 12*(4), 317–330.

Arbour, R. (2003). A continuous quality improvement approach to improving clinical practice in the areas of sedation, analgesia and neuromuscular blockade. *Journal of Continuing Education in Nursing, 34*(2), 64–71.

Barnason, S., Merboth, M., Pozehl, B., & Tietjen, M. J. (1998). Utilizing an outcomes approach to improve pain management by nurses: A pilot study. *Clinical Nurse Specialist, 12*(1), 28–36.

Bousfield, C. (1997). A phenomenological investigation into the role of the clinical nurse specialist. *Journal of Advanced Nursing, 25*, 245–256.

Brooten, D., Youngblut, J. A. M., Brown, L., Finkler, S. A., Neff, D. F., & Madigan, E. (2001). A randomized trial of nurse specialist home care for women with high-risk pregnancies: Outcomes and costs. *American Journal of Managed Care, 7*, 793–803.

Brooten, D., Youngblut, J. M., Deatrick, J., Naylor, M. D., & York, R. (2003). Patient problems, advanced practice nurse (APN) interventions, time and contacts among five patient groups. *Journal of Nursing Scholarship, 35*(1), 73–79.

Capasso, V. (1998). The theory is the practice: An exemplar. *Clinical Nurse Specialist, 12*(6), 226–229.

Carroll, D., Robinson, E., Buselli, E., Berry, D., & Rankin, S. H. (2001). Activities of the APN to enhance unpartnered elders for self efficacy after myocardial infarction. *Clinical Nurse Specialist, 15*(2), 60–66.

Charles, A., Le Vasseur, S. A., & Castle, C. (1999). Suturing of minor lacerations by clinical nurse specialists in the emergency department. *Accident & Emergency Nursing, 7*, 34–38.

Conger, M., & Craig, C. (1998). Advanced nurse practice: A model of collaboration. *Nursing Case Management, 3*(3), 120–127.

Crimlisky, J., Bernardo, J., Blansfield, J., Loughlin, M., McGonagle, E., McEachern, G., et al. (1997). Endotracheal reintubation: A closer look at a preventable condition. *Clinical Nurse Specialist, 11*(4), 145–150.

Darmody, J. (2005). Observing the work of the clinical nurse specialist: A pilot study. *Clinical Nurse Specialist, 19*(5), 260–268.

De Jong, S., & Veltman, R. (2004). Effectiveness of a CNS led community based COPD screening and intervention program. *Clinical Nurse Specialist, 18*(2), 72–79.

Dickerson, S. S., Wu, Y. W. W., & Kennedy, M. C. (2006). A CNS facilitated ICD support group. *Clinical Nurse Specialist, 20*(3), 146–153.

Doran, D. M. (2003). Functional status. In D. M. Doran (Ed.), *Nursing-sensitive outcomes: State of the science* (pp. 27–64). Sudbury, MA: Jones and Bartlett.

Doran, D. M., O'Brien-Pallas, L., Sidani, S., McGillis Hall, L., Petryshen, P., Hawkins, J., et al. (2003). An evaluation of nursing sensitive outcomes for acute care hospitals. *Journal International Nursing Perspectives, 3*(3), 109–125.

Forster, A. J., Clark, H. D., Menard, A., Dupuis, N., Chernish, R., Chandok, N., et al. (2005). Effect of a nurse team coordinator on outcomes for hospitalized medicine patients. *The American Journal of Medicine, 118*, 1148–1153.

Fowler Byers, J., & Brunnell, M. L. (1998). Demonstrating the value of the advanced practice nurse: An evaluation model. *AACN Critical Issues, 9*(2), 296–305.

Froggatt, K., & Hoult, L. (2002). Developing palliative care practice in nursing and residential care homes: The role of the clinical nurse specialist. *Journal of Clinical Nursing, 11*(6), 802–808.

Gaston-Johansson, F., Fall-Dickson, J., Nanda, J., Ohly, K. V., Stillman, S., Krumm, S., et al. (2000). The effectiveness of the comprehensive coping strategy program on clinical outcomes in breast cancer autologous bone marrow transplantation. *Cancer Nursing, 23*(4), 277–285.

Graveley, E. A., & Littlefield, J. H. (1992). A cost-effectiveness analysis of three staffing models for the delivery of low-risk prenatal care. *American Journal of Public Health, 82*(2), 180–184.

Gurka, A. M. (1991). Process and outcome components of clinical nurse specialist consultation. *Dimensions of Critical Care Nursing, 10*(3), 169–175.

Hall, I. P., Callow, I. M., Evans, S. A., & Johnston, I. D. A. (1994). Audit of a complete home nebulizer service provided by a respiratory nurse specialist. *Respiratory Medicine, 88*, 429–433.

Harrington, L., & Smith, J. P. (2005). Program development: Role of the clinical nurse specialist in implementing a fast-track postanaesthesia care unit. *AACN Clinical Issues, 16*(1), 78–88.

Hays, R. D., Sherbourne, C. D., & Mazel, R. M. (1993). The RAND 36-item health survey 1.0. *Health Economics, 2*(3), 217–227.

Hegyvary, S. T. (1991). Issues in outcomes research. *Journal of Nursing Quality Assurance, 5*(2), 1–6.

Hegyvary, S. (1993). Patient care outcomes related to management of symptoms. *Annual Review of Nursing Research, 11*, 145–168.

Hurwitz, B., Jarman, B., Cook, A., & Bajekal, M. (2005). Scientific evaluation of community-based Parkinson's disease nurse specialists on patient outcomes and health care costs. *Journal of Evaluation in Clinical Practice, 11*(2), 97–110.

Irvine, D., Sidani, S., & McGillis Hall, L. (1998). Linking outcomes to nurses' roles in health care. *Nursing Economic$, 16*(2), 58–64, 87.

Jacavone, J. B., Daniels, R. D., & Tyner, I. (1999). CNS facilitation of a cardiac surgery clinical pathway program. *Clinical Nurse Specialist, 13*(3), 126–132.

Jenkinson, C., Peto, V., Fitzpatrick, R., Greenhall, R., & Hyman, N. (1995). Self-reported functioning and well-being in patients with Parkinson's disease: A comparison of the short-form health (SF-36) and the Parkinson's disease questionnaire (PDQ-39). *Age and Ageing, 24*, 505–509.

Jennings, B. M., Staggers, N., & Brosch, L. R. (1999). A classification scheme for outcome indicators. *Image: Journal of Nursing Scholarship, 31*, 381–388.

Lacko, L. A., Dellasega, C., Salernon, F., Singer, H., Delucca, J., & Rothenberger, C. (2001). The role of the advanced practice nurse in facilitating a clinical research study: Screening for delirium. *Clinical Nurse Specialist, 14*(3), 110–115.

Laschinger, H. K., & Almost, J. (2003). Patient satisfaction as a nurse-sensitive outcome. In D. M. Doran (Ed.), *Nursing-sensitive outcomes: State of the Science* (pp. 243–281). Sudbury, MA: Jones and Bartlett.

Linck, C., & Phillips, S. (2005). Fight or flight? Disruptive behavior in medical/surgical services. *Nursing Management, 36*(5), 47–51.

Lohr, K. N. (1985). *Impact of Medicare prospective payment on the quality of medical care: A research agenda.* Santa Monica, CA: The Rand Corporation.

Martin, P. J. (1999). An exploration of the services provided by the clinical nurse specialist within one NHS trust. *Journal of Nursing Management, 7*, 149–156.

McAlpine, L. (1997). Process and outcome measures for the multidisciplinary collaborative projects of a critical care CNS. *Clinical Nurse Specialist, 11*(3), 134–138.

McCorckle, R., Benoliel, J. Q., Donaldson, G., Georgiadou, F., Moinpour, C., & Goodell, B. (1989). A randomized clinical trial of a home nursing care for lung cancer patients. *Cancer, 64*, 1375–1382.

McCreaddie, M. (2001). The role of the clinical nurse specialist. *Nursing Standard, 16*(10), 33–38.

McDowell, I., & Newell, C. (1996). *Measuring health: A guide to rating scales and questionnaires* (2nd ed.). New York: Oxford University Press.

Mick, D., & Ackerman, M. (2000). Advanced practice nursing role delineation in acute and critical care: Application of the Strong Model of Advanced Practice. *Heart & Lung, 29*(3), 210–221.

Mitchell, P. H., Armstrong, S., Simpson, T. F., & Lentz, M. (1989). American Association of Critical-Care Nurses demonstration project: Profile of excellence in critical care nursing. *Heart & Lung, 18*, 219–237.

Mitchell, P. H., & Lang, N. M. (2004). Framing the problem of measuring and improving healthcare quality. Has the Quality Outcomes Model been useful? *Medical Care, 42*(2 Suppl.), II-4–II-11.

National Association of Clinical Nurse Specialists. (2004). *Statement on clinical nurse specialist practice and education* (2nd ed.). Harrisburg, PA: Author.

Naylor, M. D., Bowles, K. H., & Brooten, D. (2000). Patient problems and advanced practice nurse interventions during transitional care. *Public Health Nursing, 17*(2), 94–102.

Naylor, M. D., Brooten, D., Campbell, R., Jacobsen, B. S., Mezey, M. D., Pauly, M. V., et al. (1999). Comprehensive discharge planning and home follow-up of hospitalized elders: A randomized clinical trial. *Journal of the American Medical Association, 281*(7), 613–620.

Phillips, J. (2005). Neuroscience critical care. The role of the advanced practice nurse in patient safety. *AACN Clinical Issues, 16*(4), 581–592.

Prevoo, M. I. L., van't Hof, M. A., Kuper, H. H., van Leeuwen, M. A., van de Putte, L. B. A., & van Riel, P. L. C. M. (1995). Modified disease activity scores that include 28 joint counts. Development and validity. *Arthritis Rheumatology, 38*, 44–48.

Raja-Jones, H. (2002). Role boundaries—research nurse or clinical nurse specialist? A literature review. *Journal of Clinical Nursing, 11*(4), 415–420.

Rankin, S. H., & Butzlaff, A. (2005). FAMISHED for support for recovering elders after cardiac events. *Clinical Nurse Specialist, 19*(3), 142–149.

Roberts-Davis, M., & Read, S. (2001). Clinical role clarification: Using the Delphi method to establish similarities and differences between nurse practitioners and clinical nurse specialists. *Journal of Clinical Nursing, 10*(1), 33–43.

Ryan, S., Hassell, A. B., Lewis, M., & Farrell, A. (2006). Impact of a rheumatology expert nurse on the wellbeing of patients attending a drug monitoring clinic. *Journal of Advanced Nursing, 53*(3), 277–286.

Savage, L. S., & Grap, M. J. (1999). Telephone monitoring after early discharge for cardiac surgery patients. *American Journal of Critical Care, 8*(3), 154–159.

Scott, R. (1999). A description of the roles, activities, and skills of clinical nurse specialists in the United States. *Clinical Nurse Specialist, 13*(4), 183–190.

Sidani, S., & Braden, C. J. (1998). *Evaluating nursing interventions: A theory-driven approach.* Thousand Oaks, CA: Sage.

Sidani, S., Doran, D. M., & Mitchell, P. (2004). A theory-driven approach to evaluating quality of nursing care. *Image: Journal of Nursing Scholarship, 36*, 60–65.

Siegert, C. D., Vleming, L. T., Vandenbroucke, J. P., & Cats, A. (1984). Measurement of disability in Dutch rheumatoid arthritis patients. *Clinical Rheumatology, 3*, 305–309.

Spielberger, C. G., Gorsuch, F., & Luchene, R. (1971). *STAI manual for the state trait anxiety inventory.* Palo Alto, CA: Consulting in Psychiatry Press.

Tijhuis, G. J., Zwinderman, A. H., Hazes, J., Breedveld, F., & Vliet, V. P. M. (2003). Two-year follow-up of a randomized controlled trial of a clinical nurse specialist intervention, inpatient, and day patient team care in rheumatoid arthritis. *Journal of Advanced Nursing, 41*(1), 34–43.

Tranmer, J. E., & Parry, M. J. E. (2004). Enhancing postoperative recovery of cardiac surgery patients: A randomized clinical trial of an advanced practice nursing intervention. *Western Journal of Nursing Research, 26*(5), 515–532.

Tsay, S. L., Lee, Y. C., & Lee, Y. C. (2005). Effects of an adaptation training programme for patients with end-stage renal disease. *Journal of Advanced Nursing, 50*(1), 39–46.

Tugwell, P., Bombardier, C., & Buchanan, W. W. (1987). Rehabilitation in people with rheumatoid arthritis. *Best Practices and Research Clinical Rheumatology, 17*(5), 847–861.

Vrijhoef, H. J. M., Diederiks, J. P. M., Spreeuwenberg, C., & Wolffenbuttel, B. H. R. (2001). Substitution model with central role for nurse specialist is justified in the care for stable type 2 outpatients. *Journal of Advanced Nursing, 36*(4), S46–S55.

Weisman, A. D., & Worden, J. W. (1976). The existential plight in cancer significance of the first 100 days. *International Journal of Psychiatry in Medicine, 7*(1), 1–15.

Wheeler, E. C. (2000). The CNS's impact on process and outcome of patients with total knee replacement. *Clinical Nurse Specialist, 14*(4), 159–172.

White, C. (1999). Changing pain management practice and impacting on patient outcomes. *Clinical Nurse Specialist, 13*(4), 166–172.

Willoughby, D., & Burrows, D. (2001). A CNS managed diabetes foot care clinic: A descriptive survey of characteristics and foot care behaviours of the patient population. *Clinical Nurse Specialist, 15*(2), 52–57.

Wojner, A. W., & Kite-Powell, D. (1997). Outcomes manager: A role for the advanced practice nurse. *Critical Care Nursing Quarterly, 19*(4), 16–24.

York, R., Brown, L., Samuels, P., Finkler, S. A., Jacobsen, B., Persely, C. A., et al. (1997). A randomized trial of early discharge and nurse specialist transitional follow-up care of high-risk childbearing women. *Nursing Research, 46*(5), 254–261.

Designing and Evaluating Nursing Interventions

Clinical Reasoning Model: A Clinical Inquiry Guide for Solving Problems in the Nursing Domain

Brenda L. Lyon

In watching disease, both in private houses and in public hospitals, the thing which strikes the experienced observer most forcibly is this, that the symptoms or the sufferings generally considered to be inevitable and incident to the disease are very often not symptoms of the disease at all, but of something quite different—of the want of fresh air, or of light, or of warmth, or of quiet, or of cleanliness, or of punctuality and care in the administration of diet, of each and all of these . . . If a patient is feverish, if a patient is faint, if he is sick after taking food, if he has a bed-sore, it is generally the fault not the disease, but of the nursing. (Nightingale, 1860/1969, p. 8)

The ability to engage in rational and deliberate reasoning or clinical inquiry to effectively solve clinical problems in the *nursing* domain is one of the cornerstones of clinical nurse specialist (CNS) practice. Clinical reasoning is often thought to be synonymous with diagnostic reasoning; however, clinical reasoning as used in this chapter is more inclusive and encompasses: (1) the differential diagnostic process to identify etiologies requiring nursing intervention, also known as diagnostic reasoning; (2) therapeutic/interventional reasoning to select predictably effective interventions to alter the target etiology(ies); and (3) evaluation of outcomes. Although focused on the patient sphere of

influence in this chapter, the clinical reasoning model (CRM) also has heuristic problem-solving value in both the nursing and system CNS spheres of influence because it is anchored on the identification of etiologies of problems.

CNS practice is focused on nursing's unique contributions to patient care while integrating, as appropriate, the care of other health care disciplines such as medicine. CNSs must be able to assess patient problems from a holistic *nursing perspective* to enable the accurate identification of problems that have etiologies requiring nursing interventions/therapeutics to achieve desired outcomes (National Association of Clinical Nurse Specialists [NACNS], 2004).

Knowledge informs perspective, that is, the perceptual lens through which clinicians assess, diagnose, and treat. Students often come to graduate programs preparing CNSs with a knowledge base grounded in and developed from educational as well as work/practical experiences that are predominantly disease-focused. Knowledge and practical expertise regarding disease and the safe and therapeutic implementation of medical therapeutics is critically important to caring for patients who have a condition requiring medical care. However, when knowledge of patient problems is principally embedded in knowledge about disease and disease-focused care, the result is that the "medical" perspective becomes the foreground of the nurse's perceptual lens. Consequently, nursing care needs can go unnoticed or

*Dr. Lyon gratefully acknowledges the permission from Wendy Unger, MSN, to use one of her CRM exemplars to demonstrate application of the CRM.

thought to be of little importance. Additionally, without adequate knowledge of patient problems that require nursing interventions/therapeutics, it is not possible to accurately rule in/out etiologies that require nursing interventions/therapeutics.

Effective CNS practice requires a highly developed perspective or perceptual lens that puts the nursing care needs of patients, when present, in the foreground of clinical reasoning, with medical problems and disease-focused care as critical background context. Central to the nursing perspective is the understanding that disease and illness are distinctly different phenomena and, furthermore, that the prevention and alleviation of illness experiences promoting the experience of wellness is the essence of nursing.

The purpose of this chapter is to present the CRM developed for the pedagogical purpose of enhancing CNS students' clinical reasoning ability in identifying etiologies to solve clinical problems in the nursing domain. Prior to presenting the CRM, background information is presented, including brief discussions about clinical reasoning from a nursing perspective, phenomena of concern to nursing, nursing required etiologies, wellness as the target outcome of nursing care, and disease and illness as distinctly different phenomena. Then, the CRM is presented with an explanation of each of its components. The chapter concludes with a summary and implications for CNS education.

Although there are other clinical reasoning models, such as the outcome-present state-test (OPT) model of clinical reasoning developed by Pesut and Herman (1999), it is not the purpose of this chapter to present an overview of those models. Models such as the OPT rely heavily on the North American Nursing Diagnosis Association (NANDA), Nursing Intervention Classification (NIC), and Nursing Outcome Classification (NOC) language. Although identifying and using nursing language is important to make the work of the discipline visible, to date, the explicit link between problems, corresponding etiologies, and how etiologies determine what interventions are required is neglected. It is the insufficient attention to the criticality of identifying etiologies that require nursing interventions to effectively treat illness experiences and to promote wellness that compelled the development of the CRM.

CLINICAL REASONING FROM A NURSING PERSPECTIVE

What distinguishes clinical reasoning in nursing and CNS practice, in particular, from other disciplines such as medicine is not the reasoning process per se but the grounding in nursing's ontological and epistemological perspective with its focus on *phenomena of concern to nursing within a holistic contextual lens* (see chapter 3). Additionally, what distinguishes clinical reasoning for CNSs from clinically skilled nurses prepared at the basic level is the expanded theoretical and research-based knowledge, including knowledge generated by basic science disciplines, pertinent to the phenomena of concern and to intended effect of nursing interventions. Knowledge about phenomena of concern to nursing along with the clinical expertise of the CNS in terms of patient population clinical experiences and outcomes, and skill in evaluating evidence and applicability to a patient population in terms of how evidence should be integrated into clinical decisions, informs CNS practice (Higgs & Jones, 2000). The personal experience and clinical expertise of the CNS substantially contributes to the professional judgment required in the appropriate use of evidence in sound clinical reasoning.

Clinical reasoning from a nursing perspective has two focal points: (1) the types of problems that are of concern and (2) the types of etiologies of those problems. In the nursing perspective, the problems are expanded beyond disease, medical therapeutics, and/or side effects of medical therapeutics and are unique foci when compared with other health care providers such as physicians, physical therapists, psychologists, pharmacists, nutritionists. "Diagnosing is discipline specific. Its focus derives from the categories of the phenomena central to that discipline. Thus, diagnoses are not medical because they are made by a physician but because they deal with phenomena in the medical domain. Similarly nursing diagnoses are those which deal with phenomena central to the nursing domain" (Carnevali, 1987, p. 9). Likewise, the etiologies of phenomena or problems central to nursing are expanded beyond disease and iatrogenic effects of treatments for disease to include other physical, psychosocial, and/or environmental etiologies that require nursing therapeutics/interventions to be altered. For the sake of conciseness, these etiologies for which nursing interventions are required are referred to as nursing required etiologies, or NREs, verses non–disease-based etiologies.

Phenomena of Concern to Nursing

Nursing has struggled for years to clearly articulate its unique perspective and contribution to society—its phenomena of concern. As the pioneer of nursing, Nightingale (1860/1969) defined nursing as "[putting] the patient in the best condition for nature to act upon him" (p. 33). She was clear that different knowledge bases informed nursing practice and medical practice. Since Nightingale, there have been multiple conceptual frameworks developed to capture nursing's discipline-specific perspective and phenomena of concern (Henderson, 1966; Johnson, 1980; King, 1989; Leininger, 1988; Neuman, 1989; Newman, 1986; Orem, 1985; Parse, 1989; Peplau, 1988; Rogers, 1970; Roy, 1984). Each framework reflects the respective author's conceptualization of phenomena that are of unique concern to nursing as well as implications for nursing actions in the context of the phenomena. Although every framework presents a somewhat different view, common threads consistent with Nightingale and the themes identified in chapter 3 are: (1) viewing the patient from a holistic perspective rather than a disease-focused perspective; (2) caring; (3) connecting, at some level, with the subjective or lived experience of the patient; and (4) meeting patients' needs for assistance in achieving wellness or well-being.

Examples of phenomena of concern to nursing articulated in the American Nurses' Association's (ANA) *Social Policy Statement* (2003) and, not surprisingly, consistent with phenomena identified in Nightingale's *Notes on Nursing* (1860/1969) include but are not limited to: self-care limitations; impaired functioning in the areas of rest, sleep, and breathing (e.g., shortness of breath); circulation problems; activity/inactivity problems (muscle weakness, balance problems, risk for falling, activity intolerance); nutritional problems including dehydration; elimination (urinary incontinence, constipation, diarrhea); skin breakdown; sexuality problems; discomfort (pain); emotional problems such as anxiety, loss, loneliness, and grief; deficiencies in decision making; self-image changes; dysfunctional perceptual orientations to health; strains related to life processes such as birth, development, and death; and problematic affiliative relationships.

Nursing Required Etiologies

Importantly, phenomena central to the nursing domain are not grounded in disease or pathology but rather in the symptoms or sufferings and functional problems caused by or contributed to by factors other than disease-based etiologies, including physical, psychosocial, and environmental factors that require and are amenable to nursing interventions. NREs necessitate nursing interventions or therapeutics to be altered (lessened or alleviated). To be clear, disease and/or injury can cause symptoms or functional problems; however, on many occasions, even when caused by disease or injury, symptoms or functional problems are often intensified by NREs, thus requiring nursing interventions. Such is the case when awkward positioning strains an incision site or when extended dependent positioning of an extremity increases edema in a patient with congestive heart failure. Categories of NREs are outlined in Table 5.1.

In addition to intensifying symptoms or functional problems triggered by disease or injury, NREs are often the trigger for symptoms or functional problems in the absence of disease or injury. Some common examples of such experiences are: (1) back pain caused by muscle strain resulting from lifting a heavy object using improper body mechanics, (2) back pain resulting from being in a supine position that strains back muscles, (3) headache caused from tensing neck and shoulder muscles while doing computer work, and (4) falling as a result of deconditioning while in the hospital. It has been estimated that 60% of all physician office visits are for illness experiences not caused by a disease, even in instances where there are multiple comorbidities (Fries, Koop, & Beadle, 1993; Hughner & Kleine, 2004; Sobel, 1995). There are also abundant examples in the literature of NREs that cause disease, complications, repeated hospital admissions, repeated

5.1 | Example Categories of Nursing Required Etiologies (NRE)

PERSON-RELATED NRE CATEGORIES	ENVIRONMENTAL-RELATED NRE CATEGORIES
■ immobility	■ inadequate resources
■ improper positioning	■ noise
■ lack of knowledge	■ air pollution
■ inadequate nutrition	■ extreme temperatures
■ inadequate hydration	■ allergens
■ inappropriate body mechanics	■ social isolation
■ poor self-care	■ sources of friction
■ learned ineffective breathing pattern	■ dampness
■ stress	■ absence of self-care assistive devices
■ negative emotions	■ barriers, hazards
■ ineffective coping	

These lists are not exhaustive.

visits to emergency rooms, and even death (e.g., lack of cleanliness, improper positioning, inadequate nutrition, over or under hydration, immobility; Mokdad, Marks, Stroup, & Gerberding, 2004).

Nursing is concerned with preventing or alleviating NREs of symptoms and functional problems so as to promote the experience of wellness or well-being in the presence or absence of disease/pathology. Specifically, nursing's unique domain and, therefore, nursing's unique contribution to patient care is the focus on diagnosing and treating phenomena (problems/conditions) caused or contributed to by NREs.

Wellness/Well-Being

"Nursing is concerned with the human processes of well-being that are inherent among all human systems, whether individual, family or community" (Arslanian-Engorin, Hicks, Whall, & Algase, 2005, p. 318). What is well-being, wellness, or the subjective experience of health? The terms *wellness* and *health* are often used interchangeably. An integrative review of the literature from 1983–2003 on lay views of health found that two critically important themes in describing the experience of health were the absence of symptoms and being able to function at an expected level (Hughner & Kleine, 2004). Unlike the medical perspective on health and wellness as objective phenomena, the subjective experience of health or feeling "healthy" is proposed here to be synonymous with the subjective experience of wellness. *Wellness* is defined as the subjective experience of somatic comfort (physical and psychological) consistent with the person's normalized expectation level and functional ability at or near perceived capability or expected level (Lyon, 1990).

Importantly, the experience of wellness is dynamic and can occur in the presence or absence of disease (Barsky, 1981, 1988). It is common for persons with chronic debilitating diseases such as rheumatoid arthritis to adapt to lower levels of function and comfort where the new levels become the expected normal. This is why it is also common to find that persons with long-standing chronic diseases will often describe themselves as very healthy or well (Faull et al., 2004; McKague & Verhoef, 2003). Wellness is the target goal of nursing care in the presence or absence of disease (Lyon, 1990, 2005).

When wellness or health are defined as the absence of disease, disability, or symptoms, as it was by nurse researchers from 1977–1987 (Hwu, Coates, & Boore, 2001), then the logical extension is that persons with chronic diseases cannot experience wellness or health. Needless to say, this creates a practical problem for nurses because "health" is one of the major components of nursing's metaparadigm—and what to do if persons with a chronic disease cannot have it? Such usage also,

in a practical sense, means the person with a chronic disease cannot experience wellness. Fortunately, nurse researchers from 1988–1998 increasingly recognized the subjective nature of health and, therefore, the experiences of both illness and wellness as well as the nonmedical causes of illness (Hwu et al., 2001). An understanding that disease, illness, and wellness are distinctly different phenomena is fundamentally important to nursing's unique perspective, unique contribution to patient care, and the CRM.

Disease and Illness as Distinctly Different Phenomena

In common lay and professional vernacular, the terms *disease* and *illness* are often used interchangeably. When nurses view disease and illness as synonymous, the practical result is a limited search for potential etiological factors contributing to or causing symptoms and functional problems from any other model except the traditional medical model.

Disease

Disease is an abnormal condition including pathology of organ function or structure and abnormal behavior. *Disease* is defined in Dorland's Medical Dictionary as "a definite pathological process having a characteristic set of signs and symptoms. It may affect the whole body or any of its parts and its etiology, pathology, and prognosis may be known or unknown" (2007, p. 469). Disease is an objective phenomenon with an identifiable group of signs and symptoms: It is observable and can be objectively measured. Therefore, the characteristics of a disease are the same across persons who have the disease, in other words, *diseases are normative phenomena*. Although there are a few exceptions, such as the attempt to label all obesity as a disease, for the most part the defining characteristic of disease is pathology (McConnell, 2007). Because each disease has a normative set or template of signs and symptoms, the differential diagnosis of disease is principally accomplished through data collection (history, physical, lab tests), to identify patterns of signs and symptoms or "illness-scripts," and then "pattern-matching" of the revealed signs and symptoms to a prespecified template for a disease (Bowen, 2006; Norman, 2006; Schmidt, Norman, & Boshuizen, 1990). Thus, the differential diagnosis process in medicine is focused on identifying the pathology or disease that is causing symptoms and/or functional problems.

Medicine's social mandate and service to society is focused on the diagnosis and treatment of disease and the generation of knowledge regarding disease and its treatment. The physician's perspective, therefore, is necessarily focused on disease. That is, disease as the etiology or causal explanation of signs and symptoms is necessarily in the foreground of the physician's perceptual lens when working with patients.

Nursing's responsibility in the medical domain is to make judgments about the medical condition of the patient and to implement the delegated (authorized via physician orders, approved protocols or guidelines) medical therapeutics safely and therapeutically (see chapter 6). Similar to physicians, research has demonstrated that expert critical care nurses make rapid judgments about the need for intervention on physiological status problems (actual or potential) by quickly processing and grouping patient data/cues and then "pattern matching" with learned cues/indicators of physiological status (Baumann & Deber, 1987).

Illness

Illness is a distinctly different phenomenon than disease (Boorse, 1975; Eisenberg, 1976, 1980; Jensen & Allen, 1994; Long & Weinert, 1992; Loomis & Conco, 1991; Wikman, Marklund, & Alexanderson, 2005)) and can have both disease-based and NRE causes (see Figure 5.1). Importantly then, illness can be experienced in the presence or absence of disease. Illness, like wellness, is a subjective experience. Specifically, it is the experience of discomfort (physical and/or emotional) greater than the person's normalized or expected level and a functional ability (e.g., activities of daily living [ADLs], social role functioning, memory, decision making) below perceived capability or expected level (Lyon, 1990).

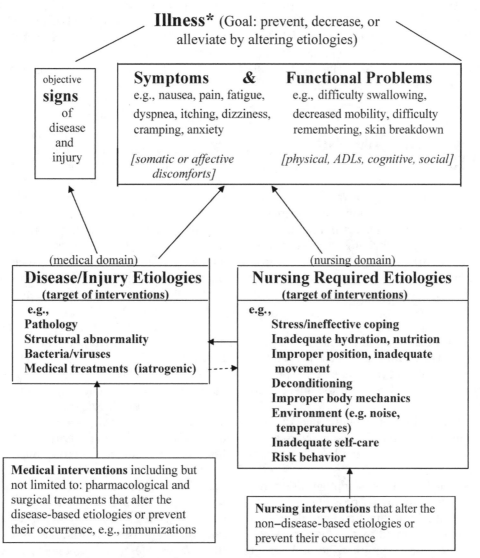

Figure 5.1 Etiologies of illness linked to treatment categories. The context in which a person is experiencing illness includes factors such as age, gender, development, and culture that may moderate or exacerbate etiologies or the illness experience. Used with permission from Brenda L. Lyon, Copyright © 1998.

Even for patients who are unconscious, nurses are concerned with the subjective experience of symptoms and functional problems. As a subjective experience, illness is not normative like disease but instead is dynamic and often varies uniquely from person to person. Therefore, the differential identification of NREs that may be triggering or intensifying symptoms and functional problems is particularly challenging. Unlike medicine, where the differential diagnosis focus is on identifying the disease that is causing symptoms and/or functional problems, the differential diagnosis focus in nursing is on the identification of NREs causing symptoms and functional problems, often without pre-established templates. Thus, the CNS's advanced knowledge about phenomena of concern to nursing and possible etiologies, along with the ability to effectively search pertinent science-based literature to assist in identifying possible etiologies, is critical to the reasoned speculation about possible NREs. The evidence-based differential diagnosis and treatment of illness caused by etiologies other than disease in the presence or absence of disease is identified as one of the hallmarks of CNS practice (Dayhoff & Lyon, 2009; NACNS, 2004).

EXPLANATION OF THE CRM AND ITS ELEMENTS

The CRM is used by the faculty in the Adult Health Nursing Department at Indiana University School of Nursing to facilitate CNS students' learning of the process of clinical inquiry while helping them shift their diagnostic perspective from a medically focused to a nursing-focused perspective. As an analytical heuristic model, the CRM is multidimensional. That is, it facilitates CNS students in:

1. Differentiating diagnostic and interventional reasoning primarily informed from a medical perspective versus a holistic or context rich nursing perspective that integrates disease and medical therapeutics as appropriate;
2. Appreciating that a clinician's knowledge of phenomena delimits the range of potentially relevant etiologies that can be hypothesized by the clinician to be ruled in or out;
3. Expanding their view of patient symptoms and functional problems by searching for possible NREs;
4. Valuing the critical role of target NREs in determining the intervention required to alter or change the NRE and therefore effectively treat the problem or prevent a potential problem;
5. Evaluating evidence and developing a theory/research-based rationale for selection of and implementation of interventions;
6. Validating that the intervention acted as intended (manipulation check); and
7. Evaluating the efficacy of the intervention in achieving desired outcome(s).

Clinical problems in the patient sphere that need solving through nursing interventions typically focus on actual or potential symptoms, functional problems (including problems with skin integrity), and/or risk behaviors. The following examples represent common clinical problems: (1) how to decrease pain intensity that is not sufficiently relieved by analgesics in the context of disease or pathology, such as tissue/organ swelling or surgical incisions; (2) how to decrease the experience of dyspnea for a person with congestive heart failure or when weaning patients from ventilators; (3) how to prevent falls in persons who are at risk for falling; (4) how to reduce nausea in postoperative patients; and (5) how to prevent skin breakdown in persons who are at risk or how to treat early skin breakdown (Gordon, 1987; Lyon, 1990).

The CRM guides the reasoning process in a stepwise fashion, facilitating the identification of NREs of problems in the context of disease and medical therapeutics when present, the rational selection of interventions to alter or resolve the etiologies, and the evaluation of intervention efficacy. The reasoning steps involved in diagnostic, therapeutic/interventional, and evaluation decisions contained in the CRM require the use of knowledge (theory/research/practical) about phenomena of concern to nursing. It is not possible for anyone to diagnose or recognize something that he/she does not understand (Carnevali, Mitchell, Woods, & Tanner, 1984). For example, if a registered nurse does not possess theoretical and evidence-based knowledge of symptoms and functional phenomena of concern to nursing and the corresponding NREs, his/her perceptual lens will be limited to disease or iatrogenic affects of medical therapeutic as etiologies of patient problems.

It is imperative that the CNS be skilled in evaluating evidence. The challenge in applying evidence, particularly research evidence, into practice is that the scientific method focuses on a very limited number of variables at specified periods of time across many homogeneous subjects for the purpose of identifying generalizable findings. Clinical practice, on the other hand, deals with a multitude of variables at a time within one patient in order to optimize a mix of outcomes intended to satisfy the particular patient's current needs and desires. It is, therefore, imperative that the CNS's professional judgments about the appropriate application of evidence be informed by the CNS's clinical expertise.

A pictorial representation of the CRM with exemplar content is presented in Figure 5.2. To promote

understanding of the CRM, it is discussed here as a linear model. It is important to recognize that multiple problems often coexist and clinical situations are typically complex so that clinical reasoning must be appreciated as a complex iterative process. The components of the CRM are defined and discussed along with examples used in teaching the model including content from an exemplar developed by Wendy Unger, MSN, when she was a student enrolled in the first Adult Health CNS course where pain is the symptom focus. Pain is used as the exemplar phenomenon because it is commonly experienced across populations of patients and is considered a nurse sensitive outcome (Doran, 2003; see chapter 4). Additionally, focusing on one common phenomenon as an exemplar gives students the opportunity to appreciate that a thorough under-standing of what is known about a symptom or functional problem is essential to identifying the full range of potentially relevant etiologies, thus guiding assessment in a meaningful manner.

Pertinent pain-related altered physiology, pharmacology, and assessment are integrated throughout the course. Each student selects a pain phenomenon that is common for their specialty area, for example, incisional pain, pain with endotracheal tube, pain from chest tubes on deep breathing, skin itching in dialysis patients, mobility-related pain, pain with turning, or pain in an extremity from dependent positioning.

Students learn, in depth, the physiology of pain and identify the pain pathway(s) for the particular type and context of pain experienced by patients in the specialty population. The learning experiences of students

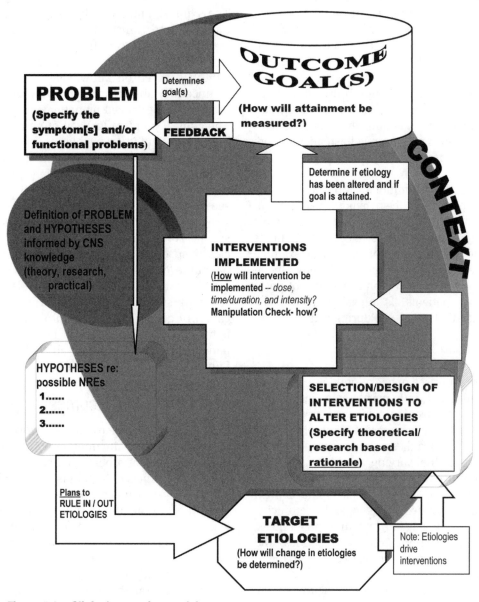

Figure 5.2   Clinical reasoning model.

regarding the altered physiology of pain is enriched by the sharing of the commonalities of pain physiology across populations, while also gaining knowledge from pain experiences unique to specialty populations (e.g., pain of mucositis in patients receiving chemotherapy, incisional pain in patients who have undergone a liver transplant, positional pain in a person undergoing a cardiac catheterization, back pain after lumbar surgery, pain experienced while deep breathing with chest tubes in place, phantom pain post amputation, incisional pain post surgery, back pain during heart catheterization, pain on turning after hip replacement). Additionally, the students acquire an advanced understanding of the pathophysiology of any disease process or injury (e.g., incision) the patient may have along with the pharmacodynamics of pharmacological agents. For example, a student focused on mucositis in patients receiving chemotherapy must understand the nature of each patient's cancer and related pathophysiology along with the action, timing, and perfusion dynamics of the chemotherapeutic agent(s) so that appropriate interventions (e.g., use of popsicles, ice chips, or saline mouth washes) can be selected and appropriately implemented (timing, dose, duration). Knowledge of the pharmacodynamics of analgesics plays an important role in evaluating the separate effects of nursing interventions on pain relief as patients more often than not are appropriately receiving analgesics for pain.

As students acquire additional knowledge of the phenomenon of pain they begin hypothesizing about possible NREs that could be triggering or intensifying pain in the context of all that is relevant to patients experiencing the selected type of pain. The example shared in Figure 5.2 and developed by Wendy Unger, MSN, was focused on the common experience of post–open heart surgery patients of "intensified pain at the Triple Lumen Insertion (TLC) site during activity."

Context

The "context" is comprised of background information/data that, in addition to nursing domain knowledge, informs CNS clinical reasoning, while also assuring patient-centered care that encompasses all aspects of the person (Institute for Healthcare Improvement, 2008). The context contains nonvarying or slowly changing historical or current characteristics of the person and situation (Gordon, 1982). Dimensions of the context include, but are not limited to, age, gender, ethnicity, culture, education, patient and/or family preferences, personality/values, disease, medical therapeutics, and the situation (e.g., patient in critical care, outpatient, loss of loved one, loss of job).

The contextual background information provides the foundation for each of the remaining components of the model. Contextual variables for a patient often delimit the range of problems from a universe of possibilities. For example, there are some problems experienced by adults that are not experienced by children and some problems experienced by women that are not experienced by men. Older adults may be more prone to certain types of problems than young adults. Likewise, persons who have diabetes are more prone to certain types of clinical problems than persons with arthritis. Context also influences the selection and implementation of a particular nursing intervention in terms of patient/family preferences, appropriateness, timing, dose, and frequency. The situational context for the exemplar presented here is adult patients in critical care post–open heart surgery.

Problem

The clinical problem, that is, the actual or potential symptom, functional problem, or risk behavior, is identified in the initial assessment. Clinical problems for patients who are unable to communicate are identified based on knowledge of the common types of uncomfortable sensations/symptoms or functional problems experienced by patients in a certain context. The clinical problem focused on in the CRM is caused by or contributed to by one or more NREs. That is, it is something that requires nursing interventions to alleviate or lessen and for which nursing is autonomously responsible and accountable (Gordon, 1987; see chapter 27).

It is important that the clinical problem be precisely stated. For example, pain post-surgery needs to be clearly specified as incisional pain, or positional back pain at level 8, or mouth pain in the context of receiving chemotherapy stated as mucositis pain at level 6. A clearly stated clinical problem informs the identification of goals. The clinical problem focused on here is the common experience of post–open heart surgery patients of "intensified pain above level 3 at the Triple Lumen Insertion (TLC) site during activity."

Goals (Desired Outcomes)

Goals are the predicted and desired outcomes (including indicators) of an intervention, which, if accomplished, represent a beneficial change in the problem. For example, incisional pain is alleviated or reduced to a 2 pain level or mucositis pain is reduced to a 2 pain level. It is also helpful to specify a timeframe for when it is expected that the goal will be accomplished. For interventions that will not have an immediate effect, the time frame is critical because this affects the timing for evaluation. The goal in the exemplar was to alleviate pain at the TLC site during activity during movement.

Hypotheses Regarding NREs (Differential or Diagnostic Reasoning About Etiologies)

Hypotheses are reasoned speculations about possible etiologies that could be contributing to the problem. The speculations are tentative until validated (Carnevali, 1987). Unlike medical diagnoses that are normative and, therefore, only need to specify the disease, clinically relevant nursing diagnoses must identify the etiology(ies) causing or contributing to clinical problems so that interventions can be effectively targeted to individual patients. The CNS's search for etiologies in a holistic assessment is expanded to include all relevant factors within the patient's context.

The essential question that is asked repeatedly during the speculation process about NREs is: "What could be causing or contributing to this patient's symptom or functional problem other than disease or the iatrogenic effects of medical therapeutics?" For example, for a patient who is 24-hours post-op from open heart surgery who experiences breakthrough pain at the insertion site of chest tubes when using the incentive spirometer, what could be contributing to the pain over and above medically related causes? Identifying etiologies contributing to this pain is clinically important because the discomfort can preclude being able to deep breathe and could then result in complications. Is it possible that the pain is being substantially contributed to the patient not knowing how to do diaphragmatic deep breathing and as a result is moving the chest wall more than necessary?

Once the etiologies are hypothesized, the CNS moves to systematically collect data to rule in and rule out the probable etiologies. During the differential or diagnostic reasoning process, disease-based etiologies including the iatrogenic effects of medical therapeutics (e.g., pharmacological agents) must be attended to because if the cause of the problem *is* limited to the pathology of the disease or injury (e.g., incision) or iatrogenic effects of medical therapeutics, then interventions must be surgical, complex mechanical, or pharmacological in nature. The CNS's ability to effectively identify probable etiologies and to conduct targeted assessment to rule in or out an etiology is delimited by the CNS's knowledge or evidence-based understanding of the phenomenon that is the problem. The accurate identification of etiologies is critical because there must be a good fit between the etiologies causing the problem and the interventions implemented, or the etiologies will not be altered or eliminated by the interventions. Implementing interventions to solve clinical problems without specifically identifying the etiologies to be targeted is like throwing darts at a dart board blindfolded.

A practical analogy is that upon trying to start your car to go home from work you discover that your car will not start. Your knowledge of the phenomenon "upon turning the key the car will not start" delimits the range of etiologies or causes that you can identify and rule in or out. If your knowledge is limited to two etiologies, such as "dead battery" and "out of gas," then those are the only two etiologies that you are capable of reasoning about. To rule out/in dead battery, if you understand that etiology, you might try to turn on the radio or notice if lights come on. If neither happens then you "rule in" dead battery and get a jump start. Furthermore, in problem solving about the dead battery, you would most likely ask yourself, "Why did the battery die?" Upon reflection, you may also remember that you did not fully close the back door because you were in a hurry to grab your lunch bag—therefore, it's likely that the light was on during your entire 12-hour shift. Knowing that, a jump start would likely be sufficient, and you probably don't need a new battery. During the diagnostic reasoning process, if you discover that the radio plays and lights come on, then you might turn to the "out of gas" etiology and pay attention to the gas gauge—something that could be done simultaneously with the possibility of "dead battery." Remembering that you were running on fumes when you pulled into the parking lot at work, you think you will have to call to get someone to bring you some gas. If your gas tank is full and it is not a dead battery, your limited knowledge about the phenomenon does not permit you to diagnostically reason about a "bad starter" or "water in the carburetor," and therefore, you can not identify the needed intervention and must refer the problem to someone else who has more knowledge.

There are times when the causal relationship between the etiology and the problem is clear. As in the previous simplistic example, when a car is out of gas there is a clear causal chain focused on one proximal cause. However, many times symptoms and functional problems are part of a complex set of etiologies, some of which are based in disease/pathology. For example, when there is a surgical incision, there is an obvious pathology in terms of tissue damage that is stimulating nerve endings and triggering the experience of "incisional pain," which requires pharmacological intervention. However, it is not uncommon for there to be breakthrough pain caused by other factors, such as improper positioning or mobilization that puts a strain on the incisional site causing "intensified incisional pain."

Target Etiologies

Target etiologies are the validated, "ruled-in," likely causes or contributors to the problem and are amenable to nursing interventions. The ruling in or out of observable etiologies involves data collection and analysis and should be done prior to implementation of an intervention. Plans to rule in or out hypothesized etiologies are specified.

Clearly identifying the etiology (causative mechanism) is a requisite to guiding the clinician in choosing or designing an intervention that will most likely remedy the problem (Adelman, 1986; Eisenhauer, 1994). However, for an etiology that is not observable or cannot be validated a priori, the causative or contributing factors can only be confirmed with the implementation of an intervention intended to alter the etiologies and then evaluating the effectiveness of the intervention. When the deliberative intervention is effective in remedying the problem, the "action" of the intervention indirectly validates the presence of the hypothesized etiology. An example of hypothesized etiologies that cannot be validated prior to implementing an intervention would be a less than 30-degree head of bed elevation and inadequate mouth care as etiologies for ventilator acquired pneumonia (VAP). These etiologies can only be confirmed when it is demonstrated that correcting them consistently eliminates the incidence of VAP.

> Wendy's knowledge-based assessment searching for etiologies causing pain at the TLC site revealed that the catheter and sutures moved in the insertion site during activity and were likely causing mechanical tension/ irritation at the TLC insertion site. It was hypothesized that the movement of the catheter and sutures was caused by *lack of securement of the TLC and increased weight of unused claves and stopcocks.* The presence of these etiologies was ruled in as the cause of the pain by applying a securement device and removing the unused claves and stopcocks and confirming the absence of discomfort with movement.
>
> The physiological explanation for intensified pain from the tissue irritation caused by movement of catheter and increased weight of claves and stopcocks as a whole is that initial tissue injury occurs with the insertion of the TLC during surgery, causing initial nociceptor firing and sensitization. The catheter is left in place during and after surgery. Its presence leads to the inflammatory process and additional chemical release, nociceptive sensitization, and nociceptor recruitment. At the 48-hour post-operative mark, patients become more active, moving from bed to chair, and from chair to walking. When patients move, the lumens of the catheter fall, creating tension at the site, causing the sensitized nociceptors to fire, release more chemicals, and become further sensitized, and further irritation and inflammation occurs. Resulting pain impulses travel along A-delta fibers to the dorsal horn of the spinal cord and through tracts to the thalamus and cortex where a sharp pain sensation is experienced. After the stimulus (tension) has been discontinued, the C fibers are involved in transmitting the burning, inflammatory pain that outlasts the stimulus (phase 2 pain). Each tension episode leads to further chemical release,

sensitization, and inflammation, putting the patient at risk for wind-up, hyperalgesia, and allodynia.

The diagnostic statement includes the validated problem and corresponding etiologies. For Wendy's exemplar, the diagnostic statement was: *Pain at TLC site due to lack of securement of TLC and increased weight of unused claves and stopcocks.* Data regarding the effectiveness of using the securement device and removing unused claves and stopcocks in reducing or eliminating discomfort at the TLC site could contribute to the development of a "best practice" protocol for care of TLC sites.

Selection/Design of Interventions to Alter Etiologies

Sidani and Braden (1998) focus on a theory-driven approach to evaluating nursing interventions when doing interventional research. Although their work is focused on research, it offers an excellent overview of important factors to consider when selecting and/or designing nursing interventions. *Interventions* are planned actions (treatments, therapies, procedures) into the life or environment of an individual that are intended to bring about beneficial changes for the individual with minimal risk of adverse outcomes (McCloskey & Bulechek, 2004; Synder, Eagan, & Najima, 1996; Thomas, 1984). Assessment or monitoring activities are not interventions. The purpose of an intervention is aimed at altering the etiologies contributing to or causing a problem or preventing etiologies to prevent a potential problem. A few examples of nursing interventions are turning, repositioning, use of cold/warm, pre-operative teaching, range of motion exercises, breathing exercises, counseling, and dietary management.

The selection or design of interventions is driven by the target etiology(ies) of the problem *and* the theoretical/research rationale indicating that the planned action should alter the etiology. Comfort measures of choice, such as a wet wash cloth to the forehead for nausea or pain, are often selected by registered nurses based on tradition and used on a trial-and-error basis without an understanding of the scientific rationale for why the intervention should work—that is, what is it that the intervention is altering?

The interventions should fit the etiologies. For example, if the etiology of your "car won't start" is that it is out of gas, then the intervention is to put gas in the car. If the target etiology of intensified incisional pain is straining the abdominal area and incision cite because of turning technique, the intervention is to teach the patient a different technique for turning to avoid straining muscles in the incisional area. If a patient is unable to turn self, the nurse turns the patient using a known technique to avoid straining involved muscles.

Therapeutic/interventional reasoning encompasses the appropriate matching of the intervention(s) with the validated target etiology(ies), selection of contextually appropriate implementation of the intervention, and evaluation of the intervention with respect to efficacy in achieving the desired outcome (Gordon, 1982, 1987). In addition to the target etiology, the selection of the intervention is grounded in a theoretical/research/practical or evidence-based rationale for being able to predict that the action will alter or remove the etiology, thereby linking the causal chain. The rationale is the logical basis for selection of the intervention; it makes use of the intervention legitimate, while avoiding anything that would be a contraindication for use of the intervention (Sidani & Braden, 1998).

In addition to matching the intervention to the etiology, it is imperative that consideration also be given to the potential for the intervention to create complications or unintended consequences. It is important to assure that use of the intervention will not counteract the intended effect of another intervention. An example would be not using cold on the skin or mucosal surface if a chemotherapeutic agent is intended to perfuse through dermal tissue.

Intervention Implementation

The implementation specifications include the "how" of delivery, including strength or dosage, when, and where. The specifications of a selected intervention are informed by theory/research (when available) or other evidence in addition to contextual factors (Sidani & Braden, 1998). Specifically, specifications identify the explicit activities of the intervention; detail the procedures, including timing, frequency and duration; and identify patient preferences as well as specify the resources that would be needed to carry out the intervention.

The concept of *strength* of an intervention corresponds to the concept of *dose* of a medication. An example of strength of dosage is how cold a wash cloth needs to be to effectively interrupt a pain pathway. *Timing* refers to when a treatment is done. An example would be waiting until the peak action of a pain medication to occur prior to implementing a mobility intervention. *Frequency* refers to how often an intervention needs to be done to either effectively treat the problem and/or maintain the desired effect. The duration of an intervention is the length of time the intervention takes or is applied (e.g., 15 seconds, 1 minute, 30 minutes, over a week). Many times the specifications for intervention implementation are informed through theory and empirical evidence; however, consistent with levels of evidence in evidence-based practice, expert opinion can guide the CNS.

After implementation of the intervention, or during if the duration is long, it is important to validate that the intervention was implemented as intended. If it is not possible to implement the intervention with an adequate dose or frequency, then it is quite probable that the intended effect will not occur.

Nursing interventions used by Wendy in her exemplar with patients were directed at preventing or reducing mechanical tissue tension at the TLC insertion site (aligning intervention with hypothesized etiology). The first intervention was use of a securement device. A Stat-Lock brand TLC securement device was applied per the manufacturer's instructions to achieve securement of the TLC and its lumens. Manufacturer's instructions indicate to place the device, which is a piece of adhesive foam with four small plastic prongs on top of it, to achieve securement, which may vary given differing patient anatomy (usually 2.5 to 3 inches from insertion site). Securement is indicated when patient can turn head left to right without causing tension and when all lumens are in place and immobile between prongs on the device. Dose: NA; Amount: 1 device; Frequency: Once and as needed if device soiled; Duration: As long as TLC in place. The second intervention was removal of superfluous claves and stopcocks from TLC lumens. All claves and stopcocks were removed until only one clave per lumen existed. Dose/Amount: Removal of all claves and stopcocks until only one clave per lumen exists; Frequency: Once; Duration: As long as TLC in place. The interventions were implemented at the peak action time of any pain medication that had been administered.

Manipulation Check

A manipulation check is done to determine if the intervention acted as intended. That is, was the wash cloth really cool, did the music really distract the patient, or did the wedge under the knees when the patient was lying flat really tilt the pelvis up to a 30-degree angle? It cannot be assumed that an intervention created the effect for which it was intended. If patient-selected music was used for the intended effect of distracting the patient because the etiology of his intensified pain is that he is focused on the pain, then it cannot be assumed that the patient experienced the music as a distraction. To be able to draw a valid conclusion about whether or not the intervention worked to alleviate or lessen the target etiology, the effective action of the intervention must be validated because there might be myriad reasons why the music did not work as a distraction. The patient must be asked if the music helped him take his mind off the pain to validate that the music acted as intended.

Wendy's manipulation check for securement involved examining all devices after application and during activity to determine if they did indeed *secure* the TLC and its lumens. For removal of superfluous claves and stop-cocks, it *was* ascertained that extra claves and stopcocks are indeed removed.

Evaluation of Outcomes

Absence of a problem (actual or potential) is the generic goal or desired outcome of nursing interventions. Outcomes of nursing interventions are referred to as nurse-sensitive outcomes. Outcomes can be objective or subjective in nature (see chapter 4).

To effectively evaluate the impact of nursing interventions on outcomes, the evaluation plan (data collection plan) should be set a priori to implementation of the intervention and should include the what (desired outcome), when it is measured, where it is measured, and how it is measured. Some outcomes are immediately evident, while others take time to evolve. The specifications of the intervention and the theoretical/research-based causal chain of how the intervention should work will inform the timing of the evaluation. Consideration needs to be given to ensure as much as possible that the data (e.g., measurement tool) has construct validity and will be reliable and sensitive enough to pick up the desired change, for example, assessing physical functioning outcomes resulting from a cardiac exercise program (Sidani & Braden, 1998).

> For Wendy's patients the outcome goal was elimination of intensified pain at TLC insertion site during activity in the population. Achievement of the outcome was measured by comparing the pre-intervention pain intensity rating on a valid pain scale ranging from 0–10 with the post-intervention pain intensity rating on the same scale before and during activity.

Additional considerations in the evaluation of interventions are particularly important when considering patient population needs and developing best practice guidelines for populations to prevent or alleviate NREs. These considerations include: objective capability, adequacy of the intervention procedure, unintended consequences, and ethical suitability. Objective capability encompasses considerations in terms of the objective nursing work requirements (time and effort) and cost considerations in terms of material resources and nursing time. Adequacy of the intervention procedure, in addition to answering the question of whether or not the intervention is effective, includes considerations discussed earlier, such as strength/dose and frequency, that would be applicable across patients. It is important to anticipate and prevent unintended consequences of interventions such as possible interference with a medical therapeutic or creation of unrealistic patient expectations for adherence. Ethical suitability entails ensuring that patients are fully informed about the intervention and that they participate, when able

and as appropriate, in decisions pertinent to the intervention.

> Wendy informed patients regarding the application of the securement device and the removal of unnecessary claves and stopcocks; there were no risks involved in implementing the interventions. The interventions were easy to administer and would not burden the nursing staff. The securement device was readily available and the cost was minimal, and the interventions are applicable across patient populations with a TLC.

Additionally, it is imperative to inform patients of any risk or possible negative consequence of the intervention and to seek verbal consent (Thomas, 1984). As always, adherence to the American Nurses Association Code of Ethics is of paramount importance (ANA, 2001).

SUMMARY

Graduate programs preparing CNSs have a societal obligation to prepare graduates in the *advanced practice of nursing*. The focus of this chapter has been on the use of a CRM as a guide for solving clinical problems in the nursing domain. The CRM is anchored in the differential diagnosis of etiologies (NREs) for clinical problems that require nursing interventions.

Critical to the advanced practice of nursing by CNSs in the nursing domain is the understanding that disease and illness are different phenomena and that illness can be caused or contributed to by etiologies other than disease or the iatrogenic effects of medical therapeutics. Use of the CRM facilitates learning the process of clinical inquiry in the patient sphere focused on nursing's unique contribution to patient care. Furthermore, experience with using the CRM helps students to shift their perceptual lens so that disease and medical therapeutics are viewed as critical parts of the "context" or background of the patient's experience and NREs are moved to the foreground in differential diagnosis. The importance of disease and its treatment are not minimized, just placed in the background and incorporated as appropriate in the differential determination of etiologies. Students often describe the experience of conducting a clinical inquiry using the model as transformational.

For patients to benefit from multidisciplinary practice, members of each discipline, while open to the perspective of other disciplines, must bring to the clinical situation a discipline-related bias in clinical reasoning—thereby collectively expanding the range of etiologies addressed. The emphasis by some organizations to require that curriculums include for all APNs, including CNSs, the generic and primary care focused 3 "Ps" (physical assessment, pathophysiology, and pharmacology) without mention of other content areas critical to informing CNS practice focused on phenomena of concern to nursing limits the acquisition of essential knowledge for CNS practice. "For too long, CNS education has included courses on physical assessment, physiology, pathophysiology, and pharmacology inconsistent with CNS practice—focusing not on illness and risk behaviors but on primary care diagnosis and management of disease" (Fulton, 2006, p. 114). Although many physical symptoms have corresponding altered physiology, the pathology of disease does not help us understand what is happening with phenomena of concern to nursing. The CNSs knowledge of phenomena of concern to nursing enables the types of clinical inquiries that will result in the identification of best practice guidelines that will promote the experience of wellness.

How to language the results of clinical reasoning in terms of diagnostic statements and inclusion of target etiologies that guide interventions is particularly challenging. Although there are substantial benefits to the use of standardized nursing language, including ease of documentation in computerized records, communication of nursing care nationally and internationally, and reimbursement of nursing care services (Rutherford, 2008), the profession has not yet identified how to identify target etiologies within standardized diagnoses or interventions. There is still considerable work to be done.

DISCUSSION QUESTIONS

1. Identify common symptoms and functional problems within your specialty populations that might be caused or contributed to by NREs, and discuss with your peers.
2. Select one symptom or functional problem that is experienced across different patient populations and identify contextual factors that would influence both NREs and what type of nursing interventions might be effective. Identify theory and research-based sources that would need to be retrieved and evaluated to explain how the NRE may be causing or contributing to the problem and that would contribute to the rationale for the type of intervention needed.

EXERCISE

1. Conduct your own clinical inquiry using the CRM as a guide to resolve a clinical problem frequently experienced by patients in your specialty population.

REFERENCES

Adelman, H. S. (1986). Intervention theory and evaluating efficacy. *Evaluation Review, 10*(1), 65–83.

American Nurses' Association. (2001). *Code of ethics for nursing with interpretive statements.* Washington, DC: Author. Retrieved January 21, 2009, from: http://nursingworld.org/books/anps earchdetail.cfm?PubNum = 9781558101760&thedesc = Cod e%20of%20ethics%20for%20n&DisNum = 10&StartRow = 1

American Nurses' Association. (2003). *Nursing: A social policy statement* (2nd ed.). Washington, DC: Author. Retrieved January 21, 2009, from: http://nursingworld.org/books/anps earchdetail.cfm?PubNum = 9781558102149&thedesc = Socia l%20Policy%20Statement&DisNum = 10&StartRow = 1

Arslanean-Engorin, C., Hicks, F. D., Whall, A. L., & Algase, D. L. (2005). An ontological view of advanced nursing practice. *Research and Theory for Nursing Practice: An International Journal, 19*(4), 315–322.

Barsky, A. J. (1981). Hidden reasons some patients visit doctors. *Annals of Internal Medicine, 94*(Pt. 1), 492–498.

Barsky, A. J. (1988). *Worried sick: Our troubled quest for wellness.* Boston: Little, Brown and Company.

Baumann, A., & Deber, R. (1987). Decision making in critical care: Implications for future development. In K. J. Hannah, M. Reimer, W. C. Mills, & S. Letourneau (Eds.), *Clinical judgement and decision making: The future with nursing diagnosis* (pp. 371–375). New York: Wiley.

Boorse, C. (1975). On the distinction between disease and illness. *Philosophy and Public Affairs, 5,* 49–68.

Bowen, J. L. (2006). Educational strategies to promote clinical diagnostic reasoning. *New England Journal of Medicine, 355*(21), 2217–2225.

Carnevali, D. L. (1987). Diagnostic reasoning: Nursing and medicine compared. In K. J. Hannah, M. Reimer, W. C. Mills, & S. Letourneau (Eds.), *Clinical judgement and decision making: The future with nursing diagnosis* (pp. 29–32). New York: Wiley.

Carnevali, D. L., Mitchell, P. H., Woods, N. F., & Tanner, C. A. (1984). *Diagnostic reasoning in nursing.* New York: J. B. Lippincott Company.

Dayhoff, N., & Lyon, B. L. (2009). Assessing outcomes in clinical nurse specialist practice (pp. 191–218). In R. M. Kleinpell (Ed.), *Outcome assessment in advanced nursing practice* (2nd ed.). New York: Springer Publishing Co.

Doran, D. M. (2003). *Nursing-sensitive outcomes: The state of the science.* Sudbury, MA: Jones and Bartlett.

Dorland's Medical Dictionary. (2007). St. Louis, MO: Elsevier.

Eisenberg, L. (1976). Disease and illness distinctions between professional and popular ideas of sickness. *Culture, Medicine and Psychiatry, 1*(1), 9–23.

Eisenberg, L. (1980). What makes persons "patients" and patients "well." *The American Journal of Medicine, 69,* 277–286.

Eisenhauer, L. A. (1994). A typology of nursing therapeutics. *Image: Journal of Nursing Scholarship, 26*(4), 261–264.

Faull, K., Hills, M. D., Cochrane, G., Gray, J., Hunt, M., McKenzie, C., et al. (2004). Investigation of health perspectives of those with physical disabilities: The role of spirituality as a determinant of health. *Disability and Rehabilitation, 26*(3), 129–144.

Fries, J. F., Koop, C. E., & Beadle, C. E. (1993). Reducing health care costs by reducing the need and demand for medical services. *New England Journal of Medicine, 329,* 321–325.

Fulton, J. S. (2006). In search of advanced clinical nurse specialist education. *Clinical Nurse Specialist, 20*(3), 114–115.

Gordon, M. (1982). *Nursing diagnosis, process and application.* New York: McGraw-Hill.

Gordon, M. (1987). The nurse as a thinking practitioner. In K. J. Hannah, M. Reimer, W. C. Mills, & S. Letourneau (Eds.),

Clinical judgement and decision making: The future with nursing diagnosis (pp. 8–17). New York: Wiley.

Henderson, V. (1966). *The nature of nursing*. New York: Macmillan Co.

Higgs, J., & Jones, M. (2000). Clinical reasoning in the health professions. In J. Higgs & M. Jones (Eds.), *Clinical reasoning in the health professions* (2nd ed., pp. 3–14). Oxford: Butterworth Heinemann.

Hughner, R. S., & Kleine, S. S. (2004). Views of health in the lay sector: A compilation and review of how individuals think about health. *Health: An Interdisciplinary Journal for the Social Study of Health, Illness and Medicine, 8*(4), 395–422.

Hwu, Y. J., Coates, V. E., & Boore, J. R. P. (2001). The evolving concept of health in nursing research: 1988–1998. *Patient Education and Counseling, 42*(2), 105–114.

Institute for Health Care Improvement. (2008). *Patient-centered care*. Retrieved January 21, 2009, from http://www.ihi.org/IHI/Topics/PatientCenteredCare

Jensen, L. A., & Allen, M. N. (1994). A synthesis of qualitative research on wellness-illness. *Qualitative Health Research, 4*(4), 349–369.

Johnson, D. E. (1980). The behavioral system model for nursing. In J. P. Riehl & C. Roy (Eds.), *Conceptual models for nursing practice* (2nd ed., pp. 207–216). Norwalk, CT: Appleton-Century-Crofts.

King, I. M. (1989). King's general systems framework and theory. In J. Riehl-Sisca (Ed.), *Conceptual models for nursing practice* (3rd ed., pp. 149–158). Norwalk, CT: Appleton & Lange.

Leininger, M. M. (1988). Leininger's theory of nursing: Cultural care diversity and universality. *Nursing Science Quarterly, 1*(4), 152–160.

Long, K. A., & Weinert, C. (1992). Descriptions and perceptions of health among rural and urban adults with multiple sclerosis. *Research on Nursing and Health, 15*, 335–342.

Loomis, M., & Conco, D. (1991). Patients' perceptions of health, chronic illness, and nursing diagnoses. *Nursing Diagnosis, 2*(4), 162–170.

Lyon, B. L. (1990). Getting back on track: Nursing's autonomous scope of practice. In N. Chaska (Ed.), *The nursing profession: Turning points* (pp. 267–274). St. Louis: CV Mosby.

Lyon, B. L. (2005). Reflecting on "Getting back on track": Nursing's autonomous scope of practice. *Clinical Nurse Specialist, 19*(1), 25.

McCloskey, J. C., & Bulechek, G. M. (2004). *Nursing Intervention Classification (NIC)* (4th ed.). St. Louis: CV Mosby.

McConnell, T. (2007). *The nature of disease: Pathology for the health professions*. Baltimore, MD: Lippincott, Williams & Wilkins.

McKague, M., & Verhoef, M. (2003). Understandings of health and its determinants among clients and providers at an urban community healthy center. *Qualitative Health Research, 13*(5), 703–717.

Mokdad, A. H., Marks, J. S., Stroup, D. F., & Gerberding, M. D. (2004). Actual causes of death in the United States, 2000. *Journal of the American Medical Association, 291*(10), 1238–1245.

National Association of Clinical Nurse Specialists. (2004). *Statement on clinical nurse specialist practice and education* (2nd ed.). Harrisburg, PA: Author.

Neuman, B. (1989). *The Neuman systems model* (2nd ed.). Norwalk, CT: Appleton & Lange.

Newman, M. A. (1986). *Health as expanding consciousness*. St. Louis: Mosby-Year Book, Inc.

Nightingale, F. (1860/1969). *Notes on nursing*. New York: Dover Publications.

Norman, G. (2006). Building on experience—The development of clinical reasoning. *The New England Journal of Medicine, 355*(21), 2251–2252.

Orem, D. E. (1985). *Nursing: Concepts of practice* (3rd ed.). New York: McGraw-Hill Book Co, Inc.

Parse, R. R. (1989). Man-living health: A theory of nursing. In J. Riehl-Sisca (Ed.), *Conceptual models for nursing practice* (3rd ed., pp. 253–257). Norwalk, CT: Appleton & Lange.

Peplau, H. E. (1988). The art and science of nursing: Similarities, differences and relations. *Nursing Science Quarterly, 1*, 8–15.

Pesut, D. J., & Herman, J. (1999). *Clinical reasoning: The art and science of critical and creative thinking*. Boston: Delmar Publishers.

Rogers, M. E. (1970). *An introduction to the theoretical basis of nursing*. Philadelphia, PA: F.A. Davis.

Roy, C. (1984). *Introduction to nursing: An adaptation model* (2nd ed.). Englewood Cliffs, NJ: Prentice Hall.

Rutherford, M. A. (2008). Standardized nursing language: What does it mean for nursing practice? *The Online Journal of Nursing Issues, 13*(1). Retrieved January 19, 2009, from http://www.nursingworld.org/MainMenuCategories/ANAMarketplace/ANAPeriodicals/OJIN/TableofContents/vol132008/No1Jan08/ArticlePreviousTopic/StandardizedNursingLanguage.aspx

Schmidt, H. G., Norman, G. R., & Boshuizen, H. P. S. (1990). A cognitive perspective on medical expertise: Theory and implications. *Academic Medicine, 65*(10), 611–621.

Sidani, S., & Braden, C. J. (1998). *Evaluating nursing interventions: A theory-driven approach*. Thousand Oaks, CA: Sage.

Sobel, D. S. (1995). Rethinking medicine: Improving health outcomes with cost-effective psychosocial interventions. *Psychosomatic Medicine, 57*, 234–244.

Synder, M., Egan, E. C., & Najima, Y. (1996). Defining nursing interventions. *Image: Journal of Nursing Scholarship, 28*(2), 137–142.

Thomas, E. J. (1984). *Designing interventions for the helping professions*. Thousand Oaks, CA: Sage.

Wikman, A., Marklund, S., & Alexanderson, K. (2005). Illness, disease, and sickness absence: An empirical test of differences between concepts of ill health. *Journal of Epidemiology and Community Health, 59*, 450–454.

Designing Innovative Interventions

Jeannette Richardson

The clinical nurse specialist (CNS), regardless of practice setting, must always be alert to the need for maintaining or improving the quality of care for his/her defined population, whether it be individual patients, families, groups, or communities (National Association of Clinical Nurse Specialists [NACNS], 2004). Continual surveillance activities and focused assessments can help identify the need for practice changes. Once a need is identified, a detailed and methodical approach is utilized to establish the current evidence base, set a goal for future practice, and create a plan for how to achieve this change.

A critical component of any planned project for change is the choice of optimal intervention strategies. An inappropriate intervention could result in failure to effect the practice change and, ultimately, suboptimal patient care. The CNS, as project leader, is responsible for the outcome of the project and any resulting impact on patient care. Consequently, s/he must be knowledgeable about which interventions apply best to different practice situations.

Interventions may follow tried-and-true methodologies familiar to those in the targeted practice setting. Alternatively, an intervention might be based on an innovative idea specifically created to address the project goal, personnel, and/or setting. Rogers, who has done an extraordinary amount of work on change theory and the innovative implementation of change, describes an innovation as an idea perceived as new by the individual (Rogers, 2003). An innovative intervention, therefore, would be an application of a new strategy or a new twist on an old intervention for the purpose of achieving desired outcomes. It presents an intriguing combination—to take a standardized base of clinical knowledge and apply it to a specific practice setting in a way that has been tapered to work best in that practice arena. Use of highly innovative interventions may help to improve the chance for success and endurance of a practice change in our current complex health care environment (Strom, 2001).

Given the leadership responsibility, how does the CNS best guide the project team in choosing implementation strategies for their project? Which methods would be most effective and enduring? And what does it mean to be innovative in choosing interventions? This chapter explores how the CNS plays a key role in planning, developing, and encouraging innovative interventions for better patient care outcomes.

BACKGROUND/LITERATURE REVIEW

The current health care system in the United States encourages a culture of evidence-based practice (EBP) in all aspects of patient care. Nursing, medicine, pharmacy, and other disciplines are using similar methodologies to examine traditional and intuition-driven practice and move toward a culture based on research-gleaned evidence. Numerous guidelines and practice statements have been established based on meta-analyses of clinical research studies, and the strength of a recommendation is related to the strength of the research.

As the diligent CNS strives to examine practice in his/her area of expertise, s/he will note that many validated, published guidelines exist that articulate exactly what is needed for optimal patient care in specific clinical scenarios. However, in many cases, health care team members have not successfully achieved either compliance with the recommended process, or desired patient outcomes. Transitioning research into practice is a complex science and should be based upon scientific evidence.

Moving from the current state of health care to a desired state requires a change in practice; multiple factors related to clients, the health care team, and the setting must be considered. Many different interventions may be available for the CNS to use to change practice, but it is most efficient and reasonable to choose strategies that have been formally researched and shown to have positive outcomes. This philosophy of investigating and choosing specific interventional strategies on the basis of research-related evidence is relatively new. Consequently, the body of knowledge is limited and incomplete. Some interventions have been examined and studied, others are chosen by virtue of expert opinion. Over time, published anecdotes followed by more rigorous research studies will generate further information. In the meantime, the CNS can use the evidence that is available in addition to some recognized generalities to provide assistance when choosing optimal interventions for a given project.

Several researchers have found that the strength of evidence based on published guidelines and clinical trials alone cannot be expected to change behavior—in fact, disagreement with the interpretation of reported trials is a key barrier to implementation (Rello et al., 2002). Likewise, a passive approach, such as targeted mailing of guidelines, was not likely to result in a behavior change. Didactic lectures were also generally ineffective (Grimshaw et al., 2001; Grol & Grimshaw, 1999).

One critical strategy for success lies in assembling a valuable team of key individuals who are dedicated to the project and considered thought leaders amongst their peers. Creating a workgroup of these exceptional people increases the probability of the social acceptance of change. With a strong team and appropriate marketing, the change can be perceived as almost irresistible (Gladwell, 2002).

Educational outreach sessions have also proved successful and involve having a trained topic expert with setting-specific information meet with health care team members within their practice arena. Providing clinicians with face-to-face conversation, the ability to ask and answer questions, and real-time problem solving improves the likelihood of project acceptance. Additionally, the use of multiple, varied, and targeted strategies to enhance compliance and avoid specific potential barriers was generally effective (Grimshaw et al., 2001).

Some health care team members are motivated to change practice through the use of a rewards system. These incentives may be either financial or of a non-financial nature such as paid time off or professional recognition (Joshi & Bernard, 1999). The CNS who wishes to provide rewards may need to negotiate with administrative personnel regarding budgetary or union concerns, staffing levels, and so forth. To be accepted, a change strategy must deliver some type of perceived benefit—enough benefits to make change worthwhile. It may be that the benefit is altruistic in nature and reflected in improved patient care outcomes. It is the responsibility of the CNS to guide the health care team members to recognize and value the benefit of the specific project implementation.

Electronic medical records systems and informatics-based approaches to improving patient care can assist in working with both individual patients and large patient populations. Innovative strategies have included the use of population registries, decision support at the time of a patient visit, and Web-based communication between patients and providers. Some research has shown that identification of patients at risk coupled with a Web-based alerting system for physicians has not impacted patient outcomes (Grant & Meigs, 2006). Alternatively, other trials have indicated that intensive, protocol-driven, nurse practitioner–run clinics have resulted in significant improvement in risk factor modification for hyperglycemia, hypertension, or hyperlipidemia (New et al., 2003). Suggestions for future trials recommend consideration for the use of clinical support staff (such as nurses), administrative staff (such as secretaries), or even direct patient-centered outreach to maximize interventional impact (Grant & Meigs, 2006).

Providing for clinical decision support in real time at the point of care through an electronic or even a paper mechanism can provide support for change with immediate and round-the-clock access to necessary information in multiple formats (protocols, published guidelines, pocket cards, intranet information, telephone hotlines, etc.; Joshi & Bernard, 1999). Other potential interventional strategies could include the use of the following (White, 2004):

1. Clinical reminders and prompts
2. Feedback on performance
3. Interactive computer based learning
4. A continuous quality improvement process

Continuous quality improvement (CQI) is a formal and structured process involving the use of data analysis tools and change strategies to bring about ongoing, positive outcomes. Many facilities utilize specific CQI processes (e.g., Six Sigma and Lean methodologies) for ensuring the quality of care for their patient populations; to enhance multidisciplinary and multidepartment communication, the CNS should be aware of and utilize those strategies sanctioned by their employer. CQI principles provide a powerful framework for project planning and have been used in health care over the last several decades to provide a systematic approach to health care reform. CQI methodologies emphasize a number of principles to enhance success, including (Joshi & Bernard, 1999):

1. Commitment by leadership
2. Recognition and focus on the customer
3. An interdisciplinary team approach
4. Use of data for decision making
5. A reasonable method for measurement of performance
6. Integration of management systems

Although the use of multiple, targeted interventions simultaneously can improve the chance for success, this process should be used cautiously and accompanied by sound rationale. It has been noted by several investigators that implementing *all* interventions at the same time is neither desirable nor practical. Furthermore, the evaluation of the interventions will be challenging due to the inability to determine which strategy caused the practice change. Making several small changes in a care process can be more easily effected and more effective than one larger action (Strom, 2001). Additionally, the innovation strategy should be accessible, useful, and dependable. Cost must be considered—if the intervention does not yield the desired results, then the strategy has been both costly and useless (Crow, 2006).

Examples of innovative thinking and strategies exist throughout health care and in other industries. The Institute for Healthcare Improvement (IHI) is credited with the conception and initial implementation of improving clinical outcomes through the use of care bundles. A *bundle* is a collection of interventions related to a specific disease process that are implemented together to significantly improve patient care outcomes. Each bundle is generally made up of three to five specific interventions. Each intervention must be supported by irrefutable scientific evidence, and all elements of the bundle have to be executed in the same space and time to ensure that clinical improvement occurs (The Joint Commission on the Accreditation of Healthcare Organizations [JCAHO], 2006). This concept of achieving quality by reducing variation has been widely established in industry (Strom, 2001). Since its creation, the bundle concept has helped to implement critical care EBP in facilities throughout the United States, and it is spreading to multiple other patient care projects in other settings.

In other industries, innovative thinking in resource management has led to the advent of *crowdsourcing*—a method of Internet advertising to locate talent outside immediate company walls. Challenges in software programming, business, chemistry, engineering, life sciences, math, and physical sciences are posted, and Internet users of all backgrounds, talents, and specialties are encouraged to submit innovative solutions to the prescribed problems. Various levels of financial compensation are rewarded to the consultants who compete with and expand upon each others' work. Crowdsourcing was created to capitalize on the limitless talent provided by the Internet (Brabham, 2008; Tapscott & Williams, 2007; Tedeschi, 2008). Bench level pharmaceutical and basic science medical research are both currently making tentative steps into the world of crowdsourcing. This strategy may one day prove to be a highly successful means for promoting quality and cost-effectiveness of health care in our country.

In addition to considering those items that promote innovation, it is equally important to examine those characteristics that limit innovation. Once identified, effort can be channeled toward reversing or working around these obstacles. Potential barriers to innovation include (Idea Champions, 2007):

1. Lack of a shared vision
2. Lack of commitment/ownership by leaders
3. Constantly shifting priorities
4. Short-term thinking
5. Focus on intervention rather than customer
6. Focus on past successes
7. Unwilling to change without significant benefit
8. Political barriers protecting entrenched interests
9. Reactive rather than proactive philosophy

By recognizing and working with or around potential barriers, the CNS can improve his/her potential for a positive and enduring change.

CONCEPTUAL FRAMEWORK

A Model for Planned Change and Innovative Interventions

Change theory concepts encourage use of a step-by-step methodology to plan for, implement, and maintain an intervention in order to achieve specific goals. Use of a detailed plan can help break down a complex and overwhelming project into bite-sized manageable pieces. Additionally, it can help to set a realistic timeline, which is helpful not only for the workgroup team, but also for administrators who might be anxious to see the project reach fruition.

There is no single "best" way to understand change management because each individual brings their own experiences and worldviews to each unique project. But many change agents find that the use of a model can assist in planning and following through with the various aspects of a change project (Shanley,

2007). Rosswurm and Larrabee (1999) have presented a formalized model for change toward evidence-based practice that integrates well with CNS practice, particularly in its subroles of project manager and change agent. This model was created to guide health care practitioners through the entire process of synthesizing empirical and contextual evidence and integrating evidence-based changes into practice. It can be adapted for use in multiple health care settings (Rosswurm & Larrabee, 1999).

The CNS as team leader or change agent for the project is critical to choosing EBP innovational strategies for change. A review and plan for project progression through all six stages of this model includes intervention-related components at numerous times throughout project planning, implementation, and evaluation.

Assess the Need for a Change in Practice

During this stage, the CNS needs to collect any information available on the practice in question. Patient preferences and dissatisfaction, quality improvement data, practitioner queries, evaluation data, or new research data all need to be considered. Barriers and potential obstacles should be identified. Data on current internal practices should be collected and compared to external sources to benchmark any differences noted from community or more global standards (Pipe, 2007). The problem must be clearly identified and defined. Any and all stakeholders should be invited to participate to clarify the scope of the problem. Health care providers, administrators, and even patients may be involved. Including strategic individuals from the onset may help implement or maintain changes at a later stage; in particular, evidence indicates that successful organizational change requires senior leadership support (Gustafson et al., 2003). Group members may need dedicated time and resources to participate in the required work sessions, and these will require administrative sanctioning. During group meetings, the CNS should utilize group process techniques such as

brainstorming, flowcharts, and multivoting for group ownership and buy-in.

Link the Problem With Interventions and Outcomes

At this time, the CNS and his/her workgroup should consider and clarify potential interventions and activities while identifying the impact of barriers. The group should be encouraged to "think outside the box" and to be creative and innovative in their approach to various options. Examples of innovations may be provided by the CNS to help jump-start idea formation, which will be based primarily on clinical judgment, systems priorities, and resources.

Innovative thinking itself can be fostered by the CNS through a model based on encouraging childlike creativity of expression. The KIDS approach to innovative thinking gives the CNS general principles as guidance to foster creative thinking among staff (Shirey, 2007):

Kindle a culture of innovative thinking and doing

Inspire others to discover and utilize the available tools of innovation

Disseminate innovation by using tested frameworks

Sustain the momentum for innovation—for innovation to be sustainable, it requires attention, focus, and the allocation of resources

The workgroup also has the responsibility to select potential outcome indicators at this time. The CNS can help the team decide what the project goals might be in terms of specific practice changes and patient outcome measurements. When facilitating group discussion and decisions regarding planned outcome measurements, the CNS should encourage the use of standardized classification systems and language whenever possible. By adhering to customary patient identifiers/descriptors such as diagnosis-related groups (DRGs) or nursing classifications systems such as nursing interventions

---

EXHIBIT 6.1   STEPS TOWARDS EVIDENCE-BASED PRACTICE

Steps	Description
1. Assess	The need for a change in practice
2. Link	The problem with interventions and outcomes
3. Synthesize	Best evidence
4. Design	The practice change
5. Implement and evaluate	The change in practice
6. Integrate and maintain	The change in practice

From "A Model for Change to Evidence-Based Practice," by M. A. Rosswurm and J. H. Larrabee, 1999, *Image: Journal of Nursing Scholarship, 31*(4), 317–322.

classifications (NICs), for instance, the ability for different individuals to communicate on the same terms is greatly enhanced. In addition, the ability to compare like data with outside facilities will be improved.

Synthesize Best Evidence

The next stage toward incorporating EBP involves a thorough review of the research relating to (1) the identified problem, (2) the potential intervention(s), and (3) the outcome indicators. The CNS has experience in the use of systematic literature reviews either through the course of academic study or in the work setting. S/he can draw upon this expertise to help guide team members to the appropriate databases and/or guideline clearinghouses. The medical librarian in many larger health care organizations is an invaluable ally and should be consulted for assistance if available.

Once evidence on the identified problem is collected it must be evaluated for its usefulness. An inexperienced team can benefit greatly from the use of a structured worksheet for literature review. This worksheet should include criteria for reference inclusion and strengths and weaknesses of the publications.

Analysis of the literature review is completed by synthesizing the best evidence and combining that information with contextual data and the potential for project viability in the current practice setting. All possible benefits, risks, and costs should be considered. Finally, the group must decide whether or not sufficient evidence exists to support the practice change in the proposed setting.

Design the Practice Change

Once the decision has been made to proceed with a practice change, clear articulation of that change is needed. All stakeholders should be involved in the description of all the detailed steps of how that change will influence practice for the specified population. This process improves the likelihood that all the necessary steps and personnel who may be affected by the change have been included. It also keeps the team members engaged and focused on the specific practice change. The step-by-step process that has been clarified is often written in the format of a protocol, procedure, or standard and can be presented visually as a flowchart or algorithm. All components of the document must be supported by the evidence base.

Any resources that may be needed, either in the implementation process or for the practice change itself, should be identified. Costs of any type—personnel, equipment, and/or capital expenditure—must be presented to administrators for clarification and support.

At this point, the CNS can propose a plan for implementation of the planned intervention. If the proposed change is large, a pilot study can help with adaptation to practice settings and enhance ownership by team members for a smoother transition. The team will need to define both desired and undesired outcomes and any specific goals for a pilot study. Creation of an evaluation form to be used along with or after implementation can help clarify process and outcome criteria and increase interrater reliability through the use of objective performance measure.

Approvals from institutional review boards, quality improvement forums, research oversight committees, and other regulatory bodies may be necessary and need to be pursued prior to implementation. Waivers and expedited reviews can often be utilized in CQI-style projects to decrease workload.

Implement and Evaluate the Change in Practice

Finally, it is time for implementation of the planned intervention. If a pilot study is to be used, that will be the initial step. The CNS must closely monitor the progress of the pilot and must be available to answer questions for successful implementation. Evaluation of the implementation process and the specified outcomes should occur at the desired stages of project implementation. Occasionally, patient and staff opinion surveys and CQI methods can be used to collect evaluation data. After the evaluation data is collected, the CNS should coordinate data analysis. Computer graphics such as charts and bar graphs can be used to visually present the results back to the workgroup.

Based on results of the project, the team now needs to decide to adapt, adopt, or reject the practice change. The following questions should be considered: Did the intervention result in the desired practice change as expected? What were the patient outcomes? What were the costs and feasibility data? What was the feedback from the stakeholders?

Integrate and Maintain the Change in Practice

Once the recommended practice change is accepted as appropriate, it needs to be communicated to all stakeholders. The CNS should consider which methods for communication are appropriate to each practice setting. S/he should consider the culture of the practice setting and the optimal strategy for enacting a change; some organizations function through top-down enforcement of change, others value multilevel collaboration. Shared governance organizations will most likely require formal committee approval of the change. The CNS must consider which mechanisms exist in the setting to permanently integrate the new practice. Formal policies, procedures, and standards of care can help to maintain the change.

The CNS can enhance ownership and encourage professional development by enlisting the help of the workgroup to present staff inservice education on the practice change. This also helps to reinforce the value of a health care culture based on EBP. Incorporating the practice into orientation manuals and processes for new staff helps to establish ongoing education of the practice.

Depending upon the practice change, ongoing monitoring of process and outcome criteria may be warranted. Intermittent or continuous CQI data collection can be used to evaluate continued compliance or the need for reinforcement strategies. Either upon the completion of project implementation or while maintaining the change, the CNS can consider incentives or rewards for performance.

Despite the fact that it can be both effective and efficient to view a plan for change in a rational and linear fashion, the successful CNS must appreciate the complex nature of change. S/he should be aware that the aforementioned processes are not truly linear; there is much overlap and backtracking and certain items might be omitted, while other unexpected aspects are included (Shanley, 2007).

Conceptual Approaches to Interventions

When considering innovative interventions as part of a specific practice change, the CNS should consider the complex individual and group professional behaviors in their practice setting in addition to the project plan. Different theoretical approaches can help elucidate rationale for behavior change and can assist the CNS in choosing appropriate interventions. Categorizing an intervention as related to a specific approach while planning for a varied group of approaches may provide a strategy that would appeal to multiple people on different levels. Some of these approaches overlap, but each has a slightly different emphasis (Grol & Grimshaw, 1999).

1. Educational Approach—Includes learning in small interactive groups and problem-based strategies. This strategy appeals to individuals who are internally motivated to strive for professional excellence and achievement. It enhances the feeling of "ownership" of the process. By choosing a project team as a resource workgroup, the CNS can maximize the empowerment aspect as well as outreach potential of an educational strategy.
2. Epidemiologic Approach—Includes the development and dissemination of evidence-based guidelines or decision-making tools. This "common sense" approach assumes that humans will make rational decisions when given information on costs, benefits, harms, and preferences.
3. Marketing Approach—Focuses on the development and marketing of an attractive product or message that is tapered to the targeted group. Innovative approaches that address various needs should be spread through multiple channels (use of key opinion leaders, mass media, etc.).
4. Behaviorist Theory Approach—Based on behavior modification through conditioning, which emphasizes that most people seek reinforcement and rewards. Review of performance, provision of feedback, and various other incentives or sanctions act as positive reinforcement.
5. Social Influence Approach—Learning and changing is often achieved through interactions within social networks. The CNS who follows the tenets of this approach will use respected peers, opinion leaders, and role models to promote use of the innovation.
6. Organizational Approach—Based upon the belief that the system guides the practices within it. Systemwide CQI strategies, including assessment of organizational barriers, are used to promote change.
7. Coercive Approach—Change occurs through regulatory pressure and control. Contracts, licensure, and standards provide authoritative power and may provide the impetus to change in a setting of organizational inertia.

Conceptualizing that a change in professional behavior can be linked to a theoretical approach can assist the CNS in guiding the choice of a related innovative interventional strategy. In addition, the project team may better understand the rationale for a particular intervention when framed by one or more of these approaches.

APPLICATION TO CNS PRACTICE

The CNS is uniquely poised to effect change throughout and across the health care continuum. Within a health care organization, s/he is often charged with directly or indirectly monitoring for the quality of patient care and acting on discrepancies. CNS educational curricula provide coursework on change theory and program development (NACNS, 2004). The CNS can integrate advanced knowledge on change theory, adult learning principles, organizational psychology, expertise in clinical specialty area, managing electronic information systems, patient safety organizations, evidence-based practice, regulatory bodies, and stress/coping theories to plan for change.

Historically, CNS practice was broken down into the subroles of expert practitioner, educator, researcher, change agent, administrator, and consultant (Hamric, 1989). These subroles are now conceptually integrated throughout the three spheres of CNS practice: (1) direct client care, (2) nurses and nursing practice, and (3) organizations and systems (NACNS, 2004). The change agent role remains an important part of CNS practice, and awareness of the characteristics of successful change agents can assist the CNS in achieving successful project implementation (Sullivan & Decker, 2001; White, 2004).

The CNS as change agent must consider the impact on all three spheres of influence. This conceptual model not only describes the focus of CNS practice as centering on clients, nurses, and systems, but it also elucidates the challenges in fulfilling this role (NACNS, 2004). When planning for a complex multidisciplinary quality improvement project or simply a reinforcement of current practice regimens, it is not unusual to strategize interventions that need to address direct client care, nurses and nursing practice, and organizations and systems sequentially or simultaneously.

Much of this chapter has described working with clients and their primary caregivers. However, the CNS–nurse interface is not only critical to patient care but is a major source of personal and professional satisfaction for the CNS. In addition to being one of the spheres of influence, nurses are often the largest group of employees in many different types of health care settings. They represent a population that has a key role in steering the health care industry on many fronts, including the use of health information technology (Geibert, 2006). The relationship between the CNS and the staff nurse is based upon common interests and practice and can be a strong influence for change (Rogers, 2003).

When considering the systems perspective, the CNS must be aware that certain organizational factors can be major determinants for project success. Multiple different qualities of the practice setting need to be considered. In today's health care environment, a flexible and participative climate is most likely to yield the desired results. Other organizational characteristics that are associated with positive change include (Crow, 2006):

1. Openness to change
2. Level of staff support for the change
3. Ease of past change implementation
4. Flexibility and adaptability
5. Optimism
6. The organization's capacity to cope over time

The CNS is often charged with ensuring the quality of patient care and the use of EBP in many different practice settings, and so s/he frequently functions as a combination of team leader, change agent, and project manager. Treating all members as valuable contributors and collaboratively troubleshooting helps in team-building. The CNS is responsible for keeping the project on schedule, while still allowing for flexibility to adjust plans as needed and to allow for creative thinking. It behooves the CNS to encourage an environment of intellectual curiosity. Working within a team that questions traditional methods of care and the rationale that "we have always done it that way" creates a mindset for positive and innovative change.

Encouraging innovation might seem to be at odds with the detail work of project management, but it is possible for the CNS to fulfill both criteria. Innovation in diagnosis and treatment to improve practice is considered to be a hallmark of CNS practice (NACNS, 2004). Individuals who utilize innovative strategies share certain qualities. The CNS who wishes to cultivate an innovative style can consider the following attributes (Ditkoff, 2004).

The successful CNS incorporates gained experiential knowledge, literature, outcomes, and benchmarking data to promote teamwork and creative thinking for innovative change techniques (Kaplow, 2007). S/he is aware that monumental organizational changes are often interdisciplinary and team-oriented in nature and that they arise from people straying outside the normal bounds of their specialties (Gleick, 1987).

EXHIBIT 6.2 CHARACTERISTICS OF SUCCESSFUL CHANGE AGENTS

Characteristics
1. Ability to combine unrelated ideas
2. Ability to energize others
3. Skill in human relations
4. Integrative thinking; big-picture focus, and detail-oriented
5. Flexibility to modify ideas
6. Persistence to resist nonproductive tampering
7. Confidence; not easily discouraged
8. Realistic thinking regarding timelines
9. Trustworthiness; history of previous successes
10. Ability to articulate a vision
11. Ability to handle resistance

Qualities
- Flexible/adaptive
- Curious
- Visionary
- Persevering
- Playful
- Makes new connections
- Recognizes patterns
- Balances intuition and analysis
- Risk taker
- Self-motivated
- Collaborative
- Resilient
- Self-accepting
- Reflective
- Committed to learning
- Articulate

Following a well-designed and comprehensive template for change (as described in the conceptual framework), the CNS helps the team to set reasonable timelines and to visualize their progress (Strom, 2001). Structured agendas should be created and followed for each meeting, and minutes should be distributed afterward to reinforce any work assignments. Meeting times should be established early on, and each session should be used efficiently (Strom, 2001). Supervising for follow-up and holding people accountable for their individual responsibilities help keeps the team positive-minded and moving forward. Finishing the feedback loop with administrative recognition for individual accomplishments and pride in performance can serve to keep staff interested in progressive improvements in their work arena.

The CNS who takes on this challenging role as change agent, team leader, and project manager often serves as the cornerstone to effective and lasting change within dynamic systems and multidisciplinary groups. Although the project workload can feel Herculean at times, expertise and skills earned by experience and developed over time can serve to flatten subsequent learning curves and decrease project anxiety. Professional, interpersonal, and economic rewards reinforce job satisfaction and prepare the CNS for the next project at hand.

> Genius is one percent inspiration and ninety-nine percent perspiration. Accordingly, a "genius" is often merely a talented person who has done all of his or her homework.
>
> Opportunity is missed by most people because it is dressed in overalls and looks like work.
>
> —Thomas Edison

EVALUATION

Leading change efforts can be a frustrating challenge that might sometimes feel as if you will never be finished. After considerable experience with project leadership and change management, the CNS can still be surprised by the fact that even when an innovation appears to have obvious advantages, it can still prove difficult for the strategy to be adopted. Change takes time—innovations may take many years from the time they become available until they are widely adopted (Rogers, 2003).

Different rates of adoption may be due to any or all of five characteristics of innovations (Rogers, 2003):

1. *Relative advantage*: The "perceived" value of an innovation has more to do with its adoption than the "objective" value. Each individual will ask, "What is in it for me?"
2. *Compatibility*: Adoption of an innovation is related to the degree that individuals perceive the idea to be consistent with their values, past experiences, and needs.
3. *Complexity*: Innovations perceived to be more complex or require the development of new skills will be adopted more slowly.
4. *Trialability*: Implementing an innovation in a phased approach may allow for enhanced value and decreased complexity of the strategy.
5. *Observability*: When individuals can easily see the results of an innovation, it is more likely to be adopted.

Evaluation of a project is necessarily done upon project completion. If very complex, use a pilot study first—evaluate—then move to the next phase.

As noted in Rosswurm and Larrabee's (1999) model for change toward EBP, evaluation of an innovative intervention begins with the initial planning for the change itself. Data should be collected on both the process used for implementation and the outcome of the intervention. As noted earlier, building in a method for objective evaluation of both process and outcome can aid in data analysis by increasing interrater reliability. Additionally, the use of standardized nomenclature will improve the ability to compare data between practice areas and even different facilities.

According to Gawlinski (2007), evaluation criteria of both process and outcome should include:

1. The outcomes that are expected to change after implementation of the innovation or practice change,
2. The outcomes or dependent variables evaluated in prior research on the issue, and
3. The outcome data already available in the institution (accessible without expending more time, energy, and money).

As alluded to earlier, multifaceted interventions are often more successful than one individual strategy. Unfortunately, it is difficult to separate the outcomes related to any specific intervention when multiple processes are applied simultaneously, so the group will need to be evaluated as a grouped intervention. One difficulty associated with implementing multiple interventions within the CQI approach is identifying which intervention had the greatest impact on improving outcomes (Strom, 2001).

In addition to using evaluation data to make determinations on the current project, the CNS will be able to use every interventional experience when planning for future changes. Publishing both process and outcomes from planned interventions for EBP can add to the body of knowledge regarding process and program effectiveness.

ADVANCED PRACTICE NURSING

In a recent role delineation study (Kenward, 2007), CNS respondents rated the following as those professional activities that they practiced most often:

1. Demonstrate critical thinking and diagnostic reasoning skills in clinical decision making.
2. Assess, plan, implement, and evaluate health care with other health care professionals/primary care providers to meet the comprehensive needs of patients.

3. Identify and analyze factors that enhance or hinder the achievement of desired outcomes for patients and family members.

The CNS carries out these activities within the context of ensuring the quality of care for his/her targeted patient or population. Critical thinking, individualizing a plan for care, and analysis of factors influencing outcomes all could contain quality improvement initiatives.

The ability of CNSs to act as leaders is also influential in determining their ability both to facilitate change and to encourage others to regard best practice statements as a priority for implementation. Nurses who were most effective in promoting local implementation of best practice statements adopted facilitator and leadership roles within their organizations. It would appear that nurses who act as local facilitators and leaders are most effective in promoting evidence-based practice (Ring, Malcolm, Coull, Murphy-Black, & Watterson, 2005).

CNSs do not typically have supervisory responsibility for employees and so may not be able to mandate changes. But consistently partnering with the nurse manager can greatly enhance the potential for success in any project. In addition, the CNS can capitalize on this nonauthoritative relationship to coach staff nurses in activities that improve patient care. Coaching, which provides a focus on improving skills rather than providing education, can be a very rewarding and productive role for the CNS. Clinical coaching has been proposed as a comprehensive approach to achieve and maintain a culture of evidence-based practice (Ervin, 2005). The literature offers some additional guidance on specific actions to consider when creating an evidence-based practice culture (Crow, 2006).

Barriers to EBP include lack of access to relevant research evidence, inadequate database searching skills, difficulty understanding research articles, time and

---

EXHIBIT 6.4 SPECIFIC ACTIONS TO CONSIDER WHEN CREATING AN EVIDENCE-BASED PRACTICE CULTURE

Specific Actions
1. Build an intricate understanding of the business side of health care and nursing.
2. Manage and lead from the future.
3. Create relentless discomfort for the status quo in administrative and clinical practice.
4. Rearrange the power and authority structure using Velcro hooks (easily rearranged again as required).
5. Frame all activities before taking action.
6. Manage the emotions of change.
7. Ensure that commitment for the change is abundant in both administration and staff.
8. Keep the changes simple and concrete.

From "Diffusion of Innovation: The Leaders' Role in Creating the Organizational Context for Evidence-Based Practice," by G. Crow, 2006, *Nursing Administration Quarterly, 30*(3), 236–242.

resource constraints, lack of mentoring and organizational support, and lack of authority to change practice (Oman, Duran, & Fink, 2008).

The CNS should also consider the emotional impact of a practice change on the staff. The potential for sustained change depends on the clinician's responses to project efforts. The change itself is not usually the problem; it is the reaction to the change. Organizations are emotional environments. Research suggests that individuals make choices based on estimates of what they expect to experience with any given change. Anxiety and fear can lead to inertia and distrust of leaders and change agents. Emotions can often be interpreted as resistance and lead to further breakdown of trust (Crow, 2006).

Eight lessons learned regarding overcoming resistance to change and on strategies and practices to facilitate improvement include (Joshi & Bernard, 1999):

1. *Don't reinvent the wheel.* Clinical guidelines and best practice techniques are widely published, so don't waste time in program development.
2. *Start with the usual suspects.* Look for areas that are ripe for improvement and where it will be easy to demonstrate substantial impact on patient outcomes.
3. *Pilot programs should be just that, pilots.* The focus of a pilot should be on content and process, not outcomes. Programs should be piloted for 3 months or less.
4. *Research data can sometimes be a barrier, not an enabler.* Do not wait for results from studies to implement a current best approach to care; expert opinion is an acceptable way to establish practice until research data is available.
5. *Guidelines by themselves have little impact in changing behavior.* Intensive effort and energy must be placed on effective strategies.
6. *One-on-one academic detailing is very effective, but resource intensive.* Use sparingly in appropriate situations.
7. *Clinical champions are instrumental in leading change.* Key thought leaders play a critical role in influencing colleagues.
8. *Change is constant!*

ETHICAL CONSIDERATIONS

The CNS who leads initiatives that improve the quality of patient care must always have an eye toward patient protection and privacy. Diligent appraisal of planned changes for the appropriate evidence-base and application site are required to ensure that translation is put into the correct practice setting. If project outcomes are not met or are suboptimal, an immediate change in care processes may be necessary for safe patient care.

Although projects for improvement need to be scrutinized for any ethical dilemmas, in many cases it is not acceptable for those improvements NOT to happen. In fact, members of the health care team are ethically responsible to participate in CQI initiatives for their patient population in order to improve care. Consider known effective interventions that can save lives, prevent disabilities, and improve quality of life. It would not be appropriate for a patient care area to withhold clinical practices supported by an evidence base.

In the course of project implementation and evaluation, structured collection and analysis of individual patient data elements is often required. Additionally, some information on clinicians may also be needed to fully evaluate a process. All this data must be treated in a highly confidential manner. The data must be completely deidentified prior to any discussions and presentations of project information. All individuals involved in the collection and analysis of the data most likely will need facility-specified education on patient privacy and human subject research. In addition, confidential data must be stored in a locked location and destroyed after a designated use date.

It is not always clear which activities are classified as quality improvement (QI) and which are considered human subjects research. Most QI activities are not human subjects research and do not require review by an institutional review board. However, because such activities may still put patients at risk, some other review may be necessary.

Specialists in the conduct of human subjects research believe that it involves the "intent" of the project. The general belief is that QI projects are created to bring about immediate improvements in health care activity and, as such, are an intrinsic normal part of health care operation. Usually, the knowledge resulting from QI activities is most applicable to the local practice arena as an effort to improve care in that particular setting.

Studies classified as research are designed to develop or contribute to generalizable knowledge and applicable to other people or situations (Lynn et al., 2007). It may require the institutional review board (IRB) within a facility to determine whether or not a project qualifies as QI or research. Some facilities have created worksheets to help project leaders determine whether or not a project should be submitted to the IRB.

DISCUSSION QUESTIONS

1. Consider a practice change that has occurred recently in your work environment. Who were the leaders of the change? Which interventions did they use? Were the interventions novel and innovative or did the team choose tried and true strategies? Do you

think that the change will still be in effect a year from now? Why or why not?

2. You may have heard the expression "If we continue to do what we've always done, we will get the results we have always gotten." Can you think of a situation in health care in which a practice change was desired but just never happened? Were interventions attempted but ultimately proved unsuccessful? What were the barriers in that situation? Do you think that another intervention might have been more successful?

3. By its very nature, innovation can be inefficient. During economic downturns, health care systems often downsize by laying off those personnel who are not considered necessary for direct patient care. This might include the CNS and other leaders who are experienced change agents. Do you think that this is a fiscally responsible strategy? If you were the CNS, how might you justify the retention of your position?

ANALYSIS AND SYNTHESIS EXERCISES

1. Think about a clinical question in your field of expertise. Perform a literature search to determine the level of evidence and any patient care recommendations that exist. Is the care in your health care system consistent with the recommendations? Design a plan to make any necessary changes and choose interventions based on the characteristics of your practice arena.

2. The Institute of Medicine (IOM) estimates that the time that it takes to integrate research findings into routine practice can be as long as 17 years (IOM, 2001). Although this may be hard to believe, the change agents within many facilities can understand why this is true. Engage a CNS in a discussion on this topic to brainstorm strategies to increase the rate of research translation into practice.

3. Various health care disciplines have turned to industry and engineering/informatics as sources of important and emerging innovations. Search the internet for examples of industrial research that has now been applied to nursing and/or medicine. (Hint: the airline industry has heavily influenced our current practices for avoiding errors to enhance patient safety.)

REFERENCES

Brabham, D. C. (2008) Crowdsourcing as a model for problem solving. *Convergence: The International Journal of Research into New Media Technologies, 14,* 75–90.

Crow, G. (2006). Diffusion of innovation: The leaders' role in creating the organizational context for evidence-based practice. *Nursing Administration Quarterly, 30*(3), 236–242.

Ditkoff, M. (2004). *Qualities of an innovator.* Retrieved January 11, 2009, from http://ideachampions.com/downloads/qualities_of_an_innovator.pdf

Ervin, N. E. (2005). Clinical coaching: A strategy for enhancing evidence-based nursing practice. *Clinical Nurse Specialist, 19*(6), 296–301.

Gawlinski, A. (2007). Evidence-based practice changes: Measuring the outcome. *AACN Advanced Critical Care, 18*(3), 320–322.

Geibert, R. C. (2006). Using diffusion of innovation concepts to enhance implementation of an electronic health record to support evidence-based practice. *Nursing Administration Quarterly, 30*(3), 203–210.

Gladwell, M. (2002). *The tipping point.* New York: Little, Brown and Company.

Gleick, J. (1987). *Chaos: Making a new science.* New York: Penguin Books.

Grant, R. W., & Meigs, J. B. (2006). Overcoming barriers to evidence-based diabetes care. *Current Diabetes Reviews, 2,* 261–269.

Grimshaw, J. M., Shirran, L., Thomas, R., Mowatt, G., Fraser, C., Bero, L., et al. (2001). Changing provider behavior: An overview of systematic reviews of interventions. *Medical Care, 39*(8 Suppl. 2), II2–II45.

Grol, R., & Grimshaw, J. (1999). Evidence-based implementation of evidence-based medicine. *Joint Commission Journal on Quality Improvement, 25*(10), 503–513.

Gustafson, D. H., Sainfort, F., Eichler, M., Adams, L., Bisognano, M., & Steudel, H. (2003). Developing and testing a model to predict outcomes of organizational change. *Health Services Research, 38,* 751–776.

Hamric, A. B. (1989). History and overview of the CNS role. In A. B. Hamric & J. A. Spross (Eds.), *The clinical nurse specialist in theory and practice* (pp. 3–18). Philadelphia: W. B. Saunders.

Idea Champions. (2007). *Culture of innovation.* Retrieved January 11, 2009, from: http://www.ideachampions.com/downloads.shtml

The Joint Commission on the Accreditation of Healthcare Organizations. (2006). Raising the bar with bundles. *Joint Commission Perspectives on Patient Safety, 6*(4).

Joshi, M. S., & Bernard, D. B. (1999). Classic CQI integrated with comprehensive disease management as a model for performance improvement. *Joint Commission Journal on Quality Improvement, 25*(8), 383–395.

Kaplow, R. (2007). Synergy model: Guiding the practice of the CNS in acute and critical care. In M. G. McKinley (Ed.), *Acute and critical care clinical nurse specialists: Synergy for best practices* (pp. 29–47). St. Louis: Saunders Elsevier.

Kenward, K. (2007). *Report of findings from the role delineation study of nurse practitioners and clinical nurse specialists* (Research Brief Vol. 30). Chicago: National Council of State Boards of Nursing, Inc.

Lynn, J., Baily, M. A., Bottrell, M., Jennings, B., Levine, R. J., Davidoff, F., et al. (2007). The ethics of using quality improvement methods in health care. *Annals of Internal Medicine, 146*(9), 666–673.

National Association of Clinical Nurse Specialists. (2004). *Statement on clinical nurse specialist practice and education* (2nd ed.). Harrisburg, PA: Author.

New, J. P., Mason, J. M., Freemantle, N., Teasdale, S., Wong, L. M., Bruce, N. J., et al. (2003). Specialist nurse-led intervention to treat and control hypertension and hyperlipidemia in diabetes (SPLINT): A randomized controlled trial. *Diabetes Care, 26*(8), 2250–2255.

Oman, K., Duran, C., & Fink, R. (2008). Evidence-based policy and procedures. *The Journal of Nursing Administration, 38*(1), 47–51.

Pipe, T. B. (2007). Optimizing nursing care by integrating theory-driven evidence-based practice. *Journal of Nursing Care Quality, 22*(3), 234–238.

Rello, J., Lorente, C., Bodi, M., Diaz, E., Ricart, M., & Kollef, M. H. (2002). Why do physicians not follow evidence-based guidelines for preventing ventilator-associated pneumonia? *Chest, 122*(2), 656–661.

Ring, N., Malcolm, C., Coull, A., Murphy-Black, T., & Watterson, A. (2005). Nursing best practice statements: An exploration of their implementation in clinical practice. *Journal of Clinical Nursing, 14*, 1048–1058.

Rogers, E. M. (2003). *Diffusion of innovations.* New York: Free Press.

Rosswurm, M. A., & Larrabee, J. H. (1999). A model for change to evidence-based practice. *Image: Journal of Nursing Scholarship, 31*(4), 317–322.

Shanley, C. (2007). Management of change for nurses: Lessons from the discipline of organizational studies. *Journal of Nursing Management, 15*, 538–546.

Shirey, M. R. (2007). Leadership and organizational strategies to increase innovative thinking. *Clinical Nurse Specialist, 21*(4), 191–194.

Stanley, D. (2006). Role conflict: Leaders and managers. *Nursing Management, 13*(5), 31–37.

Strom, K. (2001). Quality improvement interventions: What works? *Journal for Healthcare Quality, 23*(5), 4–14.

Sullivan, E., & Decker, P. (2001). *Effective leadership and management in nursing.* Upper Saddle River, NJ: Prentice Hall.

Tapscott, D., & Williams, A. D. (2007). Innovation in the age of mass collaboration. *Business Week.* Retrieved January 11, 2009, from: http://www.businessweek.com/innovate/content/feb2007/id20070201_774736.htm

Tedeschi, B. (2008). Putting innovation in the hands of a crowd. *The New York Times.* Retrieved January 11, 2009, from: http://www.nytimes.com/2008/03/03/technology/03ecom.html?_r=1&scp=1&sq=Putting%20innovation%20in%20the%20hands%20of%20a%20crowd&st=cse

White, A. (2004). Change strategies make for smooth transitions. *Nursing Management, 35*(2), 49–52.

Evaluating Interventions

Kelly A. Goudreau

EVALUATING INTERVENTIONS

> The process of disciplined evaluation permeates all areas of thought and practice . . . It is found in scholarly book reviews, in engineering's quality control procedures, in the Socratic dialogues, in serious social and moral criticism, in mathematics, and in the opinions handed down by appellate courts . . . it is the process whose duty is the systematic and objective determination of merit, worth or value. Without such a process, there is no way to distinguish the worthwhile from the worthless.
>
> *(Scriven, 1991, p. 4)*

Evaluation of nursing interventions is a key component of what nursing does in each and every practice, process, or procedure, yet, in many instances it is left to interpretation rather than definitive discussion. Typically in practice, nursing interventions are poorly documented and are not described in measurable terms, making it almost impossible to evaluate them effectively. Additionally, the process of evaluation is haphazard and poorly documented at best, or nonexistent at worst. As an action-oriented discipline, we often move very quickly to identify an intervention from our repertoire, implement it, and then change the plan of care and subsequent interventions due to a perception that the intervention was not working as intended. But have we determined exactly what the etiology of the problem was in the first place? Do we know for certain that the intervention was not effective, or was it just that the cause of the problem was different than we initially thought, making the intervention inert? This action without thought or thorough evaluation is the plague of our profession. Evaluation is given short

shrift in spite of the increasing focus on evidence-based practice. How is it that we can implement an intervention without truly taking the time to think about, reflect on, and evaluate its effectiveness?

The documentation to affirmatively support what we are doing is also often lacking. The rigor, reliability, and validity of what we are doing is not measurable due to the fact that we have not documented what we were doing in a sufficient manner and, therefore, cannot link the causal chain and *prove* that the intervention was either working or not working. We simply move to act and change the intervention even before we have thoroughly considered the etiology of the need that requires intervention, the effect of the intervention, and its outcome. It is time to change that perspective and bring to bear the tools that have been created over the last number of years in support of the work of nurses and nursing. Tools added to that list include such things as research, evidence-based practice, and the science of evaluation. It is time to be proactive rather than reactive, and it is the role of the clinical nurse specialist (CNS) to do this.

The nursing process has been in place for as long as many can remember (Orlando, 1961). It is an integral component of the manner in which nurses function and understand one another as they communicate regarding patient care initiatives and programs. Unfortunately, evaluation is also the least documented, effectively utilized, and understood component of the nursing process. According to the W. K. Kellogg Foundation (1998), evaluation should be more than just a step in a process, it should "document impact and demonstrate accountability, it should also lead to more effective programs, greater learning opportunities, and better knowledge of what works" (p. I). Many times the focus of the nursing and health care professional staff and the CNS is the assessment of the needs of the patient, their family or support system, and the health care environment in which the care is being provided. In the flurry of activity surrounding establishment of a new care plan that is assumed will meet identified needs, or ensuring that the assessment is thorough and evidence-based, evaluation of a measurable intervention is not well established. As a result, from the outset, evaluation of the interventions is often not well-documented either. Although evaluation may be done informally or is evidenced indirectly through actions taken to modify the plan of care when interventions do not demonstrate the desired outcomes, it is not clearly documented and thoroughly examined. As nurses and CNSs, we do, of course, evaluate the care given and modify the care given in order to increase the likelihood that the patient will achieve the intended outcomes. What we do not do frequently is fully document what the intervention consisted of and the outcomes and reasons for changes in the plan of care.

Although the direct patient interaction is the foundation of evaluation for both nursing and CNS practice, the CNS is expected to take evaluation to an advanced level as he or she interacts with all three spheres of influence: the patient, the nursing and health care professional staff, and the system (National Association of Clinical Nurse Specialists [NACNS], 2004). It is in the interaction with all three spheres that the CNS enacts the advanced nature of his or her role. It is up to the CNS to bring the thought process back into the selection or creation of an intervention, documentation of the intervention in measurable steps, and evaluation of the outcomes of that intervention. The CNS is the bridge between research, evaluation, and application to practice in every environment he or she touches.

Interventions performed by CNSs must include all three spheres of influence (NACNS, 2004) and are, therefore, broader than just direct application to patients. The work that is done with the nursing and allied health personnel and the system interventions is equally important. It is the synergy that is created by the interaction of all three spheres that creates the greatest impact to the patient and the outcomes of care that meet their needs. Evaluation of the outcomes of care is essential in today's health care environment, as is the evaluation of the effectiveness of interventions conducted within the nursing/health care personnel sphere of influence (educational programs and product evaluation) and systems sphere interventions (projects and quality improvement) that are implemented in an effort to increase patient safety.

This chapter provides a brief overview of nursing interventions and how an intervention should be designed in order to facilitate effective evaluation. It also discusses the background and history of evaluation

processes, including the theoretical foundation both within and external to nursing and the application of evaluation to interventions within the patient sphere of CNS practice. Interventions in the nursing/health care workers sphere have been discussed to some extent in the chapter by Doran, Sidani, and DiPietro (chapter 4) and Pacini (chapter 9). Doran et al. also discuss evaluation of systems level/systems sphere interventions as does O'Malley in her discussion of product evaluation (chapter 23) and Benton in her discussion of quality improvement (chapter 12). Although Lyon touches on the evaluation of interventions in her chapter on the clinical reasoning model (chapter 5), what has not been thoroughly discussed is the work of the CNS in evaluation itself. The CNS plays a specific role in working directly with the patient/client and his or her family, the nursing and health care worker, and the system as interventions are thoroughly evaluated. This chapter provides background to all three spheres (the patient, the nursing and health care professional staff, and the system) but focuses on the patient/client and the interventions nurses and CNSs develop and ultimately should evaluate.

BRIEF HISTORICAL BACKGROUND

In order to truly provide a frame of reference for evaluation of interventions it is important to first give voice to the intervention itself. In chapter 6, Richardson outlines the means by which the CNS develops innovation, change, and interventions in a very practical sense through the collaborative efforts of the change process. By taking interventions of the past and using change theory to create innovation she describes an "on the ground" approach to how the CNS can innovate and generate changes in the clinical environment through application of evidence-based practice and changes in interventions over time. How does one develop an intervention in the first place, however, and then subsequently bring to bear the needed evaluative measures in order to determine its effectiveness?

According to Conn (2007), interventions must be clearly defined in measurable terms for two reasons: (1) so that they may be used in a replicable way and effectively in practice, and, more importantly, (2) so they can be studied for their effectiveness. The measurability of the intervention is often lost on the day-to-day practitioner and is a concept that we struggle with on a constant basis. How can we slow down enough to truly incorporate the concepts of research and evaluation into the day-to-day practice when patients are so much more complex with comorbidities and care issues that previously would have placed them in an intensive care environment but now are in the home or nursing skilled care units? This increased complexity creates an aura of urgency in provision of care and, therefore, it could be argued, does not allow as much time for consideration and reflective thought as interventions are developed and implemented (Resnick et al., 2005).

The theory of the nursing process was first articulated by Orlando in the 1950s (Faust, 2002) with first discussion of the theory in the literature in 1961 (Orlando, 1961). In the nursing process theory, Orlando does not clearly delineate the use of the five-step process of assessment, diagnosis, planning, implementation, and evaluation, which we know today as the nursing process. Instead, she described her observations of the manner in which nurses interacted with their patients. Orlando (1961) discussed three elements in every nursing encounter: the behavior of the patient, the reaction of the nurse, and the nursing action undertaken to benefit the patient. It is an iterative process whereby the nurse clearly modifies his/her behavior based on the behavior of the patient. Orlando's theory is seen as a middle-range theory by some (Fawcett, 1995) because it does not clearly define the four elements of the metaparadigm of nursing: person, environment, nursing, and health. What it does, however, is set the tone and expectation that the scientific process will be used in the day-to-day operations of nursing, and it is considered a seminal work in the foundations of nursing practice. It is a concept that is unfortunately lost in today's hustle and bustle of daily care.

Years later these foundational concepts were taken by other nursing theorists, such as Abdellah, Henderson, and Orem, and developed over time as an adaptation of the scientific process for experimentation (Meleis, 1991). The theory was immediately seen as a way to frame the manner in which nurses thought about the care they provided to patients in all settings. The universality of the nursing process as an explanation for the way in which nurses thought and then interacted with their patients provided a scientific basis for their day-to-day activities. When the American Nurses Association (ANA) adopted the model and integrated it into all documents that defined the professional role of nursing, it became a fundamental way in which to describe what nurses do. Now, the implementation of evidence-based practice emphasizes even further the need to thoroughly evaluate the interventions that are being used with various patient populations and to question why a method has been used, whether or not it should continue to be used, and what evidence supports its continued use. This daily application of the scientific method brings to light the increasing need for nursing and all health care staff to understand how to thoroughly evaluate the care they are providing.

The purpose of evaluation is, of course, broader than just nursing and the nursing process. Stufflebeam and Shinkfield (2007) describe evaluation as a distinct profession with specific models and theories that guide and support the appropriate implementation of the specific discipline. Ultimately, evaluation should determine whether or not an intervention (individual, group, or regional/national) has achieved the desired outcome.

Within nursing, *evaluation* has been defined as the final step in an iterative process where an assessment of needs was conducted, a diagnosis and a plan were formulated and implemented, and then an assessment was conducted to determine the effectiveness of the intervention. Any intervention at any level needs to be evaluated. This general description can equally apply to any of the three spheres of CNS influence: the nursing and health care staff, the system, or the patient.

Nursing/Health Care Staff

There are key areas that the CNS evaluates when working with the nursing and health care staff. These areas include product evaluation, cost-to-benefit ratio savings measures across interventions conducted by the staff, evaluation of aggregate clinical care outcomes, and direct educational interventions.

Product evaluation is the consideration of various types of products that the staff will be using in day-to-day operations and interactions with patients. The CNS performs the function of seeking stakeholder input, feedback, and buy-in for any new products that will be used in the clinical environment (Busch, 2001; Caley & Scharf, 1992; Monahan & Donius, 1991; Simpkins, Halduven, & Stevens, 1995). Will this particular product provide the safest, most efficient, and cost-effective method of care for the patients in the context in which it is intended to be used? Product evaluation must take into consideration many factors, including the ergonomics of the environment, the demographics of the staff in terms of educational preparation, age, gender, and demographics of the patient population to be served. The CNS often uses his or her knowledge of evaluation processes to create a tool that outlines the criteria to be evaluated and then provides the summation of the outcomes for those who will make the final decisions.

This assessment of stakeholder feedback on the proposed product and buy-in to its use in the clinical environment must also include the cost/benefit ratio and analysis of both the objective and subjective data relative to a product and how the staff interacts with the product. If a product is cost-effective and efficient but is not used by the staff, it can be as costly or more costly than a product that is a little more expensive but is used effectively by the staff. Safety considerations and the costs associated with injury management must also be factored into the cost/benefit ratio if the data is to present a full and comprehensive picture of the overall effectiveness and efficiency of a particular product.

The evaluation of interventions by the health care staff in aggregate form for overall assessment of attainment of desired outcomes for patients is a data analysis component of the CNSs interaction with the health care staff. The CNS must identify overall patterns and trends in care outcomes so that the staff can take further action or can be lauded for the efforts made to improve care (Dickerson, Wu, & Kennedy, 2006). Examples of this are explicitly detailed in the Institute for Healthcare Improvement (IHI) "bundles" and measures of clinical outcomes (IHI, 2007). Issues such as ventilator associated pneumonia (VAP) are known to be impacted and prevented as a result of the very specific nursing interventions of mouth care and positioning. The CNS can increase the awareness of the nurses related to these relatively simple nursing interventions and their overall impact to the patient care outcomes.

From these aggregate analyses of outcomes come the focused educational interventions that are developed, implemented, and evaluated by the CNS. These educational interventions with the nursing staff can range from new procedures to information about illness states that are new to the staff in the patient population they care for or existing knowledge that needs to be reinforced. The evaluation of an educational intervention must take into consideration the adult learning principles and learner preferences in the clinical and educational environments or the context of care for these populations; it typically includes measurements of the learning achieved through pre- and post-testing of knowledge, as well as value judgments and informal observation of behavior in the post-educational intervention period by the CNS, the learner's self-reflection on their learning, and peer review of changes in activities and behaviors (Miller, Linn, & Gronlund, 2008). The role of the CNS is to collect this data and analyze the outcomes of the educational intervention so that it can continue to be reinforced or so that it can be modified to attain the desired results.

The System

Within the system sphere of influence CNSs can have broad-reaching effects and should, therefore, have strong evaluative effects. Evaluation of programs at a unit, facility, regional, or national level is in many instances the driving factor behind CNS practice. The assessment of specific needs on a unit can often be identified and acknowledged as essential across an entire facility. The CNS uses his or her skills to address the needs of the staff and patients from a broad perspective, which can frequently extend across multiple care units and environments. The current acknowledged fractioning of the health care system is increasing the demand for use of systems-level skill sets that are inherent in CNS practice (Institute of Medicine, 2001). As a result CNSs are in greater demand than ever before. These skills are even more important as individuals look to redesign systems and increase patient safety in all aspects

of care. CNSs have a clear role in guiding, leading, and facilitating the change efforts that must take place in today's health care system in order to increase patient safety and the quality of nursing care. Systems or programmatic level evaluation has been discussed in the literature for many years (Casper, Kenron, & McDaniel, 2005; Daponte, 2008; Rossi & Freeman, 1993; Wood, 1998). Unfortunately, however, although systems level interventions are key to the CNS role and evaluation is a key component of CNS practice, evaluation of systems level interventions has had little attention in the nursing or CNS literature.

The W. K. Kellogg Foundation (1998, 2008) describes a process whereby project-level evaluation needs to take into consideration the context of the project or program, evaluation of the implementation of the program or project in its various stages of implementation, and the final outcomes assessment whereby the intended outcomes are compared to the actual outcomes. This logical flow model can best be described in a pictorial manner and allows for action-oriented changes to the plan as the intervention unfolds and both intended and unintended outcomes are realized. Kellogg (2008) identified that "a logic model presents program information and progress toward goals in ways that inform, advocate for a particular program approach, and teach program stakeholders" (p. 5). Perhaps this is a tool that can and should be added to the CNS toolkit when looking at the development, implementation, and subsequent evaluation of programs and system-level interventions. Through the description of factors (resources or barriers to implementation of a program), activities (including products, services, and infrastructure needed to implement the program), outputs (direct results of the program), outcomes (changes in behaviors as a result of the program), and finally impacts (the ripple effect in the targeted community as a result of the program), the logic model provides both a framework for the establishment of a program or project as well as the evaluative model. By describing specifically the outputs, outcomes, and intended impacts at the beginning of a project or program, the CNS can clearly identify the evaluative measures that will be used as the program unfolds and is completed. The framework also provides the logical model for reporting the results of the program to stakeholders, thereby reducing the potentially duplicative work involved in trying to reframe evaluation information for reporting purposes.

Stufflebeam and Shinkfield (2007) identify a number of theoretical foundations for evaluation that would most likely be considered midrange theories if they were within nursing. Stufflebeam's Context, Input, Process, and Product (CIPP) model of evaluation is described along with Stake's 1967 responsive/client-centered evaluation, Patton's utilization-focused evaluation, and

Scriven's 1967 model of formative and summative evaluation processes (cited in Stufflebeam & Shinkfield, 2007). Each of the described models defines a specific process for evaluation that would inform the CNS of the outcomes of system-level programs or educational processes if used within the context of health care. Each has its strengths and weaknesses and so it is left to the CNS to explore the feasibility of use within their specific environment.

The Patient

The interaction of the patient and the nursing intervention is a key focus and essentially a primary raison d'être for the function and role of the CNS. The influence of the CNS in day-to-day practice and interventions with the patient and the staff who support the patient derives from the focus of CNS practice origination, "from nursing and for nursing."

Unfortunately, much like the nursing staff that the CNS works with, the documentation of the evaluative process is not always easily traced in the charting system or in documents that clearly articulate the outcomes of care from a nursing perspective. Typically, evaluation is not documented in a formal process but instead is reflected in the changes to the plan of care in an implicit versus explicit manner. When a notation is made to change the plan of care from one nursing intervention to another, it is assumed that the nurse evaluated the impact of the initial or previous intervention and determined that it was either ineffective or not working as well as intended and, therefore, needed to be modified or removed in lieu of an alternative intervention that will subsequently be evaluated for its effectiveness.

Documenting the effectiveness of an intervention requires a thoughtful process of establishing the etiology of the issue or need that is the indication for an intervention, crafting an intervention that is measurable and will meet that issue or need, and then evaluating the effectiveness of that intervention in addressing the issue or need. It must be based on subjective evidence that is contained within the data collected. The evidence must be validated with the patient and added to objective evidence that is available both in the chart and through observation of the patient in the context of their care. Key to all of these elements is that the need or problem can be addressed through the application of a nursing intervention and not a medically delegated intervention. Many times the nurse will look to the medical interventions that are easily pulled from a list of delegated tasks rather than look to the ways in which the nurse can use his or her skills to meet the patient's needs. For some reason, the nursing skill set and ability to intervene is downplayed or seen as less important than the delegated medical tasks that nurses carry out.

It is not clear why that happens, and the issue has been a constant struggle for nurse educators for many years (Fulton, 2003).

The difficulties with the articulation of the nursing plan of care and subsequent concurrent updating and modification of the nursing interventions on the plan of care are well-known throughout the history of nursing. The reality of nursing care on a day-to-day basis mixed with the need to document that care in a manner that is unobtrusive to the care process itself is nearly impossible. Some consider the nursing care plan to be a purely academic exercise not based in reality. How, then, does nursing reconcile the need to document and provide evidence for the foundations of care and the actual provision of care in an extremely active environment while still staying true to the fact that our autonomous focus for nursing interventions should not be only the delegated medical tasks ordered by our physician peers?

CONCEPTUAL AND/OR THEORETICAL FRAMEWORKS FOR EVALUATION OF NURSING INTERVENTIONS

The foundation of evaluation of interventions is difficult to determine because evaluation has been a component of the research process for generations. Aside from the background within nursing (Meleis, 1991; Orlando, 1961) that defines evaluation from the perspective of nursing interventions and assessment of outcomes, there are many different disciplines that have clearly defined the process of evaluation (Fitzpatrick, Worthen, & Sanders, 2003; Rossi & Freeman, 1993; Sanders, 1994; Stufflebeam & Shinkfield, 2007).

It is clear, however, that in order to get beyond the day-to-day volatility of the nurses' world one needs to slow down and think about the process of intervention and subsequent evaluation. Truly, evaluation should be the foundation of clinical practice for all nurses, but it is especially important in the advanced practice role that the CNS carries. It tends to be lost, however, in the flurry of activity that is patient care, working with the nursing and allied health staff, and "fixing the system," which is the day-to-day reality of the CNS in clinical practice. Frankly, most CNSs would indicate that they do not have time to be thoughtful and methodical in the evaluation of interventions. However, it is through this thoughtful application of evaluation that mirrors the research process that we can attain the best understanding of the interventions we are carrying out.

CNSs and nurses must look at the interventions they are implementing and assess whether or not they are *nursing* interventions, whether or not they are measurable, and whether or not they can be reliably and accurately evaluated for their effectiveness. The intervention should be grounded in theory and should have a conceptual framework that supports the foundation of the intervention. Finally, in addition to the intervention having a conceptual framework, the evaluation itself must have a conceptual framework upon which it is based.

Conn, Rantz, Wipke-Tevis, and Maas (2001) describe the attributes needing consideration when designing or selecting interventions, including: What is the conceptual basis of the intervention? Have there been previous descriptive studies conducted on the intervention? What does the related intervention research show? Has the intervention been designed for a specific population? Is the specificity or generality of the intervention consistent with the conceptual framework? Are the interventions singled or bundled, and if either, is this consistent with the conceptual framework? What is the method of delivery of the intervention? And finally, what is the dose of the intervention, and is it also supported by the conceptual framework? In each case, the intervention must be consistent with the literature and the conceptual framework that supports it. If these attributes are not in alignment with the framework, then it is extremely difficult to draw any conclusions in the evaluative stage as to effectiveness of the intervention (Sechrest, West, Phillips, Redner, & Yeaton, 1979). In this era of evidence-based practice, it is extraordinarily important to the CNS and the staff nurse alike that the selection or design of the intervention is grounded in a conceptual framework founded on subjective and objective data gained from research, as well as the patient/client and their particular context at the time that the intervention is needed. This foundation is essential if the nurse wants to be able to predict that the action will alter or remove the etiology, thereby linking the causal chain and upholding their hypothesis as to the etiology of the actual or perceived need.

Sidani and Braden (1998) also identified this point when they concluded that "knowledge of the critical inputs (component, mode of delivery, and dosage) and the chain of processes linking the intervention to outcomes are necessary for delineating the outcomes' pattern of change" (p. 141). Clearly, one cannot evaluate an intervention effectively without first designing the intervention to be measurable and linking those measures through a conceptual framework back to the interventions. In other words, in order to look at the conceptual framework for evaluation, it is also necessary to look at the intervention and the conceptual framework for the intervention (Conn et al., 2001). In many instances, the conceptual framework of the evaluation is a mismatch to the interventions, and therefore, it is not possible to measure effectively the outcomes attained. As an example, Lyon states in chapter 5 that a nursing intervention is proposed only to alter the hypothesized etiologies contributing to or causing a problem. Alternatively,

an intervention is intended to prevent etiologies and, therefore, prevent a potential problem from becoming an actual problem. It is up to the individual who is attempting to determine the most effective intervention and then measure the effectiveness of that intervention to ensure that it has been constructed in such a way as to be measurable in the evaluation phase. If it has not been constructed effectively, it will be difficult at best to determine whether or not it was the intervention that actually created the outcome that was noted and/or desired.

This thoughtful processing of interventions is often lacking in the day-to-day hustle and bustle of work on the unit, in the facility overall, and in general in the practice of the nursing and health care worker today. It is the role of the CNS to bring it back to the fore where it belongs.

APPLICATION TO CNS PRACTICE

With so many potential midrange theories on evaluation, where does a CNS begin to assist the patient and the staff who care for them to ensure that the intervention has been constructed in such a way as to facilitate the evaluative process? It is important to think about whether or not there is a conceptual framework for the care being provided when looking at and thinking about innovative ways to interact with patients/clients within the practice environment. If there is a framework that can be used in the care of a patient, then it is the role of the CNS to bring the theoretical perspective back to the day-to-day work of the nursing and health care staff. It is the role of the CNS also to increase the visibility of the evidence base in the care of patients and to bring their experience and expertise in the field to the care of each patient/client and population.

A focus on the nursing aspects of care is an essential aspect of the overall management of the patient that is often lost in the daily activities of a busy unit. It is up to the CNS as the advanced practice nurse to bring the spotlight back onto the aspect of nursing care, which is essential to the improved outcomes that patients achieve while in the health care system.

According to Thomas (1984), "the fashioning of an intervention plan calls for consideration of suitable alternatives, given available methods, as well as new approaches that might be adopted to meet the problem in question" (p. 21). Daponte (2008) outlines a specific process that can be used fairly universally and incorporates many of the previously described evaluation theories (Stufflebeam & Shinkfield, 2007). Although not specifically designed for nursing care or CNS practice, Daponte describes an evaluation framework that can be modified to meet nursing needs as follows:

- Assess whether or not there is a conceptual framework that has either been explicitly or implicitly used to create the intervention. Make it explicit if it is not.
- Determine whether or not the intervention will likely impact the etiology of the problem that the patient is articulating or that the nurse has identified and validated with the patient.
- Identify whether any current evaluative activities are formative (focused on improvement of the intervention as it is being enacted) or summative (conclusions regarding the outcomes).
- Define all the possible questions that could be asked about this intervention and its effectiveness.
- Rigorously describe the intervention by developing the theory and using a logic model that is interactive and iterative.
- Revisit the evaluation questions that could be asked.
- Only after the previous steps have been completed, develop the evaluation plan.
- Collect the data, analyze it, and write the evaluative report.

This modification of the research process specific to evaluation of interventions can be implemented fairly quickly. With easier access to nursing databases and literature searches, the CNS can role model these behaviors for the nurses and health care workers.

Key to evaluation of interventions is not only that the intervention has been clearly articulated and that the evaluation is outlined very specifically as it relates to the conceptual framework of the intervention but also that the manner in which the data is collected is reliable (consistent and replicable) and valid (able to clearly address the original problem, show change that can be attributed to the intervention, and be validated by more than just one measure; C. Beausang, personal communication, February 12, 2009).

A final consideration for evaluation in action is the potential of the Hawthorne Effect. In any formal evaluation there will be an effect simply because you are formally evaluating the care being provided. The staff will become more acutely aware of the processes and, therefore, will improve their processes, whether that was the intent or not. A notable change will take time, but by incorporating the processes and procedures into daily activities within the unit or area, the overall outcomes of care will ultimately be impacted in a measurable, reliable, and valid manner.

It is possible to implement a formal evaluation process for the care provided on a unit or with a patient population as demonstrated by Allen, Bockenhauer, Egan, and Kinnaird (2006). These administrative nurses described a 10-year process whereby nursing practice was tied directly to patient outcomes. The result was increased satisfaction from the nursing staff, an increased awareness of how their practice impacts the patient care and an ability to critically analyze the data from patient care outcomes, and most importantly, increased patient satisfaction with the care provided.

ETHICAL CONSIDERATIONS

Ethics have always been an important aspect of care for nurses and health care workers. Fortunately, in today's society, ethics are becoming an explicit component of care and are being discussed freely and openly in the context of care. Evaluation of interventions has a key ethical component and should be focused on the aspects of care that are intended to provide benefit to the patient/client. When any intervention is being developed there needs to be consideration for three key things: (1) the patient/client is fully informed of the implications of the intervention, both positive and negative, and gives consent to the treatment; (2) the benefits must be assumed to outweigh the risks associated with the intervention; and (3) the patient/client is assured of confidentiality in all aspects of the care (Thomas, 1984).

Further, nurses are bound by the ANA code of ethics as a statement of values for the profession. The ANA has clearly articulated key ethics statements in the care of patients/clients across the continuum of care provided by nurses in general, inclusive of CNS practice.

Because the evaluative process mirrors the research process in many aspects, it is important to take into consideration the needs of the patient/client and the issue of whether or not there would be potential harm to the patient/client as a result of the intervention or the evaluation being proposed. It is important to consider all aspects of the treatment and care of patients/clients from the perspective of the protection of human subjects in spite of the fact of whether or not the treatment is part of a research protocol.

SUMMARY

Evaluation of nursing interventions is an area of nursing that has been considered for generations but poorly implemented within the day-to-day activities of the nursing and health care staff. The reality of the busy unit or large number of patients/clients that the nurse or allied health worker must see on a daily basis means that there is often a loss of the reflective thought process that needs to be elemental to the care provided.

It is the role of the CNS as the advanced practice nurse to role model the behaviors that all nurses and health care workers should be exhibiting as we care for our patients/clients and populations. Key to this is the establishment or clear articulation of the evidence base and conceptual framework supporting the interventions that are carried out and the evaluations that must be enacted. Only through clear statement of the intervention in measurable terms can we then in turn evaluate the care provided and determine whether or not the intervention carried out was in fact effective in ameliorating the problem articulated and validated by the patient/client and the data collected by the nurse.

Not only does the intervention need to be clearly articulated and measurable, but it also must be linked appropriately to the etiology of the problem that the patient/client is experiencing. Nursing too often falls into the perception that the best intervention is one that has been delegated by medicine to nursing. Delegated medical interventions such as medications to manage pain rather than nursing interventions of positioning, distraction, or touch and presence are often used and assumed to be within the realm of nursing as interventions. There is a need to reclarify the role of nursing and the autonomous domain of nursing interventions and their overall value and worth. There is a need to evaluate the care provided by nurses other than the delegated medical authority that seems to be forefront. CNSs have a primary role in assisting nursing and health care workers to shift their perspective and evaluate the care they are providing.

As a result of the loss of focus on nursing interventions, so too has the documentation of interventions and the evaluation of them suffered. Orlando (1961) first articulated the role of the nurse in providing that supportive and relationship-based interface between the health care system and the patient/client. We now have many more tools we can bring to bear on further describing that unique contribution of nursing to the health care system. Evidence-based practice, midrange theory, and a far better understanding of the research process and how it can be applied to daily activities of nursing are just a few examples of what we have today that our predecessors did not.

CNSs must lead the way for the nursing staff and through doing so can impact the overall satisfaction of the staff, the patients/clients, and the patient/client outcomes. Evaluation is key to attaining those outcomes.

DISCUSSION QUESTIONS

1. Discuss the differences between nursing interventions and medically delegated interventions. Do you think there is greater value to one versus the other? How well do we document the medical interventions? The nursing interventions? Does nursing need to re-evaluate nursing interventions as a process and outcome?
2. The author has proposed that in order to have evidence of outcomes that are causal from the intervention to the evaluation there needs to be concrete

evidence that the intervention has created the outcome. Discuss how that does or does not apply to your current practice as a nurse or CNS.
3. Discuss how you use evaluation at present time in the three spheres of influence of CNS practice.

ANALYSIS AND SYNTHESIS EXERCISES

1. A CNS working with a staff nurse has noted that the patient who has a chest tube is complaining of pain to the chest wall when breathing and states he cannot do the deep breathing and coughing exercises that are needed to maintain and expand his lung tissue. Describe the potential etiologies of the pain (include physiologic, psychologic, and medical reasons). Describe potential *nursing* interventions that are specific, measurable, and based on a conceptual framework. Define how you would evaluate these interventions.
2. It was noted that staff were having difficulty with identifying cardinal signs of impending failure in patients on a cardiac unit. The CNS determined that there was need for a case-based high fidelity simulation (HFS) exercise to improve recognition of the cardinal signs and ultimately improve the staff response to those signs. Outline the conceptual framework you would use to ground this intervention. What would be some of the measurable interventions used in this case? What would be measurable outcomes that could be attributed to the HFS? What other issues/evaluative measures would you need to consider?

REFERENCES

Allen, D. E., Bockenhauer, B., Egan, C., & Kinnaird, L. S. (2006). Relating outcomes to excellent nursing practice. *Journal of Nursing Administration, 36*(3), 140–147.

Busch, A. H. (2001). The clinical nurse specialist and product evaluation. *Oregon Nurse, 66*(4), 10.

Caley, L. M., & Scharf, L. (1992). Protecting patient safety in new product evaluation. *Nursing Management, 23*(11), 49–50, 52–53.

Casper, G. R., Kenron, D. A., & McDaniel, A. M. (2005). Information technology and the clinical nurse specialist: A framework for technology assessment. *Clinical Nurse Specialist: The Journal for Advanced Nursing Practice, 19*(4), 170–174.

Conn, V. S. (2007). Intervention? What intervention? *Western Journal of Nursing Research, 29*(5), 521–522.

Conn, V. S., Rantz, M. J., Wipke-Tevis, D. D., & Maas, M. L. (2001). Focus on research methods: Designing effective nursing interventions. *Research in Nursing and Health, 24*, 433–442.

Daponte, B. O. (2008). *Evaluation essentials: Methods for conducting sound research.* San Francisco: Jossey-Bass.

Dickerson, S. S., Wu, Y. B., & Kennedy, M. C. (2006). A CNS-facilitated ICD support group. *Clinical Nurse Specialist: The Journal of Advanced Nursing Practice, 20*(3), 146–153.

Faust, C. (2002). Orlando's deliberative nursing process theory: A practice application in an extended care facility. *Journal of Gerontological Nursing, 28*(7), 14–18.

Fawcett, J. (1995). *Analysis and evaluation of conceptual models of nursing* (3rd ed.). Philadelphia: F. A. Davis.

Fitzpatrick, J. L., Sanders, J. R., & Worthen, B. R. (2003). *Program evaluation: Alternative approaches and practical guidelines.* New York: Addison Wesley Longman.

Fulton, J. S. (2003). Nursing interventions vs. interventions delivered by a nurse: Similar words, different meanings. *Clinical Nurse Specialist: Journal for Advanced Nursing Practice, 17*(5), 227–228.

Institute of Medicine. (2001). *Crossing the quality chasm: A new health system for the 21st century.* Washington, DC: Author.

Kellogg, W. K. (1998). *W. K. Kellogg Foundation evaluation handbook.* Battle Creek, MI: Author.

Kellogg, W. K. (2008). *W. K. Kellogg Foundation evaluation handbook & logic model development guide.* Battle Creek, MI: Author.

Meleis, A. I. (1991). *Theoretical nursing: Development and progress* (2nd ed.). New York: J. B. Lippincott.

Miller, M. D., Linn, R. L., & Gronlund, N. E. (2008). *Measurement and assessment in teaching* (10th ed.). New York: MacMillan Publishing Co.

Monahan, R. S., & Donius, M. (1991). Product evaluation: Research for practice. *Geriatric Nursing, 12*(6), 305–308.

National Association of Clinical Nurse Specialists. (2004). *Statement on clinical nurse specialist practice and education* (2nd ed.). Harrisburg, PA: Author.

Nielsen-Bohlman, L., Panzer, A. M., & Kindig D. A. (Eds.). (2004). *Health literacy: A prescription to end confusion.* Washington, DC: National Academies Press.

Orlando, I. J. (1961). *The Dynamic nursing-patient relationship: Function, process and principles of professional nursing practice.* New York: G. P. Putnam's Sons.

Resnick, B., Inguito, P., Orwig, D., Yahiro, J. Y., Hawkes, W., Werner, M., et al. (2005). Treatment fidelity in behavior change research. *Nursing Research, 54*(2), 139–143.

Rossi, P. H., & Freeman, H. E. (1993). *Evaluation: A systematic approach* (5th ed.). Newberry Park, CA: Sage.

Sanders, J. R. (2003). *The program evaluation standards* (2nd ed.). Thousand Oaks, CA: Sage.

Scriven, M. (1991). Beyond formative and summative evaluation. In M. W. McLaughlin & D. C. Phillips (Eds.), *Evaluation and education: At quarter century* (pp. 19–64). Chicago: National Society for the Study of Education.

Sechrest, L., West, S., Phillips, M., Redner, R., & Yeaton, W. (1979). Some neglected problems in evaluation research: Strength and integrity of treatments. In L. Sechrest, S. West, M. Phillips, R. Redner, & W. Yeaton (Eds.), *Evaluation studies review annual* (vol. 4, pp. 15–35). Newberry Park, CA: Sage.

Sidani, S., & Braden, C. J. (1998). Outcomes related factors. In S. Sidani & C. J. Braden (Eds.) *Evaluating nursing interventions: A theory driven approach* (pp. 138–160). Thousand Oaks, CA: Sage.

Simpkins, S. M., Halduven, D. J., & Stevens, D. A. (1995). Safety product evaluation: Six years of experience. *American Journal of Infection Control, 23,* 317–322.

Stufflebeam, D. I., & Shinkfield, A. J. (2007). *Evaluation theory, models and applications.* San Francisco: Jossey Bass.

Thomas, E. J. (1984). *Interventions for the helping professions.* Beverly Hills: Sage.

Wood, M. J. (1998). Evaluative designs. In P. J. Brink & M. J. Wood (Eds.), *Advanced design in nursing research* (2nd ed., pp. 124–141). Thousand Oaks, CA: Sage.

Promoting Innovation, Change, and Diffusion in Practice

Using Complex Adaptive Systems Theory to Guide Change

Kathleen Chapman

Clouds are not spheres, mountains are not cones, coastlines are not circles, and bark is not smooth, nor does lightening travel in a straight line.

—*Benoit Mandelbrot (n.d.)*

USING COMPLEX ADAPTIVE SYSTEMS THEORY TO GUIDE CHANGE

This chapter focuses on the transformational role of the clinical nurse specialist (CNS) at the systems and organizational level. Transforming practice requires adeptness in change management. The tools of change include the competencies of persuasion, influence, and negotiation. The focus of many articles and books about change is on the tools, rather than on the foundational step of thoroughly evaluating as many of the aspects of the involved system as possible. An appreciation of the myriad parts affected by the systems and their real or potential impact on the change is an essential first and ongoing step. This discernment will make the formulation of strategies that enhance the positives and mitigate the negatives possible so the desired change can be accomplished.

The goal of this chapter is to stimulate introspection and awareness of the questions that need to be answered while the CNS engages in the various phases of change management. To apply the tools of change effectively, the dynamics of the system to which the tools are applied must be fully evaluated and well understood.

Using complex adaptive theory as a framework for posing questions, the CNS will be positioned to groom the environment for successful and enduring change.

CHANGE AGENT

The advanced practitioner educates, challenges policy with new evidence, takes on clinical issues that are in search of a solution, and innovates, that is, effects change. Opportunities for change occur on many levels within the health care environment (Porter-O'Grady & Malloch, 2003). Change might be reactionary, that is, a necessary response to maintain equilibrium when other things change (e.g., economic downturns and upturns, system mergers, war, evolving patient demographics, presence of new disease entities, and staff shortages), or it may be an intentional disruption of equilibrium so that continuous improvement can occur (e.g., new technology, emerging evidence, new health care roles, and new scopes of practice).

Change has been defined as the product of the interactions or interconnections between different systems or different people from which new behaviors emerge (Penprase & Norris, 2005). The definition is expressive of the daunting task involved in successfully managing the process of change. Interactions and interconnections imply many potential paths to simultaneously consider, control, empower, enhance, and mitigate.

CNSs achieve systemic change in many ways. They lead multidisciplinary teams through the selection and implementation of new technology; develop new approaches to the care of patient populations with new clinical guidelines and new staff roles; chair magnet steering committees; organize colleagues to form new professional organizations; change medical center policies, procedures, and by-laws; and form local and university partnerships with physicians and nurses to enhance the education of students and residents.

Practice is transformed through specialist involvement in the clinical, professional, political, and educational arenas. The human and health care systems the CNS interacts with are complex, the variables are many, and the subsequent potential outcomes are diverse. To be successful, many elements need to converge harmoniously so that change is adopted and sustained. Complex adaptive systems theory provides a framework within which change can be anticipated, understood, embraced, and designed (Zimmerman, Lindberg, & Plsek, 2001).

COMPLEX ADAPTIVE SYSTEMS

Three principles central to complex adaptive systems (CAS) are *relationships, self-organization*, and *nonlinear predictability*. Several definitions of CAS appear in the literature. A definition provided by Plsek and Greenhalgh (2001) is that a CAS is a collection of individual agents "whose actions are interconnected" (web of relationships) "so that one agent's actions changes the context for other agents" (self-organization) "with freedom to act in ways that are not always totally predictable" (*nonlinear*).

Relationships

CAS theory emerged from the physical sciences of mathematics and physics in three phases. The first phase occurred in the early decades of the 20th century with the description of the principle of relationships. It is the concept that the whole is more than merely the sum of its parts. A CAS is made up of a web of relationships. Everything impacts everything else.

While exploring the subatomic world, physicists discovered that matter could not be adequately described just by naming its parts, that is, protons, neutrons, and electrons. They found that the same combination of subatomic particles did not guarantee the same physical outcome. Instead, identical ratios of the same protons, neutrons, and electrons existed in varying forms.

Capra (1982) observed that whether an electron was a wave or a particle depended on the electron's relationship with other subatomic particles. He said that as we penetrate into matter, nature does not show us any isolated basic building blocks, but rather appears as a complicated web of relations between the various parts of a unified whole.

Self-Organization (Emergence)

The second phase emerged from the science of thermodynamics. Scientists discovered that heating a thin layer of liquid resulted in the organization of new structures. They found that if enough energy flowed from the outside, a new pattern of complex structures spontaneously organized.

Experimentation demonstrated that as heat reached a certain critical value, convection replaced conduction and a pattern of hexagonal, honeycomb-shaped cells appeared. Heating the liquid moved it from equilibrium. There no longer was a uniform temperature throughout. The unstable form reorganized into an ordered hexagonal pattern. This principle was defined as self-organization (Capra, 1996). In more contemporary literature, the principle is also referred to as emergence (Penprase & Norris, 2005).

In self-organization, order is created without direction from the top; there is no focal point, no "centralized" clearinghouse for ideas. The ability of a system to self-organize is a function of the number of agents included within it and the intensity of its connections.

Nonlinear Predictability (Coevolution)

The third phase involved the concept of nonlinear relationships and actions, also referred to as chaos. CAS have multiple positive and negative feedback loops, the influence of external constraints, and exquisite sensitivity to initial conditions. Because of this nonlinearity and sensitivity to initial conditions, the details of the new behavior are inherently unpredictable (Penprase & Norris, 2005).

To illustrate, Holden (2005) describes meteorology experiments in which only a few decimals in a weather modeling computer program were changed. Even though the changes were minimal, the resulting weather prediction was very different. Small changes in the initial characteristics of an active system were found to dramatically affect the long-term behavior of that system.

CAS coevolve. Coevolution means that small changes can have a large impact. When one thing changes, it all changes. The system boundaries are open or fuzzy, not fixed. Depending on what the system is, they are open to the flow in or out of matter, energy, and information. Members in a system are not static. Each can be members of different systems at the same time (Minas, 2005).

Living Systems vs. Machines

Prior to these scientific discoveries, the world was described in a mechanical, predictable, cause-and-effect manner. Machines move in a consistent way, are made up of consistent parts, and remain static in size and function. Living systems behave differently than

EXHIBIT 8.1   KEY FEATURES OF COMPLEX ADAPTIVE SYSTEMS

Key Features

1. Complex adaptive systems will be self-organizing, and new elements will emerge at various points. These changes may be incremental or dramatic as they adapt to reactions between subsystems and with other systems.
2. Uncertainty is inevitable in an evolving system, rendering top-down control impossible. The views and experiences of those at a variety of points in an organization are necessary to gain an understanding of it.
3. Spontaneous change occurs more readily where there are a range of different behavior patterns (microdiversity).
4. Agents within an organization act according to their own internal rules or mental models. Attractor patterns within the system will "frame" and limit change.
5. Simple rules or guiding principles can lead to innovative emergent changes.
6. Change can be stimulated by the encouragement of new generative relationships. These can produce new insights and solutions into complex problems.
7. There will be simultaneous stability and instability at the edge of chaos, this being a requirement for the emergence of novelty.

Adapted from Zimmerman et al., Olsen and Eoyang, and Stacey, as appears in "Use of Complex Adaptive Systems Metaphor to Achieve Professional and Organizational Change," by A. Rowe and A. Hogarth, 2005, *Journal of Advanced Nursing, 51*(4), 396–405.

machines. Living systems flow and move and adapt and become and burst and morph. They are complex and adaptive.

There are many examples from nature, for example, flocking birds, ant colonies, and schools of fish. Cilliers (1998) described fish behavior to illustrate the concept of nonlinear relationships. He said that the condition of the fish being observed would depend on a large number of factors, including the availability of food, the temperature of the water, the amount of oxygen and light, the time of the year, and so forth. As these conditions varied, the size of the school of fish adjusted itself optimally to suit prevailing conditions, despite the fact that each individual fish could only look after its own interests. The system of the school of fish as a whole organized itself to ensure the best match between the system and the environment.

This organization of fish was also adaptive in the same sense that the school would be sensitive to changing conditions in the light of past experience. There was no agent that decided for the school what should happen, nor did each individual fish understand the complexity of the situation. The organization of the school emerged as a result of the interaction between the various constituents of the system and its environment.

Within a framework of CAS, health care organizations and systems of care are characterized as living entities. Health care systems are adaptive. Unlike mechanical systems, they are composed of individuals who have the capacity to learn and change as a result of experience. The components (individuals) react to internal and external stimuli, and adapt in response (Plesk, 2001; Rowe & Hogarth, 2005).

Health care systems, like all living systems cannot be broken into simple parts. The complex cannot be made simple, cannot be understood in simple terms, and cannot be solved in simple ways (Lindstrom, 2003). Complex systems are nonlinear and not completely predictable. It is not known whether the complex system will unfold in a trajectory, a bifurcation, self-organize, emerge, or coevolve. The causal incident is a change in the value of one or more parameters. Even at the point of bifurcation, as an example, there is unpredictability as to which branch the system will follow.

Systems with even a minute amount of uncertainty in their current condition are likely to behave unpredictably in their next condition due to different reactions to negative and positive feedback. In addition, the behavior of a CAS is time dependent. The direction the system may take at any point is a function of how it behaved in the past, but it is not possible to predict the trajectory based on its past behavior alone.

USING CAS THEORY TO INFORM CNS PRACTICE IN MANAGING CHANGE

Observations from nature can be applied to human behavior and organizational systems. Advanced practice nurses learn to view the health care environment through a number of lenses, including the system and policy-setting level that drives the quality of patient care. To ensure success, the change agent must consciously step back and up, always viewing the issue from the balcony and through the added lens of complexity science.

Minimum Specifications (Self-Organization)

It may seem counterintuitive, but complexity science research demonstrates that relatively simple rules lead to complex, innovative system behavior. Plesk cites studies of the flocking of birds and the schooling of fish to avoid predators: "These studies and computer models have confirmed that a few simple rules can guide complex behavior toward a goal. Such systems move toward their goals by having (1) a common purpose (avoiding predators), (2) internal motivation (surviving another day) and (3) some simple rules that guide behavior (keeping up with the group, moving toward the center of mass of the group, and avoiding collisions)" (2001, p. 63).

The tendency is to do the opposite, that is, to specify in great detail what is to be done at all levels of the system so the desired goal (the change) is accomplished. This overspecification can result in inefficiency, that is, steps that are not necessary, unnecessary additional hand-offs, lower quality, lower satisfaction, and higher costs.

Minimum specifications, on the other hand, leave room for self-organization and emergence, creativity and innovation. Rather than lengthy, defined process and implementation steps, the system undergoing change is given a few simple and flexible rules and a statement of desired outcome.

Minimum specifications invite discussion about how the change is to be achieved and, in so doing, increase connectedness and a shared vision among the component parts. If minimum specifications focus on broad outcomes, they will encourage generative relationships and the emergence of solutions that are relevant to local conditions (Minas, 2005).

Attractors vs. Resistance

Resistance is often cited as the reason change comes slowly, or not at all. Minas (2005) asserts that if resistance is seen as the reason, then the concluded solution is to battle against, and to overcome, resistance wherever it is found. CAS theory, however, informs us that behavior follows the attractors in a system. Managing change within the context of CAS involves a paradigm shift. In CAS, change is viewed as a "drawing toward" rather than as a "pushing against."

To be successful, the CNS must understand how a change in system parameters can shift the system from one attractor pattern to another that is more desirable. In other words, what are the nonpunitive incentives for changing behavior? The change agent needs to deliberately set the stage by making compelling, evidence-based arguments for the desired outcome in a way that will be viewed as deserving of the time and effort of those impacted.

Considerations could include incentives that are patient-related, profession-related, process-related, or financial, as well as incentives that are individually based or team based. Something is an attractor if involved members of the change are able to meaningfully fill in the blank, "If A becomes B, the benefit will be_____."

Surprise!

The edge that lies between order and chaos is where creativity and flexibility thrive. At the edge of chaos, the environment is unpredictable, exciting, and bursting with new ideas and innovation (Penprase & Norris, 2005). It is at this edge of surprise where change occurs.

In the daily work of health care, moments of surprise occur regularly. We are surprised by our patients, by our colleagues, by our systems, and by our own reactions. Attempts to eliminate surprise are futile. The complexity lens suggests that surprise is not necessarily the result of any one factor, but it is the result of the fundamental nature of the system being observed (McDaniel, Jordan, & Fleeman, 2003). We are not machines that operate in linear and predictable ways.

We simply need to come to terms with the notion that uncertainty and unpredictability cannot be mapped out in advance. In human ecosystems, the only predictable element is lack of predictability. Therefore, surprise is inevitable because it is part of the natural order and cannot be avoided, eliminated, or controlled.

CAS allows us to capitalize on the surprises that confront our work lives using the strategies of creativity and learning. The change agent's role is to identify patterns and trends, assist staff to accept and adjust to changes, support coordination of the various elements of change, and help staff maintain focus and identity as they experience a turbulent health care environment (Begun & Kaissi, 2004). Change agents need to anticipate, develop a capacity for, and invite surprise on a daily basis. In the words of McDaniel, "It is not a question of, 'How can I keep this from happening,' but rather, 'How can I make creative use of what is happening?' " (McDaniel et al., 2003, p. 272). n fact, the system and its components need to be moved regularly to the edge of chaos so that creativity and flexibility can thrive (Kaiser Permanente, 2009). At the edge of chaos, self-organization can only result from interactions between people. As a change agent, the CNS encourages new ideas and supports risk-taking by presenting evidence, challenging rituals, and asking questions. The CNS is instrumental in contributing to an environment

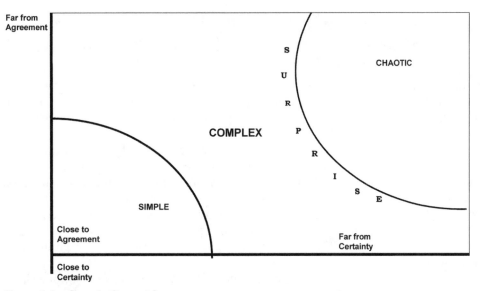

Figure 8.1 Complexity matrix.

Modified from Stacey, Hassey, and Brown as cited in "The Application of Complex Adaptive Systems Theory to Clinical Practice in Rehabilitation," by C. Brown, 2006, *Disability and Rehabilitation, 28*(9), 587–593.

in which relationships reflect trust, comfort, acceptance, inquiry, celebration, and flexibility.

Because the edge of chaos is unstable, the environment is ripe for an infinite number of new behaviors and new ideas to spontaneously emerge. The Institute of Medicine (IOM) report states: "In complex adaptive systems . . . the parts . . . have the freedom and ability to respond to stimuli in many different and fundamentally unpredictable ways . . . Such behavior can be for better or for worse, that is, it can manifest itself as either innovation or error" (Plesk, 2001, p. 322). The challenge for the CNS, of course, is to intervene with innovation.

THE VIEW FROM HERE: PREPARING FOR CHANGE

While embarking on a change process, the CNS needs to thoughtfully consider a series of questions so that the entire CAS is appreciated. The competencies defined in the *Statement on Clinical Nurse Specialist Practice and Education* provide a conceptual framework for evaluating the complexity of the environment (National Association of Clinical Nurse Specialists, 2004). Formulating answers to the questions suggested by the competencies can be used as a strategy to inform a template for action.

Assessment: Identifying and Defining Problems and Opportunities

Each and every step within the change process is equally important. The questions for assessment

presented here are neither intended to be complete, nor used once. Instead, the questions should evolve and should be asked again and again as circumstances self-organize, new relationships emerge, or surprise is encountered. Each step in the CAS change process is not a one-time event.

What organizational structures and functions exert impact?

Are levels of approval required? Does the desired change impact other functions and organizational entities? What organizational data are accessible? What are the tools available to collect additional relevant organizational data?

What are the professional climate and the level of multidisciplinary collaboration?

Is the group of stakeholders a unified team? A high-level functioning group will facilitate the change process. Is the group dysfunctional? Lack of multidisciplinary functioning will require additional preparation of the environment involving attention to communication and teambuilding.

What are the system-level variables?

What is the state of the organization's financial health? Does the desired change cost anything? What are the indirect costs? What is the opportunity cost? In what ways can the desired change be matched to the

EXHIBIT 8.2 CNS COMPETENCIES: ORGANIZATION/SYSTEM SPHERE OF INFLUENCE

Assessment: Identifying and Defining Problems and Opportunities
1. Uses/designs system-level assessment methods and instruments to identify organization structures and functions that impact nursing practice and nurse-sensitive patient care outcomes.
2. Assesses the professional climate and the multidisciplinary collaboration within and across units for their impact on nursing practice and outcomes.
3. Assesses targeted system-level variables, such as culture, finances, regulatory requirements, and external demands, that influence nursing practice and outcomes.
4. Identifies relationships within and external to the organization/system that are facilitators or barriers to nursing practice and any proposed change.
5. Identifies effects of organizational culture on departments, teams, and/or groups within an organization.
6. Monitors legislative and regulatory health policy that may impact nursing practice and/or CNS practice for the specialty area/population.

From *Statement on Clinical Nurse Specialist Practice and Education* (2nd ed.), by National Association of Clinical Nurse Specialists, 2004, Harrisburg, PA: Author.

organization's strategic plan? What are the other things that the system is dealing with that will add energy or drain energy?

What are the relationships within and external to the organization/system that are facilitators or barriers?

What is the organization's past history relative to staff cooperation and follow-through? Who are the external stakeholders—external to the CNS group, external to nursing, external to the organization? Is each a facilitator or a barrier? In what way?

What are the effects of organizational culture on departments, teams, and groups?

Does the CNS have position power, expert power, or other informal power? Does the culture expect formal designation and endorsement of a leader? Does the organization celebrate risk-taking and change? Is the culture bureaucratic? Is there a charge letter for the initiative that is widely distributed?

What legislative and regulatory health policies provide impact?

Is there scope of practice considerations, Joint Commission considerations, or payor considerations?

What are the implications for existing medical center policies and procedures?

Diagnosis, Outcome Identification, and Planning

After each assessment, the CNS is ready to interpret findings and identify options. Priorities, feasibility, and minimum specifications are considered.

What are the facilitators and barriers?

Who are the supporters of the change and who are the process owners? Are they on board? Could the initiative be considered controversial, provocative, or otherwise anxiety producing? What are the non-human facilitators and barriers, for example, time, space, location?

What are the variations in organizational culture that exert influence?

What are the values, attitudes, and beliefs of the affected group about the proposed initiative? What are the values, attitudes, and beliefs of the affected group about change, in general? Are the values, attitudes, and beliefs among the affected group of patients and/or staff homogeneous or heterogeneous? What is the impact of age and experience? What are the positive influences and the negative influences of each? How can the positives be enhanced and negatives minimized?

EXHIBIT 8.3   CNS COMPETENCIES: ORGANIZATION/SYSTEM SPHERE OF INFLUENCE

Diagnosis, Outcome Identification, and Planning
1. Diagnoses facilitators and barriers to achieving desired outcomes of integrated programs of care across the continuum and at points of service.
2. Diagnoses variations in organizational culture (i.e., values, beliefs, or attitudes) that can positively exert influence.
3. Draws conclusions about the effects of variance across the organization that influences outcomes of nursing practice.
4. Plans for achieving intended system-wide outcomes, while avoiding or minimizing unintended consequences.
5. Draws conclusions about the impact of legislative and regulatory policies as they apply to nursing practice and outcomes for specialty populations.

From *Statement on Clinical Nurse Specialist Practice and Education* (2nd ed.), by National Association of Clinical Nurse Specialists, 2004, Harrisburg, PA: Author.

What variations across the organization exert influence?

What is the organizational structure? Is it centralized, decentralized, matrix, product line? Are staff empowered to participate? Is the manager hands-on or hands-off? What are the implications for communication, socialization, and permission? How does that vary for each of the potentially affected groups? Is the platform burning equally for each of the impacted groups, that is, does everyone believe change is needed? If not, what are the strategies that can be used to turn up the heat?

What will achieve intended system-wide outcomes while avoiding or minimizing unintended consequences?

What groundwork is needed? Are the outcomes specifically defined and measurable? If the initiative fails, what is the worst-case scenario for patients, staff, and the organization? How does the initiative potentially impact the conditions of work? What are the obligations to the union, and how will they be met?

What is the impact to legislative and regulatory policy?

Are legislative stakeholders involved? What are the funding implications? Are there any role boundary or scope of practice issues? Are there state certificate of need regulations that need to be considered? Will the initiative impact the organization's scope or level of services? If so, what are the potential reporting obligations to external regulatory entities, and what are the new systems that need to be put in place to meet new regulations? Does this result in additional cost to the organization?

Intervention: Developing and Testing Solutions

An over-arching consideration in this section is whether the testing of the potential solution will be a process improvement or research. Discussion of the differences is not within the scope of this chapter. Because the distinction can be gray, it is recommended that the local nursing research resource be consulted. Depending on the intervention method and how the outcomes intend to be reported to the professional community, the initiative will require addressing the related ethical considerations and may require institutional review board approval.

What innovative solutions can be generalized across differing units, populations, or specialties?

Does the innovation have potential for application to other situations? Is the initiative under consideration generic enough to work across the continuum of care? What variations may be necessary? How can others from different units, populations, or specialties be invited to shape the intervention?

How will resulting innovations be deployed across the full continuum of care for different population groups and/or specialties?

Is it realistic for implementation in other areas? Will customization be needed? How will the innovation

Intervention: Developing and Testing Solutions

1. Develops innovative solutions that can be generalized across differing units, populations, or specialties.
2. Leads nursing and multidisciplinary groups in implementing innovative patient care programs that address issues across the full continuum of care for different population groups and/or specialties.
3. Contributes to the development of multidisciplinary standards of practice and evidence-based guidelines for care, such as pathways, care maps, benchmarks.
4. Solidifies relationships and multidisciplinary linkages that foster the adoption of innovations.
5. Develops or influences system-level policies that will affect innovation and programs of care.
6. Targets and reduces system-level barriers to proposed changes in nursing practices and programs of care.
7. Facilitates factors to effect program-level change.
8. Designs methods/strategies to sustain and spread change and innovation.
9. Implements methods and processes to sustain evidence-based changes in nursing practice, programs of care, and clinical innovation.
10. Provides leadership for legislative and regulatory initiatives to advance the health of the public with a focus on the specialty practice area/population.
11. Mobilizes professional and public resources to support legislative and regulatory issues that advance the health of the public.

From *Statement on Clinical Nurse Specialist Practice and Education* (2nd ed.), by National Association of Clinical Nurse Specialists, 2004, Harrisburg, PA: Author.

be communicated to other audiences? What are the deployment issues and options?

What are the implications for the development of multidisciplinary standards of practice and evidence-based guidelines for care, such as pathways, care maps, and benchmarks?

What additional development is needed? Does the innovation need to be tested with other patient or staff populations? What are the tools that can be developed to assure consistent implementation and permanence?

How can system-level barriers to change be targeted and reduced?

What are the identified barriers? What are the attractors? How can the attractors be enhanced and communicated? How can trust and openness be enhanced? How can necessary relationships be garnered? How can the environment be encouraged to ask questions and express concerns? What is the best way to communicate answers so everyone feels informed?

What are the paths for developing system-level policies that affect innovation and programs of care?

How should the required policies be developed, tested, and/or revised? Who should be involved? What does the evidence suggest? What amount of consensus is reasonable? Which are the minimum specifications?

How can the factors to effect program-level change be facilitated?

How will the system/organizational factors impact the change at the program level? What are the attractors at the program level? Are they consistent with the attractors at the organizational level?

What are the strategies needed to sustain and spread change and innovation?

How can change be stabilized? What will move the edge from the upper right quadrant toward the lower left quadrant? What are the structures that can be put in place to ensure continuing relationships, and how can the attractors be made more permanent?

What are the methods and processes that will ensure that evidence-based changes will be sustained?

What are the success factors? What is the plan to update the evidence over time? How will incremental success be celebrated? What are the ongoing person, money, and space resource implications? How will access to needed resources be guaranteed?

How can the CNS provide leadership for legislative and regulatory initiatives to advance the health of the public with a focus on the specialty practice area/population?

How should the innovation inform legislation, regulations, or professional standards? What is the role of the change in ensuring public safety? What are the policy issues? What are the current legislative opportunities? What is the relevant professional group that can be contacted with information about the innovation? Are professional committee membership opportunities available?

How can professional and public resources be mobilized to support legislative and regulatory issues that advance the health of the public?

What are the grants and other funding streams available to support initial, current, and developing innovation? How can colleagues be informed of relevant pending legislation and opportunities for educating policy makers? What volunteer opportunities are available to position the CNS for future influence?

Evaluation of the Effects

Evaluation tools and methods need to be considered at the beginning of the change process, much like discharge planning needs to begin at patient admission.

What are the evaluation methods or instruments that can be used to identify system-level outcomes of programs of care?

Will the evaluation be formal or informal? Are standardized tools available? Will permissions be required? Who will be responsible for the collection of data? How often? Where will the results be reported?

How will system-level clinical and fiscal outcomes of products, devices, and patient care processes using performance methods be evaluated?

Who will the audience be? How will effectiveness be defined? Is the definition the same for the patient, the nurse, the physician, the administrator, and the chief financial officer? How will modeling be used? How can a

---

EXHIBIT 8.5   CNS COMPETENCIES: ORGANIZATION/SYSTEM SPHERE OF INFLUENCE

Evaluation of the Effects
1. Selects evaluation methods and instruments to identify system-level outcomes of programs of care.
2. Evaluates system-level clinical and fiscal outcomes of products, devices, and patient care processes using performance methods.
3. Uses organizational structure and processes to provide feedback about the effectiveness of nursing practices and multidisciplinary relationships in meeting identified outcomes of programs of care.
4. Evaluates organizational policies for their ability to support and sustain outcomes of programs of care.
5. Evaluates and documents the impact of CNS practice on the organization.
6. Documents all outcomes in a reportable manner.
7. Disseminates outcomes of system-wide changes, impact of nursing practices, and CNS work to stakeholders.

From *Statement on Clinical Nurse Specialist Practice and Education* (2nd ed.), by National Association of Clinical Nurse Specialists, 2004, Harrisburg, PA: Author.

dashboard or balanced scorecard be developed to demonstrate effectiveness?

How can the organizational structure and existing organizational processes be used to provide feedback about the effectiveness of nursing practices and multidisciplinary relationships in meeting identified outcomes of programs of care?

What are the typical reporting formats and frequencies at the organization level? How can the innovation and its impact be made visible to the organization? Can updates be added to the agendas of key medical and administrative committees? How can opportunities be created to publicize the outcomes in internal and external medical center communication?

What organizational policies need to be evaluated for their ability to support and sustain outcomes of programs of care?

Are there policies that are in conflict with the innovation? Does the new evidence provide a path for revision? Who are the stakeholders of the existing policy? What additional policies are needed to provide the structure to support the desired outcome? Are there union bargaining obligations involved?

How will the impact of CNS practice on the organization be evaluated and documented?

What are the organization's stated and unstated expectations regarding the change? What are the ways the expectations can be shaped, for example, targets established, timeline identified, and work products defined. Who will evaluate the change? What did the CNS personally bring to the value equation? Where will the CNS's leadership role in the change be acknowledged and documented?

How will outcomes be documented, ensuring a reportable format?

Some of the report customization issues for the various reports include: who will read it, report details such as length, language, technical level and verbal or written format. Additional considerations include "what are the quantifiable and objective outcomes?" and "what additional calibration is needed to refine the measurement as the change process stabilizes?"

How will outcomes of system-wide changes, impact of nursing practices, and CNS work be disseminated to stakeholders?

Who are the various stakeholders? How do the attractors vary among stakeholders? What information is most compelling for each group? What were the nonlinear impacts? What was the value of the change on the system? What was the impact of the change on the nursing process?

THE BUSINESS CASE

The CNS may need the organizational hierarchy to formally embrace and endorse a change. Organizational level initiatives that require resources in the six figures, or detailed computer programming, or the establishment of a new service or program, for example, will need to compete for limited institutional resources. To compete successfully, a written proposal that demonstrates a thorough analysis of the issue, thoughtful consideration of options, data-driven recommendations, and financial projections will be required.

Each organization will likely have its own customized template for presenting the business case. CAS theory provides a firm foundation for developing comprehensive and compelling arguments. A disciplined consideration of the questions suggested in the previous section will enable the CNS to convey a comprehensive and credible proposal. The questions asked can be customized to the scope and complexity of the desired change.

An example of a business template that lends itself well to incorporating the CAS perspective is displayed in Exhibit 8.6. The Executive Decision Memorandum is an example of a formal format that has been used by the Department of Veterans Affairs to describe recommended changes and request approval for implementation.

Each of the content areas are completed, considering impact of the change on a number of complex system elements: stakeholders, dissenting opinions, impact on existing programs and facilities, legal or legislative impact, budget or financial impact, public relations or media considerations, and congressional or public officers or public agency considerations. In the example, option 1 is typically status quo. Pros and cons of each are outlined, and the recommended option is indicated.

ADVANCED NURSING PRACTICE

The advanced practice nurse is well-positioned by education and by role to exert a positive influence on the organization and on the system. Application of CAS theory to change moves the nurse beyond the realm of expert clinical practitioner to new arenas of major organizational impact. Specific outcomes of CNS practice at the organization and system level are displayed in Exhibit 8.7.

Complexity theory appears largely in the computer science, physics, biology, medicine, and management

EXHIBIT 8.6 EXECUTIVE DECISION MEMORANDUM

Executive Decision Memorandum
  I. Summary of facts/background
  II. Synopsis of significance of related issues
  III. Criteria for decision making
  IV. Stakeholder involvement
  V. Options and arguments
    A. Option 1
      1. Argument pro
      2. Argument con
    B. Option 2
      1. Argument pro
      2. Argument con
    C. Option 3
      1. Argument pro
      2. Argument con
  VI. Recommended option
  VII. Dissenting opinions regarding recommended option
  VIII. Effect of recommended option on existing programs and/or facilities
  IX. Legal or legislative considerations of the recommended option
  X. Budget or financial considerations of the recommended option
  XI. Public relations or media considerations of the recommended option
  XII. Congressional or other public official or agency consideration of the recommended option
  XIII. Implementation considerations

Department of Veterans Affairs. (n.d.). *EDM format*. Retrieved January 9, 2009, from http://www1.va.gov/nursing/docs/TNC_EDM_2007Feb15.doc

literature (Brown, 2006; Goldberger, 1996; Kernick, 2002). The lack of literature describing how CAS theory is manifest in the clinical nursing arena and in CNS practice, however, provides an abundance of research opportunities. In addition to research, it is important that the CNS contribute to CAS literature by describing successes and failures. Often the most valuable insights are gained from what did not work well and from the lessons learned.

CAS theory informs the CNS that there is no formula that guarantees successful change. Furthermore, the same combination of staff and/or resources that led to successful change in one setting does not guarantee the same results in another setting. In each case, the approach must be customized to account for all of the unique characteristics of the individuals, the situation, and the physical and emotional environment.

CAS theory challenges us to embrace uncertainty and to support self-organization. The goal is to create the environmental conditions within which an innovation can emerge, not to engineer the change. The CNS creates the conditions a number of ways, through reflection, debate, challenge, fostering development of multiple new relationships, education, and validating new skills.

CAS provides insight into how organizations are sustained, how they self-organize, and how outcomes emerge. CAS theory informs us that organizations learn, adapt, and change through behavioral processes. As an agent of change, the CNS understands and unravels relationships, fosters new interconnections, and facilitates new solutions—all at the edge of chaos.

DISCUSSION QUESTIONS

1. The following two quotes were retrieved from a complexity Web site (Plexus Institute, 2007): "Life will never surrender its secrets to a yardstick," attributed to Dee Hock, and "As humans we are complex and chaotic when healthy and rigidly orderly when ill," attributed to Stuart Davidson. What does each statement tell you about CAS theory and/or change? How do the statements relate to CNS practice?

2. Research has demonstrated that 75% of all change initiatives fail (Bunker & Wakefield, 2005). Does this figure surprise you? Why do you think this might be

EXHIBIT 8.7 ORGANIZATION/SYSTEM SPHERE OF INFLUENCE

Outcomes of CNS Practice

1. Clinical problems are articulated within the context of the organization/system structure, mission, culture, policies, and resources.
2. Patient care processes reflect continuous improvements that benefit the system.
3. Change strategies are integrated throughout the system.
4. Policies enhance the practice of nurses individually as members of multidisciplinary teams.
5. Innovative models of practice are developed, piloted, evaluated, and incorporated across the continuum of care.
6. Evidence-based, best practice models are developed and implemented.
7. Nursing care and outcomes are articulated at organizational/system decision-making levels.
8. Stakeholders (nurses, other health care professionals, and management) share a common vision of practice outcomes.
9. Decision makers within the institution are informed about practice problems, factors contributing to the problems, and the significance of those problems with respect to outcomes and costs.
10. Patient care initiatives reflect knowledge of cost management and revenue enhancement strategies.
11. Patient care programs are aligned with the organization's strategic imperatives, mission, vision, philosophy, and values.
12. Staff comply with regulatory requirements and standards.
13. Policy-making bodies are influenced to develop regulations/procedures to improve patient care and health services.

From *Statement on Clinical Nurse Specialist Practice and Education* (2nd ed.), by National Association of Clinical Nurse Specialists, 2004, Harrisburg, PA: Author.

the case? In your opinion, what are the most difficult aspects of leading change?

3. Think of an example of a well-known change that has been sustained over time and another of a well-known change that has not lasted. From a CAS perspective, what could the different outcomes be attributed to? What are the hallmarks of enduring change?

ANALYSIS AND SYNTHESIS EXERCISES

1. Using an example from your personal experience, analyze a change in terms of self-organization, emergence, and coevolution. What was the change? What was your role in the change? How did self-organization, emergence, and coevolution each present? Was the change successful? Why or why not?
2. Analyze a failed change that you experienced from the CAS principle of "web of relationships." What are the different types of relationships that you can identify in your example? How did each contribute to the change? What relationships were ignored but should have been addressed? What could you have anticipated that would have made a difference in the outcome? What relationships should have been created?

3. Visit a complexity, change, or innovation Web site. What elements of surprise did you discover there? How do the concepts relate to CNS practice at the organization level?
4. Interview a CNS about a successful change led at the organization level. Use a subset of questions suggested by CNS system/organization level competencies to form the interview tool. How did each step develop? What insights did the CNS gain? What were the lessons learned? What other questions did you formulate from a CAS and change perspective under the categories of assessment, diagnosis, intervention, and evaluation? What were the attractors? What does the CNS cite as the key success factor? How did the CNS celebrate the success?

REFERENCES

Begun, J., & Kaissi, A. (2004) Uncertainty in health care environments: Myth or reality? *Health Care Management Review, 29*(1), 31–39.

Brown, C. (2006). The application of complex adaptive systems theory to clinical practice in rehabilitation. *Disability and Rehabilitation, 28*(9), 587–593.

Bunker, K., & Wakefield, M. (2005). *Leading with authenticity in times of transition.* Greensboro, NC: CCL Press.

Capra, F. (1982). *The turning point.* Toronto: Bantam Books.

Capra, F. (1996). *The web of life.* New York: Anchor Books.

Cilliers, P. (1998). *Complexity and postmodernism: Understanding complex systems.* London: Routledge.

Department of Veterans Affairs. (n.d.). *EDM format*. Retrieved January 9, 2009, from www1.va.gov/nursing/docs/TNC_EDM_2007Feb15.doc

Goldberger, A. (1996). Non-linear dynamics for clinicians: Chaos theory, fractals, and complexity at the bedside. *The Lancet, 347*(9011), 1312–1314.

Holden, L. (2005). Complex adaptive systems concept analysis. *Journal of Advanced Nursing, 52*(6), 651–657.

Institute for Healthcare Improvement. (n.d.). *Transforming care at the bedside*. Retrieved January 9, 2009, from http://www.ihi.org/IHI/Programs/StrategicInitiatives/TransformingCareAtTheBedside.htm

Kaiser Permanente. (n.d.). *The Sidney R. Garfield Health Care Innovation Center*. Retrieved January 9, 2009, from http://xnet.kp.org/innovationcenter

Kernick, D. (2002). Complexity and healthcare organizations. In K. Sweeney & F. Griffiths (Eds.), *Complexity and healthcare, an introduction* (pp. 93–121). Abingdon, UK: Radcliffe Medical Press.

Lindstrom, R. (2003). Evidence-based decision-making in healthcare: Exploring the issues through the lens of complex adaptive systems theory. *Healthcare Papers, 3*(3), 29–35.

Mandelbrot, B. (n.d.). Retrieved January 9, 2009, from http://www history.mcs.st-andrews.ac.uk/Quotations/Mandelbrot.html

McDaniel, R., Jordan, M., & Fleeman, B. (2003). Surprise, surprise, surprise! A complexity science view of the unexpected. *Healthcare Management Review, 28*(3), 266–278.

Minas, H. (2005). Leadership for change in complex systems. *Australasian Psychiatry, 13*(1), 33–39.

National Association of Clinical Nurse Specialists. (2004). *Statement on clinical nurse specialist practice and education* (2nd ed.). Harrisburg, PA: Author.

Penprase, B., & Norris, D. (2005). What nurse leaders should know about complex adaptive systems theory. *Nursing Leadership Forum, 9*(3), 127–132.

Plexus Institute. (2007). Retrieved January 9, 2009, from http://www.plexusinstitute.org

Plesk, P. (2001). Redesigning health care with insights from the science of complex adaptive systems. In Committee on Quality of Health Care in America & Institute of Medicine, (Eds.), *Crossing the quality chasm: A new health system for the 21st century* (pp. 61–88). Washington, DC: National Academies Press.

Plsek, P., & Greenhalgh, T. (2001). The challenge of complexity in health care. *British Medical Journal, 323*, 625–628.

Porter-O'Grady, T., & Malloch, K. (2003). *Quantum leadership: A textbook of new leadership*. Boston: Jones and Bartlett.

Rowe, A., & Hogarth, A. (2005). Use of complex adaptive systems metaphor to achieve professional and organizational change. *Journal of Advanced Nursing, 51*(4), 396–405.

Zimmerman, B., Lindberg, C., & Plsek, P. (2001). *Edgeware: Insights from complexity science for health care leaders* (2nd ed.). Irving, TX: VHA, Inc.

Engaging Staff in Learning

Christine M. Pacini

Change in health care as a microcosm of the broader universe is occurring at a rate that makes it almost impossible to keep up. Mechanisms for delivering service, generating relevant products and processes, and reconfiguring systems are becoming increasingly complex. Some of the most formidable characteristics of these systems are that they are inherently uncontrollable and unpredictable, thereby requiring new models and approaches for responsive intervention. For example, concepts such as shared leadership, healing sanctuaries, servant leadership, communities of caring, and self-managed work teams are evolving in support of values related to patient-family centrality, customer-focused behavior, process improvement, safety, and high-quality clinical and behavioral outcomes.

One of the key problems is that past approaches to leading, managing, and learning are far less relevant in environments characterized by values associated with newer knowledge about how change occurs and how individuals think and behave (Goleman, 1998; Greenleaf, 1996; Porter-O'Grady & Malloch, 2003). In particular, traditional practices of teaching and learning with regard to aims, content, and methods may now serve as impediments to organizational growth and understanding models of transformation. The content of transformation requires a movement away from industrial, linear thinking toward a focus on integration, outcome, flexibility, responsiveness, holism, contingency thinking, and anticipatory openness to possibility.

As has been the case for several decades, CNSs engage and function within this dynamic context providing "expertness representing advanced or newly developed practices [in nursing]" (Peplau, 1965/2003).

The *Statement on Clinical Nurse Specialist Practice and Education* (National Association of Clinical Nurse Specialists [NACNS], 2004) clearly articulates a practice paradigm whereby the application of clinical expertise may occur either directly or by influencing nurses and nursing personnel through evidence-based standards and programs of care. As such, CNSs, in addition to their foundational obligation to provide expert nursing practice in the patient/client sphere, further advance nursing practice and improve patient outcomes through role modeling, consultation, education, and advocacy as they engage in work with other nurses (nursing and nursing practice sphere) and the broader organization or system.

As is evident in the description of outcomes and competencies (NACNS, 2004), the work of translating clinical expertise may take many forms in the daily life of a CNS. However, the obligation to consistently and creatively transmit knowledge and skill development is most clearly apparent in the sphere of influence dedicated to nurses and nursing practice. Therein, key outcomes represent the dimension of CNS performance necessarily dedicated to the functions of instruction and facilitation of learning:

- Knowledge and skill development needs of nurses are delineated.
- Nurses engage in learning experiences to advance or maintain competence.
- Career enhancement programs are ongoing, accessible, innovative, and effective.
- Educational programs that advance the practice of nursing are developed, implemented, evaluated, and linked to evidence-based practice and effects on clinical and fiscal outcomes.

Furthermore, specific competencies demonstrate expectations that the CNS:

- Utilizes and designs appropriate methods and tools to assess knowledge, skills, and practice competencies of nurses and nursing personnel to advance the practice of nursing;
- Identifies desired outcomes of continuing or changing nursing practices;
- Mentors nurses to critique and apply research evidence to nursing practices;
- Develops and implements educational programs that target the needs of staff to improve nursing practice and patient outcomes; and
- Evaluates the ability of nurses and nursing personnel to implement changes in nursing practice.

CONCEPTUAL/THEORETICAL SUPPORT

The Context of Change

Several organizing frameworks serve to enhance an understanding of the trajectory for facilitating learning in the service of nurses and nursing practice. Foundational to all tenets of instruction and education is the incorporation of a meaningful context about change. In the 21st century, the work of teaching and learning in our health care settings consistently occurs within environments characterized by complexity, variety, activity, variability, patterned chaos, and ever-present change. As soon as one has the time to consider the nuances and details of the most recent changes, new changes transpire. Porter-O'Grady and Malloch (2003) vividly depict the context wherein health care and clinical practice occur. They describe a "new vessel" where leaders, clinicians, educators, and others must exercise their intellect and demonstrate productivity in entirely new ways. Using quantum theory as the basis for their analysis, they further explicate that change is not a thing or an event, but rather a "dynamic that is constitutive of the universe" (p. 6). As such, it is entirely impossible to avoid change because it is everywhere. Instead, the appropriate work or response is to influence the circumstances and consequences of change. Providing direction is the work of leading change. As Steven Hawking has stated, "Change is." Chaos, complexity, and change are not things but forms of dynamic activity, and they are the only constants in the universe. This represents a substantive paradigm shift from previous change models that prescribed a movement to and away from "freezing" (Lewin, 1951; Millay, 1995; Reinhard, 1988).

Incorporation of this current perspective regarding change should transform and revolutionize processes that de facto impede or delay innovation. It is

imperative that creativity, applied knowledge, responsiveness, and openness are expected and prevail as normative behavior. It is a fundamental requisite of life to be able to adapt to ever-changing conditions. Science and technology are altering every aspect of our lives. The challenge is to embrace the new circumstances and then sort out their implications and applications as we go.

Principles of Teaching and Learning

As change represents a major contextual entity for the function of education, several principles of teaching and learning serve to frame the actual work of engaging with others to accomplish knowledge transfer and skill development. The literature is replete with a variety of philosophical perspectives and theories related to learning (Clark, 1993; Cross, 1981; Dewey, 1938; Galbraith, 1990; Knowles, 1980; Maslow, 1970; Merriam & Brockett, 1997; Skinner, 1974; Thorndike, Bregman, Tilton, & Woodyard, 1928). Rather than providing summative descriptions of the various theories, several principles are delineated that have been derived from an analysis of several key references (Abruzzese, 1996; Alspach, 1995; Avillion, 2001, 2004; Bastable, 2003; Billings & Halstead, 1998; Spath, 2002). In particular, focused consideration is directed toward principles that address the requirements of adult learners.

Adults Need a Reason for Learning and Are Problem-Centered Learners

Adult learners want to know why it is important for them to participate in an educational activity. They more readily engage in work-related learning activities to solve anticipated or actual problems. Their interests tend to focus on immediate application of that which has been learned in order to more effectively fulfill required role expectations or responsibilities. Motivation and readiness are enhanced to the degree that adult learners perceive that the instruction is relevant to their work. Furthermore, adults more readily place a high value on their time given their many personal and professional obligations.

Most Adults Are Self-Directed in Their Pursuit of Learning

It is commonly observed that adults demonstrate a preference to exercise some degree of control over what they learn and how they learn it. In addition, they typically exhibit both the need and desire to participate in determining when and where they will engage in learning activities and what kinds of activities those will be.

Adults Bring a Variety of Life and Work Experiences to Any Learning Situation

One's personal and professional experiences enhance any learning situation and, even if not directly relevant, may serve to compliment the learning process. Adults place value on their own experiences, as well as those of others. Furthermore, adults expect that others, most notably the individual(s) engaged in the work of teaching/instruction, will recognize and value those past and current experiences.

An Adult Is Not an Adult, Is Not an Adult

Adults are heterogeneous as learners and deserve respect as mature individuals. Unlike school-age children who experience a strong pressure to conform, adults more commonly value their independence in thought and behavior. In addition, adult learners have considerably more diverse backgrounds and, as such, may require varying degrees of support in learning. Developmental stages vary across the trajectory of the adult life span and flexibility may fluctuate concomitantly. For example, habits, attitudes, values, and behaviors evolve over many years of life experience and may be more deeply embedded in the older adult learner than in those who are younger.

Adults Are Voluntary Learners

The option of seeking employment and subsequently engaging in required learning activities may occur for any number of reasons. Some individuals will present with altruistic motivation and high levels of professional commitment. Others may primarily be interested in securing a paycheck, obtaining improved benefits, or changing to a new employer after having been downsized from a more prestigious position. The possibilities and motivations are almost limitless. Nonetheless, the essential understanding is that learner engagement is likely affected by the situation that precipitates voluntary entry into the learning process.

Having given consideration to the reality that adults are the key recipients of learning interventions in the sphere of influence related to nurses and nursing practice, it is also necessary to delineate other evidence-based learning principles that need to be incorporated as CNSs exercise their leadership in the development of others. These fundamental precepts represent a synthesis of theoretical and empirical literature that presently guides best practice in the realm of instruction and facilitation of learning (Abruzzese, 1996; Alspach, 1995; Avillion, 2001, 2004; Bastable, 2003; Billings & Halstead, 1998).

Learning Occurs as a Consequence of Self-Activity

Learners will learn more, retain more, and achieve more effectively when they are actively involved in the learning experience. Thus, learning requires active participation by the learner. Dewey's (1916) axiom that "we learn by doing" is as true today as it was when first documented in the early 20th century. Learning is a dynamic process that requires active participation in order to more readily accomplish educational aims.

Learning Is Influenced by the Environment Within Which It Occurs

Both physical surroundings and psychological climate impact instruction and learning. Understandably, the process may be further influenced by virtue of the nature of clinical environments wherein CNSs and their clinical colleagues practice. Pace, volume, and acuity provide the context for new learning and application of principles in real time. Complexity and variability in processes, environment, and personnel further complicate one's trajectory for learning, whether new to the profession, new to the organization, or new to the focus for requisite instruction.

Empirical evidence demonstrates that physical environment can facilitate learning when it includes adequate lighting, temperature control, and acoustics; when media can be readily seen and heard; and when learners are comfortable in their seating and workspace (Bastable, 2003; Galbraith, 1990). The dilemma of crafting this type of ideal environment in the midst of a clinical reality characterized by "just-in-time" learning needs, complexity, and extraordinary demands to preserve patient safety and sustain high-quality outcomes becomes readily evident.

Learning Is Social and Interactive

Similar to the perspective that links learning outcomes with environmental appropriateness, it is also essential to understand that the psychological environment impacts learning as well. Learning is substantively enhanced in an environment characterized by consistent and supportive interpersonal interactions, engaged responsiveness, acknowledgement of existing knowledge and competence, and a spirit of inquiry, fairness, and openness. Learning is a shared responsibility between teachers and learners. Thus, CNSs can facilitate learning by way of their social interactions with staff by relating to them as trustworthy colleagues who deserve recognition and by welcoming them to the process of growth and enhanced understanding.

Learning Is Intentional and Is Influenced by the Motivation and Readiness of the Learner

In concert with the understanding that adults are most commonly self-directed in their pursuit of learning, it stands to reason then that learning is most effective when it is directed at objectives or aims that the learner interprets as being meaningful and useful. Motivation is enhanced when learners can participate in identifying their needs and in the planning activities that would meet those needs. It is important to note that motivation to learn is not a constant, no matter how eager an individual may customarily be. Motivation waxes and wanes in response to stress, fatigue, demands, hassle factors, and/or perception about the relevance (or lack thereof) of learning activities. Evidence further suggests that positive intrinsic motivators (e.g., a personal sense of accomplishment, self-satisfaction, feelings of competence, and subsequent role security) enhance the process of learning more than negative extrinsic motivators (e.g., threats, criticism, punishment for "noncompliance"). As the old adage suggests: "Success breeds success." Thus, one of the strongest motivators for continued interest and engagement in learning is the experience of success. Similarly, readiness to learn is shaped by an individual's personal and complex state of physical, psychological, social, and intellectual preparedness for learning and is an intrinsic characteristic that influences learning outcomes.

Learning Is Facilitated by Positive and Immediate Feedback

As noted previously, successful performance of a newly learned or improved skill provides a strong motivating stimulus for continued learning. Thus, timely recognition of successful achievement of a learning outcome is critical to sustain the momentum for ongoing growth and development. The impact of positive feedback is well described as a critical element that serves to enforce optimal performance (Alspach, 1995; Fitzgerald, 2003; Wlodkowski, 1990). It may take many forms, including verbal recognition, encouragement, or written comments.

Learning Is Retainable and Can Be Transferred to New Situations

Despite the pressure exacted by many learners requiring new information or knowledge, retention and transference of learning is best accomplished by preliminarily introducing general principles (e.g., standards, guidelines, concepts, norms) before exceptions to general principles are introduced. The habit of eagerly introducing a new learner to all the "shortcuts" or exceptions that one has acquired over years of previous experience provides no added value whatsoever to the attainment of an appropriate understanding of the phenomenon of interest. The ability to tolerate ambiguity or variance requires a higher level of cognitive interpretation and evolves as one acquires more *experiential* knowledge accumulated over time. Thus, it is reasonable to expect that as one is learning a new process, it is easier to learn the *usual* process before attempting to learn how the process may differ for emergent situations, atypical patients, or some other type of variable. Premature instruction related to exceptions or variation tends to provoke a sense of personal distress about limited capacity or evoke a crisis of trust about others and their level of understanding or support. At the very least, precipitous attention to variation and exceptions tends to confuse learners who may experience a sense of being overwhelmed by unnecessary details provided too soon.

Learning Is Inferred Rather Than Observed

The fundamental manifestation that learning has occurred is the subsequent observation that behavior has changed. These changes may be demonstrated in actual work performance (which is ideal and preferred), in a simulated experience, in documentation, or by way of verbal or written evidence. Embedded in this premise is the understanding that there are three essential domains of learning: cognitive, affective, and psychomotor. As such, observations of behavioral change as a consequence of learning are correlated with these domains. That is, psychomotor performance related to fine motor, manual, or gross motor skills is best assessed in a situation that requires demonstration of the ability to manipulate equipment, coordinate physical movements around a task, or exercise gross body movement to accomplish a requirement. Evidence that affective learning has occurred is revealed when learners manifest attitudes, beliefs, and values that are compatible with the aims of the learning experience or, more broadly, with the philosophy of the sponsoring organization. Thus, observation of individual performance *in context* is more likely to provide verification of affective learning, though that is not the only method to confirm that values or beliefs have been changed as a consequence of an instructional intervention. Behavioral changes in the cognitive domain are manifested in a variety of ways. Often written tests are used to determine if learners possess adequate knowledge requisite for their position. It is important to note, however, that distinction among levels of cognitive performance (e.g., knowledge, comprehension, application, analysis, synthesis, and evaluation) may mandate different approaches to verify integrated/internalized behavioral manifestation of learning.

Learning Is Influenced by the Nature of the Learning Experience

Given that learning is a continual and dynamic process of integrating new information or skills with existing knowledge or competence, learners are continually adding, subtracting, modifying, or changing what they previously held to be true. As such, it is critical that instructional interventions be suitable for the content and skills that are to be learned and vary in response to learners' progress and development. The burden of success rests with the instructor's sensibility about the relevance and utility of the learning experience and their correlated response to modify learning experiences in order to sustain the momentum of discovery and accomplishment. There is nothing less helpful than iterating and reiterating the same message or technique in light of evidence that suggests that the experience is not moving learners to change anything. The fun part of the work of instruction and learning is engaging in the interactive and dynamic exchange with learners and implementing creative instructional solutions to accomplish learning outcomes. It is also important to note that the business of *unlearning* also is relevant to this analysis. That is, as organizational change precipitates new performance requirements or new technology or any other phenomenon that generates a necessity for new learning, it may also render obsolete previous customary procedures or standards of care. Thus, experienced learners may have considerable amounts of knowledge to unlearn if new procedures, products, or processes differ considerably from what they have been accustomed to. This reality may also provoke a stance of resistance when new learning expectations conflict with prior experience or understanding. Correspondingly, less experienced staff have less of a need to unlearn because their experience is limited.

Finally, it is evident that learning proceeds best when it is organized and clearly communicated (Alspach, 1995). Instructional organization of principles to be delivered facilitates the transfer, acquisition, and integration of knowledge to new situations. Furthermore, clear communication of the purpose, aims, objectives, and outcomes of the learning experience establish the context and expectations for behavioral change, performance, and normative standards. It is also important to note that every learning experience should be targeted and focused toward accomplishing a delineated set of outcomes. Often there is tendency to be sure that every possible nuance of a learning topic is "excavated" and addressed. Retention and mastery of content is enhanced when clear delineation of realistic expectations are articulated and instructional interventions correlate with a sensible scope of expectation.

Novice to Expert

An extraordinarily useful developmental framework of how individuals come to know and engage in clinical practice has been developed and empirically validated by Patricia Benner (1984) and colleagues (Benner, Tanner, & Chesla, 1996). This paradigm has substantive implications for reforming instructional interventions in the clinical world. A fundamental construct is that practice without theory cannot alone produce fully skilled behavior in the complex working situations experienced by nurses. This is a common professional belief that is well understood and valued in nursing. The critical consideration articulated by Benner et al. (1996) that leads to a more accurate understanding of the nature of progression in practice is that theory without practice experience has even a lesser chance of producing fully realized success in the field. Thus, it is critical to understand that theory and experience intertwine in a mutually supportive process as nurses continually develop their skills. Only when both dimensions are cultivated and valued can full expertise be realized.

Five stages of development have been described: novice, advanced beginner, competent, proficient, and expert. Each stage is characterized by manifestations that should direct those charged with instruction and development to respond and design appropriate interventions that make sense and have logical congruity with the prevailing behaviors and learning needs exhibited at that stage. For example, the term *novice* is typically and mistakenly used to describe anyone who is new to a situation. More accurately, the term refers to individuals who have virtually no background, understanding, or experience of a given clinical situation. Thus, the term more appropriately describes the stage of practice manifested by nursing students who have no previous experiential or practical knowledge upon which to base their judgments or interventions. Thus, through instruction, the novice requires and acquires *rules* for drawing conclusions or determining actions based upon facts of the situation that are recognizable without experience in the skill domain that is being learned. For example, if one is learning to drive a car and has never done so before, the novice driver is given a standard or formula for the safe distance at which to follow another car at a given speed. From an experiential perspective, instructional time is not spent describing what a car looks like because this knowledge is assumed to have been already acquired. Rather, the emphasis is placed on the targeted rule that will frame safe performance. It is important to note that nuances related to safe distance and safe speed as they are applied in varying environmental conditions (e.g., snow, sleet, rain) cannot be fully understood or learned until there is a concomitant experiential learning event where the three interactive variables occur simultaneously.

In contrast to the context-free rules that are taught to novices, advanced beginners require extensive, guided experiences with patients so that they can readily identify components of recurring patient situations. Clinical situations present to advanced beginners as a set of tasks that must be accomplished. The task requirements are central at this stage, and all other aspects of the clinical situation, such as the patient's changing condition or the family's concerns or distress, form the background for their focus. It is critical to understand that this is not a flaw in the individual. This is a normal developmental stage in the journey to acquiring expertise across a broad range of aspects of practice. It is suggested that everyone who engages in staff development of any kind reflect back on their early practice and recall how personal success was perceived and measured. Recall the thrill and relief associated with getting through a shift, completing every task that needed to be done, finishing report on time, and managing to avoid incurring the wrath of a more seasoned colleague. This represents an appropriate trajectory and focus for individuals early in their career. Personal distress is rampant during this stage and is only exacerbated by arrogant and insensitive posturing by more experienced individuals who express concerns about progression and expectations that are unrealistic and unfair.

Competence in practice is typically demonstrated by nurses who have been in the same or similar clinical practice for 18 months or more. Nurses practicing at this level differ from advanced beginners in their improved organizational ability and technical skills. This increase in skill opens up possibilities for noticing and developing new clinical knowledge so that in familiar situations they have an increased ability to anticipate a likely course of events and respond appropriately. The work of the nurse at this stage is typically organized around the work of planning for and anticipating likely events in the given course of a patient situation. The language of the nurse is more process-focused, and one detects a commitment to setting and accomplishing goals. It is at this stage that one also begins to see the manifestation of disillusionment because the nurse is more able to detect the fallibility of other providers and recognize gaps in scientific knowledge. This can provoke a sense of crisis as the realization grows that not everyone is as competent or supportive as was previously thought. Furthermore, at this stage, nurses realize that they are not only responsible for task accomplishment but also for subsequent outcomes. This growing awareness that one has actual authority for a defined scope of practice and is accountable for patient outcomes can provoke a sense of personal distress about limited capacity.

Proficiency is a stage of transition between competency and expertise. Practice is transformed in five major ways:

1. Development of engaged reasoning in transitions,
2. Emotional attunement to a situation—doing what needs to be done,
3. Ability to recognize changing relevance of aspects in the clinical situation,
4. Socially skilled sense of agency, and
5. Improved and more differentiated skills of involvement with patients and families.

Increased perceptual acuity and responsiveness to a particular situation are hallmarks of this stage. Performance at this level requires an experiential base with a particular patient population because the skills noted previously depend on having a perceptual grasp of qualitative distinctions, which can only be acquired by seeing and contrasting patterns of clinical manifestations in a variety of situations as they evolve over time.

Expert nurses have extensive experience and possess an intuitive grasp of clinical situations. They identify critical problem areas without having to review multiple alternatives. They are smooth and fluid in the initiation of appropriate interventions. Expert nurses detect subtle changes, and their performance is characterized by a fusion of thought and action. They are able to see the big picture and accurately derive salient features from the clinical situation, and they demonstrate embodied know-how. The practice of expert nurses is further characterized by strong moral agency and an overt commitment to the preservation of personhood, patient attunement, and respect for the dignity and integrity of patients and families.

Leadership Principles

The NACNS *Statement on Clinical Nurse Specialist Practice and Education* (2004) clearly identifies that leadership is an essential CNS characteristic required for effective practice in all spheres of influence. In order to accomplish an educational agenda and facilitate learning outcomes, the NACNS statement articulates a set of leadership skills that are critical for problem delineation and analysis, formulation of a strategic vision and plan, deriving creative solutions and possibility for change, and inspiring others to action. These include:

■ Interpersonal skills of listening, validating, reflecting, providing constructive feedback, and conveying a caring attitude;
■ An ability to formulate and logically convey ideas while being sensitive to the needs and feelings of others;

- Utilization of nursing science and knowledge generated by related disciplines;
- Creating innovations in patient care;
- An ability to think critically, make decisions, and synthesize scientific knowledge for application to practice;
- Participation in research, clinical inquiry projects, and research utilization, including cost analysis;
- Creation and implementation of evidence-based change to improve safety, quality, and cost-effectiveness;
- Collaborative systems thinking that detects that which is working well, that which requires revision, and that which will best predict the successful accomplishment of high-quality and cost-effective outcomes;
- A shared decision-making philosophy that encourages strong working relationships among nurses and other multidisciplinary health care providers.

As a corollary to these identified skills, it is also important to recall the perspective advanced by Porter-O'Grady and Malloch (2003). It is their thesis that leadership is mainly concerned with adapting to change. Given the assumptions and realities exhibited in the present-day health care arena, leaders need to be fluid and adaptable because their role changes in concert with the ever-changing conditions. "Leaders are aware that it is in the pursuit of meaning that the direction of change can best be discerned. They continually look past the real and the present toward the unformed and potential to better evaluate the present and the direction of transformation. The subtle themes and ebbs and flows that lie just beneath the surface of events and experiences have more to say to leaders than the events themselves" (p. 36).

This represents a vastly different paradigm from that espoused less than one generation ago when leadership meant being a good manager, guiding one's peers and subordinates like a good parent, and directing their activities in the interest of the organization. The critical skills were those required for planning, organizing, directing, and controlling. In the current context of complexity and change, authentic leaders are motivated by the connections that give meaning and value to the current reality. For example, motivated leaders focus on potential, share the work, understand that new kinds of work are evolving and requisite, and do different work differently. Unmotivated leaders focus on the present, wallow in the negative, project that things consistently are getting worse, and manifest a disengaged stance.

Leadership skills are learned, and their mastery does not require extraordinary intellectual capability. As is evident from even a cursory review of world history, leaders emerge in a wide variety of circumstances and manifest an extensive range of talents and personalities. There is no one "correct" pattern of behavior or personality type

that is most suitable for the leadership role. What leaders have in common, however, is the ability to understand the complexities and nuances of human interactions and relationships. They appreciate patterns revealed in chaos and are able to "straddle" that which is now and that which is evolving. Furthermore, they are optimistic and able to engage others in the journey of progress toward an unimagined and preferred future.

STRATEGIES FOR ENGAGING STAFF IN LEARNING: APPLICATIONS TO CNS PRACTICE

It is essential to preface the subsequent discussion with the fundamental disclaimer that educational intervention is absolutely *not* the universal solution to every problem or practice gap that may be detected in a clinical setting. Far too often the standard response to any demonstrated need, less than desirable clinical outcome, or performance gap is to first and foremost set out on a quest to "educate them." Perhaps even more distressing is the notion that gathering nurses together in some kind of a collective herd for a staff development program is necessarily the preferred method for imparting wisdom and leading the masses to the "promised land." Wright (2004) reports that only 10%–15% of all problematic issues are due to knowledge or skill deficits. She identifies that several other factors may better serve to explain undesirable variance in outcomes, such as system problems, communication barriers, attitudinal issues, individual performance patterns, unavailability of necessary tools or equipment, or departmental barriers.

In any case, it is clearly the obligation of those exercising clinical leadership to participate in the careful analysis of these problems and to accurately assess why they occurred. An educational intervention should be designed and implemented only when there is clear evidence that a lack of knowledge or skill was the underlying reason for the problem.

Facilitating Learning by Creating Opportunity

In light of the conceptual and theoretical support presented thus far, the development of strategies to engage staff in learning must necessarily be framed within a context of creativity and encouragement. As a clinical leader and expert, the CNS's role is to create opportunity that encourages employees' personal and professional growth. The American Nurses Association (2000) has outlined the scope and standards of practice for nursing professional development. Several philosophical statements direct one to interpret that the creative work of professional development requires a substantive commitment far beyond obligations associated with meeting regulatory or task-focused requirements. The work of facilitating the development of fully engaged nursing professionals transcends a notion of something "nice to do" to something essential and necessary to do. Again, there exists an abundance of literature that recommends and describes a wide range of strategies to accomplish staff learning outcomes (Abruzzese, 1996; Alspach, 1995; Avillion, 2001, 2004). The subsequent focus is targeted to address those strategies that are most consistent with a realistic picture of current practice environments where one is essentially "building the bridge as one walks on it" (Quinn, 2004).

Mentoring and Coaching

There is substantial evidence that supports and prescribes mentorship and coaching as strategies that facilitate the development and transformation of nurses in practice (Benner et al., 1996; Cunningham & McNally, 2003; Dracup & Bryan-Brown, 2004; Ervin, 2005; Robinson-Walker, 2004; Waddell & Dunn, 2005; Wilson & Porter-O'Grady, 1999). The NACNS (2004) standards specifically identify mentoring as a necessary competency in the sphere of influence related to nurses and nursing practice.

Merriam-Webster's Online Dictionary (2003) defines *mentor* as a "trusted counselor or guide," *preceptor* as a "teacher, tutor," and *coach* as "one who instructs or trains a performer, or team of performers." The role of *preceptor* is usually limited in time, to orientation or validation of competency for a specific required skill. In contrast, a *mentor's* role is ongoing and requires a higher level of knowledge and expertise because a mentor not only serves as a role model and resource but also assists an individual in acquiring new knowledge and skills. The role is formalized when the mentor also creates a formal educational plan with an individual to assist him or her in developing their practice, including a range of competencies or aspects of practice. The mentor and protégé meet regularly to discuss progress toward identified goals and any new needs that have arisen.

Coaching can be either formal or informal. It is characterized as a process in which the *learner* sets the agenda, identifies the challenges or needs that are present, and postulates about strategies and pathways that will facilitate growth and accomplishment. At its root, coaching is about change. The coach is a partner who can enhance the learner's understanding of their present reality. The coach is a "guide on the side" or a "guide from behind" who is skilled in the process of sorting out what is working well, letting go of what is no longer serving well, and assisting in the development of new skills and practices that are required for future success.

Coaching provides "just in time" learning. It is listening and focused facilitation that is 100% dedicated to the agenda of the staff member in transition. In the healthiest of situations, the coach is somewhat like a friend in that he or she is dedicated to the learner's needs and is genuine in their interest and care. The coach is unlike a friend in that he or she is guided by objectivity, is external to or "outside" of the personal experience, and has a primary stake in the outcome of the relationship such that the learner demonstrates forward progress and expresses satisfaction thereof. Given the span of responsibility that is embedded in the definition of the CNS role (NACNS, 2004), it is apparent that coaching as a behavior is requisite and foundational to interactions and relationships with nursing staff. The actions and intent associated with coaching and mentoring should be obvious and prevalent in the day-to-day practice of any CNS.

Facilitating Development Around Stages of Practice

Advanced Beginners

In most instances, the work of developing the practice of advance beginners is assigned to preceptors. However, there are common misconceptions about how best to frame the learning experience of our newest colleagues in practice. The strategies described may be directly applied by CNSs as they make rounds and encounter orientees in practice. Another possibility is that the strategies could be reinforced among preceptors who most likely assume the bulk of responsibility for local orientation. In either instance, the principles are critical for ensuring an appropriate learning intervention that facilitates the transition toward competence (Benner et al., 1996).

Beginners require a historical context and possible future course of a patient situation. They simply have not had adequate experience to see a given population of patients with varied disease processes through complete illness trajectories. Thus, it is useful to provide a context for presenting symptoms as they arise and to let the learner know what is and is not to be expected with particular categories of patients or illnesses.

Because the clinical world of the advanced beginner revolves around tasks and procedures and the patient situation more frequently shows up as background, it is helpful then to assist the learner by linking together the sometimes disjointed components of report, the chart, and clinical presentation of the patient into a meaningful whole. This will facilitate the learner's ability to detect some kind of order in the immense and sometimes conflicting information that exists for each patient and fluctuates from moment to moment.

Providing care in other ways than "by the book" requires practical reasoning gained by experience over time. Thus, it is not helpful to divert beginners away from the rules or standards by which they were taught. Instead, it is more affirming and encouraging to recognize that the learner is replicating the standard process and to acknowledge their accomplishment when they have completed it.

Advanced beginners live in a world of insecurity and concern about the adequacy of their performance overall. They can be assisted by offering opportunities to review and contemplate over situations that did not go particularly well. Questions about why a particular patient died or why certain actions were or were not taken frequently go unanswered. It is useful to review complex or interesting cases by specifically examining the decisions and actions that were documented in a patient chart. This approach distances the learner from some of the emotion faced in the situation and provides an opportunity to learn from experience that is grounded in a specific case.

It is critical to assist the advanced beginner in knowing how to safely "delegate up." Sadly, everyone in a clinical setting is not motivated to be supportive and helpful to new employees or learners. Similarly, not all experienced individuals demonstrate sufficient competency around all of the skills and knowledge required for clinical practice. Thus, a key strategy early in the trajectory of development for the beginner is to identify safe, knowledgeable, and willing persons who will assist them through any dilemmas they may encounter. In this capacity, it is the obligation of every CNS to assume a stance of availability and openness that welcomes the questions and accepts the vulnerability of someone new to a setting.

There is a substantial teaching role in helping advanced beginners manage aspects of nursing that occur away from direct patient care. Included in this are issues such as obtaining appropriate physician response and managing interactions with other services such as laboratories, dietary, and pharmacy. Because the advanced beginner is characteristically so focused on patient care (e.g., getting through the shift, task completion), the smooth acquisition of skill related to problem resolution with the larger system should not be the focus of instruction at this phase. Rather, interventions should be targeted toward assisting this learner with requisite skills associated with working with physicians. Learners benefit from information about fundamental situations that require questioning. It is helpful to reinforce beginners' correct judgments about situations when they conflict with physicians' assessments or plans. Most importantly, it is essential to coach the learner in formulating a "script" for proposing something that will more likely evoke a responsive action. For example, the utilization of the situation-background-assessment-recommendation (SBAR) communication approach provides a useful framework for organizing one's thoughts during a situational briefing (Institute for Healthcare Improvement, 2006).

It is imperative that advanced beginners work in environments where they feel secure asking questions. In order to maintain a safe clinical experience for patients, it is essential that beginners' inexperience not be judged as personal inadequacy but recognized as an expected phase in the development of clinical judgment. Most hazardous to patients are environments that are interpersonally threatening, that punish early mistakes, or that set up barriers to the free exchange of questions from advanced beginners. Despite the reality that "official" orientation may conclude after 6, 8, 10, or 12 weeks, it is crucial to sustain some type of mentoring or coaching relationship for at least 6 months. Giles and Moran (1989) discovered that the option of maintaining a recognized relationship between each advanced beginner and one experienced nurse for the full duration was most efficacious. In reality, the need for support and continuing orientation does not automatically end on the day that someone is counted in staffing.

Becoming Competent

Benner and colleagues (1996) note that nurses practicing at the competent stage differ primarily from advanced beginners by their increased clinical understanding, technical skill, organizational ability, and the ability to anticipate the likely course of events. This stage is further characterized by a degree of disillusionment because nurses begin to detect fallibility in the system, gaps in scientific knowledge, and the existence of nonaltruistic motivation in others. Unfortunately, it is common to observe that responses to nurses at this stage may be dismissive in nature and suggestive that their concerns are a symptom of adjustment problems rather than legitimate observations of systems issues that require intervention and resolution. One of the most supportive strategies at this stage is to truly listen to their struggles rather than insisting that they cope or get along. This can be a mechanism for creating institutional renewal that can break the cycle of disillusionment and departure from the profession. It is personally very compelling to recall the extreme pain and disillusionment expressed by a competent nurse about 2 years into her practice in a large perioperative service where she routinely observed and experienced verbal abuse secondary to an excessive system of authority gradient. More tragic was the complacency of others and their inability to take action to bring a halt to this long-standing pattern of violence. Needless to say, this nurse with exceptional intellect and potential left the setting and struggled with her career decision thereafter. Fortunately, a CNS and clinical educator on her new unit collaborated to debrief and design an intervention that combined instructional requirements with consistent interpersonal support that facilitated her transition to proficient practice after another period of 18 months.

As one reflects on typical instructional patterns in clinical settings, it is common to observe a monumental investment in orientation and staff development during the early phase of employment or internal transfer. Additional instructional investment is routinely provided in order to accomplish mandatory competency requirements on an annual basis. Despite evidence that suggests that the stage of competency represents a highly vulnerable period in the transition to proficiency and expertise (Benner et al., 1996), one rarely hears of interventions designed to manage this developmental stage of skill acquisition in terms of debriefing disillusionment, clarifying manifestations of hyper-responsibility, or learning about skill of involvement with patients and families. CNSs are uniquely prepared to facilitate this type of intervention given their expert grasp of clinical phenomena, ability to see the larger picture, and aptitude for providing nurses with a venue for articulating their concerns. More importantly, because the CNS is engaged in the organization and system sphere, he/she can advocate for appropriate reform and resolution of issues at a higher level.

Because competent nurses rely heavily on goal setting and planning, they can further benefit from ongoing practice in problem identification. Exercises in determining which of many competing problems is the most salient can increase their capability with respect to discernment. Similarly, practice in seeing the big picture, through detailed case analysis or following patterns of patient responses as depicted in the record or flow sheet, can enhance understanding of the relationship between patient response and related therapy. It is also useful at this stage to share personal narratives, stories, or exemplars that reveal mistakes or things that went wrong. Often dramatic and emotional, yet very memorable, these types of shared experiences can be more effective in modifying behavior than procedural accounts of standard practice or that which *should* be done.

Proficiency: A Transition to Expertise

Benner et al. (1996) suggest that new kinds of staff development be implemented for nurses who are becoming proficient. Narratives of learning told in small groups that focus on changing one's perspectives and expectations in a clinical situation can be very instructive and support the advancement of skill development in problem identification and responsiveness to salient

patient manifestations. It is important for the individual who is leading this exercise to publicly sanction the learner's recognition of changing clinical relevance and legitimize the correlated thinking as being astute and flexible. This is a very different instructional stance than being critical that the individual had the incorrect perception or plan from the outset. Instead, the developmental and instructional work is to flesh out the thinking and judgment exhibited by the nurse that ebbs and flows with evolving and changing clinical data.

At this stage of practice, it is critical that nurses become more skilled at negotiating with physicians. As they become more adept at detecting changing relevance in the patient's circumstances, the capacity to adequately communicate that to those who are often functioning away from the actual situation becomes ever more essential. Negotiating clinical knowledge requires interpersonal skill, trust in one's own grasp, and a capacity to see the situation from a different vantage point. That being the case, instructional strategies that simulate responses characterized by skepticism, intellectual challenge, acceptance, or complacency can assist the learner in targeting their communication so that the risk to patients is minimized. Again, saliency is a key phenomenon of interest in communication.

Perhaps the most important consideration in facilitating learning with proficient nurses or those transitioning to that level of practice is the reality that one's authentic engagement, support, acceptance, and receptivity can actually contribute to the individual's formation around moral agency. This is a very powerful obligation, and the work of assisting nurses to know what things can and cannot wait has substantive implications for the well-being of patients and families. The courage associated with exercising appropriate judgment and intellect for the benefit of others, and sometimes with some degree of real risk, can only be achieved when nurtured by those who are similarly attuned and committed to role modeling their own response-based practice in concrete situations.

Expertise in Practice

Perhaps the most important intervention related to working with nurses at this stage is to study and learn from their expert practice. Implications from this type of analysis should arm the CNS with information to bring forward in larger organizational venues. Narrative evidence suggests that all too often expert nurses must engage in Herculean efforts to overcome organizational impediments to their practice (Benner et al., 1996). Typically, structures and processes are geared toward minimal expectations, "pushing excellence to the unacknowledged and unaccommodated margins" (p. 169). Gearing organizational structures and policies to the minimal standards of performance only serves to mask the very examples of excellence that should be highlighted and extended in practice. Consequently, this handicaps leaders in the organization by forcing an emphasis on shoring up deficits rather than designing for excellence. Simple compliance is not the manifesto for movement toward fully engaged and empowered practice. It is essential then to study the patterns of expert nursing practice revealed in our organizations and to redesign systems and infrastructures that remove barriers and facilitate a reality whereby these nurses are able to exercise the full compliment of their skills and knowledge.

Instructional Strategies

Role Modeling

Alspach (1995) suggests that CNSs are ideally suited for effectively demonstrating their expertise by role modeling key behaviors, especially in complex patient/family situations. They are able to exemplify through behavior and observable action how a particular role is assumed. Other nurses then can enhance their clinical competence by observing and emulating the practice that was observed. For example, complex communication with several players exhibiting a range of intellect and emotion is a common reality in practice. Think of insecure, frightened, and frustrated families who have difficulty navigating the environment and the phenomena impacting their loved one. Add to the mix a group of service line physicians who may have a different agenda or demands and may be perceived to be in a hurry or not adequately attentive. This has the potential for evoking strong responses and interactions that only further compromise the well-being of the family. In these types of situations, it is common to call upon a CNS to facilitate the management of this type of encounter. However, the key developmental intervention is to purposely bring a staff nurse to the encounter and subsequently engage in a moment or two of debriefing about the key communication principles that were operationalized in the situation. This facilitates an ability to link principles with action, behavior, and outcome.

Rounds

There are many conceivable purposes for engaging in clinical rounds. Often CNSs function as partners in multidisciplinary rounds where case presentations occur and plans are crafted for moving patients/families toward desirable outcomes. In these instances, it goes without saying that the CNS should include the staff nurse in the process and engage them in participation while preserving their integrity and safety if the

individual is at a stage where he/she is just beginning to demonstrate agency in the context of multidisciplinary communication.

More importantly, however, it is recommended that CNSs, in the course of their routine individual rounds and interactions with patients, staff, and families, use this opportunity as a vehicle for detecting exceptional practice and acknowledging progress thereof. These circumstances provide wonderful options for extending growing practice to the next stage of development. Positive feedback and reinforcement are strong motivators for continued personal investment in ongoing practice improvement. The credibility of one's expertise in the field is enhanced by relating and applying knowledge in concrete and visible ways. Concomitantly, as one engages in what may be considered to be an "environmental scan," trends, themes, and patterns of less than desirable practice may be detected as well. It is critical to confront the practice, relate the observed variance to the applicable standard/principle, provide instruction regarding the appropriate alternative, and offer concrete rationale.

Mini In-Service

In the present world of clinical practice characterized by high acuity, staffing demands, and fast pace, it is almost impossible to implement planned instructional in-services where nurses leave their environment and engage in a more formal learning encounter. However, almost every day a challenging patient/family situation will reveal itself as an opportunity for development. Because one may be required to implement a complex intervention, use this as a just-in-time occasion to bring a few staff together for a few minutes to demonstrate a particular skill or engage in a creative solution. Subsequently, patients will benefit from staff learning, and learners benefit because they can see the immediate application of principle/theory to practice. Needless to say, patients and families must agree to participate in this exercise.

Family as "Faculty"

The mini in-service mechanism can also set the stage for engaging patients or family as "faculty." Many patients present with long-term chronic conditions where they have achieved mastery around their ability to manage devices, navigate the health system, and vividly depict the experience of being a recipient of health care and nursing services, some that is good and some that is problematic. The personal account of a patient or family member as an instructional intervention can be extraordinarily powerful and profound. Furthermore, their acquired psychomotor skills in light of their own unique characteristics can provide nurses with enhanced understanding about modifying interventions.

Critical Incident

Davis (1995) describes this strategy as being useful for the purpose of exploring events in the learner's own life that have relevance to a particular clinical situation. Commonly, learners initiate this type of opportunity when they reveal a personal experience that provokes a response, emotion, or crisis. In this instance, it is essential to assess the degree to which this revelation and response may impact patient care. More often, this situation affords an opportunity for learners to share clinical information and apply previously learned knowledge to the current situation. The CNS can take advantage of this by framing differences and similarities or deriving principles that are transferable to the current patient situation.

In light of the big-picture thinking that characterizes CNS practice, it is more reasonable to expect that the clinical leader will *initiate* a critical incident intervention in the face of tragic outcomes. For example, the sudden and unanticipated loss of a hospitalized child can provoke much personalization and emotion. Many nurses in the setting may be parents, and their attunement to the pain and suffering experienced by another parent will enhance their ability to connect and engage in extraordinary ways. Others at earlier developmental stages of practice may not yet have the capacity to respond in such a sensitive and involved manner. In those instances, the CNS must extend outward to include individuals in dialogue about the trajectory of engaging with patients and families in crisis. Timely, responsive, flexible, and sensitive coaching around critical incidents can foster an engaged stance required for humane and personalized care.

Strategies and Activities Linked to Principles of Adult Learning

Previously, several general learning principles and others more specific to adult learning were delineated as a theoretical/conceptual frame of reference for implementing the instructional or developmental role in CNS practice. Table 9.1 serves to correlate these principles with relevant learning strategies and activities that could be applied in practice.

EVALUATION

There is an abundance of literature regarding the importance of evaluating learning outcomes in practice (Abruzzese, 1996; Alspach, 1995; Avillion, 2001, 2004; Bastable, 2003; Billings & Halstead, 1998; Kirkpatrick,

1999; Snow, 2002; Spath, 2002). The critical elements about evaluation in practice reside in an ability to detect in real terms and in real time the learners' capacity to apply principles in practice. Recall that learning is evidenced only when one observes a change in behavior. Alspach (1995) describes four steps in an evaluation process that confirm the learner is able to translate principles into action: (1) measurement, (2), comparison, (3), appraisal, and (4) decision.

For example, at the first level, one could evaluate performance by detecting a learner's ability to simply measure. Using body weight as an example, it is easy to think about ways that one could evaluate a learner's ability to accomplish that skill. The second step of the process suggests then that the learner would be able to compare a measured outcome against an established standard for weight that is expressed in pounds or kilograms for different heights and ages. Next in the process, one would evaluate to determine if the learner can appraise the outcome. For example, he/she would interpret that the measured weight renders a patient overweight, underweight, or within normal range for their height and age. At the final stage of the process, the learner would be able to utilize the information acquired through the first three steps to make a decision or take some action about the finding. For example, they would decide that someone needed to gain weight and subsequently take action to establish a nutritional consult or engage in patient teaching.

Kirkpatrick (1999) provides another framework for guiding evaluation. This model is useful in that it directs the evaluator to get to a level of validating behavioral change and impact on outcomes. There are four levels of evaluation described by Kirkpatrick: reaction, learning, behavior, and results. Table 9.2 summarizes the key elements and characteristics of each level.

LEADING TO OUTCOME: THE UNIQUE MANIFESTATIONS OF CNS LEADERSHIP IN THE DEVELOPMENT OF OTHERS

One of the most unique features of the CNS role is the prevailing requirement and expectation that all action leads to outcome. Every assessment, plan, intervention, and consultation is directed toward enhancing quality, patient safety, and evidence-based practice. Thus, the work of engaging staff in learning is necessarily driven by these obligations and responsibilities.

Quality

The identification of nursing sensitive and multidisciplinary quality indicators has reframed the context of practice over the past few decades. Initially, the emphasis was placed on the study of processes and improvement

| Teaching/Learning Strategies and Activities Correlated With Principles of Adult Learning

PRINCIPLE	STRATEGIES AND ACTIVITIES
Adults need a reason for learning and are problem-centered learners.	■ Ask adult learners to identify problems that they perceive as most important and immediate in their work. ■ Focus instruction on that which is essential for successful job performance. ■ Initially, attend to learning needs and issues that are likely to be experienced on a daily basis; limit content to those areas with immediate applicability. ■ Use realistic case studies and actual work scenarios. ■ Provide meaningful rationale that substantiates the purpose for acquiring any given skill or knowledge.
Most adults are self-directed in their pursuit of learning.	■ Provide resources and learning aids that are readily available and support the learner's quest for "just-in-time" information. ■ Use a contract or timetable that articulates clear learning outcomes, yet allows the learner flexibility and options for accomplishing those aims.
Adults bring a variety of life and work experiences to any learning situation.	■ Use critical incident methodology to link personal experience with actual learning foci. ■ Design methods using small group discussion, rounds, case studies, or simulated role play to enable learners to link their past experience with current learning and facilitate transfer of understanding. ■ Contrast past and present working experience.
Adults are heterogeneous as learners and deserve respect as mature individuals.	■ Expect differences in opinions, interpretations, values, and viewpoints. Use this rich diversity of thinking to progress to nonlinear or creative learning options. ■ Avoid taking a dogmatic stance. ■ Relate to learners as adults and avoid hierarchical positioning as teacher over students. ■ Limit the use of arbitrary or unnecessary rules and policies in instructional venues.
Adults are voluntary learners.	■ Engage in conversation about what an individual aspires to accomplish by working in a given setting or organization.
Adults are voluntary learners *(continued)*	■ Engage in conversation about what an individual aspires to accomplish by working in a given setting or organization ■ Detect behavioral cues (e.g., apathy, failure to complete required assignments, etc.) that suggest that the learner's needs may not be adequately addressed. The default interpretation is that there is something wrong with the learner. Instead, probe to detect the utility of the instructional intervention. ■ Collaborate with the learner to brainstorm other options to accomplish the learning outcome
Learning occurs as a consequence of self-activity	■ Whenever possible be sure to use active learning methods ■ Avoid overutilization of passive observational learning experiences ■ Facilitate action, thinking, reflecting, doing, practicing, talking, utilizing repetitive opportunities for psychomotor skill acquisition, etc.
Learning is influenced by the environment within which it occurs	■ Encourage staff to ask questions and challenge current practice ■ Avoid the "blunting" phenomenon by suppressing enthusiasm that comes with accomplishment. It is not helpful to suggest that a newly acquired task or skill is really "no big deal" or to suggest that "after 100 times," one will get disenchanted or jaded. ■ Portray an impression of openness, acceptance, sensitivity and care ■ Adopt a nonjudgmental stance in working with learners. Avoid threatening language. ■ When engaged in an instructional activity, minimize distractions and fully attend to the learner

(continued)

| Teaching/Learning Strategies and Activities Correlated With Principles of Adult Learning (*continued*) |

PRINCIPLE	STRATEGIES AND ACTIVITIES
Learning is social and interactive	■ Use realistic case studies that require learners to think, apply principles, detect subtle changes, problem-solve, etc. ■ Bring together a small group of staff at differing stages of practice to interact around an interesting or challenging patient
Learning is social and interactive *(continued)*	■ Bring together a small group of staff at differing stages of practice to interact around an interesting or challenging patient ■ Exercise patience ■ Be constructive when delivering a critique ■ Use humor, have fun!
Learning is intentional and is influenced by the motivation and readiness of the learner	■ Suggest that learners keep a "tic" card in their pocket to jot down any intriguing findings for future instructional follow-up or dialogue ■ When rounding, ask about employee learning goals as well as their patient care goals. Correlate any potential learning opportunities with their assignment. ■ Influence assignment-making that fosters intrinsic motivation by assuring that learners achieve some consistent degrees of success
Learning is intentional and is influenced by the motivation and readiness of the learner	■ Counsel learners to keep performance expectations realistic. The work of the advanced beginner is a normal developmental trajectory and one should not ever be made to feel badly about their practice.
Learning is facilitated by positive and immediate feedback	■ Be generous in offering support, approval and praise ■ Provide criticism by first noting that which was done accurately/properly and then clarifying how to improve other aspects of performance ■ Plan or interject opportunities for learners to experience as much success as possible. This requires an ability to detect learner strengths and manipulate within the clinical environment to provide unique and interesting options. ■ Remember that development does not end when individuals complete orientation. It is affirming to detect progress and accomplishment among all levels of staff.
Learning is retainable and can be transferred to new situations	■ Review new concepts shortly after introduction ■ Summarize key instructional messages frequently and before proceeding to a new concept ■ Limit content to that which is necessary in a given situation. Do not overwhelm learners with unwarranted detail ■ Provide for adequate practice ■ Build learning activities on previous experiences. ■ Progress from simple to complex; or from concrete to abstract
Learning is inferred rather than observed	■ Use existing tools to document observations of learning accomplishment
Learning is influenced by the nature of the learning experience	■ Avoid reliance on any one instructional method, especially passive activities ■ Include learners' suggestions and preferences regarding learning activities and options ■ Inquire about discrepancies that may exist between old and new practices. Provide rationale for local differences. Avoid adopting a defensive posture.
Learning proceeds best when it is organized and clearly communicated	■ Use appropriate sequencing principles: easy to hard, simple to complex, concrete to abstract, first to last step. ■ Use retrievable learning aids to supplement content ■ Develop small units of instruction that are organized around one major principle or construct

| A Summary of Leveled Evaluation Approaches

LEVEL OF EVALUATION	CHARACTERISTICS OF THE EVALUATION APPROACH
Reaction	■ Reaction data is a measure of customer satisfaction. ■ Data have applicability for improving instructional methods and program revision. ■ End-of-program evaluation instruments are frequently used to assess what is commonly referred to as the "happiness factor." ■ Evaluation questions address presenter requirements (i.e., style, use of instructional aids, class timeliness, etc.). ■ Data are often gathered to assess the degree to which the instructor met the learning objectives. ■ Open-ended questions are included to solicit additional comments and suggestions. ■ Posttraining measurement may also be designed to occur several weeks after training has been conducted. This allows the learner to evaluate the instruction using their subsequent experience in practice as a context for satisfaction.
Learning	■ Serves to detect if the learner has actually learned anything as a consequence of the instructional activity. ■ Common methods include paper and pencil tests to validate cognitive knowledge, skill performance validation to assess psychomotor competency, or field observation to discern application of values or organizational beliefs/standards. ■ Best practice requires that there be a pre- and posttest; ideally validated with a control group.
Behavior	■ Determines whether learned knowledge and skill are actually applied in the workplace; also known as knowledge transfer. ■ Chart reviews and audits serve to verify if learned behaviors actually occur and are documented. ■ Other resources for data regarding behavior include: measurement of employee performance during drills and simulations; performance measured by 360-degree surveys; performance reported on annual evaluation instruments; or review of other records such as code cart checklists, quality control logs, etc.
Behavior *(continued)*	■ Best practice requires that baseline data are collected and compared with measures subsequent to instruction. ■ Unscheduled observations provide a more realistic evaluation of internalized behavior.
Results	■ Common indicators include: time savings, better quantity, improved quality, or personnel data (e.g., fewer injuries, less absenteeism, etc.). ■ Results evaluation can only be linked to instructional intervention when an appropriate and relevant terminal program objective is imbedded in the program. ■ Best practice requires that baseline data are collected and compared with measures subsequent to intervention.

thereof. Presently, the concern of providers, health care organizations, insurers, payers, recipients of health care, and others is focused on outcomes. This reality manifests its impact every day and in every setting where nursing and health care are delivered. Significant debate continues to persist concerning the appropriate identification and measurement of quality indicators. The numerous ways of considering indicators can lead to confusion and frustration with quality-improvement activities, especially as it relates to measurement and resource utilization. Yet, the prevailing interest among all involved parties is that the quest for quality is essential.

It is further understood that nursing makes a profound contribution to the well-being of patients and families.

Then, how does the CNS transcend the chasm between true interest and motivation toward improvement and the often prevailing sense of threat or frustration associated with measurement, tracking, and auditing? The dissonance represented by this question provides a focus for developmental intervention on the part of the CNS. Duffy (2002) articulates that, with clinical expertise, the CNS is viewed as a credible practitioner. From this power base, team members will be more apt to follow recommendations and suggestions. CNSs can set the tone for expected behaviors of team members in terms of open-mindedness and professionalism by way of their own demeanor (Saks, 1998). It is suggested that through mentoring, the CNS can help staff nurses develop the skills to take on additional responsibilities in the continued identification of quality indicators.

Evidence-Based Practice (EBP)

Nothing appears more essential to the CNS competencies than exhibiting a fully realized commitment to the utilization of evidence in practice. Repeatedly, the NACNS (2004) statement articulates the obligation to translate clinical expertise into nursing care provided either directly or via influence of nurses and nursing personnel through evidence-based nursing. This emphasis is a key feature that distinguishes the practice of CNSs from other clinical experts.

Several papers describe this critical obligation to enhance patient care by way of research utilization (Ervin, 2005; Ferguson & Day, 2004; Heitkemper & Bond, 2004; Newhouse, Dearholt, Poe, Pugh, & White, 2005; Stevens, 2005). Inherent therein are suggestions and direction with respect to the corollary developmental requirements that accompany the implementation of EBP strategies. Ervin (2005) identifies that CNSs typically have staff positions in which they interact with nurses in everyday practice. Because they usually do not have supervisory responsibilities for employees, this organizational relationship may be capitalized on to assist individual nurses to improve their skills through the mechanism of coaching and for the purpose of enhancing the use of empirical rationale for practice. Ervin suggests that a CNS can assist individuals or groups of nurses to establish plans for review of current literature. Another approach is for the CNS to organize a group of nurses to read a specific article or journal each month and prepare a written summary for the entire staff. It is also the role of the CNS to assist staff nurses in discriminating between evidence that has been accumulated using sound methods and analysis from that which is not as robust. In this capacity, the CNS may ask targeted questions that guide thinking about the implications of information for practice within the context of patients in the particular setting. CNSs serve as role models and motivators for others to become interested in seeking answers to complex problems. Analyzing and synthesizing literature are approaches to address these problems and enhance critical thinking and judgment. Any exercise that fosters healthy discourse and debate around evidence and best practice serves to enhance the intellect of those caring for patients. Embedding a stronger sensibility around asking better questions rather than sustaining an ideology of "dogma worship" will go far to facilitate the development of an informed workforce motivated by consistent attention to inquiry. Wisdom and improved intellectual capacity is not an outcome associated with being right at all times. Instead, wisdom is fostered by open dialogue and intellectual exchange of thoughts, ideas, and informed propositions.

Safety

One of the most compelling and current requirements in clinical settings across the country is the necessary attention and effort required to ensure that patients are safe while they are recipients of nursing and health care. Ebright and colleagues (Ebright, Patterson, Chalko, & Render, 2003; Ebright, Patterson, & Render, 2002) have provided some convincing evidence to suggest that a major developmental domain for CNS leadership is essential in four key areas: changing to a nonpunitive culture, learning about system complexity, learning about health care worker resiliency, and introducing change. They suggest that the CNS is in an excellent position to change the traditional culture of blame that typically surrounds error. An essential behavior in CNS practice is building and maintaining trust through relationships on a daily basis with patients, staff, and leadership. These relationships can serve to increase understanding from near miss or adverse events. The objective is to learn from these events and work collaboratively to eliminate those systems issues that precipitate the probability for error.

It is readily apparent that there exist gaps and disconnections that contribute to a practice environment characterized by complexity, hazards, and work-arounds. Identification of these gaps at the point of care is essential for improving safety. To accomplish this, the CNS can contribute by leading near-miss and adverse-event investigations. In this capacity, the CNS can influence others to view these processes as opportunities for learning rather than assigning blame. He/she can role model for all health care staff the acknowledgement and then the setting aside of hindsight and bias. Multidisciplinary collaboration should incorporate human factors science and the New Look Model (Ebright et al., 2002), which provides an easy-to-use framework for educating others about concepts related to complex system failure, as well as new approaches to safety.

CNSs are well positioned in organizations to study and detect how staff manages to navigate the complexity of the actual work environment. In the course of leading near-miss or adverse-event investigations, data can be derived that explains how staff react effectively and successfully to prevent an adverse event or minimize negative outcomes. These data can be used to design educational interventions or forums that highlight practitioner thinking, recognition, and actions. The utilization of storytelling, especially as the stories relate to successful "rescues," provide a powerful basis for studying the interface of systems processes.

Finally, it is suggested that CNSs are in a key position to not only respond to data and events but to anticipate and articulate the potential contribution of planned organizational changes that carry some degree of risk for creating new system gaps or latent failures (Ebright et al., 2002). Anticipating and preparing for how change might introduce new forms of complexity or latent failures is also needed to maintain safe environments.

SUMMARY

Given the current demands of the health care environment, CNSs are optimally positioned to apply their leadership, collaboration, and consultative competencies to the work of staff development. This work is consistent with standards set forth by the NACNS. The obligation to consistently and creatively transmit knowledge and skill development is most clearly apparent in the sphere of influence dedicated to nurses and nursing practice.

Theoretical and conceptual models related to the context of change, principles of teaching and learning, and leadership serve to frame strategies for engaging staff in learning as it relates to unique dimensions of CNS practice. Key interventions related to creating opportunities, coaching, mentoring, facilitating development around stages of practice, and utilization of specific strategies derived from fundamental adult learning principles are introduced to provide options for targeted learning needs. Two frameworks for evaluation are provided that validate learning outcomes and applicability in practice. Finally, the essential work of "leading to outcome" is described as a phenomenon that distinguishes CNS practice in health care settings.

DISCUSSION QUESTIONS

1. How does transformation differ from or relate to change?
2. Chaos theory and complexity science require leaders to alter their understanding of how change works. In this context, how does the CNS operationalize his/her role in relationship to change, the larger system, the staff, and the challenges that lie ahead? Frame the discussion in light of engaging staff in learning.
3. Identify at least three current educational practices or common instructional interventions that are counterintuitive to facilitating learning among advanced beginners.
4. How can the CNS collaborate with education specialists, clinical educators, and expert nurses to accomplish learning outcomes?
5. What factors commonly contribute to an outcome where education is used inappropriately to resolve a problem, issue, need, or gap?

6. What three evaluation strategies are least likely to be utilized in practice? How can the CNS go about implementing those strategies more effectively?

ANALYSIS/SYNTHESIS EXERCISES

1. Relate CNS competencies as described in the NACNS (2004) statement to the work of facilitating learning among clinical staff. What are the priorities in this domain of practice?
2. Reflect on the current environment where you work. Analyze the physical surroundings and psychosocial climate in terms of facilitating a successful learning encounter. Identify modifications or adjustments that are requisite for accomplishing meaningful learning outcomes.
3. Identify two different circumstances where you would engage in the work of mentoring or coaching. Analyze how the relationships would differ in each circumstance.

CLINICAL APPLICATION CONSIDERATIONS

1. Using the principles of teaching and learning, develop a learning intervention to resolve observed variability in the nursing care of a circumscribed population of patients. Assume that there exists a knowledge or skill deficit. For example, design a just-in-time learning intervention that reduces variability in the management of nausea.
2. Reflect on the talents and competencies of the nursing staff where you currently practice, and apply novice-to-expert theory to managing observed disillusionment among competent nurses.
3. Apply relevant learning principles that would enhance the development of a proficient nurse in terms of improving communication with physicians.
4. Construct a collaborative rounding model including a CNS and a nursing administrator that would serve to facilitate learning outcomes for new graduates.

REFERENCES

Abruzzese, R. S. (1996). *Nursing staff development: Strategies for success* (2nd ed.). St. Louis: Mosby.

Alspach, J. G. (1995). *The educational process in nursing staff development*. St. Louis: Mosby.

American Nurses Association. (2000). *Scope and standards of practice for nursing professional development*. Washington, DC: Author.

Avillion, A. E. (2001). *Core curriculum for staff development* (2nd ed.). Pensacola, FL: National Nursing Staff Development Organization.

Avillion, A. E. (2004). *A practical guide to staff development: Tools and techniques for effective education*. Marblehead, MA: HCPro.

Bastable, S. B. (2003). *Nurse as educator: Principles of teaching and learning for nursing practice* (2nd ed.). Boston: Jones and Bartlett.

Benner, P. (1984). *From novice to expert: Excellence and power in clinical nursing practice*. Menlo Park, CA: Addison-Wesley.

Benner, P., Tanner, C. A., & Chesla, C. A. (1996). *Expertise in nursing practice: Caring, clinical judgment, and ethics*. New York: Springer.

Billings, D. M., & Halstead, J. A. (1998). *Teaching in nursing: A guide for faculty*. Philadelphia: Saunders.

Clark, M. C. (1993). Transformational learning. In S. Merriam (Ed.), *An update on adult learning theory* (pp. 47–56). San Francisco: Jossey-Bass.

Cross, K. P. (1981). *Adults as learners: Increasing participation and facilitating learning*. San Francisco: Jossey-Bass.

Cunningham, L., & McNally, K. (2003). Improving organizational and individual performance through coaching. *Nurse Leader, 1*(6), 46–49.

Davis, B. G. (1995). *Tools for teaching*. San Francisco: Jossey-Bass.

Dewey, J. (1916). *Democracy and education*. New York: Macmillan.

Dewey, J. (1938). *Education and experience*. New York: Collier.

Dracup, K., & Bryan-Brown, C. W. (2004). From novice to expert to mentor: Shaping the future. *American Journal of Critical Care, 13*(6), 448–450.

Duffy, J. R. (2002). The clinical leadership role of the CNS in the identification of nursing-sensitive and multidisciplinary quality indicator sets. *Clinical Nurse Specialist, 16*(2), 70–76.

Ebright, P. R., Patterson, E. S., Chalko, B. A., & Render, M. L. (2003). Understanding the complexity of Registered Nurse work in acute care settings. *The Journal of Nursing Administration, 33*(12), 630–638.

Ebright, P. R., Patterson, E. S., & Render, M. L. (2002). The "new look" approach to patient safety: A guide for clinical nurse specialist leadership. *Clinical Nurse Specialist, 16*(5), 247–253.

Ervin, N. E. (2005). Clinical coaching: A strategy for enhancing evidence-based nursing practice. *Clinical Nurse Specialist, 19*(6), 296–301.

Ferguson, L. M., & Day, R. A. (2004). Supporting new nurses in evidence-based practice. *Journal of Nursing Administration, 34*(11), 490–492.

Fitzgerald, K. (2003). Instructional methods. In S. B. Bastable (Ed.), *Nurse as educator: Principles of teaching and learning for nursing practice* (2nd ed., pp. 355–388). Boston: Jones and Bartlett.

Galbraith, M. W. (1990). *Adult learning methods*. Malabar, FL: Kreiger Publishing.

Giles, P. F., & Moran, V. (1989). Preceptor program evaluation demonstrates improved orientation. *Journal for Nurses in Staff Development, 5*(1), 17–24.

Goleman, D. (1998). *Working with emotional intelligence*. New York: Banatam.

Greenleaf, R. K. (1996). *On becoming a servant leader*. San Francisco: Jossey-Bass.

Heitkemper, M. M., & Bond, E. F. (2004). Clinical nurse specialists: State of the profession and challenges ahead. *Clinical Nurse Specialist, 19*(3), 135–140.

Institute for Healthcare Improvement. (2006). *SBAR*. Retrieved January 12, 2009, from: http://www.ihi.org/ihi

Kirkpatrick, D. L. (1999). *Evaluating training programs: The four levels*. San Francisco: Berrett-Koehler.

Knowles, M. S. (1980). *The modern practice of adult education: From pedagogy to andragogy* (Rev. ed.). New York: Associated Press.

Lewin, K. (1951). *Field theory in social science*. New York: Harper & Row.

Maslow, A. H. (1970). *Motivation and personality*. New York: Harper and Row.

Merriam, S. B., & Brockett, R. G. (1997). *The profession and practice of adult education: An introduction*. San Francisco: Jossey-Bass.

Merriam-Webster's Online Dictionary. (2003). Retrieved January 12, 2009, from http://www.merriam-webster.com/dictionary/coach

Merriam-Webster's Online Dictionary. (2003). Retrieved January 12, 2009, from http://www.merriam-webster.com/dictionary/mentor

Merriam-Webster's Online Dictionary. (2003). Retrieved January 12, 2009, from http://www.merriam-webster.com/dictionary/preceptor

Millay, C. S. (1995). Planned change. In A. Marriner-Tomey (Ed.), *Case studies in nursing management: Practice, theory and research* (2nd ed., pp. 93–116). St. Louis: Mosby.

National Association of Clinical Nurse Specialists. (2004). *Statement on clinical nurse specialist practice and education* (2nd ed.). Harrisburg, PA: Author.

Newhouse, R., Dearholt, S., Poe, S., Pugh, L. C., & White, K. M. (2005). Evidence-based practice. *Journal of Nursing Administration, 35*(1), 35–40.

Peplau, H. (1965/2003). Specialization in professional nursing. *Clinical Nurse Specialist, 17*(1), 3–9.

Porter-O'Grady, T., & Malloch, K. (2003). *Quantum leadership: A textbook of new leadership*. Sudbury, MA: Jones and Bartlett.

Quinn, R. E. (2004). *Building the bridge as you walk on it: A guide for leading change*. San Francisco: Jossey-Bass.

Reinhard, S. C. (1988). Managing and initiating change. In E. J. Sullivan & P. J. Decker (Eds.), *Effective management in nursing* (2nd ed., pp. 93–119). Menlo Park, CA: Addison Wesley.

Robinson-Walker, C. (2004). Coaching: A tool for excellence in nursing leadership. *Voice of Nursing Leadership, 2*(11), 8–9.

Saks, N. (1998). Developing an integrated model for outcomes management. *Advanced Practice Nursing Quarterly, 4*(1), 27–32.

Skinner, B. F. (1974). *About behaviorism*. New York: Knopf.

Snow, C. (2002). Evaluation of staff education programs. In JCAHO (Ed.), *The Joint Commission guide to staff education* (pp. 53–63). Oakbrook Terrace, IL: Author.

Spath, P. L. (2002). *Guide to effective staff development in health care organizations*. San Francisco: Jossey-Bass.

Stevens, R. R. (2005). *Essential competencies for evidence-based practice in nursing*. San Antonio, TX: Academic Center for Evidence-Based Practice.

Thorndike, E. L., Bregman, E. D., Tilton, J. W., & Woodyard, E. (1928). *Adult learning*. New York: Macmillan.

Waddell, D. L., & Dunn, N. (2005). Peer coaching: The next step in staff development. *The Journal of Continuing Education in Nursing, 36*(2), 84–89.

Wilson, C. K., & Porter-O'Grady, T. (1999). *Leading the revolution in healthcare: Advancing systems, igniting performance* (2nd ed.). Gaithersburg, MD: Aspen.

Wlodkowski, R. J. (1990). Strategies to enhance adult motivation to learn. In M. W. Galbraith (Ed.), *Adult learning methods: A guide for effective instruction* (pp. 97–117). Malabar, FL: Kreiger Publishing.

Wright, D. (2004). Is education the answer? *Trend Lines, 15*(1), 1, 8.

10

Shaping Practice: Evidence-Based Practice Models

Lisa Hopp

Evidence-based practice (EBP) has become the mantra of health care in the first decade of the 21st century. In fact, some authors have declared that EBP is one of the most significant themes to ever develop in global health care (Rycroft-Malone, Bucknail, & Melynk, 2004). The forces driving the world's preoccupation with EBP include recognition that large margins of people do not receive recommended care and that more than a decade can pass before new discoveries become routine practice, as well as a number of sociopolitical factors. These include:

- Governments need to contain escalating health care costs.
- Recognition that reform must occur to change care processes and human resource management.
- Systems need to change to enable the way clinical knowledge is produced, critiqued, implemented, and evaluated in practice.
- Refocus on patient safety and patient-centeredness.

Like many movements, there are true, pseudo, and false claims of health care providers "doing evidence-based practice." Because of their skills and competencies in the patient, nurses/nursing practice, and organization/ system spheres of influence, clinical nurse specialists (CNSs) are particularly well-suited to authentically implement evidence in their own and others' practice.

Many authors and disciplines have defined EBP, but most definitions include three elements that inform and contribute to making decisions in clinical practice. That is, EBP occurs when clinicians make decisions using the best available evidence, their clinical expertise, and

patient preferences. Sackett, Rosenberg, Gray, Haynes, and Richardson (1996) wrote that evidence-based medicine is "the conscientious, explicit, and judicious use of current best evidence in making decisions about the care of individual patients. The practice of evidence-based medicine means integrating individual clinical expertise with the best available external clinical evidence from systematic research" (p. 71). DiCenso, Cullum, and Ciliska (1998) expanded upon this definition to include four elements that should inform clinical decision-making in nursing practice: best available evidence from research, patient preferences, clinical expertise, and available resources. Each element of this definition provides opportunities for CNSs to influence the health outcomes of patients. They need to develop competencies in the systematic search, retrieval, appraisal, synthesis, transfer, implementation, and evaluation of the best available evidence while integrating their tacit clinical knowledge and the preferences of the patient.

HISTORICAL BACKGROUND

EBP has both a long and short history beginning with Florence Nightingale but taking on "movement" status in the mid-1990s. For nursing, its origins can be attributed in part to Nightingale's work in the years after the Crimean war. She advocated for the proper generation, interpretation, and implementation of findings from research. Her knowledge of the scientific method and statistical procedures informed her efforts to influence how policy makers could use epidemiologic data to make decisions. She complained that the governmental ministers' lack of proper understanding of how the data they collected contributed to their failure to use the results to make decisions (McDonald, 2001).

The next significant activity occurred in the late 1970s and '80s when nursing leaders focused on models of research utilization. The CURN and WICHE projects were large-scaled efforts aimed at increasing nurses' use of research, but they did not emphasize exhaustive search and synthesis of the best available evidence, nor did they stress the integration of patient preferences and clinical expertise in the equation.

Nightingale's frustration with decision makers' neglect of the evidence was echoed some 80 years later when Archie Cochrane, a British epidemiologist and physician, criticized the medical community for its failure to use rigorous systematic reviews of available evidence to inform the decisions (Cochrane Collaboration, n.d.). Like Nightingale, he recognized that preventable infant deaths could be improved on a large scale if physicians based their decisions on the unused, but consistent, findings from several randomized controlled trials. Indeed, the subsequent efforts of the collaboration named after Cochrane were first aimed at assembling a registry of trials involving perinatal health. Cochrane emphasized the supremacy of the randomized controlled trial for determining the effect of treatments, publishing two hard criticisms of medicine in 1972 and 1979. He campaigned for the wide availability of systematic reviews and meta-analyses of multiple randomized controlled trials to inform treatment decisions (Cochrane Collaboration, n.d.). (Although he died in 1988 before his ideas became reality, the Cochrane Center, later renamed as the Cochrane Collaboration, launched in 1992. It has rapidly grown to be a multinational collaboration that includes the largest library of systematic reviews of effect, a database of controlled trials, and a variety of entities working to support EBP. During the same time period, York University established the Center for Research Dissemination [CRD] with a similar purpose of developing systematic reviews of evidence of treatment effectiveness. The CRD has continued to grow and has close links with the Cochrane and Campbell Collaborations, a collaboration aimed at evidence synthesis relevant to the social sciences).

While the Cochrane library contains some evidence that is directly related to the effects of nursing interventions, another organization evolved to more directly address problems relevant to nursing and nurse midwifery. In 1996, Alan Pearson and colleagues founded the Joanna Briggs Institute (JBI) in Adelaide, South Australia. JBI is an operational unit of the Royal Adelaide Hospital, the teaching hospital associated with the University of Adelaide. The institute was so named to pay homage to the first matron of nursing of the facility that provided the institute's initial funding

and continued support (Joanna Briggs Institute, n.d.). Like the Cochrane collaboration, JBI's purpose was to develop a worldwide collaboration to address global health priorities through synthesis and dissemination of systematic reviews of evidence. But the founders took a broader view of what constitutes legitimate evidence that included findings from rigorous research as well as from experience and expertise. They advocated that health care and nursing practice would benefit from syntheses of studies of feasibility, appropriateness, and meaningfulness as well as effectiveness. The collaboration now includes centers and members distributed throughout six continents of the world in both developed and developing nations. The work of the institute and collaborating centers continues its strong focus on nursing and nurse midwifery but embraces multiple health care disciplines. All of the JBI centers are developed on a framework of academic–clinical partnerships within their regional jurisdictions as well as research and development linkages among the international collaboration (JBI, n.d.). CNSs can consult the JBI Web pages to find a center near their area; at the time of this publication, five centers exist in North America.

In 1997, the Agency for Healthcare Research and Quality (AHRQ) began its initiative to support EBP in the United States. While the mission of AHRQ is broad and includes all aspects of supporting health care quality and safety, it began awarding 5-year contracts to EBP centers in the United States and Canada to produce technology assessment, health reports, and systematic reviews that have particular clinical, social, or economic importance. The completed electronic reports are freely available on the AHRQ Web site (http://www.ahrq.org/clinic/epcindex.htm).

The Institute of Medicine (IOM) series of reports about the safety of patients in the hospital had profound impact on accelerating interest in EBP in the United States. The authors estimated that on the whole, only about 55% of Americans received recommended care, that inadequate care resulted in 18,000 unnecessary deaths annually from myocardial infarction, and on the average, it takes 17 years before a new discovery becomes routine practice (IOM, 2003). Subsequent to these reports, the IOM and other organizations have called for significant changes to accelerate the integration of evidence into practice.

CNSs are poised to play a significant role in the next chapter of EBP in North America and other countries where this model of advance practice exists. Many health care agencies continue to struggle with the transfer of evidence from its generation and synthesis to the everyday practice of clinicians. CNSs practice nursing at the intersections of disciplines, of science, clinical expertise, patients, and other nursing professionals; thus, they are the ideal candidates to accelerate the complex and messy process of evidence utilization.

CONCEPTUAL/THEORETICAL SUPPORT FOR EBP AND CNS PRACTICE

Many models have emerged to guide EBP. Most of them reflect five basic steps—posing a question, searching for evidence, critically appraising the evidence, implementing the recommendations of the evidence, and evaluating the outcomes. These steps are parallel to the nursing process (see Table 10.1).

The models can be differentiated based on their focus and scope, their degree of conceptual and empirical support, and how they can be operationalized (see Table 10.2).

Two of these models, Promoting Action on Research Implementation in Health Services (PARIHS) and JBI, are particularly fitting for CNS practice and are discussed in more depth here. To learn more about other models, readers can refer to the original publications or descriptions in texts focused specifically on EBP.

Promoting Action on Research Implementation in Health Services

Kitson, Harvey, and McCormack (1998) introduced the PARIHS model in an effort to describe the complexities of implementing evidence into practice. They argued that superficial, linear models were inadequate to help clinicians successfully drive the change process. The research and development team at the Royal College of Nursing Institute in London have continued to refine the model based on a series of concept analyses addressing each of the elements of the model, retrospective data analysis, and a descriptive study to evaluate its content validity (Rycroft-Malone, 2004). In addition, a number of investigators, including Health Services Research and Development Services project teams within the U.S. Veterans Affairs, have used the model to frame evidence implementation studies (Brown & McCormack, 2005;

Doran & Sidani, 2007; U.S. Department of Veterans Affairs, 2006).

The model predicts that successful implementation of research is a function of a dynamic relationship of three elements: evidence, context, and facilitation. These elements exist on a low to high continuum within a health system; success is more likely when all three elements are strong. CNSs can impact all three elements and their subelements if they employ competencies to shift or maintain evidence, context, and facilitation toward the high end of the continuum.

Rycroft-Malone, Seers, et al. (2004) conducted a concept analysis of evidence and presented a convincing argument that legitimate evidence includes not only the findings from research but also local data, professional knowledge and clinical experience, and patient experience and preference. The interaction among these forms of evidence is complex and untidy. Rycroft et al. stressed that nurses must assess the value and weight of each information source according to criteria before entering them into the decision-making process in order to legitimize each source. In addition, health care providers must strive to use the most robust evidence to inform practice.

Research is generally regarded as the most important source of information for EBP. Indeed, some equate EBP with research-based practice and regard the randomized controlled trial as the only believable source of evidence. Rycroft-Malone, Seers, et al. (2004) and many others have argued for a far more pluralistic view that endorses many other forms of research evidence. Nonetheless, health care providers must critically appraise and weigh the quality and strength of the research and its applicability. Examples of criteria embedded in the PARIHS model characteristic of low-level research-based evidence criteria include poorly conceived, designed, or executed research or when research is seen as certain or unequivocal proof. On the other hand, examples of high-level research-based evidence criteria

10.1 | Comparison of the Nursing and EBNP Process

NURSING PROCESS	EBNP PROCESS
Assess	Formulate question based on baseline data/situation analysis
Diagnose	Formulate question based on baseline data/situation analysis
Plan	Transfer evidence by designing interventions and systems based on best available evidence, patient preference, and clinical expertise
Implement	Implement these interventions using evidence-based strategies
Evaluation	Measure outcomes

Comparison of Select EBNP Models Developed or Revised Since 1990

MODEL	FOCUS/SCOPE	EMPIRICAL/THEORETICAL SUPPORT	OPERATIONAL TOOLS	COMMENTS
ACE Star		Used to guide clinical implementation projects but limited published empirical or theoretical support.	EBP competency statements derived from iterative consensus process of invited U.S. clinical and academic experts in progress. Testing of an inventory of EBP readiness in progress.	A practical model that describes the steps commonly associated with the evidence-based process. Competency statement and inventory may be helpful in guiding CNSs in their own and others' development. Model would be stronger with greater empirical and theoretical support available.
Iowa	■ A schematic algorithm that begins with problem or knowledge-focused triggers and decision algorithm leading to development and implementation of guidelines. ■ Aimed at facilitating decisions of teams.	Developed based on experiences; pragmatic approach that has been used extensively to run unit-based projects and to guide development activities.	Toolkit available for purchase.	A practical model that helps structure the decisions relevant to evidence implementation; represents process in a highly linear manner. Model would be stronger with greater empirical and theoretical support available.
Stetler	■ Refinement of research utilization model to include individual and groups as well as organizational use of evidence. ■ Phased approach with focus on critical thinking throughout the process and a greater emphasis on synthesis.	Pragmatic model that integrated a variety of theoretical underpinnings; refined in collaboration with CNSs and reflects the shift from research utilization (RU) to EBP; broad application to all forms of practice.	Detailed explanation and tips for each phase included in publication.	Assumptions well-explicated; revised model reflects evolution of thinking about RU; bears the wisdom of experiences long involved in bridging research-practice gap.
Rosswurm & Larrabee	■ Blends steps of EBP process and Roger's diffusion of innovation theory. ■ Aimed at organizational diffusion of change.	Theoretical support based on Roger's Diffusion theory; used to guide implementation projects.	Critical Appraisal worksheet cited provided in original article.	This model appeals to many who understand Roger's Diffusion of Innovations model; has been used in evaluation work.
Dobbins et al.	■ Aimed at dissemination and utilization of research findings in clinical decision making and health policy. ■ Built on Roger's five-stage Diffusion of Innovations model.	Incorporates Roger's theoretical work with evidence from systematic reviews of research implementation.	Lists of strategies based on systematic reviews.	Model appealing for changing health policy; strength is in the incorporation of synthesized evidence from implementation research.

PARIHS	■ Comprehensive organizational model aimed at describing interactions and complexities of changing practice and moving evidence into practice. ■ Weighs factors that contribute to the relative strength and relationships among evidence, context, and facilitation.	Extensive concept analyses for the three major elements of the model; validation study; used to guide a variety of implementation studies and practice development.	Self-assessment tool under development to aid strategy planning.	This model has particular appeal for CNS practice and warrants consideration. CNSs are prepared to move organizations toward the high end of evidence, context, and facilitation; model fits how CNSs advance nursing practice via the three spheres of influence.
JBI	■ Comprehensive, cyclical model that reflects the iterative nature of EBP. Incorporates diverse types of evidence to answer many types of clinical questions. ■ Aim is to improve global health through tools available to aid EBP implementation at multiple levels from individuals to countries.	Based on examination of literature and broad experience in leading global efforts in the research and development of EBP; research in progress to evaluate the effectiveness of tools.	Robust, comprehensive tool set for each stage of the EBP process, including software for systematic reviews, critical appraisal, preappraised sources of evidence, systematic reviews, best practice sheets, implementation and evaluation tools, and searching and providing evidence sources to evaluation of evidence utilization.	

ACE = Academic Center for Evidence-Based Practice Web site (http://www.acestar.uthscsa.edu/), Iowa.
Iowa is from "Infusing Research Into Practice to Promote Quality Care," by M. Titler, C. Kleiber, V. Steelman, C. Goode, B. Rakel, J. Barry-Walker, et al., 1994, *Nursing Research, 43,* 307–313; Stetler is from "Updating the Stetler Model of Research Utilization to Facilitate Evidence-Based Practice," by C. Stetler, 2001, *Nursing Outlook, 49,* 272–279;
Rosswurm & Larrabee is from "A Model for Change to Evidence-Based Practice," by M. A. Rosswurm and J. H. Larrabee, 1999, *Image: Journal of Nursing Scholarship, 31,* 317–322.
Dobbins et al. is from "A Framework for the Dissemination and Utilization of Research for Health-Care Policy and Practice," by M. Dobbins, D. Ciliska, R. Cockerill, J. Barnsley, and A. DiCenso, 2002, *The Online Journal of Knowledge Synthesis for Nursing, 9,* 7.
PARIHS = Promoting Action on Research Implementation in Health Services, is from "The PARIHS Framework—A Framework for Guiding the Implementation of Evidence-Based Practice," by J. Rycroft-Malone, 2004, *Journal of Nursing Care Quality, 19,* 297–304.
JBI = Joanna Briggs Institute, is from "The JBI Model of Evidence-Based Healthcare," by A. Pearson, R. Wiechula, A. Court, and C. Lockwood, 2005, *International Journal of Evidence Based Healthcare, 3,* 207–215.

include studies that are well-conceived, designed, and executed and studies in which research evidence is seen as one part of a decision, when it is judged as relevant, and when investigators acknowledge the lack of certainty inherent in research (Rycroft-Malone, 2004).

Even muddier than research-based evidence is the role and critical appraisal of the clinical expertise and patient/client preference. Rycroft-Malone (2004) acknowledged that the discipline is in the early stages of explicating and testing the meaning of clinical expertise. In order for individual expertise to be considered credible, this knowledge needs to be consciously explicated, analyzed, exposed to external sources of critique, and affirmed by consensus.

Like clinical expertise, the discipline does not yet fully understand the role of patient/client preferences as a source of evidence or its influence in evidence-based decision making. Nurses and CNSs have the moral and ethical obligation to meld the patient/client's interest into the design of any assessment, intervention, or evaluation process, but the mechanisms to do this are more reliant on the expertise of the caregiver than hard and fast rules. In addition, CNSs can use syntheses of qualitative studies of patient experiences to inform their understanding of patient preferences. In some countries, mechanisms exist to engage consumers in the development of clinical practice guidelines (CPGs) and systematic reviews. As CNSs analyze and appraise CPGs, they should judge the degree that patients as stakeholders have been involved in the construction of the guideline (AGREE Collaboration, 2004). PARIHS model criteria indicating a low level on the patient preference continuum include patient preferences not valued as evidence or seen as the only type of evidence; those indicating a high level include multiple biographies used, partnerships with health care professionals in place, and patient preferences judged as relevant and importance weighted.

The second major theme of the PARIHS model is context, which is defined as the setting where people receive their health care services or where individuals and teams implement the EBP change. In their concept analysis, McCormack et al. (2002) contended that when organizations are strong in culture, leadership, and evaluation they more likely support getting evidence into practice. For example, cultures will be more successful if they promote learning; can self-define prevailing beliefs and values; allocate human, financial, and equipment resources; and align initiatives with strategic goals. Leadership rated on the high end of the continuum would be characterized by transformational styles; role clarity; effective teamwork; effective organizational structures; democratic decision making; and enabling and empowering in the teaching, learning, and managing processes. Similarly, leaders who are autocratic, unclear about roles, lack teambuilding

skills, and are didactic in their teaching, learning, and management skills will be less successful in evidence implementation. The third component of context is evaluation. Organizations that use multiple sources and methods (clinical, performance, economic, experience evaluations) to give feedback to individuals, teams, and systems will be more successful than those that use narrow, single-method approaches or none at all (Rycroft-Malone, 2004). The model suggests that CNSs who lead and support other leaders to move toward the high end of the leadership continuum will promote a culture conducive to getting evidence into practice.

The third theme of the PARIHS model is facilitation, defined as enabling others or making easier the process of implementing evidence (Harvey et al., 2002). CNSs can directly act as facilitators to implement evidence into practice. The model predicts that they will be most successful when they act more holistically (as opposed to focused on a specific task) to enable others through sustained partnerships and use adult learning approaches to teaching and a wide range of skills to support and enable others. Skilled facilitators adjust their role based on the needs of the learners and the phase of the project (Rycroft-Malone, 2004).

In summary, the PARIHS model suggests that CNSs will be more successful when they select the most robust evidence to inform practice; support a learning culture that is characterized by strong, transformational leadership with a capacity to appropriately evaluate outcomes of change and implementation; and act to facilitate implementation of evidence in a skillful, fluid, and holistic manner (see Table 10.3) (Rycroft-Malone, 2004).

Joanna Briggs Institute (JBI) Model

The second model that merits further discussion is the JBI model. This model is quite different from the PARIHS framework because it aims to improve global health rather than implement evidence in a local situation and has multiple tools to make the model operational. Its developers define EBP in a manner consistent with previously stated definitions. That is, EBP is clinical decision making that incorporates the best available evidence, the context of care, client preference, and professional judgment (Pearson, Wiechula, Court, & Lockwood, 2005). The model represents the EBP as a four-component process of evidence generation, synthesis, transfer, and utilization to achieve global health. Clinicians and/or consumers identify questions, concerns, or interests relevant to health care, and evidence and knowledge are generated to effectively meet these needs in feasible and meaningful ways. The evidence is then synthesized and transferred to health care providers who use and evaluate the impact on health outcomes. CNSs can play a role in each phase of the cycle,

10.3 | Strategies for CNS Implementation of Evidence—Application of PARIHS Model

EVIDENCE

- Select questions that are highly relevant to the population and/or care unit
- Seek highest quality synthesized evidence sources when available
- Consider all legitimate sources of evidence (feasibility, applicability, meaningfulness, and effectiveness), matching type of evidence and clinical question
- Use standardized tools to appraise all sources
- Provide preappraised sources to front-line staff
- Consider the magnitude of the evidence
- Develop mechanisms to incorporate patient preference into decision making, including evidence from systematic reviews of meaningfulness
- Maintain an openness to discussing tacit clinical knowledge; seek critique from and consensus with others

CONTEXT

- Participate and advocate for transformational leadership models
- Advocate for adequate staff access to computers and the Internet
- Build relationships with nurse researchers to facilitate a climate of investigation
- Develop programs that are keenly relevant to staff to ignite their interest in EBP
- Use audit and feedback to build a culture of evidence and evaluation
- Advocate for and request information system support to enable data mining prospectively and retrospectively
- Develop EBP skills of key leaders
- Collaborate with administrators to develop appropriate skill mixes to support EBP
- Provide outcome feedback to nursing leaders to demonstrate capacity and outcomes of EBP
- Advocate for information systems that have the capacity to bring evidence summaries to the point of care as well as cues and prompts within electronic plans of care

FACILITATION

- Use multiple strategies to build staff skills that are highly interactive; avoid passive didactic strategies
- Assess and enhance search skills of databases that are appropriate for the point of care
- Build mechanisms to enhance access to librarian resources and professional services of library scientists
- Develop peer experts that are recognized for their EBP skills
- Provide concise preappraised summaries of evidence on the burning topics, making the evidence quality and source explicit
- Incorporate cues and prompts to remind providers of key interventions
- Build policies that incorporate the best available evidence; make the evidence source and quality explicit

from generating knowledge through research; synthesizing research through systematic reviews; transferring knowledge through education; advocating for and planning information systems; and facilitating evidence utilization through practice change, evaluation of process, systems, and outcomes, and embedding changes within the system. The model is based on the premise that consumers and health care providers are interested in questions that relate to the feasibility, appropriateness, meaningfulness, and effectiveness of interventions (Pearson et al., 2005).

APPLICATION TO CNS PRACTICE

According to all conceptual models, the EBP process begins when health care providers question the usual and standard approaches to practice. Regardless of the sphere of influence or stage in the nursing process, CNSs continuously reflect upon their practice and look for opportunities for improvement. One can argue that nearly every stage of the nursing process and most of CNS competencies can be related to EBP. For example, when conducting assessments of the patient, nursing personal, or organizational problems, CNSs use tools and methods based on the best available evidence of sensitivity, specificity, positive and negative predictive value, and reliability. Their choices are also affected by the feasibility and understanding of the resources and context. The interventions that they choose are based on the best available evidence from research, their clinical expertise, and the patient or client preferences. In the nursing personnel and organizational spheres of influence the meaning of client preferences includes the preferences and needs of nurses and the system. When they implement the evidence-based interventions directly or indirectly, they consider the evidence that supports particular strategies to facilitate change, the context that influences the probability of success, and the tools and skills to facilitate changing practice. Finally, they use valid and reliable measurements of outcomes and generate local data to feedback into the EBP cycle (see Table 10.4).

Both the PARIHS and JBI models provide a framework and tools that are compatible and useful to this cycle of evidence-based improvement and innovation.

An Attitude of Inquiry and Asking Questions

This attitude of clinical curiosity and skepticism is critical to advanced nursing practice. Examples of CNS patient/client sphere competencies that relate to clinical inquiry include identifying the need for new assessments, selecting evidence-based nursing interventions that target etiologies, and choosing appropriate methods to evaluate outcomes. Similarly, the nurse and organizational spheres of influence require CNSs to question standard and usual practice. Examples of nurses and nursing practice–related competencies include using/designing methods and instruments to assess outcomes related to nursing practice within and across units of care; using/designing appropriate methods and instruments to assess knowledge, skills, and practice competencies of nurses; and identifying needed changes in equipment or other products based on evidence, clinical outcomes, and cost-effectiveness. Examples of organization and system sphere of influence competencies include using and designing system-level assessment methods and instruments to identify organization structures and functions that impact nursing practice and nurse-sensitive outcomes, diagnosing variations in organizational culture that positively or negatively affect outcomes, and developing or influencing system-level policies that affect innovation and programs of care. These competencies require that CNSs first pose questions that lead to the search, selection, and application of evidence in order to use the best assessment tools to assess, intervene, and evaluate outcomes.

CNSs employ an attitude of clinical inquiry to formulate a specific question that will drive the rest of the EBP process. These so-called foreground questions are those that are searchable and lead to particular types of evidence sources. Foreground questions address issues related to diagnosis, prognosis, harm, effects of interventions, and economic impact. Background questions are those that are broader, more descriptive in nature and more likely addressed by information found in textbooks or similar resources. For example, a background question related to the patient sphere of influence might be, "How does smoking lead to chronic bronchitis and emphysema?" and a foreground question might be, "What is the effect of inspiratory muscle training verses general exercise on inspiratory muscle strength and endurance in patients with chronic bronchitis and emphysema?" The CNS would most likely answer the background question with a summary of the basic science and theory about how smoking leads to destruction of lung parenchyma and the subsequent mechanical impact of thoracic hyperinflation. However, the foreground question about effectiveness of treatments is best answered by a systematic review with meta-analysis of randomized controlled trials. Questions related to the effect of interventions can be specified using a PICO format, where P corresponds to the population of interest, I represents the intervention or exposure in question, C is the comparison intervention or control, and O is outcome.

Other foreground questions relate to the meaning of health and illness as experienced by patients. These questions are best answered with metasyntheses of qualitative studies or within a comprehensive systematic review. An example of a meaningfulness question might be, "What is the meaning of breathlessness in patients with chronic obstructive pulmonary disease who experience an exacerbation?" These questions are best formed using a PIC format, where P represents participants, I corresponds to the phenomena of interest, and C represents context or, alternatively, a two-part approach framed by situation and population (Dicenso, Guyatt, & Ciliska, 2005). Readers can consult many excellent textbooks and other references for templates to help formulate searchable questions.

Searching and Appraising the Evidence

The next phase of the EBP process is to search and critically appraise the evidence. The PARIHS model predicts that when the evidence from research is strong, evidence is more likely to become part of practice. Therefore, CNSs need to know what types of evidence will answer their questions, where and how to search for the evidence, and how to critically appraise the evidence to inform their selection. The search strategy is structured by keywords and synonyms derived from the PICO question and conducted in a step-wise manner that will most likely lead to the highest level of

10.4 Select *CNS Outcomes and Competencies Related to EBP

CNS OUTCOMES	CNS COMPETENCIES	EBP APPLICATION/EXAMPLES
Patient/Client Sphere		
1. Diagnoses are accurately aligned with assessment data and etiologies.	Conducts comprehensive, holistic wellness and illness assessments using known or innovative evidence-based techniques, tools, and methods.	Selects and uses (e.g., fall, pressure ulcer, venothrombosis) risk assessment tools based on critical appraisal of measurement qualities (sensitivity, specificity, positive and negative predictive ability).
2. Nursing interventions target specified etiologies.	Selects evidence-based interventions that target etiologies of illness or risk behaviors.	Identifies specific modifiable risk factors (e.g., balance, gait, immobility) based on application of risk assessment tool.
3. Prevention, alleviation, and/or reduction of symptoms, functional problems, or risk behaviors are achieved.	Incorporates evidence-based nursing interventions within a specialty population.	Selects interventions (e.g., medication modification, bed surface, mobility program) to modify specific risk based on a critical appraisal of sources, transparency in methods, and fit with patient preferences.
4. Unintended consequences and errors are prevented.	Develops interventions that enhance the attainment of predicted outcomes while minimizing unintended consequences.	Uses internal and external data (e.g., documentation of risk modification or observational data) to identify common rates and sources of errors or complications to develop preventative approaches.
5. Predicted and measurable nurse-sensitive patient outcomes are attained through evidence-based practice.	Before designing new programs, identifies, collects, and analyzes appropriate data on the target population that serve as the basis for demonstrating CNS impact on program outcomes.	Identifies a need for change and establishes a baseline by conducting a baseline audit of process and outcome or analyzing available baseline data (e.g.., used JBI's PACES and POOL audit/feedback tool to identify nursing process and patient outcomes related to falls, pressure ulcer, catheter-related infections). Compares institutional data with available external data or benchmarks (e.g., compare fall, pressure ulcer and catheter infection rates with national and international benchmarks).
	Selects, develops and/or applies appropriate methods to evaluate outcomes of nursing interventions.	Uses valid, reliable, specific, and sensitive measures of outcomes (e.g., CDC criteria for hospital-acquired infections, National Pressure Ulcer Prevention Advisory Panel staging criteria).
	Documents and disseminates the results of innovative care.	Presents poster/paper in collaboration with staff at local, regional, national, or international event to share findings. Writes publication based on project.

(continued)

Select 'CNS Outcomes and Competencies Related to EBP (*continued*)

CNS OUTCOMES	CNS COMPETENCIES	EBP APPLICATION/EXAMPLES
Nurses/Nursing Practice Sphere		
1. Evidence-based practices are used by nurses.	Uses/designs methods and instruments to assess patterns of outcomes related to nursing practice within and across units of care.	Gathers process and outcome data using valid and reliable tools; develops charts and data displays to determine patterns (e.g., develops run-charts to relate process and outcome trends related to venothrombosis, pressure ulcers, etc.).
2. The research and scientific base for innovations is articulated, understandable, and accessible.	Mentors nurses to critique and apply research evidence to nursing practice.	Conducts EBP rounds with small groups of nurses to specify PICO questions; uses rapid appraisal checklists to appraise synthesized sources of evidence or individual reports of research when synthesized sources are unavailable; advocates for Internet access and/or creates space on intranet for staff access to preappraised sources, such as JBI's Best Practice Sheets.
	Anchors nursing practice to evidence-based information to achieve nurse-sensitive outcomes.	Attends systematic review training and conducts a systematic review related to a relevant problem; collaborates with others to design policies based on synthesized evidence; imbeds sources and levels of evidence with policy recommendations; conducts audit and feedback cycles to determine care unit's effectiveness.
3. Educational programs that advance the practice of nursing are developed, implemented, evaluated, and linked to evidence-based practice and effects on clinical and fiscal outcomes.	Develops and implements educational programs that target the needs of staff to improve nursing practice and patient outcomes. Assists staff in the development of innovative, cost-effective patient/client programs of care. Creates an environment that stimulates self-learning and reflective practice. Mentors nurses to acquire new skills and develop their careers. Disseminates results to stakeholders.	Uses an "academic detailing" approach to engage staff in learning evidence-based practice innovations (e.g., offering one-on-one and small group sessions based on unit of care needs, providing short summaries of evidence and tips for implementation via a monthly EBP newsletter). Provides consultation on costs/benefits of changing a nursing practice based on a comprehensive systematic review that includes an economic evaluation. Designs a merit-based system of reward that includes recognition of staff's participation in self-learning activities (e.g., criteria include participation in PICO and EBP rounds, rapid appraisals of evidence sources, evidence-based policy development, etc.); designs or makes accessible distance learning self-learning modules about EBP (e.g., collaborates with librarian to create an online module about searching for evidence). Mentors small groups of nurses of varying expertise to develop EBP skills; leads team to develop, implement, and evaluate an EBP quality improvement practice change and helps them publish and present their findings.

Organization/System Sphere

1. Patient care processes reflect continuous improvements that benefit the system.	Contributes to the development of multidisciplinary standards of practice and evidence-based guidelines for care, such as pathways, care maps, and benchmarks. Evaluates multidisciplinary EBP resources; collaborates to develop a proposal to integrate information systems to enhance access to EBP resources at the point of care; implements plan to integrate these EBP systems into daily decision-making processes (e.g., considers systems such as JBI Connect™, InfoPOEMS™, and Pepid™).
2. Evidence-based, best practice models are developed and implemented.	Develops or influences system-level policies that will affect innovation and programs of care. Develops system-wide guideline for policy development that requires transparency in methods and information sources; advocates that developers of major practice changes study the impact of the change on nursing work flow and patterns before sustaining the change (e.g.., pilot test and evaluate impact of evidence-based hand-off process change before implementing it system-wide).
3. Change strategies are integrated throughout the system.	Implements methods and processes to sustain evidence-based changes to nursing practice, programs of care, and clinical innovation. Develop a proposal for a EBP practice council within a shared governance model to influence implementation of EBP within a system; frame implementation of the EBP practice council with a model such as PARIHS and/or JBI.

*Outcomes and competency statements are verbatim from the *NACNS Statement on Clinical Nurse Specialist Practice and Education* (2nd ed.), by National Association of Clinical Nurse Specialists, 2004, Harrisburg, PA: Author; statements and examples are selected as illustration and are not meant to be a comprehensive list.

evidence. That is, they would first search for a high-quality clinical practice guideline based on meta-analyses or systematic reviews. If no high-quality guideline exists, they would search for a systematic review. If no synthesized sources exist, they would seek individual reports of research.

Unfortunately, no single search strategy or database exists to find the best available evidence. Rather, CNSs need to know where to look and how to search. CPGs are inventoried at the Agency for Healthcare Quality's Web site, http://www.guidelines.gov/. Because these guidelines vary in their quality, users must take care to critically evaluate them by first screening the many guidelines that may exist for a particular condition or problem using the "compare" tool to screen, and then closely appraising those they select from the first-pass screening. The Registered Nurses of Ontario have published many high-quality CPGs relevant to both general and specialized nursing practice, and electronic versions are freely available to the public at http://www.rnao.org under their best practice guideline pages. Other global organizations produce quality CPGs, such as the National Institute for Clinical Excellence in the United Kingdom (http://www.nice.org.uk/) and the New Zealand Guidelines Group (http://www.nzgg.org.nz/index.cfm). In the United States, many professional societies create guidelines that can be found online. However, because these organizations have no standard criteria or approach, readers must critically appraise the rigor of these CPGs. Links to many organizations that produce guidelines throughout the world can be found on the links page of the JBI Web site (http://www.joannabriggs.edu.au). CNSs can look for systematic reviews using bibliographic databases or at sites that publish systematic reviews such as Cochrane, JBI, and AHRQ Web sites.

Both the PARIHS and JBI models of EBP stress a pluralistic view of what constitutes legitimate evidence. However, both models address the need to be both comprehensive in the search and to judge the strength of the evidence in order to determine the *best available* evidence. They both underline the importance of selecting and blending the types of evidence that will appropriately answer a particular question. For example, questions related to effectiveness of an intervention will best be answered by a systematic review of randomized controlled trials (usually ranked at the top of any evidence hierarchy), but questions related to the appropriateness of an intervention may be better answered with local data in conjunction with the consensus of local experts. Regardless of the type of best available evidence, it is imperative that the methods, source, quality, and strength of the evidence are transparent to the users.

Because evidence sources vary widely in their quality, CNSs need to use standardized approaches to critically appraise the evidence they find. Clinical practice guidelines can be evaluated using the Appraisal of Guidelines Research and Evaluation (AGREE) instrument developed by an international collaboration of researchers and policy makers (AGREE Collaboration, 2004). Systematic reviews and individual reports of research can be appraised with tools developed by the Joanna Briggs Institute Rapid Appraisal Program (RAPid) (http://www.joannabriggs.edu.au/services/rapid.php) or the Critical Appraisal Skills Programme (CASP) tools developed by the Public Health Research Unit of the United Kingdom National Health Service (http://www.phru.nhs.uk/Pages/PHD/resources.htm). Essential criteria for any synthesized source are that the methods are transparent and there is evidence of the evidence. For example, if an organization or author makes a claim of "best practice" or that they have published a guideline but do not include a discussion of the protocol for the search or mention criteria for including and excluding evidence, the source cannot be judged for how it could be considered "best available." Similarly, if a guideline does not identify the level of the evidence using a ranking system, one cannot judge the quality information supporting the guideline.

Evidence Synthesis and Transfer

If the search and appraisal process has produced an excellent CPG or systematic review the next step is to transfer the evidence to practice. If the search does not net a synthesized source, CNSs may rely upon the next best available source or plan to conduct a systematic review. In order to conduct systematic reviews, CNSs and other investigators should seek appropriate training and will likely need software to aid the process. The Joanna Briggs Institute and its collaborating centers offer periodic systematic review training. In addition, JBI has published a suite called the System for the Unified Management of the Review and Assessment of Information (SUMARI), which allows users to develop a protocol; manage bibliographic references; and analyze quantitative, qualitative, and economic evidence, and text and opinion through its four analytical applications. If users wish to submit protocols for peer review and publish systematic reviews through JBI, they must first be certified by successfully attending a training workshop. The Cochrane Collaboration also has freeware available to conduct meta-analyses of randomized controlled trials with an accompanying user's manual and resources. Visitors can find links to a variety of workshops and resources on the Cochrane Web site. Alternatively, JBI includes use of the Cochrane freeware, Review Manager (RevMan), in its training. In order to conduct a Cochrane review, authors must submit protocols and reports for peer review to a specific Cochrane Review Group. Other entities produce and publish high-quality systematic reviews using other methods and tools.

The transfer of evidence into practice is one of the more challenging aspects of EBP. Tools for transfer include clinical practice guidelines or other condensed information sources such as the Oncology Nursing Society's Putting Evidence into Practice (PEP) series, JBI's Best Practice Information Sheets, the American Association of Critical Care Nurse's Practice Alerts, or other commercially available products such as POEM™—Patient-Oriented Evidence that Matters. These transfer tools must meet quality criteria, including transparency in methods and evidence quality ratings, but they help solve the issue of putting the evidence in the hands of clinicians at or near the point of care—a key issue in moving EBP forward. CNSs may find that having clinical practice guidelines available via a hand-held device is helpful to inform their practice. This has yet to become a broadly used technology by frontline nurses.

CNSs play a key role in the transfer of evidence. They fit the role of "knowledge broker" through multiple competencies. A CNS incorporates evidence into nursing interventions within specialty populations (patient sphere); draws conclusions about the evidence-base and outcomes of nursing practice that require change, enhancement, or maintenance (nurses and nursing practice sphere); and contributes to the development of multidisciplinary standards of practice and evidence-based guidelines of care (organization/system sphere; National Association of Clinical Nurse Specialists [NACNS], 2004). CNSs can advocate for technological solutions to help transfer evidence to the point of care. For example, they can advocate for Internet access for frontline nurses; participate in planning information systems that support easy access to condensed, preappraised evidence; evaluate quality of information sources; work in transdisciplinary teams to examine the impact of information systems on workflow, and so forth.

Implementation/Utilization

Implementation of evidence makes or breaks the EBP process. This step may be most dependent upon CNS facilitation skills and is likely highly dependent upon context. However, the empirical evidence to support what nursing organizational infrastructure best supports implementation of evidence is underdeveloped. Foxcroft and Cole (2000) conducted a systematic review of randomized controlled trials, controlled clinical, and interrupted time series (updated to include literature through 2002) aimed at determining the effectiveness of nursing organizational infrastructures on promoting EBP. They defined nursing infrastructure as the "underlying foundation or basic framework through which clinical care is delivered and supported" (p.3). They classified elements in a taxonomy that included

management framework, work patterns, skill mix, information strategies, nurse development structures, research infrastructure, clinical supervision programs, quality monitoring systems, and "other." They were unable to make any recommendations because of the poor quality of the research that they found. That is, none of the studies met the rigor of their original criteria. They relaxed selection criteria to include any study that included an evaluation of infrastructure on outcomes in order to describe the baseline science. They found that authors tended to make claims of success without providing adequate evidence to support their conclusions. They made no recommendations for practice but concluded that investigators need to conduct more research using high-quality interrupted and complex interrupted time series designs.

Meijers et al. (2006) conducted a systematic review aimed at assessing the relationships between contextual factors and research utilization in nursing, using the PARIHS model to frame the review. They used less conservative criteria in order to capture existing research, albeit lacking sufficient controls to make cause-effect claims. They excluded studies of poor methodological quality using a standardized set of appraisal criteria and found 10 papers that met their inclusion criteria. They found statistically significant relationships between research utilization and multiple modes of research education and training; access to library resources, CNSs, or nurse researchers; extent of research-related role responsibility and sustained involvement in change teams; the degree of research climate; perceived support of colleagues, physicians, and key administrators; time spent studying while on and off duty; support for involvement in research and data collection; and material support.

Other systematic reviews of CPG implementation studies have examined interventions aimed at increasing physician use of guidelines. The interventions that showed the more consistent improvements in provider compliance with guidelines included reminders (median improvement of 14.1% improvement in 14 randomized cluster comparisons), dissemination of educational materials (8.1% improvements in 4 randomized cluster comparisons), audit and feedback (7.0% improvements in 5 randomized cluster comparisons), and multifaceted interventions involving educational outreach (6.0% improvements in 13 randomized cluster comparisons) with no relationship between the number of components and the effects of multifaceted interventions (Grimshaw et al., 2006).

While there may be no evidence from experimental designs, descriptive data exist that point to barriers to implementing evidence in nursing practice. CNSs can address these barriers within a conceptual framework such as PARIHS or JBI to facilitate and strengthen the context for EBP. Pravikoff, Tanner, and Pierce (2005) surveyed 3,000 American nurses using a stratified random sample with a net response rate of 37%. There were 760 clinical nurse respondents with 39% holding baccalaureate degrees, 51% holding diplomas or associate's degrees, and only 9% with master's degrees. They found that the most common method of seeking information was from a colleague, and respondents seldom sought journal articles, research reports, or hospital libraries to answer their questions. Only 46% were familiar with the term *evidence-based practice.* Among the top 10 individual barriers (other than time) were lack of value for research in practice, lack of understanding of the structure of electronic databases, difficulty accessing research materials, lack of computer skills, difficulty understanding research articles, lack of access to a computer, lack of library access, and lack of search skills. The top institutional barriers included other goals took higher priority, difficulty recruiting and retaining staff, organizational budget for acquisition and training in information resource use, organizational perception that nursing staff are not eager to incorporate or pursue EBP, and a persistent perception that EBP is not achievable in the real world.

These findings and the theoretical frameworks suggest a number of implications for CNS practice (see Table 10.3). When designing interventions within the patient sphere of influence, CNSs implement the recommendations from the best available evidence from research but negotiate these interventions in collaboration with the patient/client and other providers, while blending their clinical expertise with the decision.

When influencing nursing practice and personnel, CNSs use facilitation skills to break barriers. When educating nurses, they need to conduct interactive sessions rather than passive, didactic sessions and use an "academic detailing" approach where they engage in development through EBP rounds and one-on-one sessions in the midst of care delivery as the context allows. They should preassess the staff's information management skills and build them where necessary and provide them with concise, straightforward summaries of the best available, preferably synthesized, evidence sources. They can increase access to evidence by providing it at the point of care and helping nurses interpret the findings so they may be empowered to negotiate with patients and other disciplines.

CNSs influence context via the system/organizational sphere. These interventions are complex and require collaboration with others. CNSs can provide transformational leadership through direct and indirect strategies. Though the evidence is evolving, the theoretical framework suggests that when CNSs occupy line administrative roles they can have profound impact by building the skill mixes that support EBP, building relationships with nurse researchers in academic settings if none exist in their own settings, and promoting a culture of evidence. CNSs in traditional roles contribute to context by building teams to address EBP in their settings.

These teams need to include key stakeholders such as the frontline staff. CNSs can advocate for staff to have time on the job to participate in evidence-based initiatives by exploring innovative strategies to cover staffing needs for patient care while releasing staff to engage in evidence-based initiatives. CNSs can work with information system workers to develop data-mining systems to gather both prospective and retrospective data to enable diagnosis of problems and their etiologies as well as outcome measurements.

EVALUATION AND OUTCOME MANAGEMENT

Evaluation is the final step of both the nursing and EBP process. Most of the CNS outcomes listed in the NACNS Statement relate to the impact of EBP. But those that explicitly address EBP are:

- Predicted and measurable nurse-sensitive patient outcomes are attained through EBP (patient sphere)
- EBPs are used by nurses
- Evidence-based, best practice models are developed and implemented (NACNS, 2004)

In order for evaluation of outcomes to be meaningful, CNSs need to select measurement tools that are valid and reliable and fit the question at hand. Both process and outcome measurements are necessary to enable analysis of the effects of evidence-based initiatives. The reality of the clinical setting can pose barriers to obtaining these data. For example, electronic documentation methods may not provide adequate data to monitor critical aspects of a care process or even to capture the outcome precisely. Though proxy measures may be the more feasible, they usually come at some cost to measurement quality.

CNSs should strive to capture data in a way that is simple to understand but revealing. A complete discussion of how best to represent data is outside the scope of this chapter. However, the metric must allow for adequate precision to detect differences. For example, infrequent events may be better tracked by measuring days between occurrences rather than rates. When tracking rates, the denominator needs to provide a meaningful metric. For example, when measuring catheter-related infections, it is more meaningful to index incidence with those at risk, that is, those with catheters inserted, than all patients regardless of exposure.

Finally, like any quality management process, outcomes need to be fed back into the cycle of improvement. In addition, key stakeholders must be informed of performance and engaged in the continuous cycle of improvement. Particularly successful and unsuccessful approaches to implementation merit dissemination via journals, agency events, and national and international meetings.

ADVANCED NURSING PRACTICE

CNSs often address practice issues that are quite fundamental to nursing practice, but the methods of advancing the practice of nursing and using evidence to support for these fundamental practices are complex. Pravikoff et al. (2005) concluded that nurses in the United States are not ready for EBP. Very few respondents in Pravikoff's sample were master's prepared nurses, so it is unlikely that this conclusion can be extended to CNSs. Certainly, nursing educators need to prepare their graduates at all levels of practice to move from a tradition-based discipline toward an evidence-based discipline. The data underline a great need for frontline nursing staff development, and CNSs are already positioned to move this agenda forward through facilitation and context building. This will happen best in the midst of practice where CNSs work with their sleeves rolled up, side by side with the bedside nurse.

Not all nurses are or will be prepared for every step of the EBP. Nurses prepared at the technical level can collaborate with professional and advanced practice nurses to identify clinical issues and assist with the practical aspects of evidence implementation. Professional nurses prepared at the baccalaureate level have the skill to search literature and do rapid appraisals of research and clinical practice guidelines, recommend practical solutions for implementation, and participate in evaluation audits. CNSs participate and lead all aspects of EBP, including conducting systematic reviews. Their critical appraisal skills are more sophisticated, and they understand the complexities of the implementation process. They use data to diagnose and specify etiologies of problems within all three spheres and manage all aspects of using evidence to solve these problems. These competencies set them apart from nurses prepared at the undergraduate levels.

ETHICAL CONSIDERATIONS

EBP is aimed at "doing the right thing." That is, it is about acting with beneficence to achieve the best possible patient outcomes. The ethical principles of beneficence, justice, and respect all play a role in evidence-based decision making (Ledbetter, 2000).

In some cases, data exist to quantify the benefit of treatment to help inform decisions related to beneficence and harm. In fact, the probability of benefit and harm can be estimated by calculating the numbers needed to treat (NNT) from frequency data and the potential harm of a treatment using numbers needed to harm (NNH;

DiCenso et al., 2005). For example, if an intervention has a NNT of 5 (95% confidence interval [CI], 3–7), then 5 people would need to receive the intervention to benefit 1 person, with the true value falling between 3 and 7 (DiCenso et al., 2005). Similarly, a NNH of 100 (95% CI, 90–120) means that 100 people would need to receive a treatment before 1 more person would be harmed by the adverse effects of a treatment, with the true number falling between 90 and 120. When these data exist, they may help systems and individuals weigh the benefits and harm of interventions and their adverse effects. The magnitude of the treatment effect, the type and probability of adverse effect, and the nature of the decision itself will contribute to how CNSs engage patients' autonomous preferences. CNSs can learn more about using patient decision aids to help staff use these aids (DiCenso et al., 2005).

The principles of justice, beneficence, and respect must be upheld when CNSs make decisions about what type of EBP efforts require human subject committee oversight. CNSs should seek institutional review board (IRB) approval for projects when they plan to collect data and disseminate the findings of the project. If they are involved in quality improvement cycles where all data are deidentified, the project may not require IRB approval, but they should discuss the project with the chair of the human subjects committee before launching any EBP project.

Ethical issues are likely to dominate discussions related to evidence-based health policy and new health care resource allocation schemes. CNSs need to remain actively engaged in these deliberations, advocating for the responsible use of health care dollars as well as for patient interests.

SUMMARY

EBP is the burning issue of the decade. Since the advent of advanced nursing practice, CNS practice and education has focused on using theory and research to advance the practice of nursing. CNSs use evidence in their individual clinical decisions in the patient sphere of influence and facilitate and lead other nurses, and organizations use evidence to achieve the best outcomes. They are uniquely positioned to ask the questions, find and appraise the evidence, and design, implement, and evaluate innovations. In short, they are and will be the catalyst for evidence-based nursing practice.

DISCUSSION QUESTIONS

1. What are the key elements of the definition of evidenced-based nursing practice? What are the implications of these elements for CNS practice?

2. How has the EBP movement developed throughout the world? How have sociopolitical factors influenced EBP among nations that have largely private-pay health care systems and those that are largely nationalized?

3. What are some examples of false, pseudo, and authentic claims of EBP that you have seen in your practice or education? What factors differentiate these claims?

4. How do the nursing process and EBP process compare?

5. What requirements are necessary for a model to help CNSs implement EBP in all spheres of influence? How do the various EBP models compare in their support of CNS implementation of evidence?

6. What CNS competencies and outcomes as described in *NACNS's Statement on Practice and Education* speak directly to promoting EBP among the three spheres of influence? Which address EBP indirectly?

7. How and why do the following sources of evidence compare in terms of their breadth, strength of control of bias, and role in EBP: systematic reviews of RCTs, systematic reviews of non-RCTs, clinical practice guidelines, single RCTs, cohort studies, before and after single group studies, consensus statements by a specialty organization, and metasynthesis of qualitative studies. In what circumstances might these be the "best available evidence"?

8. According to Rycroft-Malone, Seers, et al. (2004), clinical expertise needs to be consciously explicated, analyzed, exposed to external sources of critique, and affirmed by consensus. How might CNSs affirm their clinical expertise to meet these criteria?

9. According to the PARIHS model, what conditions should the CNS promote to increase the probability of successfully implementing an evidence-based innovation?

10. Based on the findings of Pravikoff et al. (2005) and evidence from systematic reviews of implementation strategies, how can CNSs influence nursing personnel to further EBP in the United States?

11. What tools will facilitate getting evidence into practice, and where might they be found? What type of approaches to implementation are ineffective? How can CNSs promote technical solutions to break down barriers to evidence implementation?

ANALYSIS AND SYNTHESIS

1. Search for a systematic review on a particular topic of interest to your specialty practice. Find a single research study about the same issue. Compare the findings from the systematic review and the individual study. Are the conclusions similar or different? How does your confidence in the bottom line recommendation compare?

2. Select a clinical topic of interest to your specialty practice. Go to http://www.guidelines.gov/ to search for clinical practice guidelines. Use the "compare" tool to compare three of them at a time. How do the guidelines compare in terms of the rigor of their development, the transparency in methods, and supporting evidence? Select one and apply the AGREE instrument to complete the critical appraisal. Would you consider facilitating its implementation? Why or why not?

3. Select a model to consider in depth. How does the model fit the complexity of EBP? How does it help direct CNS practice in the three spheres of influence?

4. Find five different systems for ranking levels of evidence (e.g., Centers for Disease Control, U.S. Preventative Services Task Force, etc.). Create a comparison chart and summarize the similarities and differences. What are the implications of the lack of a standard leveling system for CNS practice?

5. Search and analyze systematic reviews related to implementation of guidelines or other sources of evidence (begin by searching the Effective Practice and Organization of Care [EPOC] database of systematic reviews at http://www.cochrane.org). Create three lists—strategies that consistently work, strategies that may work, and strategies that consistently do not work. How might you use this list to design implementation interventions?

CLINICAL APPLICATIONS

1. Develop a clinical implementation project in collaboration with a clinical team; use a conceptual model to frame the process to include the following:
   a. Identify a potential problem.
   b. Brainstorm potential etiologies, and gather assessment data to support or refute the diagnosis.
   c. Generate a PICO question related to the effectiveness of an intervention to target the etiology.
   d. Search for best available synthesized evidence; if a synthesized source is unavailable, find primary evidence.
   e. Appraise the evidence source using a standardized tool to decide on applicability.
   f. Generate recommendations for implementation.
   g. Implement and gather data to evaluate outcomes.
   h. Generate further recommendations for improvement.

2. Conduct "PICO" rounds:
   a. Round with nursing staff in small, brief sessions.
   b. Ask them to identify current, relevant clinical issues. If they have difficulty identifying an issue, ask them to recount the types of patients and interventions they have provided. Ask questions about how they made their clinical decisions, and solicit possible alternative decisions.

c. Help them identify each element of the question—population, intervention, comparison, and outcome.

d. Find evidence that relates to the questions and provide short, key point summaries of synthesize evidence if it is available.

3. Organize a journal club to critically appraise CPGs or systematic reviews relevant to issues identified by nursing staff.

4. Participate in a product analysis team. Search for evidence related to the type of technology and gather user requirements through focus groups. Conduct a cost analysis and provide a recommendation of the product in collaboration with the team.

5. Meet with nursing leaders to explore their vision for EBP and the role of CNSs in that vision.

REFERENCES

Agency for Healthcare Research and Quality. (2008). *Overview of evidence based practice centers.* Retrieved June 24, 2009, from http://www.ahrq.gov/clinic/epc/

AGREE Collaboration (2004). *Agree instrument.* Retrieved January 9, 2009, from: http://www.agreecollaboration.org/instrument/

Brown, D., & McCormack, B. (2005). Developing postoperative pain management: Utilising the promoting action on research implementation in health services (PARIHS) framework. *Worldviews on Evidence-Based Nursing, 2,* 131–141.

Cochrane Collaboration. (n.d.). *Chronology of Cochrane collaboration.* Retrieved January 9, 2009, from http://www.cochrane.org/docs/cchronol.htm

Dobbins, M, Ciliska, D., Cockerill, R., Barnsley, J., & DiCenso, A. (2002). A framework for the dissemination and utilization of research for health-care policy and practice. *The Online Journal of Knowledge Synthesis for Nursing, 9,* 7.

Doran, D. M. & Sidani, S. (2007). Outcomes-focused knowledge translation: A framework for knowledge translation and patient outcomes improvement. *Worldviews on Evidence-Based Nursing, 4,* 3–13.

DiCenso, A., Cullum, N., & Ciliska, D. (1998). Implementing evidence-based nursing: Some misconceptions. *Evidence Based Nursing, 1,* 38–40.

DiCenso, A., Guyatt, G., & Ciliska, D. (2005). *Evidence-based nursing: A guide to clinical nursing.* St. Louis: Mosby.

Foxcroft, D. R., & Cole, N. (2006). Organisational infrastructures to promote evidence based nursing practice. *Cochrane Database of Systematic Reviews, 3.* Art. No.: CD002212. DOI: 10.1002/14651858.CD002212.

Grimshaw, J. M., Thomas, R., Maclennan, G., Fraser, C., Ramsay, C. R., Vale, L., et al. (2006). Toward evidence-based quality improvement: Evidence (and its limitations) of the effectiveness of guidelines dissemination and implementation strategies (1966–1998). *Journal of General Internal Medicine, 21,* S14–20.

Harvey, G., Loftus-Hill, A., Rycroft-Malone, J, Tichen, A., McCormack, B., & Seers, K. (2002). Getting evidence into practice: The role and function of facilitation. *Journal of Advanced Nursing, 37,* 577–588.

Institute of Medicine. (2003). *Patient safety: A new standard of care.* Washington, DC: National Academies Press.

Joanna Briggs Institute. (n.d.) *About JBI.* Retrieved January 9, 2009, from http://www.joannabriggs.edu.au/pdf/about/AboutJBI.pdf

Kitson, A, Harvey, G., & McCormack, B. (1998). Enabling the implementation of evidence based practice: A conceptual framework. *Quality Health Care, 7,* 149–158.

Ledbetter, C. A. (2000). Evidence-based best practice: The common knowledge of ethical clinical scholarship. *Online Journal of Nursing Synthesis, 7.*

McCormack, B., Kitson, A., Harvey, G., Rycroft-Malone, J., Tichen, A., & Seers, K. (2002). Getting evidence into practice: The meaning of "context." *Journal of Advanced Nursing, 38,* 94–104.

McDonald, L. (2001). Florence Nightingale and the early origins of evidence-based nursing. *Evidence Based Nursing, 4,* 68–69.

Meijers, J. M. M., Janssen, M. A. P., Cummings, G. G., Wallin, L., Estabrooks, C. A., & Halfens, R. Y. G. (2006). Assessing the relationships between contextual factors and research utilization in nursing: Systematic literature review. *Journal of Advanced Nursing, 55,* 622–635.

National Association of Clinical Nurse Specialists. (2004). *Statement on clinical nurse specialist practice and education* (2nd ed.). Harrisburg, PA: Author.

Pearson, A., Wiechula, R., Court, A., & Lockwood, C. (2005). The JBI model of evidence-based healthcare. *International Journal of Evidence Based Healthcare, 3,* 207–215.

Pravikoff, D. S., Tanner, A. B., & Pierce, S. T. (2005). Readiness of U.S. nurses for evidence-based practice. *American Journal of Nursing, 105,* 40–51.

Rosswurm, M. A., & Larrabee, J. H. (1999). A model for change to evidence-based practice. *Image: Journal of Nursing Scholarship, 31,* 317–322.

Rycroft-Malone, J. (2004). The PARIHS framework—A framework for guiding the implementation of evidence-based practice. *Journal of Nursing Care Quality, 19,* 297–304.

Rycroft-Malone, J., Bucknail, T., & Melnyk, B. M. (2004). Editorial. *Worldviews on Evidence-Based Nursing Practice,* 1–2.

Rycroft-Malone, J., Seers, K., Tichen, A., Harvey, G., Kitson, A., & McCormack, B. (2004). What counts as evidence in evidence-based practice? *Journal of Advanced Nursing, 47,* 81–90.

Sackett, D. L., Rosenberg, W. M. C., Gray, J. A. M., Haynes, R. B., & Richardson, W. S. (1996). Evidence based medicine: What it is and what it isn't. *British Medical Journal, 312,* 71–72.

Stetler, C. (2001). Updating the Stetler Model of research utilization to facilitate evidence-based practice. *Nursing Outlook, 49,* 272–279.

Titler, M., Kleiber, C., Steelman, V., Goode, C., Rakel, B., Barry-Walker, J., et al. (1994). Infusing research into practice to promote quality care. *Nursing Research, 43,* 307–313.

U.S. Department of Veterans Affairs. (2006). *QUERI implementation guide.* Retrieved January 9, 2009, from http://www.queri.research.va.gov/

11

Transformational Leadership as the Clinical Nurse Specialist's Capacity to Influence

Brenda L. Lyon

Today's demands on health care systems to improve patient care, including safety and cost-effectiveness, highlight the need for the transformational leadership of clinical nurse specialists (CNSs). The transformational leadership work of the CNS is principally focused on transforming patient care by closing the gap between what is known and what is done in practice and by resolving systems level problems that impede effective patient care.

Leadership is a hallmark of CNS practice in all three spheres of influence. The essence of leadership is fundamentally the capacity to influence. *Influence* is the "power of producing an effect without apparent exertion of force or direct exercise of command" (*Merriam-Webster Online Dictionary*, 2008). Influence and, therefore, leadership is not about having position authority; it is the ability to get others to be motivated to work toward accomplishing a vision. The importance of influence as the major avenue through which CNSs positively impact both patient outcomes and cost-effectiveness is reflected in the adoption of "spheres of influence" as the framework for the National Association of Clinical Nurse Specialists (NACNS) *Statement on Clinical Nurse Specialist Practice and Education* (2004).

The purpose of this chapter is to present leadership as a relationship-oriented capacity to influence or motivate others to work toward shared goals in improving patient outcomes and cost-effectiveness. The *capacity*

to lead is a complex quality that encompasses particular personal and relationship-focused attributes, the ability to earn and effectively use interpersonal power, and the judicious use of the principles of influence. The combination of all of these elements is necessary to enable the CNS's enactment of transformational leadership for the purpose of positively affecting others in the work of improving patient care outcomes in complex health care systems.

The chapter begins with a brief discussion of the common types of CNS work in complex systems (chapter 8) that require leadership ability. The personal and relationship-focused attributes of effective leaders are identified. Then the concepts of interpersonal power and the principles of influence, including influence strategies, are presented as foundational to understanding the features of transformational leadership in the next section. The chapter concludes with a summary and discussion questions.

COMMON TYPES OF CNS CLINICAL WORK REQUIRING LEADERSHIP

The necessity for CNSs in health care systems is omnipresent because of the endless drive to improve patient outcomes and the cost-effectiveness of care. The high incidence of infections, skin breakdown, and falls in many hospitals, coupled with the Centers for

Medicare and Medicaid Services' (CMS) initiation of new reimbursement policies resulting in nonpayment to hospitals for care resulting from these and other preventable complications, simply increases organizational incentives to provide quality patient care (Rosenthal, 2007).

CNSs are well-positioned to lead change efforts within organizations to cost-effectively improve patient outcomes. It is imperative that CNSs continually assess patient care outcomes to identify needs for practice improvement. Once identified, the CNS must visibly seize those leadership opportunities by working with nursing staff, other health care professionals, and administration in bringing about needed changes (see chapter 21).

Health care facility needs for leadership to bring about nursing practice improvement may be focused in either or both the nursing sphere and system sphere with a wide range of foci. The nursing sphere may include, but is not limited to, needs for leadership in: (1) identification of critical indicators for nurse-sensitive outcomes to enable measurement and feedback to staff regarding the effectiveness of care (Duffy, 2002), (2) bridging knowledge/skill gaps between evidence and what is done at the bedside (Dietz & Smith, 2002; Seeman, Soukup, & Adams, 2000), (3) empowerment of staff to promote assertive advocacy on behalf of patients (Green & Jordan, 2004), and (4) development and implementation of innovative programs of care for patient populations (Morissette, 2004). System leadership opportunities may include, but are not limited to: (1) identification and resolution of gaps in system supports that contribute to work complexity and hazards in patient care (Ebright, Patterson, & Render, 2002), (2) identification and resolution of clinical barriers (including norms and relationships) that negatively impact patient outcomes, (3) development of critical indictor matrices for multidisciplinary quality indicators in conjunction with other disciplines (Duffy, 2002), (4) guiding multidisciplinary groups in system solutions to clinical problems (Benedict, Robinson, & Holder, 2006), and (5) boundary management between disciplines (Foggow, Solie, Tracy, & Gjere, 2005).

ATTRIBUTES OF LEADERS

To be able to positively impact changes in a health care system, the CNS must have personal and relationship-oriented attributes that enable his/her ability to be in relationship with others in a positive way to be able to influence them. Several of the attributes important for CNSs to possess identified in chapter 2 are consistent with attributes identified through research on transformational and authentic leaders.

Personal Attributes

Research has demonstrated that personal attributes contributing to the capacity to lead include: (1) self-confidence, (2) proactive orientation, (3) trustworthiness, (4) reliability, (5) strong sense of purpose, (6) self-discipline, (7) optimistic orientation, and (8) resilience and persistence. Bass (1999) conducted a review of research on attributes of transformational leaders over a 20-year period. The two primary personal attributes necessary for a leader's ability to influence were self-confidence (a sense of security) and a proactive orientation, that is, the ability to envision a desired future and set aims. George (2003) found that authentic leaders are believable, genuine, trustworthy, and reliable. They have a strong sense of purpose, solid values, and are self-disciplined. According to George, authentic leaders possess four psychological strengths, including confidence, hope, optimism, and resiliency. Optimism is characterized by focusing on the glass as half full rather than half empty. Optimists do not take failure personally but rather look at it as an opportunity for learning and improvement. Resiliency is an important aspect of persistence, which is the ability to deal with difficult situations with determination (George, 2003). In addition to these attributes, Spinelli (2006) and Dirks and Ferrin (2001) identified charisma as an essential personal attribute of transformational leaders.

Relationship-Oriented Attributes

In addition to person-focused attributes, there are important relationship-oriented attributes of leadership. Bass (1999) found in his study of transformational leadership that a critically important attribute was the ability to initiate and maintain positive relationships with others. The attribute is characterized by a high degree of "other-orientation" rather than narcissistic desires and is manifested by a high degree of empathy and an ability to give and contribute. Being an effective listener is one manifestation of being other-oriented. Bass also found that the ability to clearly articulate a vision that unifies values and intellectually stimulates others is very important.

George (2003) found that authentic leaders focus on building on people's strengths instead of focusing on weaknesses. Authentic leaders are often able to transform an organization and/or parts of an organizational system. Building self-confidence that others will have in you requires being able to see possibilities (positive visualization) and a preponderance of positive self-talk, as well as positive situational focusing (Lyon, 2001a). Positive talk can become contagious and contribute to group confidence (Avolio & Luthan, 2006).

Reaffirming many of the personal and relationship-oriented attributes of transformational leadership in nursing are the findings of the concept analysis conducted by Grossman and Valiga (2005) to identify the essential characteristics of leadership. The results of their analysis generated nine characteristics, including: creativity, vision building, adaptability, stewardship, flexibility, risk taking, conflict management, credibility, and empowerment. These nine characteristics were used to develop The Leadership Characteristics and Skills Assessment Tool.

Importantly, all of the attributes of transformational leaders contribute to trust formation (Dirks & Ferrin, 2001; Spinelli, 2006). Basically, transformational leaders, discussed further in a later section, are able to foster a sense of trust between themselves and others and build a history of being viewed as capable in "showing the way," which is consistent with the leadership work of Kouzes and Posner (2002).

The long list of personal and relationship-oriented attributes required for leadership can seem daunting and leads some to believe that a person must be born with leadership attributes—that it is not possible to learn them. On the contrary, each of the personal and relationship-oriented attributes can be learned, developed, or enhanced over time using targeted strategies. There is an exercise at the end of this chapter focused on helping burgeoning CNSs in the development of leadership attributes.

INTERPERSONAL POWER AND INFLUENCE

The personal and relationship-oriented attributes identified previously are fundamentally important to maximize the leader's effectiveness in influencing others. Leaders are able to envision a better way and to influence people to commit to making the vision reality. The ability to influence in a noncoercive manner is dependent on a number of factors in addition to the attributes identified previously, not the least of which is having interpersonal power (Bass, 1999; Burns, 1978; Gillespie & Mann, 2004; Kouzes & Posner, 2002). The concept of *power* is intriguing. It is often thought of as a negative attribute. When power is thought to be a bad thing it is usually in the context of someone possessing control over others with the intent of causing harm or creating negative consequences. However, power in itself is not a bad thing and can be and often is used for positive/beneficial ends.

Interpersonal Power

Power is energy, that is, the "ability to act or produce an effect" (*Merriam-Webster Online Dictionary*, 2008). From a physics perspective, *energy* is the capability or force to move an object. A magnet is a good analogy to explain interpersonal power. A magnet is a compound of an element (iron, nickel, cobalt, or neodymium) that has been correctly mixed together (in the right atmosphere) with a higher weight element, such as strontium, to be able to hold a charge, then the combined mixture is infused with an electrical charge to magnetize. The result is a magnet that attracts, that is, draws or pulls other elements to it (How Stuff Works, 2008).

Change initiatives are more effective when they encompass "drawing to" or "pulling" strategies as opposed to "pushing" strategies (Eisenbach, Watson, & Rajinandini, 1999). The notion of "drawing to" rather than "pushing" differentiates two types of power—personal power (attributable to the person) and position power (attributable to the position). Pushing strategies are more reflective of position power. That is, persons with position or line authority such as administrators typically have the decisional authority to mandate direction as well as the ability to use tangible rewards and disincentives to push people in the desired direction.

Within health care organizations, CNS positions are typically salaried positions without line authority or position power. Characteristically, CNSs report directly to administrators such as the chief nursing officer (CNO) or director of advanced practice. CNSs must earn interpersonal power and purposefully use influence strategies to stimulate nursing staff and members of other health care disciplines to work toward visions focused on improving patient outcomes and cost-effectiveness.

As is evident from the previous discussion, interpersonal power and leadership are not the same constructs. Leadership is not power, per se, but is the use of power to pull others toward a goal. Power is a social construct, that is, it can only exist when there are two or more people present. Although normally not incorporated into the understanding of personal power, Emerson's (1962) classic research on "dyadic resource dependence" demonstrated that when one person in a relationship has difficult-to-obtain resources that the other needs, then the person with the resources has power in that relationship. Farmer and Aquinis (2005) integrated Emerson's resource dependence theory with identity (role) theory (Ashforth, 2001) and self-verification theory (Burke, 1991) to explain power in relationships. The new theoretical postulates are applicable to any situation where one person desires to influence another. Understanding that power is a relational concept that is in large measure affected by one person (or group) needing the resources of another person (or group) has practical implications for CNSs. It is sometimes helpful to think of it in the following manner, which is consistent with Emerson's research findings: When person or group "A" *needs* person or group "B" more than person or group "B" needs person or group "A," then group "B" has more power! It is often helpful for CNSs to understand that an important derivative of their work is creating perceived *need* for their work in the organization.

The advanced nursing knowledge and skill that CNSs possess, along with expertise in their specialty area and ability to work with groups to change practice, are greatly needed by health care organizations. Therefore, there is abundant opportunity for a CNS to gain recognition as someone who is highly valued in the organization. The ability of CNSs to influence others, including staff nurses, other members of the health care team, the CNO, and the chief executive officer (CEO) is, in significant measure, dependent on the assets they bring to help meet the *organization's needs*. These assets can be categorized into the types of power discussed in the following sections, including knowledge power, charisma power, referent power, and resources power (Huber, 2000; Roberts & Vasquez, 2004).

Knowledge Power

Knowledge power is expertise. Expertise encompasses both knowledge and skill. You've often heard the phrase "knowledge is power." Knowledge is almost universally powerful in that it is needed for almost any activity; it is universal currency. Knowledge is so valuable that if protected in the form of patents or copyright or other legal means it is actually a saleable commodity in the form of intellectual capital. CNSs have expert clinical knowledge and knowledge about how to advance the practice of nursing and patient care to improve patient outcomes and cost-effectiveness. As a CNS's knowledge in these areas becomes apparent in an organization, the *value* of the CNS to the organization and, therefore, the power of the CNS in the organization is enhanced.

Charisma Power

Charismatic power in essence is the ability to charm others. Charisma is a personal quality that is characterized by being appealing to others through a combination of factors, including pleasing appearance, enthusiasm, excellent communication skills, and the desire to be engaged with others. Charismatic people demonstrate the desire to be engaged with others by acknowledging others and remembering names and important aspects of the lives of others such as family, significant others, or pets. Being likable is important for a CNS. Different than the CNS needing to be liked by everyone, it is presenting oneself in a pleasing fashion and an engaging demeanor. It is important to recognize that being in good relationships with others establishes social capital. Groves's (2005) research findings on charisma supported the significant positive relationship between a change agent's level of charisma and general openness to initiatives targeting organizational change.

Referent Power

While knowledge and charisma power are possessed by the person having it, referent power is network power. That is, the CNS needs to nurture and maintain good relationships with people in higher levels of position power, for example, work colleagues and professional colleagues or even friends who happen to be in positions of power. It is important that CNSs be in good relationships with key stakeholders in an organization including the CEO, CNO, and chief financial officer (CFO).

Resource Power

While the persons you are in relationships with can be a source of referent power, the personal resources you have, including critical thinking and problem-solving ability, the ability to work with and lead groups, and other services you can provide, are a source of *resource* power. Resource power also includes tangible resources, such as money and property, but the most pertinent to CNSs is the provision of nontangible resources. A common example is the important service that CNSs provide in leading multidisciplinary group work within an organization.

The CNS can acquire considerable interpersonal power by continuing to develop knowledge/skill competencies corresponding to the needs of the organization, demonstrating charisma, attending to the development of positive relationships with those who have position authority and being generous in the provision of services. In addition to acquiring interpersonal power, it is important to be sensitive to the basic principles of influence.

Influence

Individual effectiveness in organizations is largely dependent on the individual's ability to influence others (Cable & Judge, 2003; Kipnis & Schmidt, 1988; Yukl & Falbe, 1990). In his classic work on influence, first published in 1984 and later updated based on additional research, Cialdini (2008) identified six principles that form the foundation for the ability to influence or to get another person to say "yes." The book is a wonderful interweaving of theory and empirical evidence, and each of the principles is summarized next.

Rule of Reciprocity

The *rule of reciprocity* is based upon the norm of desiring to pay back or repay another person for something that was provided. In other words, it is common for humans to experience an obligation to repay once something is given to them. Research has demonstrated that the rule of reciprocity is very powerful and can even spur unequal exchanges, where a person feels indebted to even do a larger favor than the one received. This is another example of social capital. An example of the rule of reciprocity is helping a staff nurse with a difficult patient by demonstrating calming strategies that soothe the patient while bathing and changing the bed, and the next week the staff nurse volunteers to be on the practice improvement team focused on caring for patients experiencing confusion.

Commitment and Consistency

The principle of *commitment and consistency* is based on the human desire to be consistent in words, attitudes, and deeds. The desire to be consistent is reinforced by a society that highly values consistency. This principle is played out by a person agreeing with or making a commitment to a stand or position, and then, based on that position, there is a greater willingness to demonstrate actions that are consistent with the prior commitment. Commitments are most effective when they are active, public, and viewed as internally motivated rather than coerced. Once a position has been taken the person is more likely to behave in ways consistent with the stand. An example of the principle of commitment and consistency is when individuals in a multidisciplinary group agree that patient safety is a priority for their respective disciplines and then later agree to a new policy on hand washing that mandates reporting actions not consistent with the policy.

Social Proof

The principle of *social proof* is based on two human tendencies. First, when people are uncertain about what behavior is viewed as most appropriate in a group, they are more likely to view the behavior of others and accept those behaviors as correct or expected. Second, people are more inclined to follow the behavior of others who are similar to them. An example of social proof is when a CNS models asking questions about why a particular problem (symptom or functional) is being experienced by patients and then openly seeks the data/evidence to identify the etiology of the problem and what nursing care is required to prevent it. Later, a staff member who has observed the CNS, makes it known that he/she is wondering why the patients on the orthopedic unit are experiencing breakthrough pain despite all of the analgesics being administered.

Liking

The fourth principle, *liking*, corresponds to charisma power discussed earlier. In general, people prefer to say "yes" to people that they know and like. There

are several factors that affect "liking," including: physical attractiveness, similarity, praise, familiarity, and association. Research has demonstrated that physical attractiveness/appearance creates an advantage in the ability to persuade and to change the attitude of others (Cialdini, 2008). Regarding similarity, we tend to like people who are like us and share common beliefs. Praise and/or the judicious use of sincere compliments can enhance liking. Repeated contact with a person can create a sense of comfort or familiarity, and when we are associated with positive things or events there is often a halo effect. How a CNS dresses can promote a sense of similarity and association, and thus, CNSs should be sensitive to their audience. When working with staff nurses, many CNSs wear scrubs or a nice lab coat over comfortable everyday work clothes, but they bring business clothes for the hospital board meeting that will be attended in the evening. Further, it is essential that CNSs acknowledge, give credit, and publicly praise staff nurses and others for their contributions to accomplishing a goal and to demonstrate gratitude—to say "thank you." In this day of high-tech communications, hand-written thank you notes stand out as something very special!

Authority

There is substantial research evidence for the principle of *authority*. There is a strong pressure in society to obey legitimate authority. Obedience to legitimate or appropriate authority is viewed as correct conduct. Research has shown that authority is demonstrated through titles (inferring knowledge), clothing, and automobiles. When a person possessed one or more of these symbols there was more deference or obedience by those who encountered him or her (Cialdini, 2008). Examples of authority are the titles of CEO, CNO, CFO, and, increasingly, the title of CNS. Another example of authority is a classy dress suit (for women or men), interestingly often referred to as a "power" suit.

Scarcity

Scarcity is the last and sixth principle. Interestingly, people tend to assign more value to an opportunity or an object or information that is less available. For example, research has demonstrated that the act of limiting access to a message may cause people to want it more. Information that is perceived to be exclusive is more highly valued (Cialdini, 2008). This is not to say that it is a good thing to control information or resources by hoarding. It is, however, one reason why hospital CEOs and CNOs tout that their hospital has Magnet status and that they have eight CNSs! There is a national shortage of CNSs demonstrated by the large number of open CNS positions continuously advertised by hospitals and recruiting agencies. Recognition of the fortunate position a hospital is in when there are CNSs employed by the hospital can influence administrators to be early adopters of CNS recommendations.

TRANSFORMATIONAL LEADERSHIP

Although transformational leadership has been a focus in nursing literature for the past 20 years, the importance of transformational leaders has been recognized for more than 30 years. Burns (1978), who first defined transformational leadership, asserted in his classic book on leadership that transformational leaders are able to appeal to the followers' sense of values, help them see a higher vision, and encourage them to exert themselves in helping to achieve the vision. The personal and relationship-oriented attributes along with earned interpersonal power and the judicious use of the principles of influence covered previously form the foundation for effective transformational leaders.

Transformational leaders motivate others to work on behalf of an organizational vision/mission and related goals. Transformational leaders inspire others to believe that the goal is both significant and attainable. They are able to intelligently articulate the rationale for and evidence undergirding the need for the goal, while inviting discussion and dialogue in refining the goal and encouraging others to be curious and to take risks. Similar to the approach advocated for leaders in the principles of complex adaptive systems is the importance of viewing difficulties as opportunities to be curious about solutions and to take risks in discovering new solutions. Taking risks is easier when members of a group share the same values because that fosters a higher level of trust (Gillespie & Mann, 2004). Transformational leaders are also able to reduce uncertainty and to reduce the experience of apathy by being visible and being positive (Bass, 1999).

Herold, Fedor, Caldwell, and Liu (2008) compared transformational leadership with change leadership in a study of 343 employees in 30 organizations representing a wide variety of industry sectors. Findings from the study demonstrated that transformational leadership and an employee's commitment to specific change projects were significantly positively related. That is, transformational leaders were able to get more commitment regardless of their ability to manage change well and regardless of the personal impact of the change on the employee's specific job situations (workload and relationships). *Commitment* was defined as encompassing both the attitude toward the change as well as the willingness to work on behalf of the successful implementation of change. This type of commitment is commonly referred to as "buy in." Herold's findings

were consistent with research on authentic leadership (George, 2003).

Transformational leadership skills are the most effective in providing clinical leadership in motivating and guiding others toward practice improvements (Cook & Leathard, 2004). Thus, the development of transformational leadership skills, discussed here as *practices*, is critical to the work of CNSs.

Five Practices of Transformational Leadership

The five practices of exemplary transformational leadership were identified by Kouzes and Posner (2002). Their work, initially published in 1993, is grounded in interviews of 1,100 leaders. In their study of exemplary leaders beginning in the 1980s and carried through the 1990s, they found that the attributes of leadership have not changed, but the context for leadership has changed rather dramatically. In today's world, there is a heightened degree of uncertainty and sense of chaos. Leaders must recognize: (1) the reality of the speed of change as an outgrowth of new technologies; (2) the changing workforce, where trusting organizations and experiencing a sense of commitment is not necessarily commonplace; (3) the common need to search for meaning, including the desire to make a difference; (4) the connectivity of people (social capital, in that it is human networks that make the difference); and (5) the global economy requiring global understanding (Kouzes & Posner, 2002). It is imperative that CNSs be sensitive to the realities of today's world and workforce while focusing on their own self awareness, social awareness, and interpersonal skills.

In today's context there are many challenging opportunities for leaders in health care organizations. The leadership challenge is to mobilize others to want to do extraordinary things to turn challenges into successes. The five practices of leadership to mobilize others include: modeling the way, inspiring a shared vision, challenging the process, enabling others to act, and leading with the heart (Kouzes & Posner, 2002).

Modeling the Way

In describing *modeling the way*, Kouzes and Posner (2002) make the important point that it's not titles that win you respect, it's your behavior. CNSs must model the behavior they expect from others, including talking clearly and openly about what you value, because it is important to lead from what you believe/value. For example, "The most important people in this hospital are the patients . . . our primary concern must be their well-being and safety." A true leader's behavior is consistent with those values and is evidenced by spending time with those you are leading, sharing stories that make the values come alive, being there in uncertain times, and asking questions that help to focus attention on values and priorities. You can model the way by saying to staff nurses: "You are the ones on the front line—the patients need you to feel free to question and to take action to assure the quality of their care."

Inspiring a Shared Vision

Inspiring a shared vision first requires that the leader can envision a desired and attractive future for the organization or service unit, such as an intensive care unit. With a "we can do" message that vision or dream is shared enthusiastically and in a manner and language consistent with the values and desires of those listening. In other words, CNSs must take time to listen to nursing staff to learn who they are and what they value. Tapping into those values and dreams helps to start the fire in them to take actions that will help make their hopes or dreams come alive. "Leaders cannot command commitment, only inspire it" (Kouzes & Posner, 2002, p. 15). Reality doesn't exist outside of us—we create it! The clear image of the future pulls the leader and others forward as a collective whole (Kouzes & Posner, 2002).

Challenging the Process

All of the leaders interviewed by Kouzes and Posner (2002) had in some way *challenged a process*—be that a new product, a rule, regulation, or legislation, or a way of doing business. In that manner, leaders are pioneers or innovators. Leaders listen. They encourage others to ask questions and challenge processes. "Why are we changing beds everyday?" "Why are we using these expensive mouth swabs—do we know that they are more effective than just good mouth care?"

It's the leader's job to sell a problem and to frame it as an opportunity to do better or to do something in a different way to produce better outcomes. They also recognize that venturing into new territories carries uncertainties, potential risks, and failures. A leader always treats challenges or difficult situations as learning opportunities while acknowledging the emotions of self and others. These types of efforts are adventures—discovering what works and what doesn't and helping others feel safe while affirming that everyone is in this together (Lyon, 2001b).

Enabling Others to Act

Leaders *enable others to act*. "Leadership is a team effort" (Kouzes & Posner, 2002). Leaders manufacture hope. "Together, I know we can do this!" Hope is important in enabling change (Avolio & Luthan, 2006).

Hope can be reinforced by breaking large, complex goals down into accomplishable steps and celebrating these milestones (Avolio & Luthan, 2006; Lyon, 2001a).

Good leaders foster a sense of trust and the desire for collaboration. Enabling others to act necessitates that others feel a sense of ownership and the power to take risks in trying new ways to solve problems (Lyon, 2001c). The establishment of teams that have the responsibility and authority to act on particular clinical problems, for example, skin care or ventilator acquired pneumonia, and where members can act as consultants to other nurses or other members of the health care team is a great way to enable action.

Leading With the Heart

CNSs are commonly passionate about their specialty and the power of nursing to positively improve patient outcomes, making it easier to *lead from the heart*. It has been said that the difference between a vision and a goal is passion, that is, a vision is inspired by passion. Passion is the fire for a CNS's work. When a CNS is positively passionate about his/her work, the passion is a source of enjoyment and is evident to others. It can be contagious!

It is often helpful for CNSs to tap into the value structure of staff nurses and other members of the health care team. When a staff nurse or physician person can be engaged in work that is consonant with his/her values, then it is more likely that the individual will experience satisfaction and even joy in doing the work.

As noted earlier, CNSs can be "hope" leaders focused on forward movement consistent with an organization's mission and the desire to improve patient outcomes. Recognizing and celebrating the achievement of patient care goals can bring joy to the work of nursing.

SUMMARY

Effective CNSs are transformational leaders in health care organizations who work to advance the practice of nursing and patient care in general to improve outcomes in a cost-effective manner. Transformational leaders have the personal and relationship-oriented attributes and the interpersonal power to effectively use influence strategies to motivate others to work toward shared goals. The interpersonal power to influence others within an organization is earned by being responsive to and appropriately meeting the needs of stakeholders, including staff nurses, other members of the health care team, and executive leadership.

The essential elements involved in the capacity to lead or influence others include particular personal and relationship-focused attributes, the ability to earn and effectively use interpersonal power, and the judicious use of the principles of influence. Each of these elements form the foundation for the enactment of the five practices of transformational leadership skills, modeling the way, inspiring a shared vision, challenging, enabling others to act, and leading with the heart.

Earning the power to influence and developing transformational leadership skills requires that the CNS attend to both personal and professional development to enhance the positive attributes inherent in transformational leaders and to be cognizant of the important relationship between an organization's needs and the CNS's resources. The discussion questions and exercises that follow are designed to guide the reader in the personal development of leadership attributes.

DISCUSSION QUESTIONS

1. Identify and discuss the types of interpersonal power you observe in practicing CNSs. What are the common types of interpersonal power you see in the most admired CNSs within an institution? How do you know when a CNS has garnered interpersonal power?
2. Identify and discuss the influence strategies that you have observed your CNS preceptors, faculty, and other leaders use to effect change.
3. Discuss with practicing CNSs what they found as the most difficult leadership challenge in effecting a practice change with staff nurses and with a multidisciplinary team.

CHAPTER EXERCISES

1. Make a list of the personal and relationship-oriented attributes of leadership. Conduct a personal assessment of your strengths with respect to each of these attributes, and identify areas for growth. For each area of growth, identify at least one thing you can do to enhance your personal and/or relationship-oriented attributes. The list may include such things as joining "Toast Masters," taking a course in assertiveness training or conflict management, making it a priority to write thank-you notes, taking a powerful other to lunch, seeking feedback from peers, or taking a course in listening.
2. Interview one transformational leader in an institution where you work or where you are having clinical experiences about interpersonal power, influence strategies, and transformational leadership skills. Use the content in each of these suggestions to formulate your questions.

REFERENCES

Ashforth, B. E. (2001). *Role transitions in organizational life: An identity based perspective.* Mahwah, NJ: Lawrence Erlbaum Associates.

Avolio, B. J., & Luthan, F. (2006). *The high impact leader: Moments matter in accelerating authentic leadership development.* New York: McGraw-Hill.

Bass, B. M. (1999). Two decades of research and development in transformational leadership. *European Journal of Work and Organizational Psychology, 8*(1), 9–32.

Benedict, L., Robinson, K., & Holder, C. (2006). Clinical nurse specialists within the acute care for elders interdisciplinary team model. *Clinical Nurse Specialist, 20*(5), 248–251.

Burke, P. J. (1991). Identify processes and social stress. *American Sociological Review, 56,* 836–849.

Burns, J. M. (1978). *Leadership.* New York: Harper & Row.

Cable, d. M., & Judge, T. A. (2003). Managers' upward influence tactic strategies: The role of manager personality and supervisor leadership style. *Journal of Organizational Behavior, 24,* 197–214.

Cialdini, R. B. (2008). *Influence: Science and practice* (5th ed.). Boston, MA: Allyn and Bacon.

Cook, M. J., & Leathard, H. L. (2004). Learning for clinical leadership. *Journal of Nursing Management, 12,* 436–444.

Dietz, B., & Smith, T. T. (2002). Enhancing the accuracy of hemodynamic monitoring. *Journal of Nursing Care Quality, 17*(1), 27–34.

Dirks, K., & Ferrin, D. (2001). The role of trust in organizational settings. *Organizational Science, 12*(4), 450–467.

Duffy, J. R. (2002). The clinical leadership role of the CNS in the identification of nursing-sensitive and multidisciplinary quality indicator sets. *Clinical Nurse Specialist: The Journal for Advanced Nursing Practice, 16*(2), 70–76.

Ebright, P., Patterson, E. S., & Render, M. L. (2002). The "new look" approach to patient safety: A guide for clinical nurse specialist leadership. *Clinical Nurse Specialist: The Journal for Advanced Nursing Practice, 16*(5), 247–253.

Eisenbach, R., Watson, K., & Rajinandini, P. (1999). Transformational leadership in the context of organizational change. *Journal of Organizational Change, 12*(2), 80–89.

Emerson, R. M. (1962). Power-dependence relations. *American Sociological Review, 27,* 31–41.

Farmer, S. M., & Aguinis, H. (2005). Accounting for subordinate perceptions of supervisor power: An identity-dependence model. *Journal of Applied Psychology, 90*(6), 1069–1083.

Foggow, D. J., Solie, C. J., Tracy, M. F., & Gjere, N. (2005). Clinical nurse specialist leadership in computerized provider order entry design. *Clinical Nurse Specialist, 19*(4), 209–214.

Gillespie, N., & Mann, L. (2004). Transformational leadership and shared values: The building blocks of trust. *Journal of Healthcare Management, 19*(6), 588–607.

George, B. (2003). *Authentic leadership: Rediscovering the secrets to creating lasting value.* San Francisco, CA: Jossey-Bass.

Green, A., & Jordan, C. (2004). Common denominators: Shared governance and work place advocacy—strategies for nurses to gain control over their practice. *Journal of Issues in Nursing, 9*(1).

Grossman, S. C., & Valiga, T. M. (2005). *The new leadership challenge: Creating the future of nursing* (2nd ed.). Philadelphia, PA: F. A. Davis.

Groves, K. S. (2005). Linking leader skills, follower attitudes and contextual variables via an integration of charismatic leadership. *Journal of Management, 31,* 255–277.

Herold, D. M., Fedor, D. B., Caldwell, S., & Liu, Y. (2008). The effects of transformational and change leadership on employee's commitment to a change: A multilevel study. *Journal of Applied Psychology, 93*(2), 346–357.

How Stuff Works. (2008). *Magnets.* Retrieved August 19, 2008, from http://science.howstuffworks.com/magnet.htm

Huber, D. (2000). *Power and conflict: Leadership and nursing care management.* Philadelphia: WB Saunders.

Kipnis, D., & Schmidt, S. M. (1988). Upward-influence styles: Relationship with performance evaluations, salary, and stress. *Administrative Science Quarterly, 33*, 528–542.

Kouzes, J. M., & Posner, B. Z. (2002). *Leadership: The challenge* (3rd ed.). San Francisco: Jossey-Bass.

Lyon, B. L. (2001a). Conquering frustration: REAPing the Benefits. *Reflections in Nursing Leadership, 27*(1), 38–39.

Lyon, B. L. (2001b). Positive situational focusing: Pollyanna or a powerful stress prevention strategy? *Reflections in Nursing Leadership, 27*(2), 38–39, 45.

Lyon, B. L. (2001c). Strategies to enhance positive situational focusing skills. *Reflections in Nursing Leadership, 27*(3), 36–37, 44.

Merriam-Webster Online Dictionary. (2008). Influence. Retrieved July 17, 2008, from http://www.merriam-webster.com/dictionary/power

Merriam-Webster Online Dictionary. (2008). Power. Retrieved July 17, 2008, from http://www.merriam-webster.com/dictionary/power

Morissette, J. (2004). Clinical nurse specialist as a leader of a bariatric program. *Clinical Nurse Specialist: The Journal for Advanced Nursing Practice, 19*(4), 209–215.

National Association of Clinical Nurse Specialists. (2004). *Statement on clinical nurse specialist practice and education* (2nd ed.). Harrisburg, PA: Author.

Roberts, D. W., & Vasquez, E. (2004). Power: An application to the nursing image and advanced practice. *AACN Clinical Issues, 15*(2), 196–204.

Rosenthal, M. B. (2007). Nonpayment for performance? Medicare's new reimbursement rule. *The New England Journal of Medicine, 357*, 1573–1575.

Seemann, S., Soukup, M., & Adams, P. (2000). Hospital wide intravenous initiative. *Nursing Clinics of North America, 35*(2), 361–373.

Spinelli, R. (2006). The applicability of Bass's model of transformational, transactional and laissez-faire leadership in the hospital administrative environment. *Hospital Topics, 84*(2), 11–18.

Yukl, G., & Falbe, C. M. (1990). Influence tactics and objective in upward, downward, and lateral influence attempts. *Journal of Applied Psychology, 77*, 525–535.

12

Creating a Culture of Quality

Nancy Benton

According to the National Association of Clinical Nurse Specialists' (NACNS) *Statement on Clinical Nurse Specialist Practice and Education* (2004), clinical nurse specialists (CNSs) "provide expert and independent care to promote health by promoting wellness, preventing illness, and providing expert assistance with disease care" (p. 55). Implied within this statement is that CNSs practice in their role with attention to the quality of care provided. Quality in health care, however, can be an elusive concept. The purpose of this chapter is to provide some insight into how quality in health care is defined, measured, and improved to create a culture of quality within the context of the practice and role of the CNS.

Historic approaches and perceptions of quality in health care are discussed, followed by contemporary approaches to ensuring health care quality. A definition for quality health care from the nursing perspective is also discussed. Finally, the CNSs role in creating a culture of quality is explored.

BACKGROUND

In order to understand quality as it pertains to nursing roles, it is useful to go back to the beginning of modern nursing. Additionally, there is information and insight to be gained from reviewing the medical profession's approach to quality health care.

Quality Pioneers

It could be argued that the first nurse to address quality of care was Florence Nightingale in the mid-19th century. She abhorred and fought to change the appalling conditions in which soldiers of war received medical care. By changing and improving the conditions where injured soldiers were treated, mortality outcomes were improved. This could be defined as one of the first quality outcomes in health care where nursing played a key role. Florence Nightingale may well be the first nurse who was also a health care quality improvement specialist. Not unlike today's quality professionals, Florence Nightingale used scientific methodology to gather data and employed statistical processes to identify areas in need of improvement (Neuhauser, 2003).

Later, her aspirations to improve the quality of health care led her to open the first training academy for nurses. It could be said that modern nursing has its most fundamental beginnings in the pursuit of quality health care. Florence Nightingale devoted her entire adult life to improving the quality of health care as it relates to the nursing profession. In addition to collecting data and using statistical techniques to identify improvement opportunities related to clinical practice and outcomes, she also devoted herself to improving the competence of nurses through standardized training for nurses.

In a more recent example for quality improvement in health care, a 20th-century pioneer in health care quality, Avedis Donabedian, proposed a comprehensive approach to examining quality in his landmark paper "Evaluating the Quality of Medical Care" (Donabedian, 2005). Donabedian has been called the father of quality assurance, and it is his work that is most often cited in health care quality research. Donabedian, a physician with a master of public health degree, recognized that medical care does not occur in a vacuum. The health care system and numerous health care disciplines are interwoven with each other and inextricably linked to quality outcomes. Recognizing this linkage, Donabedian proposed a structure-process-outcome model for assessing quality. *Structure* referred to the physical and organizational settings in which providers of health care practice, as well as the tools and resources they have available. *Process* referred to the manner in which health care was administered, such as patient–provider interaction, documentation of interventions, and competence of practice. Finally, *outcomes* referred to whether the desired result was achieved (Donabedian, 1980). These three dimensions of health care delivery are the framework most often used to develop methods for examining and improving the quality of health care. Measuring components of the structure, process, and outcome of health care delivery help determine what is working well and what needs improvement.

Donabedian (2005) devoted his entire career in medicine and public health to promote better understanding of quality and methods to improve the quality of health care. In a 1996 article he offered the following advice: "To my mind, the most important single condition for success in quality assurance is the determination to make it work. If we are truly committed to quality, almost any reasonable method will work. If we are not, the most elegantly constructed of mechanisms will fail" (p. 406). Donabedian was trying to tell us that passion for improvement is the necessary ingredient to successful quality improvement efforts.

DEFINING QUALITY

The word *quality* is used in health care frequently, for example, high-quality health care, quality health care organizations, improving the quality of health care, ensuring quality, quality management, and quality improvement. *Quality* as a word is easily defined, and there are many definitions. However, quality in health care is a complex concept that is not easily defined. The American Heritage Dictionary (2000) lists *quality* as an adjective: Having a high degree of excellence: the importance of quality health care. To be certain, quality in health care is important, but the question remains, what is quality in health care, and how do we know it when we see it?

The first step in understanding a complex concept such as quality in health care is to define the concept. The literature on health care quality is scant with true concept analyses as defined by Walker and Avant (1994). Nevertheless, there are some definitions available that relate to quality in health care.

In their policy statement H-450.975, the American Medical Association (AMA; 2007) defines quality of care as "the degree to which care services influence the probability of optimal patient outcomes." The Institute of Medicine (2001, p 52) defines quality as "the degree to which health services for individuals and populations increase the likelihood of desired health outcomes and are consistent with current professional knowledge." Both of these definitions seem to leave out key components of quality important to nursing, namely, caring and patient involvement. The American Nurses Association (ANA) states that quality is a changing concept and that, currently, quality in health care is "meeting the public's expectations in the delivery of clinically effective, efficient, and affordable health care services" (Kay, 2005 p.75). This definition explicitly includes the patient perspective on quality. However, the concept of safety in health care is missing from this definition of quality.

Quality is a concept that is influenced by individual perceptions. Quality in health care is not necessarily a concept that demands attention when it is present in the health care experience. Indeed, quality in health care may best be noticed and described when it is missing from the health care experience. For example, the patient who waits many hours in an emergency room only to receive the wrong treatment by overworked health care professionals in an abrupt and less than caring manner is sure to recognize the lack of quality in his/her health care experience, whereas the patient who receives timely, correct treatment from health care professionals who are compassionate and caring may consider the experience routine and expected. That patient may not necessarily think to describe the experience as quality health care.

What is quality for some may not be so for others. The indicators of quality may differ depending upon the viewpoint of the evaluator and the context in which the health care experience occurs. Patient perceptions of whether or not they have received quality health care are often very different from the health care professionals' perceptions of whether quality health care was delivered. Equally, the patient and professionals' perceptions may be very different from the health care system perspective of whether quality health care was delivered. An all-encompassing definition of quality as it relates to health care is difficult.

PERSPECTIVES ON QUALITY

As mentioned previously, perceptions of quality in health care differ depending upon the standpoint of the observer. Patients, health care practitioners, and health care systems will all have different ideas of what represents quality.

Within the category of health care providers, nursing and medicine clearly have different definitions of quality. Most prominent in medicine's literature is outcomes of clinical care as a measure of quality (IOM,

2001). In nursing, assessment, processes, planning care delivery, and a holistic focus for quality health care is evident (Attree, 1996.)

In the context of the CNSs role, quality health care demands that we examine the practice component as well as the patient perception of quality. Additionally, as an advanced practice nurse, an essential characteristic of the CNS is advanced expertise in "human and organizational factors that affect resource management, quality, and cost across the continuum of care" (NACNS, 2004, p. 14). The CNS must also be concerned with quality, not only as it relates to individual care but to populations as well as health care systems.

QUALITY AND CNS SPHERES OF INFLUENCE

The conceptual model of CNS practice includes the patient/client sphere, the nurse and nursing practice sphere, and the organization/system sphere (NACNS, 2004). The concept of quality health care and its relationship to the three spheres is the framework for the CNS role in creating a culture of quality.

Patient/Client Sphere

Today, most patients have some idea of the meaning of quality health care; however, individual perceptions of quality may differ between patients. If there is any doubt in the patient's mind about the quality of health care they are receiving, the Agency for Healthcare Research and Quality (AHRQ) has published a consumer booklet titled "Guide to Health Care Quality: How to Know It When You See It." In this guide the AHRQ places emphasis on the clinical quality of care. Did the outcome achieved match the desired outcome? There is no disagreement that outcome measures, such as whether the surgery removed all of the cancer or whether the treatment regimen improved cardiac output, are appropriate indicators of quality for patients. However, outcome measures are not the only important indicators of quality.

Age-specific quality is another consideration. A geriatric patient's view of quality health care is likely different than the young adult view, which is different, yet again, from the perspective of a pediatric patient. The pediatric patient may gauge quality by whether or not the immunization injection was painful or whether the health care staff were friendly. The young adult patient may value timeliness of the appointment and waiting room times as important indicators for quality. The geriatric patient, however, may value the provider's caring attitude and willingness to take the time to listen to them as the most important indicator of quality. The

patient viewpoint is an important measure of quality health care.

Patient satisfaction reports encompass the latest research on patient perceptions, which includes domains of satisfaction related to health care provider interactions, ancillary health care staff interactions, timeliness and responsiveness of care, and whether educational needs were met. Some satisfaction surveys also include questions regarding the environment in which care was delivered, such as whether the waiting rooms and exam rooms were clean and well-appointed.

The patient as a partner in his or her own health care is also important. Most patients today are very well-informed about health care and their particular chronic disease. Being patient-centered demands that the CNS not only demonstrate a caring attitude but also be responsive to including the patient in decision making about his/her own health care. This requires the CNS to be equally well-informed and well-equipped to answer questions and provide the latest evidence-based information to help the patient in decision making.

The patient/client sphere of nursing practice as it relates to creating a culture of quality includes two important concepts. The first concept is patient satisfaction: Does the patient/client perceive his/her needs were met in a manner that was competent, respectful, and caring? The second concept relates to CNS competence: Is the CNS well-informed regarding the latest treatment options and alternatives, and was this information shared with the patient in a way he or she could understand and, therefore, participate in the decision making?

Nurse and Nursing Practice Sphere

Most, if not all, health care professionals enter the health care profession with the intent to ease the pain and suffering caused by illness and injury and to help to restore patients to their optimal potential functioning. The successful provision of health care is most often measured by outcome indicators. Did the patient receive a timely diagnosis? Did the surgery remove all of the cancer? Did the patient live?

CNSs advance nursing practice by setting examples and providing leadership to guide nurses in the application of evidence-based practice. There is substantial evidence in the literature with regard to improved outcomes for patients that can be directly related to the quantity and quality of nursing care (ANA, 1997). The CNS role in quality with regard to the nurses and nursing practice sphere is to be well-versed in the measures of quality that relate to nursing practice and to facilitate optimal performance in those measures. Some examples of quality indicators for nursing care are pressure ulcer development, intravenous infiltration occurrences, and falls.

Organization/System Sphere

The health care system is also concerned with quality. Therefore, the CNS has a role in quality improvement from a systems perspective. Examples of system issues are access to the health care system in the form of access to care, waiting times for appointments, and waiting room times. These are three common indicators of quality from a system perspective. Reduction of cost, waste, and risk are other matters of quality from the health care system perspective.

The CNS role in quality from an organization/system perspective is to understand issues of quality that are important to the health care organization. The CNS can lend clinical and organizational expertise to improving performance on those indicators that have been defined by the organization.

In summary, quality in health care as it relates to the conceptual model of CNS practice and the three spheres of influence necessarily overlap. What is within the patient/client sphere and nursing and nursing practice sphere of influence overlaps into the organization/system sphere. The following case example illustrates how the three spheres of influence overlap.

Case Example

A 55-year-old patient is admitted to the hospital with pneumonia and chronic obstructive pulmonary disease (COPD) exacerbation. This patient has intersected the HMO health care system six times within the past year but has not received pneumococcal or influenza immunizations. The medical team is concerned with the immediate episode of care for this patient, and immunizations have not been ordered. The CNS reviews the patient record and notices that this is his third hospital admission with pneumonia and COPD exacerbation in the past 18 months. The CNS also notices that there is no record of immunizations. The CNS approaches the patient and asks about his immunization history. The patient states that influenza and pneumococcal immunizations were offered to him once, but he refused because he does not like shots. The CNS provides information to the patient regarding recent research that indicates significantly reduced COPD exacerbations and hospitalizations for patients who have had both influenza and pneumococcal immunizations. The patient agrees to be immunized, and the CNS alerts the registered nurse (RN) assigned to that patient to administer both immunizations under a recently developed protocol (developed by the CNS) for administration of immunizations without a physician order.

After the episode with the single COPD patient, the CNS considers a system approach to immunization from an acute care perspective. The CNS gathers data on admissions of patients who could benefit from immunizations. The CNS discovers that there is no system in place to identify and administer immunizations to a particular population of patients who could benefit significantly, that is, patients with admitting diagnoses of COPD or pneumonia. This issue becomes the driver for the CNS to gather a team to explore the development of a system that identifies and vaccinates all patients with an admitting diagnosis of COPD or pneumonia.

This is an example of all three spheres of influence in CNS practice coming together to improve patient outcomes: First, the ability to recognize an opportunity to deliver evidenced-based care in the form of immunizations and providing appropriate evidence-based education to the patient falls under the patient/client sphere; second, alerting the RN in charge of the care of that patient to administer the immunizations relates to the nurse and nursing practice sphere; and third, utilizing the system-level approach to identify high-risk patients who could benefit from immunizations and facilitating an organizational approach to expedient immunizations falls under the organization/system sphere.

QUALITY FRAMEWORKS

The structure, process, and outcome model of quality health care proposed by Donabedian (1996) is closely aligned with the CNS spheres of influence. The organization/system sphere relates to *structure* in the Donabedian model. The nurse and nursing practice sphere relate to *process,* and the patient/client sphere relates to *outcomes.*

With the exception of Donabedian's early and enduring works, there is a dearth of conceptual models of quality in health care. Particularly lacking are conceptual models of quality as they relate to nursing practice. This reveals the nascent nature of the science of quality health care within the context of nursing.

That is not to say that nursing has not been vocal about quality as it relates to nursing care. In 1995, the ANA published the Nursing Care Report Card for Acute Care in which they proposed 21 measures of nursing care purported to be linked to the quality and availability of nursing care in the acute hospital setting. In 1997, the ANA asked for proposals to develop and maintain the National Database for Nursing Quality Indicators (NDNQI). In 1998, NDNQI, which is now a registered trademark, began accepting data from hospitals and charging for the use of the system, including submission of data as well as reports from the database.

The NDNQI uses the structure, process, and outcomes (Donabedian, 1980) approach to measuring quality by identifying nurse-sensitive indicators of quality. Nursing-sensitive indicators are defined as those outcomes that improve in the presence of greater quantity (higher staffing ratios) or quality (educational levels and competence of nursing staff) of nursing care. As mentioned earlier, some examples of quality indicators for nursing care are pressure ulcer development, intravenous infiltration occurrences, and falls.

These nursing-sensitive measures help hospitals to analyze the quality and quantity of nursing care services. The national database provides benchmark performance with which the individual health care institution can compare their performance to similar hospitals across the nation.

Another quality model that incorporates a broad view of health care and seeks to define quality is the Quality Health Care (QHC) model (N. Benton, personal communication, 2007). It is made up of three spheres, which encompass three areas of quality that are most often considered important elements in quality health care. The intersection of the three spheres, that is, where the three elements exist together, encompasses the factors that define quality health care (see Figure 12.1).

Safe health care includes all of the processes and procedures in place to ensure health care is delivered in a safe manner. The indicators of safety include processes such as hand-washing monitors, time-out protocols for surgery, fall reduction programs, and a *do not use* list of abbreviations to name a few. The indicators of patient-centered health care include processes designed to measure patient satisfaction, such as emergency room waiting times and other patient-centered indicators of quality. Clinically competent health care includes education and competency of staff; adherence to clinical practice guidelines for chronic disease, such as annual retinal eye exam for diabetics who are insulin dependent; and adherence to prevention guidelines, such as screening for colorectal, breast, and cervical cancer and immunizations. The QHC model proposes that when all three elements come together for a particular patient or population, quality health care is achieved.

The QHC model differs from the Donabedian structure, process, and outcomes model. Donabedian's model proposed a framework to guide quality professionals in developing measures for quality. The QHC model is a conceptual model for defining quality in health care. The QHC model can also be used to categorize health care activities for identifying quality factors as well as risk factors in existing systems of health care delivery.

MEASURING QUALITY

Quality cannot be measured directly. Quality is measured by performance on identified indicators of quality. One indicator of quality is approval or accreditation from a quality oversight organization. Other indicators of quality encompass the domains of prevention, disease management, patient satisfaction, and patient safety.

Quality Oversight Organizations

One of the longest standing and well-known health care quality oversight organizations is The Joint Commission (formerly known as the Joint Commission on the Accreditation of Healthcare Organizations). This quality oversight organization has its roots firmly in the practice of medicine. The precursor to today's Joint Commission Standards was the Minimum Standards for Hospitals document created by the American College of Surgeons in 1917. However, it was not until 1953 when The Joint Commission first offered accreditation to hospitals and published the first Standards for Hospital Accreditation. Over the next 50 years, The Joint Commission expanded beyond hospital accreditation to nearly every venue in which health care is delivered, including inpatient and outpatient care. Today, all federally funded health care organizations and any health care organization that accepts federal payments for health care, such as Medicare, is required to maintain accreditation from The Joint Commission or an equivalent quality oversight group.

The list of accrediting agencies is long and includes organizations such as the National Council on Quality Assurance (NCQA), which has developed standards for health care plans and outpatient clinical care. The College of American Pathologists (CAP) has developed standards for the accreditation of diagnostic laboratories. The American Association of Blood Banks (AABB) has developed accreditation standards for blood and tissue banks. The Commission on the Accreditation of Rehabilitation Facilities (CARF) has developed accreditation guidelines and standards for medical rehabilitation facilities, as well as behavioral health, community, child, youth, and aging services. This list is not comprehensive

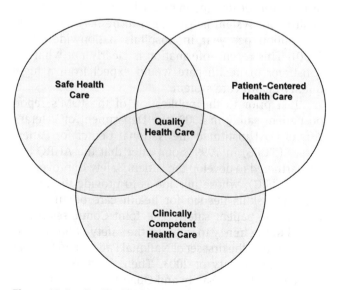

Figure 12.1 Quality health care model.

and accounts for only a handful of the quality oversight groups available to assess the quality of care provided by health care facilities and programs. In addition to national accreditation organizations, most states have quality oversight agencies (state inspectors) that periodically inspect health care facilities, most often in the long-term care arena of health care.

Quality Indicators

Whether an organization achieves and retains accreditation by a quality oversight group can be one indicator of quality. There are many other indicators of quality, such as adherence to clinical practice guidelines for chronic disease and population-specific prevention measures. Patient satisfaction has also become an indicator of overall quality.

Clinical Practice Guidelines

Guidelines for practice derive from research surrounding treatment of certain conditions, acute and chronic. For example, a patient with a diagnosis of insulin-dependent diabetes mellitus should receive very specific disease management elements of care, such as annual diabetic retinal examination, annual hemoglobin A1c laboratory testing, diabetic foot examination, renal function and lipid studies, and so forth. A patient presenting to an emergency room with a chief complaint of chest pain should receive aspirin, unless contraindicated for some other reason, and an electrocardiogram within 10 minutes.

There are literally hundreds of clinical practice guidelines that are based upon the most current research. A comprehensive and searchable database for clinical practice guidelines is provided by the AHRQ under the title of National Guideline Clearinghouse (AHRQ, 2007).

Prevention Guidelines

Although some clinical practice guidelines incorporate prevention for specific diagnoses, prevention guidelines are generally more population-based. For example, colorectal cancer screening should be done for all patients over the age of 50 and a one-time pneumococcal immunization should be given to all healthy adults age 65 and over, to name just two. The U.S. Preventive Services Task Force of the AHRQ (2006) has developed a guide for preventive services for clinicians that includes all of the recommended preventive health care services for all populations from pediatric to geriatric.

Patient Satisfaction

Another indicator of quality is patient or customer satisfaction. While the work surrounding health promotion and disease prevention was occurring in the late 1970s and early 1980s, customer satisfaction was just beginning to be explored as a potential indicator of quality (Cleary & McNeil, 1988). Until the connection between patient satisfaction and medical malpractice was made, not much attention was given to patient satisfaction in the literature. As the field of research into patient satisfaction became more active, patient satisfaction as a quality indicator emerged (Peskin, Micklitsch, Quirk, Sims, & Primack, 1995; Woodward, Ostbye, Craighead, Gold, & Wenghofer, 2000). When health care became something people sought for more than just illness or injury care and free market principles began to effect health care organizations there arose a competition for patients, particularly in the corporate for-profit hospitals and health systems. This phenomena helped focus attention on what the consumer of health care was looking for, thus, patient satisfaction as an indicator of quality became a popular research subject. Today, patient satisfaction is an important quality indicator in any health care organization.

Patient Safety

With all of the oversight of quality in health care by various accrediting organizations and the wealth of information to guide the health care system in delivering quality care, one might assume that high-quality health care is the standard in this country. However, in 2000, the IOM published *To Err is Human*, a comprehensive look at the safety of our health care system. In this publication the researchers estimated that between 44,000 to 98,000 deaths occur in the United States each year as a result of medical error. In other research it was estimated that 1.3 million nonfatal medical injuries resulted in disability or lengthened hospital stay (Bates & Gawande, 2000). The cost of medical error in the form of lost income, disability, and cost to the health care system is estimated to be between $17 to $29 billion per year in hospitals nationwide (IOM, 2000). This recent information is clearly not what the consumer of health care would expect from a high-quality health care system.

Just prior to the publication of the IOM's report on patient safety in 2000, the Department of Veterans Affairs (VA) instituted the National Center for Patient Safety (NCPS) in 1999. Soon after that the AHRQ and VA partnered to develop the Patient Safety Improvement Corps (PSIC), whose mission is to provide the knowledge and skills needed for health care organizations to improve patient safety. The Joint Commission also joined in the frenzy to improve the safety of health care by instituting the first set of National Patient Safety Goals (NPSG) in January of 2003. Then, in 2005, Congress passed the Patient Safety and Quality Improvement Act of 2005 (AHRQ, 2005), which was designed to analyze and aggregate patient safety information in an effort to identify system failures that could lead to improvement.

CNS Role in Quality Measurement

In order for something to be measured, it must be reduced to a numerical value. Quality oversight groups such as The Joint Commission issue a score or status to health care organizations. The Joint Commission has identified a cohort of universal quality measures for acute care hospitals called ORYX measures. Acute care organizations can now measure themselves against similar organizations to determine their quality standing with regard to emergent care for acute myocardial infarction, congestive heart failure, and pneumonia care, as well as nonemergent surgical care.

Beyond The Joint Commission's ORYX measures, many health care organizations who monitor their own quality measures have adopted clinical practice guidelines based upon diagnoses, prevention guidelines based upon the populations they serve, patient satisfaction scores, and patient safety goals. For each of these categories, quality indicators are developed to determine who needs the particular intervention and whether or not the intervention occurred. This results in a performance measure for that particular indicator. Most performance measures have target levels established by the organization that are based upon national data. Approximation of the target level is then translated into quality. A scorecard is developed, and the organization sets goals for the scorecard. For example, the organization will meet or exceed the target level for at least 30 of 45 targets. For targets that are not met, the organization will institute a performance improvement project to assist in reaching the target.

In addition to occasional collection of data points for quality monitoring, the CNS role in measuring quality is to understand the organizational approach to quality. The approach of the organization may differ depending upon the business model and whether it is a for-profit, corporate-owned health care delivery system or a federal- or state-funded organization. Each organization will have their own quality goals and measures defined. The CNS should be familiar with the goals and understand the measures of quality specific to that organization.

IMPROVING QUALITY

Measuring quality is a necessary and first step to quality improvement. Before something can be improved, two things must be known: Do the data indicate a need for improvement? If so, what is the baseline upon which improvement will be determined? An improvement team cannot know that their process changes have led to improvement unless they have baseline data with which to compare the postimplementation data.

Performance Improvement Methods

The basic process in performance improvement is similar to the nursing process with which all nurses are familiar: assess, plan, implement, and evaluate. However, in performance improvement the processes are named differently. There are numerous performance improvement methodologies, such as the Plan, Do Study, Act (PDSA) or the Focus, Analyze, Develop, and Execute (FADE) methodology, to name just two. What they all have in common is that they begin with identifying and analyzing the problem. This involves collecting and analyzing baseline data to determine causes and possible solutions. Based upon the analysis, a solution is identified and implemented and follow-up data are collected and compared to the baseline data to determine if the improvement was successful. If the desired performance level is not achieved, the process begins again and continues to repeat until the desired level of performance is achieved and sustained.

Quality Monitors

Once the improvement is accomplished, it may need to be monitored for a time to be sure the improvement efforts are sustained and that the processes put in place do not slide back into the preimprovement mode. Monitoring a new improvement is one type of quality monitor.

Another type of quality monitor is an ongoing monitor for quality, such as infection control monitoring or utilization monitoring. This type of quality monitoring is designed to continue indefinitely for the purpose of identifying problems as soon as possible. Statistical process control (SPC) techniques and control charts are often used to monitor and analyze the data for indicators of a quality problem. Details of SPC techniques are beyond the scope of this chapter; however, it is important for the CNS to know that SPC is a powerful tool that is often used in quality improvement.

The CNS Role in Improving Quality

Identifying opportunities for improvement that address or enhance patient safety issues, clinical competence and practice issues, and patient satisfaction issues is the primary role of the CNS in improving quality. The QHC model (Figure 12.1) can be used to guide the CNS in identifying areas where opportunities for improvement may exist. Once the need is identified, the CNS can facilitate the development of an improvement team to address the issue. The CNS role on the performance improvement team can be one of content expert, team leader, or team facilitator. The CNS must draw upon his/her leadership skills and often function in several roles on an improvement team in order to move the process forward.

CNS STRATEGIES FOR CREATING A CULTURE OF QUALITY

Strategies for creating a culture of quality can be aligned with the CNS core competencies. In Table 12.1, the CNS core competencies from the *Statement on Clinical Nurse Specialist Practice and Education* (NACNS, 2004) are listed on the left side of the table, and specific competencies for creating a culture of quality are provided on the right side of the table.

The CNS plays a pivotal role in identifying opportunities for improvement and in facilitating improvement in the health care organization. One of the most important skills a CNS must learn is multidisciplinary collaboration. Quality improvement opportunities rarely exist in a state where the CNS can identify the issue and improve the performance single-handedly or by collaborating only with other CNSs. Most quality issues are complex and require the input of several disciplines in identifying what needs to be improved in order to achieve the quality outcome.

Creating a culture of quality requires the CNS to understand the organizational priorities for quality. In the absence of clear organizational priorities, the CNS

12.1 | CNS Core Competencies and Quality Culture Strategies

CNS CORE COMPETENCY	CNS QUALITY CULTURE STRATEGY
1. Use knowledge of differential illness diagnoses and treatments in comprehensive, holistic assessments of patients within the context of disease, diagnoses, and treatments. The outcome of differential diagnosis of illness is to explicate etiologies that require nursing interventions to prevent or alleviate the illness.	Understand and use clinical practice guidelines and prevention guidelines to improve the quality of care to individual patients.
2. Design, implement, and evaluate innovative individual and/or population-based programs of care to achieve desired quality, cost-effective nurse-sensitive outcomes.	Use knowledge of performance goals related to clinical care to design and implement processes that facilitate delivery of care to individuals and populations.
3. Serve as a leader/consultant/mentor/change agent in advancing the practice of nursing among other nurses and across organizations to achieve outcomes.	Know and understand institutional performance measures and current performance for the purposes of identifying areas that need improvement and initiating process changes.
4. Advance nursing practice through innovative evidence-based interventions, best practice guidelines, and modification of professional standards and organizational policies that direct the care of nursing personnel and other providers of health care to improve outcomes.	Achieve expert understanding of prevention and clinical practice guidelines as well as patient satisfaction and patient safety to act as mentor and teacher of guidelines to other nurses.
5. Lead multidisciplinary groups to facilitate collaboration with other disciplines in the attainment of outcomes across the continuum of care.	Act as content expert in multidisciplinary teams designed to improve performance on quality performance measures.
6. Interpret the dimensions of nursing care requiring resources at the system level, and provide leadership to ensure that the system adequately supports the delivery of nursing care.	Provide leadership at the institutional or community level to develop policies and procedures that support improvement on quality performance measures and adherence to clinical practice and prevention guidelines.
7. Expand the practice of nursing through ongoing generation and acquisition of scientific knowledge and skills to maintain expert clinical competencies that leads to desired outcomes.	Facilitate the research and development of additional nurse-sensitive quality indicators and competencies to address nurse-sensitive quality indicators.
8. Demonstrate professional citizenship and fiscal responsibility in the health care system by focusing on health policy and/or resource management to ensure quality, cost-effective outcomes of nursing care.	Demonstrate knowledge of performance improvement and the linkage between quality performance measures and clinical outcomes.

may use the QHC model (Figure 12.1) to explore the realm of quality health care and identify areas needing improvement. Once the opportunities for improvement are identified, the CNS can start by collecting baseline data if none exists. Armed with accurate baseline data, the CNS can then inspire others to participate in a multidisciplinary team process to brainstorm and target processes for improvement.

DISCUSSION QUESTIONS

1. In a large HMO, a quality indicator for colorectal cancer screening is that all patients age 50 or older should be screened. The institution is performing at 58% on this quality measure, which means that of all those who should been screened, only 58% were actually screened. The U.S. Preventive Services Task Force recommends annual fecal occult blood testing (FOBT) or colonoscopy every 10 years, or sigmoidoscopy or double contrast barium enema every 5 years. During an interdisciplinary discussion of performance measures, the reason for the poor performance on the colorectal cancer screening measure is discussed, and it is revealed that there is a lack of capacity for colonoscopies and that FOBT cards are not routinely given to patients. The CNS suggests stepping up efforts to increase FOBT for all patients 50 years or older who have not previously been screened. Is this an appropriate intervention? Why or why not?

2. The gastroenterologist on staff at the institution voices loud opposition to screening all patients with FOBT. His reasons are twofold: (a) FOBT screening can produce false positives and, in his opinion, is not an accurate screen for colorectal cancer; and (b) all positive FOBTs will need to be screened with colonoscopy, and as he said earlier, they simply have no more capacity to take on additional colonoscopy workload. Screening all eligible patients with FOBT would overwhelm them with additional workload. What would be a good response to this physician's comments?

3. Clinical practice guidelines for diabetes are comprehensive. Among other numerous annual and semi-annual testing and examinations, it is recommended that diabetic patients receive an annual foot exam, which includes sensory testing. The institution collects data on performance of all of the "diabetic measures" and discovers that nearly all of the guidelines are occurring at least 80% of the time with the exception of the annual foot exam, which occurs about 40% of the time. The primary care physicians in the HMO are responsible for all of the diabetic measures, and their collective comment is that these patients are so complex that to do the foot exam, unless the patient already has his/her shoes off, takes too much valuable physician time. Further, the reason that the rest of the diabetic performance measures are only hovering around 80% is that there are just so many, and the physician providers only have a limited amount of time with each patient. The CNS recommends an improvement effort that educates the clinic nurses to perform the foot exam and suggests instituting a diabetic protocol that orders all of the laboratory blood tests for hemoglobin A1c, lipids, and renal function automatically when they are due without specific orders from the physician. The physicians agree that this is a good idea. What is the next step for the CNS? Discuss all of the elements that need to be put in place to institute the aforementioned protocol.

REFERENCES

Agency for Healthcare Research and Quality. (2005). *The patient safety and quality improvement act of 2005*. Retrieved January 9, 2009, from http://www.ahrq.gov/qual/psoact.htm

Agency for Healthcare Research and Quality. (2006). *Guide to clinical preventive services. Recommendations of the U.S. Preventive Services Task Force*. Retrieved January 9, 2009, from http://www.ahrq.gov/clinic/pocketgd.htm

Agency for Healthcare Research and Quality. (2007). *National Guideline Clearinghouse*. Retrieved January 9, 2009, from http://www.guideline.gov

American Medical Association. (2007). *Definition of quality (policy number H-450.975)*. Retrieved January 24, 2009, from http://www.ama-assn.org/ad-com/polfind/Hlth-Ethics.pdf

American Nurses Association. (1995). *Nursing care report card for acute care*. Washington, DC: American Nurses Publishing.

American Nurses Association. (1997). *Implementing nursing's report card: A study of RN staffing, length of stay and patient outcomes*. Washington, DC: American Nurses Publishing.

Attree, M. (1996). Towards a conceptual model of "quality care." *International Journal of Nursing Studies, 33*(1), 13–28.

Bates, D. W., & Gawande, A. A. (2000). Error in medicine: What have we learned? *Annals of Internal Medicine, 132*(9), 763–767.

Cleary, P. D., & McNeil, B. J. (1988). Patient satisfaction as an indicator of quality care. *Inquiry, 25*(1), 25–36.

Donabedian, A. (1980). *Explorations in quality assessment and monitoring, volume 1: The definition of quality and approaches to its assessment*. Ann Arbor, MI: Health Administration Press.

Donabedian, A. (1996). The effectiveness of quality assurance. *International Journal for Quality in Health Care, 8*(4), 401–407.

Donabedian, A. (2005). Evaluating the quality of medical care 1966. *Milbank Quarterly, 83*(4), 691–729.

Institute of Medicine. (2000). *To err is human: Building a safer health system*. Washington, DC: National Academies Press.

Institute of Medicine. (2001). *Crossing the quality chasm: A new health system for the 21st century*. Washington, DC: National Academies Press.

Kay, M. (2005). Issues update. The ANA's visionary approach: Shining the light on high-quality care—one step at a time. *American Journal of Nursing, 105*(7), 73.

National Association of Clinical Nurse Specialists. (2004). *Statement on clinical nurse specialist practice and education* (2nd ed.). Harrisburg, PA: Author.

Neuhauser, D. (2003). Florence Nightingale gets no respect: As a statistician that is. *Quality and Safety in Health Care, 12,* 317.

Peskin, T., Micklitsch, C., Quirk, M., Sims, H., & Primack, W. (1995). Malpractice, patient satisfaction, and physician-patient communication. *Journal of the American Medical Association, 274*(1), 22.

Walker, L., & Avant, K. (1994). Concept analysis. In L. Walker & K. Avant (Eds.), *Strategies for theory construction in nursing* (3rd ed.), 77–102. Upper Saddle River, NJ: Prentice Hall.

Woodward, C. A., Ostbye, T., Craighead, J., Gold, G., & Wenghofer, E. F. (2000). Patient satisfaction as an indicator of quality care in independent health facilities: Developing and assessing a tool to enhance public accountability. *American Journal of Medical Quality, 15*(3), 94–105.

13

Newer Thinking About Patient Safety

Patricia R. Ebright

At the start of the 21st century, the health care industry made dramatic changes in its approach to patient safety. Although fundamental clinical nurse specialist (CNS) competencies outlined in the *Statement on Clinical Nurse Specialist Practice and Education* (National Association of Clinical Nurse Specialists [NACNS], 2004) equip CNSs with essential core knowledge and skills for leading and participating in a variety of program efforts, it is important that CNSs understand how these competencies complement the new approach to patient safety. Interestingly, it was through learning from other industries about the need to approach safety differently that health care inadvertently found itself aligned more than ever with nursing care theories and the advanced practice of nursing defined by CNS core competencies, which focus on the uniqueness and complexity of humans and other complex systems.

This chapter includes discussion of the events leading to the shift in patient safety focus and of subsequent legislative and regulatory developments that have had an impact on work in patient safety. Concepts and information learned from other high-risk industries about several theoretical frameworks and models underpinning the changes are explained, including the epidemiology of error, human factors, complex adaptive systems, safety culture, and characteristics of high-reliability organizations. The most recent developments in the evolving knowledge about patient safety improvement are discussed as well as ongoing and future challenges in implementation and improvement efforts.

Widely used strategies and tools for assessing, improving, and evaluating safety are identified. The author has outlined important organizational behaviors

characteristic of an effective patient safety program. The chapter concludes with ethical considerations for CNS work in patient safety.

HISTORY OF THE PATIENT SAFETY MOVEMENT

The nursing profession and CNSs, in particular, have always focused on the development and implementation of standards, education, and mentoring of nurses that promote patient safety and quality (Peplau, 1965/2003). Starting in the early 1980s, before the 2000 release of *To Err is Human: Building a Safer Health System* by the Institute of Medicine (IOM) on medical error and patient safety, a series of events drew attention to injury and deaths resulting from medical error. These events included: establishment of the Anesthesia Patient Safety Foundation in 1984 for improvement of perioperative patient safety (Silker, 2006); findings reported from physician studies on the large numbers of preventable disabling injuries and deaths identified from medical records in the 1990s (e.g., Leape, 1994); 1996 regulatory and legislative activities by The Joint Commission (2009a) requiring hospital compliance with monitoring, investigation, and reporting of errors; and the creation of national organizations focused on patient safety (e.g., National Patient Safety Foundation in 1998 and the National Quality Forum in 1999).

Until the IOM report was released in 2000, most health care providers did not appreciate the magnitude of the medical error problem. Furthermore, those who were concerned about medical error tended to try traditional methods of approaching the problem with little long-term success. Reading about the tens of thousands of Americans who were dying each year from errors in medical care and the hundreds of thousands who were injured, or almost injured, during their care served as a wake-up call that more was needed to be done to prevent harm to patients and to improve quality of care. It became clear for many leaders in the health care industry that existing approaches to safety and quality were no longer sufficient to improve or even sustain the quality of care necessary to protect patients as recommended in subsequent IOM reports.

Authors of *Crossing the Quality Chasm: A New Health System for the 21st Century* (IOM, 2001) called for fundamental change to improve health care through six aims (see Table 13.1).

Health care leaders searched for solutions from industries other than health care, such as the airline, aerospace, and nuclear industries, to prevent high-stakes failures and reduce the harm resulting from error. These industries had learned long before about why errors happen, the role of human limitations in error generation, and the roles that workers and leaders play in increasing and sustaining safety (Weick & Suttcliffe, 2001).

More specifically, leaders of health care organizations began to realize that sustainable improvements in patient safety would require a switch from the traditional health care focus on individual care providers as the sole cause of error to consideration of the complex systems in which they work, and to the limited capacity within individuals themselves. This represented a change in focus from demanding perfect individual performance in imperfect situations to understanding the imperfect situations in which imperfect performers work. This change in approach to patient safety has required swift action by health care leaders related to new learning, resources, and shifts in long-held cultural norms.

Though some health care organizations have made great progress toward the recommendations from the IOM (2001), they vary widely in sustainable achievements, demonstrating the daunting task of changing an entire industry's culture surrounding failure (Leape & Berwick, 2005). The next section describes legislative and regulatory efforts that have affected the pace of needed change.

Legislative and Regulatory Focus on Patient Safety

In response to the IOM reports and starting with Minnesota in 2003 (Minnesota Department of Health, 2009), individual states have continued to enact legislation to require health care organizational reporting and public disclosure of serious errors. State reporting systems vary by whether they are mandatory or voluntary; and if mandatory, the types of information reported, and what is done with the data. Two major problems with the current effectiveness of state systems are underreporting by health care organizations and lack of funding to maintain and manage the data.

Since 2003, The Joint Commission has published an annual list of Patient Safety Goals that health care organizations must achieve to receive a successful accreditation review (The Joint Commission, 2009b). The Institute for Healthcare Improvement (IHI) sponsors clinically focused improvement initiatives to challenge health care organizations toward the realization of successful patient outcomes through specific quality and safety programs (e.g., IHI, 2009). These initiatives have resulted in thousands of lives saved. The National Patient Safety Foundation (NPSF) and the Agency for Healthcare Research and Quality (AHRQ) fund research on patient safety. The following organizations have also responded to the 2000 IOM report with efforts to improve patient safety: Department of Health and Human Services (DHHS), Center for Disease Control and Prevention (CDC), Center for Medicare and Medicaid Services (CMS), Leapfrog Group, and Healthgrades.

13.1 | Six Aims for Fundamental Change in Health Care

AIM	DESCRIPTION
Safe	Avoid injuries to patients from the care that is intended to help them.
Effective	Match care to science; avoid overuse of ineffective care and underuse of effective care.
Patient-centered	Honor the individual and respect choice.
Timely	Reduce waiting for both patients and those who give care.
Efficient	Reduce waste.
Equitable	Close racial and ethical gaps in health status.

In early 2000, work in patient safety focused on the need to move away from the traditional focus on individuals and the so-called blame culture that enveloped error situations. We moved to more understanding of complex systems, understanding of how error occurs, and ways to redesign specific aspects of the environment based on assessments of error situations. More recent efforts in attempting to improve and sustain delivery of safe patient care have turned to building resiliency in both our health care workers and care systems to prevent error and minimize poor outcomes as much as possible. We continue to learn about why things go wrong despite best intentions and to implement interventions to reduce adverse/near-miss events. These continuing efforts require leadership.

CNSs have been leaders in their organizations for many of the new legislative and regulatory activities related to patient safety. CNSs will continue to be leaders in this work because of their educational background and unique work experience in all three spheres of health care organizations (NACNS, 2004). CNS education emphasizes problem-solving strategies at the patient, nurse, and organizational system levels based on etiology-informed interventions and evaluation. This aspect of their practice and education makes CNSs very interested in the new learning about error generation, human limitations, and the complex adaptive systems (CASs) in which care is delivered. Because of the nature of their staff versus line role position in most organizations and their influencing skills, CNSs are uniquely prepared to effect change across diverse groups of care providers and workers, and they are able to accommodate cultural differences and reaction to change. Most fundamental to ongoing and dramatic change in health care, CNSs are experts in illness and disease management, which is crucial to understanding the impact of design and improvement changes on patient populations and care delivery, as well as for identification of important outcomes for measurement.

NEW LEARNING ABOUT PATIENT SAFETY

Several frameworks and models provide the backdrop for new learning related to the new approach to patient safety. One of these is *New Look* (Cook, Render, & Woods, 2000). In order to effectively lead and influence patient safety improvements, it is essential that CNSs acquire the fundamental knowledge base that supports this approach, which was introduced to health care in the late '90s and early 2000 and continues to drive the current initiatives for improvement of patient safety and quality. The following sections cover what we have learned about complex adaptive systems, evolution of error, work at the "sharp end," human limitations,

safety cultures, and finally, characteristics of high-reliability organizations.

Complex Adaptive Systems

In health care organizations, we have traditionally controlled the complexity inherent in situations and environments by assuming a simplistic pattern of decision making or causality. The benefit to this approach has been the appearance and feeling of control. A downside, however, is that such thinking includes the belief that activity is consistent and continuous and that there is one best solution for multiple situations (Suchman, 2002). Though nurses' basic educational preparation is grounded in a focus on the uniqueness of individual clients, maintaining this focus when providing nursing care very often competes with organizational priorities fitting with standardized, one-solution thinking. Our continuing attempts in nursing to solve problems following an error incident (e.g., wrong blood administration) with only the re-education of nurses about the related policy or procedure demonstrates the faulty assumption that one individual is the cause of the problem.

In contrast to traditional one-solution approaches to problem solving, approaches consistent with CAS characteristics are more compatible with today's health care environments and problems such as antibiotic-resistant diseases (Zimmerman, Lindberg, & Plsek, 1998). These complex system characteristics include unpredictability, ambiguity, time-pressure and stress-laden situations, high stakes, and decision making by teams with frequently changing members (Klein, 1998). Unlike linear explanations, explaining why things happen in light of CASs is very difficult. Causality is not unidirectional but most often bidirectional, involving the interaction of two or more entities. From these complex interactions emerge unpredictable behavioral patterns leading to small changes that may or may not lead to major widespread changes. Therefore, making change in complex environments requires recognition and appreciation for the bidirectionality and unpredictability of system relationships, including human, technical, and process. The focus for change in CAS thinking is on the ultimate goal but also on the intervening moments and processes because it is understood that each situation holds the possibility for continuation of the same, for surprises, or for new and emerging patterns. In his book *Diffusion of Innovations,* Rogers (2003) introduced us to findings about the realities and complexity surrounding implementation of change. In a complexity-based approach to problem solving or change, we understand we will not have complete control of situations or people in real work environments, just as we learned in nursing that we cannot control all aspects of individual client health situations.

What we in health care have learned from other high-stake industries, such as the airlines and nuclear power plants, about the evolution of error compliments the characteristics of CASs and challenges our traditional one-solution thinking approach to patient safety. Although this direction is new to health care, it is very consistent with the profession of nursing's holistic approach to care and its focus on the unique aspects of human beings for understanding illness and wellness. Demonstrated in the following sections is the natural fit of CNSs' advanced nursing practice focus on identification of etiologies as the basis for nursing care with the focus on system etiologies for a new approach to patient safety. This new approach to patient safety requires understanding of the details of actual work and of the actual and potential contributors (etiologies) to adverse/near-miss events.

Evolution of Error

Human factors science is a science focused on human performance in varying situations and environments, often in interaction with technology. The New Look approach (Cook et al., 2000) is a framework developed by human factors researchers based on system failure work by James Reason (1990) to explain the evolution of error or near-miss errors in health care situations. According to New Look, errors are not the result of a single failure of an unreliable component (such as an individual or piece of technology), but rather the result of multiple failures in the intended defenses of a system. New Look proponents suggest that improvements in patient safety can occur only when the five principles listed in Table 13.2 are appreciated by health care providers and leaders in a health care system (Woods & Cook, 1998).

13.2 | Five Principles Necessary to Understand for Improvement in Patient Safety

PRINCIPLE	INTERPRETATION
1. Safety is made and broken in systems, not by individuals. Adverse events result from the way work is designed and the interaction of components of the system.	1. Individuals as well as the systems in which they work are complex adaptive systems and as such reflect characteristics of complexity, including bidirectionality, relationships, and emerging and adaptive patterns.
2. Progress on safety begins with understanding technical work. Our current understanding of real work is naïve and incomplete, leading to the development of performance rules that are impossible to apply in a complex, heterogeneous, and rapidly changing world. Progress in safety depends on understanding how technical and organizational factors play out in real work.	2. Our tradition in health care is linear, and our tendency is to look for simple explanations. We must appreciate the delivery of health care work within complex environments to successfully implement and sustain improvements in safety. Detailed individual policies and procedures perfectly written and taught without consideration of actual work processes will not be sufficient to prevent adverse events.
3. Productive discussions of safety avoid confounding failure with error. Failure results from a breakdown in systems, whereas error is usually assigned to humans and relates to a social process for attributing cause.	3. The traditional culture surrounding failure and reaction to failure in health care is blame. Language following failure that reflects the traditional culture (e.g., error, blame, incident report) will lead to the same traditional reaction, or blaming, and is not a productive response in terms of improving safety.
4. Safety is dynamic and not static; it is constantly renegotiated. Complex, ever-changing systems require that people change and adapt constantly. However, adaptation is often based on inadequate information and only partly successful. Understanding this dynamic is the foundation for understanding safety. Increasing complexity makes safety harder to achieve.	4. Attention to improving and sustaining patient safety will require ongoing activities and continual adjustment.
5. Tradeoffs are at the core of safety. Complex work environments will always be characterized by uncertainty, discontinuities, and missing information. Understanding how people cope with these challenges will increase understanding of safety.	5. Understanding real work means appreciating the complexity of environments and realizing that in complex environments the resilient and most constant factor is the ability of people to adapt successfully. We need to learn how people manage in complex situations.

New Look: Using Reason's Swiss Cheese Model to Explain Failure

According to the New Look model (Cook et al., 2000) and as shown in Figure 13.1, which was adapted from Reason's Dynamics of Accident Causation model (Reason, 1990), layers of defense exist at all levels of an organization to provide guidance and boundaries around which decisions are developed and implemented. Traditionally, health care organizational defenses included but were not limited to policies and procedures, standard care guidelines, chain-of-command processes for communication and decisions, budget and resource allocations, report and hand-off mechanisms, competency standards, and technology. These defenses constituted important aspects of an organization's work in setting guidelines, standards, and boundaries for performance. However, in the past they have not allowed for either the situational or individual variation in naturally occurring events. They were intended for the "perfect" situation and, most often, for the experienced and knowledgeable provider.

Latent conditions, or *gaps,* are discontinuities in the layers of defenses in naturally occurring, or real work, environments (Cook et al., 2000). To illustrate, a gap exists when a specific patient situation does not exactly fit a policy and procedure for medication administration and following the policy or procedure would not be in the best interest of the patient. A gap exists when there is a lack of experienced personnel on a busy unit for one specific shift, resulting in less than the needed competencies and experience required to provide care

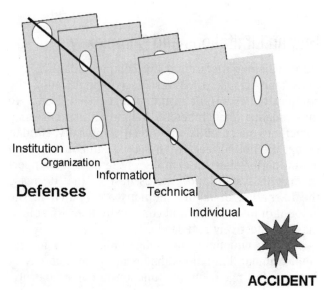

Figure 13.1   The New Look: Genesis of complex system failure.

From "The New Look: Genesis of Complex System Failure," by R. I. Cook, 1997, University of Chicago: Cognitive Technologies Laboratory. Copyright © 1997 by Cognitive Technologies Laboratory. Reprinted with permission.

for the unit's current acuity level and number of patients.

As the previous examples demonstrate, gaps do not represent overt failures, but they do constitute a type of latent condition that threatens the continuity of care and, when combined with other gaps or latent conditions, may lead to a *near miss* (an event or situation that could have resulted in an accident, injury, or illness, but did not, either by chance or through timely intervention) or *adverse event* (untoward incidents, therapeutic misadventures, iatrogenic injuries, or other adverse occurrences directly associated with care or services provided within the jurisdiction of a medical center, outpatient clinic, or other facility; adverse events may result from acts of commission or omission) (VA National Center for Patient Safety, 2009).

Active failures are errors and violations caused by acts performed by workers (e.g., nurses) closest to the "sharp end" of the system (e.g., patient care) and that affect system safety most directly (Reason, 1990). Reason suggested that most active failures are consequences of latent conditions and not principal causes of errors. For example, using a situation discussed previously, inadequate staffing (system gap or latent condition) for a specific shift may result in a nurse who is responding to time pressures to check one, but not all, patient identifiers (active failure) and then administers the wrong medication. The latent condition of inadequate staffing was a significant contributor to the error, even though not checking all identifiers also contributed.

Sometimes worker adaptation to ongoing system gaps (or latent conditions) becomes part of the routine work and goes unrecognized by the organization. As a consequence, implementation of new changes may unintentionally disrupt the efficacy of worker strategies to make up for latent conditions, or some changes may even create new gaps in the system. For example, a new technology or change in process may increase the time spent on a previously well-managed process and disrupt what has become a routine current flow of work. This type of disruption may cause decision *trade-offs* (decision resolutions that involve conflicting choices between highly unlikely but highly undesirable events and more likely but less catastrophic ones). Trade-offs are types of decisions made by nurses and other health care providers "between interacting or conflicting goals, between values or costs placed on different possible outcomes or courses of action, and between the risks of different errors" (Cook & Woods, 1994, p. 279) and more serious adverse patient outcomes. Using the medication error event described previously, the nurse "traded off" doing the more careful medication checks, probably relying on one or more other usually reliable cues (delivered medications to same patient earlier in shift, cared for the patient yesterday, capsules were same color she was accustomed to seeing, etc.) to be able to work faster and meet other organizational goals and/or patient care needs.

Leape and Berwick (2005) explained that health care lags behind other industries in safety because of its reliance on individual performance as the main key to improvement. Other industries have reduced errors by understanding that the way to be safer is to design systems so that it is difficult to make a mistake and easy to recover from mistakes that do occur (Weick & Sutcliffe, 2001).

Complexity of Work at the Sharp End Model

One of the principles stated previously for enabling progress in patient safety is about the importance of understanding actual work (see Table 13.1). Woods (1988) proposed that a major barrier to making progress in safety and quality is the failure to appreciate the complexity of work. In real work situations people anticipate, detect, and bridge gaps necessary for the delivery of safe care every day.

As Figure 13.2 (Cook & Woods, 1994) illustrates, health care workers operate at the point of care delivery (the *sharp end* and lower point of the triangle) and are involved in constantly evolving situations. Organizational resources and layers of defense from above (the *blunt*

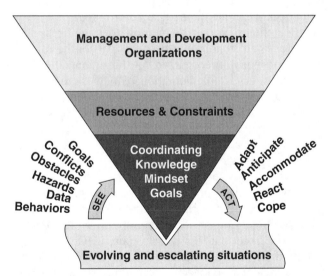

Figure 13.2 At the point-of-contact end of a complex system in which care is delivered is the health care worker (lowest point of triangle in the figure). To the left, the worker sees the factors that contribute to system complexity. To the right are the actions that resilient workers perform through coordination of knowledge, mindset, and goals to bridge gaps and achieve safety.

From "Behind Human Error: Cognitive Systems, Computers, and Hindsight," D. D. Woods, L. J. Johannesen, R. I. Cook, and N. B. Sarter, 1994. Copyright © 1994 Human Systems Ergonomic Information and Analysis Center, WPAFB. Reprinted with permission.

end) support and sometimes constrain health care workers as they continuously manage workloads using their knowledge, immediate perceptions, and own goals to handle situations. Surrounding care situations and confronting workers are multiple goal conflicts, obstacles, hazards, ambiguous and inadequate or missing data, and others' behaviors (the system complexities on the left side of the model). Workers usually prevent things from going wrong by anticipating, reacting, accommodating, adapting, and coping (characteristics of worker resiliency on the right side of the model) with system gaps and discontinuities. Furthermore, bridging these gaps involves constant compromise between multiple competing goals to make trade-off decisions in the midst of a changing environment.

The cognitive, or *invisible,* work required in complex work environments is demanding and despite best efforts may result in adverse events. Four characteristic dimensions of complex environments increase cognitive problem-solving demands and difficulty (Woods, 1988): dynamism, large numbers of parts and connectedness between parts, high uncertainty, and risk. Klein (1998) identified common characteristics across different types of complex occupations and industries that influence decision making. Time pressures, high stakes, inadequate information (missing, ambiguous, or erroneous), ill-defined goals, poorly defined procedures, dynamic conditions, people working in teams, and stress contribute to complexity in work and decision making. Yet, despite these complexities, workers learn to make decisions and act, creating and actually increasing safety most of the time by using their knowledge, attending to shifts in current situational states, and balancing interacting and sometimes conflicting goals.

Human Limitations and Complexity

Human beings themselves are complex adaptive systems, and despite their resilience in navigating the complexity of current health care environments, we must realize that inherent human limitations may sometimes succumb to situational complexity. Human beings are not perfect. Although we can educate them about performing in complex systems and support them with system and process designs that decrease the likelihood of failure, humans are limited in the amount of information and complexity they are able to manage effectively and safely.

During situations involving multitasking, for example, human limitations may result from a variety of factors affecting "cognitive function in dynamic evolving situations, especially those involving the management of workload in time and the control of attention" (Cook & Woods, 1994, p. 270). This very type of work is crucial for ensuring safe and effective care in most situations. In addition to multitasking situations, additional human limitations have been reported relative to fatigue, negative emotions, and/or illness. For example, memory capacity, attention span, distractibility, bias, physical capability, and performance limits are human factors that are challenged during these situations. Other contributors that may affect human performance include environmental factors, such as heat, cold, noise, visual stimuli, motion, and lighting; physiologic factors, including sleep loss, alcohol, and drugs; and psychological factors, including competing activities and other emotional states (e.g., boredom).

Cook and Woods (1994) described two major human performance problems related to changes in attentional dynamics during certain situations. First, *loss of situation awareness* is the failure to maintain accurate tracking of the multiple and changing interactions between parts of processes or systems. Related to this is a lack of *mindfulness,* defined by Langer and Piper (1987) as the ability to scrutinize and refine expectations based on new information and/or contextual aspects of a situation.

Secondly, *fixation* is the failure to revise assessment of a situation as new information becomes available (Cook & Woods, 1994). As individuals avoid fixation, they are demonstrating *sensemaking,* or the ability to reconstruct and interpret incoming information anew in ambiguous, complex, and evolving situations (Klein, Moon, & Hoffman, 2006). Health care providers encounter new information in clinical care settings continually that requires sensemaking to make appropriate decisions about patient care.

Recognizing and appreciating the human factors that limit individual performance in complex situations, despite the best of intentions by competent and responsible care providers, are essential to initiating efforts for improving patient safety. AHRQ's *Manual on Mistake-Proofing the Design of Healthcare Processes* (Grout, 2007) provides basic information and a guide to incorporating human factors and limitations into interventions to improve safety. The extent of our success in improving safety will always depend on our accounting for the human factors and limitations accompanying failure. Our responses to failure as well as proactive planning and design that support human performance limitations in future similar situations will create opportunities for safer care.

Hindsight Bias and Blame

Since the IOM report (2000) and as a result of learning from other industries about complex systems and human limitations, accident investigation in U.S. hospitals has begun to move from a focus on only the persons involved in an accident to more of a search for multiple potential contributors, often existing as latent conditions or gaps. Before the IOM report, investigations were often influenced by the natural tendency for

humans to look back from an adverse event and see only a simplified path of decision making related to the specific event (Fischoff, 1975). This tendency, which characterizes most investigations, is called *hindsight bias.* Despite ongoing education of health care providers and administrators regarding this tendency, hindsight bias remains a formidable challenge to the identification of actual contributors to an accident. Assigning blame is quick, often seems sufficient, the "fix" is viewed as simple, and formal or informal positive feedback to the person managing the aftermath by assignment of blame is frequently provided by those in charge.

What is lost through hindsight bias and swift assignment of blame are the complex human and environmental factors and the unavoidable trade-offs that contributed to the experience of the individual(s) involved in the actual situation. Getting stuck in hindsight bias can result in the loss of important learning about: (1) system gaps that could be redesigned and eliminated from the organization, (2) potential system supports that might be appropriate to implement given normal human limitations that contributed to the event, and (3) opportunities for increasing individual resiliency for responding to future similar complex situations.

Organizational behaviors that are core to improving patient safety are awareness of the negative effect of hindsight bias on learning and purposeful efforts toward avoiding this bias during evaluation of contributors to near-miss and adverse events. In addition to awareness of hindsight bias, other characteristics of an effective patient safety culture and safety program that result from avoidance of hindsight bias include: acknowledgement of human limitations; commitment on the part of management to, and modeling of, nonpunitive, problem-solving approaches to accident investigation; facilitation of open communication and involvement of front-line workers for learning and problem solving; design of formal systems of follow-up; and communication and training after new learning but before intended changes are developed and implemented.

The pressure on health care organizations to perform well has been increased because of the publication of patient safety "report cards," reflecting performance on patient safety goals and state medical error reporting system data where available. Compounding potential negative effects on an organization's reputation are the financial implications of reimbursement denials that involve care delivery failures related to patient safety goals. Many health care organizations' natural tendency will be to respond to this pressure by reverting to traditional blame and focus on individuals as the solution to improved performance. These types of responses to error usually are quickly visible and satisfying to leaders in the short run. These responses also usually involve punishment or evoke fear of punishment, but there is no evidence that they support sustained improvement in patient safety or the building of an effective patient safety culture. A major challenge for the CNS as leader for improvement in patient safety and development of an effective safety program is to influence others in the organization to implement effective strategies that reflect learning from other highly reliable industries that base improvement strategies on systems and human factors knowledge.

High-Reliability Organizations

Health care has learned about how to make improvements in safety from other organizations that demand high reliability because of the catastrophic nature of failure if it should occur. Key to our learning have been works by Weick and Suttcliffe (2001), who analyzed core processes for achieving high reliability across varying types of organizations. The authors identified a template of five high-reliability organization (HRO) characteristics they called *mindfulness* (in contrast to the previous more general definition in "Human Limitations and Complexity"), which they proposed increase the ability to maintain reliable performance. See Table 13.3 for the five characteristics found to be common among HROs.

Patient safety researchers proposed that studying complexities and hazards at the sharp end, how providers cope with system gaps, and how system gaps are created or avoided through operational changes is essential for understanding human performance in complex systems (Cook & Woods, 1994; Cook et al., 2000; Woods, 1988). Previous to 2000, no research was found that focused on complexity of the health care system in relation to nurses' work in actual work situations. Research conducted for the purpose of understanding nursing work, including descriptions of factors characteristic of nursing work environments, factors that influence registered

nurse (RN) decision making, and RN strategies to manage workflow in providing patient care during actual work situations, has increased since the IOM 2000 report (e.g., Ebright, Patterson, Chalko, & Render, 2003; Ebright, Urden, Patterson, & Chalko, 2004; Potter et al., 2005; Tucker & Spear, 2006). In each of these studies, the researchers used methods of direct observations of nurses during actual work and/or interview strategies to elicit details of nurses' activities, thinking, and decision making while in the process of delivering care.

Reports from these studies describe gaps and latent failures confronting nurses in the midst of care delivery (e.g., missing equipment, interruptions, waiting for access to needed systems and resources, lack of time to complete interventions that were judged necessary to reach desired outcomes, and inconsistencies in how information was communicated or could be relied on for access if needed). Other results demonstrated nurse strategies for dealing with, or adapting to, the gaps (e.g., anticipating or forward thinking, proactive monitoring of patient status to detect early warning signals, strategic delegation and hand-off decisions to maintain flow of workload, individualized paper memory aids, and "stacking" management of activities to be done).

Three types of knowledge were found that affected RN decision making: knowledge about individual patients, typical patient disease profiles, and unit workflow routines (Ebright et al., 2003). Other factors affecting decision making included patterns of goal conflict or simultaneous and sometimes competing goals that, together, were difficult to reach in a timely or expected manner. Types of competing goals included maintaining patient safety, preventing getting behind schedule, avoiding increasing complexity, appearing competent and efficient to patients/families and coworkers, and maintaining patient/family satisfaction.

13.3 Characteristics of High Reliability Organizations (HROs)

CHARACTERISTIC	EXAMPLE
Preoccupation with failure	Treat any lapse as a symptom that something is wrong. HROs focus on actual as well as near-misses for investigation.
Reluctance to simplify interpretations	Take deliberate steps to create more complete and nuanced pictures of details surrounding a failed process.
Sensitivity to operations	Maintain an ongoing concern with the unexpected. HROs look for, and deal quickly with, latent failures before an event occurs.
Commitment to resilience	Focus on detecting, containing, and bouncing back from adverse events. Adverse events do not disable HROs.
Deference to expertise	Push decision making down to the front-line and authority moves to people with the most expertise regardless of rank.

Moving forward with patient safety improvement efforts that fail to take into account the complexities of actual work flow and conditions will not result in increased reliability or sustained improvements. A focus only on increasing individuals' knowledge base, or fear of consequences from failure, will not result in consistent perfect performance given imperfect situations. A combined appreciation of human limitations and of system complexity is needed to reach the level of reliability achieved by HROs (Reason, 2000).

APPLICATION TO CNS PRACTICE

CNSs contributed to patient safety in multiple ways before the IOM report was published in 2000, and they have had a substantial impact on improvement efforts based on what we have learned since then. Health care organizations will continue to look for effective strategies to improve the quality of care and reduce error in their institutions in light of new and evolving legislative and regulatory requirements.

As outlined in the *Statement on Clinical Nurse Specialist Practice and Education* (NACNS, 2004), CNSs have the educational background, including core competencies related to complex systems and leadership for implementation of change, strategic organizational positioning, and essential expert clinical knowledge, to facilitate and lead successful and sustained patient safety improvements. The CNS is in a position to influence patient safety work in five important ways: (1) role-modeling behaviors of a nonpunitive safety culture, (2) facilitating and leading ongoing efforts to learn about system complexities, (3) facilitating and leading ongoing efforts to learn about health care worker

resiliency, (4) proactively managing potential increases in complexity with strategic introduction of change, and (5) staying current with the evolving patient safety literature and evidence for best practice.

Providing Leadership for a Nonpunitive Safety Culture

An effective culture of safety is one in which workers are willing to share details surrounding near-miss and adverse-event situations for continuous learning about gaps in the system. For an organization to sustain an effective culture of safety, health care workers must work in an environment that is nonpunitive, where they feel safe to speak up and where they are invited and encouraged to participate in the improvement process. Building a culture of safety requires relationships based on trust, open communication, and a belief that those closest to the work, specifically patient care, are most knowledgeable about the work itself and are needed in the improvement processes.

Successful CNS practice is dependent on nurturing and maintaining trust through relationships on a daily basis with patients and families, multidisciplinary health care personnel, and the organization's leadership. Thus, the nature of CNS practice is characterized by a unique combination of skills that includes communication strategies, relationship building, systems focus, and a clinical care delivery expertise, which makes the CNS a valuable resource for others in the organization. Other leaders can benefit from observing the ease with which the CNS is able to blend each of these strengths to influence people and programs to achieve change. Specific behaviors that the CNS should demonstrate to support and influence an effective safety culture are listed in Table 13.4.

13.4 | CNS Supportive Behaviors of an Effective Patient Safety Culture

BEHAVIORS

1. Open communication about, and role-modeling of responses to, adverse events and near-misses that reflects absence of hindsight bias.

2. Commitment to and role-modeling of nonpunitive, problem-solving approaches to accident investigation and follow-up interventions.

3. Open communication and acknowledgement of human limitations as a contributor to adverse/near-miss events and incorporation of response interventions and systems redesigns that support and account for identified human limitations.

4. Facilitation/leading and role-modeling of open communication and inviting of participation of front-line workers for maximum learning and creative problem solving to reduce the risk of future events.

5. Facilitating/leading the design of formal systems of adverse event/near-miss follow-up processes and dissemination of learning throughout the organization after an event.

6. Role-modeling timely open communication and reporting about own adverse/near-miss events and identified gaps and latent conditions that could result in future events.

Achieving measurable improvements in safety for patients depends on an organizational culture based on safety culture behaviors from all persons in leadership roles, as well as the front-line care providers across units, departments, and facilities. With their educational background and competencies used in everyday practice, CNSs can be instrumental in role modeling and leading others toward this important goal.

Learning About System Complexities

Fundamental to improvement in patient safety is identification of the gaps and discontinuities (latent failures or conditions) as well as active failures that contribute to complexity and hazards at the point of care (Cook et al., 2000). The CNS core competency related to differential diagnosis captures the essential critical thinking skills that allow explication of those gaps and discontinuities, or etiologies, that contribute to adverse and near-miss events (NACNS, 2004, pp. 25–26). The CNS should use this core competency for direct application to specific investigations of single events or to grouped event data; lead and role model for teams of nurses and other disciplines the application of the competency to single event or grouped event data; and interpret and articulate for other leaders in the organization the process and outcomes of differential diagnosis, including etiologies of adverse and near-miss events and the most appropriate interventions to prevent or diminish the impact of future adverse and near-miss events.

In addition, with experiential knowledge of actual work environments within which health care workers practice, the CNS brings to a variety of event investigations an informed curiosity that is essential for identification of the goals, conflicts, obstacles, hazards, data, and behaviors that contribute to the complexity surrounding care situations (Figure 13.2). Leading investigations to maintain and sustain focus on these aspects of an adverse or near-miss event provides the CNS opportunities to role model for other health care staff the acknowledgment and then the setting aside of hindsight bias, a huge barrier to safety and quality improvement. The CNS should emphasize the benefit of timely storytelling to detail the complexity surrounding adverse and near-miss event situations and for accurate identification of etiologies and potential interventions. Getting past hindsight bias and the tendency to simplify factors causing an event is paramount for learning about what is needed for improvement.

Learning About Health Care Worker Resiliency

Just as important as learning what latent failures or conditions were present in adverse and near-miss event situations is learning how practitioners anticipated, accommodated, reacted, adapted, and coped with complexities to avert or decrease the impact of the adverse and near-miss events (Figure 13.2). The CNS should investigate and document during event investigations how practitioners managed to navigate the complexity of the actual work environment, how they reacted effectively or ineffectively and successfully or unsuccessfully to prevent an adverse event, or how they were able to minimize the negative outcome. Details obtained during event investigation about practitioners' cues for recognition of a problem and subsequent sequence of actions during the situation can provide excellent information for development of future interventions. Information learned from this line of investigation can be incorporated into recommended interventions for educating staff, redesigning processes and systems to support staff, or for developing new processes or designs. The CNS should facilitate the capture of event details related to coping and adaptation by probing the storyteller for the minute information surrounding the situation that is normally lost through general questioning after an event. This detail provides the less experienced staff important knowledge that is sometimes only obtained by years of actual clinical experience.

Tools for Increasing Understanding of Actual Work

Health care organizations used quality management systems to manage, measure, and attempt to improve processes and outcomes before the IOM report (2000). With the new approach to patient safety, new quality management methods have been borrowed from manufacturing. These methods, some referred to as LEAN, are a particularly appropriate fit because they were processes developed to increase quality through identification of defects and inefficiencies leading to errors or failures. Principles of LEAN were developed by Womack and Jones in 1996. Henry Ford first pioneered some of the LEAN principles for workflow production in the automobile industry, and Toyota further developed the concepts (Womack, Jones, & Roos, 2007). Some of the LEAN tools used by industry are useful for increasing understanding of system complexity and human limitations that contribute to adverse events. CNSs need to know about these tools to be able to use them effectively in patient safety–related projects and to understand the outcome data and implications for designing and choosing appropriate patient safety interventions.

Table 13.5 lists examples of retrospective and prospective tools used in quality and patient safety work. Other methods may be called different names but are used for very similar purposes. *Retrospective* tools are useful for gathering data after an adverse

13.5 | Examples of Tools for Understanding Work Complexity and Etiologies of Failure

TOOLS	DEFINITION
Root Cause Analysis	A process for identifying the basic or contributing causal factors that underlie variations in performance associated with adverse events or near misses (http://www.va.gov/ncps/glossary.html).
Event Flow Diagram	A diagram that uses graphical symbols to depict the nature and flow of events leading up to an adverse/near miss event.
Data Mining (also can be used prospectively)	Data mining is the analysis of large amounts of data for relationships that have not previously been discovered and increase understanding of work complexity.
Healthcare Failure Mode and Effects Analysis	A prospective assessment that identifies and improves steps in a process thereby reasonably ensuring a safe and clinically desirable outcome. A systematic approach to identify and prevent product and process problems before they occur. (www.va.gov/ncps/SafetyTopics/HFMEA/HFMEAIntro.pdf)
Workflow Analysis-Process Mapping	The analysis and representation of clinical work processes from the perspective of the staff member(s).
Positive Deviance	A process whereby managers actively look for those extraordinarily successful groups and individuals, and bring the isolated success strategies of those "positive deviants" into the mainstream. (http://www.12manage.com/methods_pascale_positive_deviance.html)
Risk Resilience Assessment	Assessment of the strengths and weaknesses in the ability of an organization to manage risk (Nolan & Resar, 2008).

or near-miss event. *Prospective* tools are very helpful in analyzing systems and processes to identify opportunities for redesign to prevent adverse events or decrease the impact of failure or to prioritize improvement efforts. Used appropriately, these tools are all about understanding details of processes, including the human component, for the purpose of learning what needs to be done to increase reliability and reduce the likelihood of failure. Like any other method or tool, inappropriate application of the methods or interpretation of outcome data will produce poor results. Appropriate use and application can result in increased and sustainable quality.

Managing the Complexity Inherent in Change

With advanced clinical knowledge, a systems orientation, and strategic positioning in the organization that is directly or closely linked to the actual clinical work environment, the CNS should be prepared to anticipate and articulate the potential contribution of planned organizational changes for creating new system gaps and latent failures. As patient safety leader, consultant, mentor, and change agent, the CNS should provide guidance in appreciating how new complexities may result from even well-developed and planned change efforts. Anticipating and preparing for how change might introduce new forms of latent failure and complexity in relation to the overall actual work of practitioners is also needed to maintain safe environments. The CNS should begin the design and preparation for implementing change by asking staff to answer two crucial questions designed to elicit potential consequences of the change and listed in Table 13.6.

Each of these questions will result in the type of feedback not usually obtained from traditional general requests for feedback and can be very productive in identification of potential gaps and latent failures not anticipated by project planners.

Analysis of feedback from these questions allows adjustment or redesign of the change and also identifies solutions to be created and included in content for the educational rollout prior to the change. For example, when a computer software design administrator was asked 1 week before the implementation of a new computer system about what might go wrong, he identified a list of 10 possible failures. As a result, the staff were given specific directions about what to do if any of the 10 situations occurred. *Hoping* that none of the 10 identified possible failures would occur without back-up planning would not have been sufficient to prevent increased complexity for those involved in patient care, nor supportive of patient safety.

13.6 | Questions to Identify Potential Consequences of Change

1. Think about incorporating this new process (technology) into your actual workflow. How will this new process (or technology) in any way change the way you work, or the flow of your work?

2. As you think about incorporating this change in process (or technology) into your work, imagine that the change ends up not being successful. Why do you think that will be? What probably caused it to not be successful?

Staying Current With the Evolving Patient Safety Literature and Evidence for Best Practice

New and emerging knowledge continues to develop about the importance of communication, teamwork, and clarifying accountabilities in this new approach to patient safety as health care organizations and patient safety researchers apply other industry models to safety improvement. CNSs should become familiar with the continuing development of innovative models and research as the health care industry adopts and adapts other industry methods to health care work.

For example, those who have applied team development strategies for improving teamwork have had to acknowledge and adjust for the fact that health care teams often involve differing roles, numbers of members, and even differing members throughout a day. There is a shift of focus from building strong "teams" to developing "expert team member behaviors and competencies" that will transfer with members as team composition changes.

Failure in communication is the most frequently identified contributor to adverse and near-miss events. The multiple aspects of how, when, by whom, and in what situations information is communicated have been found to be very complex across a variety of complicated health care situations (Leonard, Graham, & Bonacum, 2004; Patterson, Roth, Woods, Chow, & Gomes, 2004). Issues related to what to standardize, how to format, or through what medium information should be disseminated by health care providers have unleashed many different models and approaches to increase accuracy and completeness. Testing and research will determine what models and critical parts of models result in successful transfer of information and in what situations. It is likely that no complicated model of information transfer will result in successful outcomes in all situations.

Early learning about new approaches to patient safety included the need to create a "nonblame culture" to increase worker reporting about adverse and near-miss events. Learning about system contributors requires worker willingness to share stories about what lead up to and surrounded actions resulting in failure. Health care leaders, as well as some providers, however, are uncomfortable with the term, thinking that *nonblame* reduces or eliminates workers' sense of accountability for safe decision making and actions. For some who are responsible for patient safety outcomes, it is difficult to separate the process of managing poor performance from the process of adverse and near-miss investigation. Tools such as Just Culture (Frankel, Leonard, & Denham, 2006) have been developed to guide managers through algorithms for determining risk behaviors in failure-related incidents and performance management actions for follow-up.

The challenge for health care organizations is to educate management on the appropriate application of these tools so that an effective culture of safety with nonblame approaches to failure investigations, separate from ongoing management of poor performance, is realized. The processes should be separated, with managing poor performance after an event only considered as a result of completed failure investigation. Some failures do not include any evidence of poor performance. Assigning blame and poor performance in the aftermath of an adverse or near-miss event but before investigations are complete may lead to bias conduct of the investigation and result in less focus on, and discovery of, system contributions (Ebright & Rapala, 2003). Managing poor performance continuously and separate from event aftermath helps to remove the blame from event investigation.

Recent literature focuses on approaches to patient safety and new frameworks concerning management of risk and risk resilience. Nolan and Resar (2008) proposed that once we reach a certain level of competency and consistency regarding identification of root causes and failure mode analysis, our attention should turn to evaluating and increasing the organization's risk resilience. Risk resilience is the assessment of an organization's strengths and weaknesses to adapt to variation. Nolan and Resar proposed use of a tool that facilitates conversations about predesigned defenses and adaptability.

Amalberti, Vincent, Auroy, and de Saint Maurice (2006) wrote about the Rasmussen/Amalberti framework for understanding violations and system migrations that occur away from standard procedures and that are sometimes necessary to maintain safety amid dynamic conditions. The authors described a continuum of safe behavior that starts with initial safe spaces of action, to creation of borderline-tolerated conditions of use, and ends with normalization of deviance and reckless individual behavior. They emphasize the need to manage risk-taking, to understand factors that influence tolerable and intolerable violations and migrations, and to understand which of these need to be supported in certain circumstances and which need to be managed.

ETHICAL CONSIDERATIONS

The CNS will continue to be involved in managing and role modeling for patient situations involving ethical aspects related to provision of safe care and the communication and decision making required. What is important and new for leadership of patient safety efforts is the commitment by the CNS to the appropriate evidenced-based application of new knowledge that health care has discovered from other industries since the IOM (2000) report. It is no longer acceptable for leaders at any level to blame individuals for error and implementation of strategies that fail to explicate the system contributions to adverse events. Just as CNSs articulate the complexity of individual patient cases, they must articulate the complexity of actual work situations that leads to adverse and near-miss events, and they must provide leadership and influence for designing efforts that incorporate the new approach.

DISCUSSION QUESTIONS

1. What was the response to the last adverse event in your organization? Was the response focused primarily on blame or details surrounding the event? How did you respond? What was your role, if any, related to event aftermath, organizational learning, or dissemination of findings after the event investigation? How could you improve on your response to the event to have influence at each of the three spheres of your practice?
2. Who is responsible for overall patient safety activities in your organization? What is your relationship with patient safety activities at each of the three sphere levels?

ANALYSIS AND SYNTHESIS ACTIVITY

1. Analyze the current patient safety efforts in your organization. Are the current activities most reflective

of: (1) traditional management of error; (2) developing systems and structure for error reporting, investigation, and redesign; or (3) beginning to systematically assess the organization's risk resilience ability?

CLINICAL APPLICATION CONSIDERATION

1. Choose a change project currently in progress (may or may not be your own). Assess through sharp end care providers the implications of the change on total workload and subsequent effect on direct patient care and patient care outcomes (e.g., new gaps or latent failure modes). Develop a response to provider input as appropriate: for example, redesign some aspects of change itself; provide helpful education for users regarding impact of change as noted by providers; and/or articulate clearly to the owner of the change initiative why new information should be considered that may alter current plans before implementation of the change.

REFERENCES

Amalberti, R., Vincent, C., Auroy, Y., & de Saint Maurice, G. (2006). Violations and migrations in health care: A framework for understanding and management. *Quality and Safety in Health Care, 15*(Suppl. 1), 66–71.

Cook, R. I. (1997). *The new look: Genesis of complex system failure.* Chicago: Cognitive Technologies Laboratory.

Cook, R. I., Render, M., & Woods, D. D. (2000). Gaps in the continuity of care and progress on patient safety. *British Medical Journal, 320,* 791–794.

Cook, R. I., & Woods, D. D. (1994). Operating at the sharp end: The complexity of human error. In M. E. Bogner (Ed.), *Human error in medicine* (pp. 255–310). Hillsdale, NJ: Lawrence Erlbaum Associates.

Ebright, R., Patterson, E., Chalko, B., & Render, M. (2003). Understanding the complexity of registered nurse work in acute care settings. *Journal of Nursing Administration, 33*(12), 630–638.

Ebright, P., & Rapala, K. (2003). Blame: Do you know it when you see it. *Outcomes Management, 7,* 3–6.

Ebright, R., Urden, L., Patterson, E., & Chalko, B. (2004). Themes surrounding novice nurse near-miss and adverse event situations. *Journal of Nursing Administration, 34*(11), 531–538.

Fischoff, B. (1975). Hindsight does not equal foresight: The effect of outcome knowledge on judgment under uncertainty. *Journal of Experimental Psychology: Human Perception and Performance, 1,* 288–299.

Frankel, A. S., Leonard, M. W., & Denham, C. R. (2006). Fair and just culture, team behavior, and leadership engagement: The tools to achieve high reliability. *Health Services Research, 41*(4), 1690–1709.

Grout, J. (2007). *Mistake-proofing the design of health care processes.* (Prepared under an IPA with Berry College.) AHRQ Publication No. 07–0020. Rockville, MD: Agency for Healthcare Research and Quality.

Institute for Healthcare Improvement. (2009). Retrieved June 26, 2009, from http://www.ihi.org/ihi/programs

Institute of Medicine. (2000). *To err is human: Building a safer health system*. Washington, DC: National Academies Press.

Institute of Medicine. (2001). Committee on Quality of Healthcare in America. *Crossing the quality chasm: A new health system for the 21st century*. Washington, DC: National Academies Press.

Klein, G. (1998). *Sources of power: How people make decisions*. Cambridge, MA: MIT Press.

Klein, G., Moon, B., & Hoffman, R. F. (2006). Making sense of sensemaking I: Alternative perspectives. *IEEE Intelligent Systems, 21*(4), 70–73.

Langer, E. J., & Piper A. (1987). The prevention of mindlessness. *Journal of Personality and Social Psychology, 53,* 280–287.

Leape, L. L. (1994). Error in medicine. *Journal of American Medical Association, 272*(23), 1851–1857.

Leape, L., & Berwick, D. M. (2005). Five years after *To Err Is Human:* What have we learned? *Journal of American Medical Association, 293*(19), 2384–2390.

Leonard, M., Graham, S., & Bonacum, D. (2004). The human factor: The critical importance of effective teamwork and communication in providing safe care. *Quality and Safety in Health Care, 13*(Suppl. 1), 85–90.

Minnesota Department of Health. (2009). Retrieved June 26, 2009, from http://www.health.state.mn.us/patientsafety/ae/background.html

National Association of Clinical Nurse Specialists. (2004). *Statement on clinical nurse specialist practice and education* (2nd ed.). Harrisburg, PA: Author.

Nolan, T., & Resar, R. (2008). *Strategic system for safety.* Cambridge, MA: Institute for Healthcare Improvement.

Patterson, E. S., Roth, E. M., Woods, D. D., Chow, R., & Gomes, J. O. (2004) Handoff strategies in settings with high consequences for failure: Lessons for health care operations. *International Journal of Quality Health Care, 16*(2), 125–132.

Pascale, R., & Sternin, J. (2009). *Positive deviance.* Retrieved June 26, 2009, from http://www.12manage.com/methods_pascale_positive_deviance.html

Peplau, H. (1965/2003). Specialization in professional nursing. *Clinical Nurse Specialist, 17*(1), 3–9.

Potter, P., Wolf, L., Boxerman, S., Grayson, D., Sledge, J., Dunagan, C., et al. (2005). Understanding the cognitive work of nursing in the acute care environment. *Journal of Nursing Administration, 35*(78), 327–335.

Reason, J. (1990). *Human error.* Cambridge: University Press.

Reason, J. (2000). Human error: Models and management. *British Medical Journal, 320,* 768–70.

Rogers, E. M. (2003). *Diffusion of innovations* (5th ed.). New York: The Free Press.

Silker, E. (2006). *APSF history overview.* Retrieved January 13, 2009, from http://apsf.org/about/brief_history.mspx

Suchman, T. (2002). Linearity, complexity and well-being. *Medical Encounter, 16*(4), 17–19.

The Joint Commission. (2009a). *A journey through the history of the Joint Commission: 1996.* Retrieved June 26, 2009, from http://www.jointcommission.org/AboutUs/joint_commission_history.htm#1996

The Joint Commission. (2009b). *National Patient Safety Goals.* Retrieved June 26, 2009, from http://www.jointcommission.org/PatientSafety/NationalPatientSafetyGoals/

Tucker, A. L., & Spear, S. J. (2006). Operational failures and interruptions in hospital nursing. *Health Services Research, 41,* 643–662.

VA National Center for Patient Safety. (2001). *The basics of healthcare failure mode effects and analysis.* Retrieved June 26, 2009, from http://www.va.gov/ncps/SafetyTopics/HFMEA/HFMEAIntro.pdf

VA National Center for Patient Safety. (2009). *Glossary of patient safety terms.* Retrieved June 26, 2009, from http://www.va.gov/ncps/glossary.html

Weick, K. E., & Sutcliffe, K. M. (2001). *Managing the unexpected: Assuring high performance in an age of complexity.* San Francisco: Jossey-Bass.

Womack, J. P., Jones, D. T., & Roos, D. (2007). *The machine that changed the world: The story of lean production—how Japan's secret weapon in the global auto wars will revolutionize western industry.* New York: The Free Press.

Woods D. D. (1988). Coping with complexity: The psychology of human behavior in complex systems. In L. P. Goodstein, H. B. Anderson, & S. E. Olsen (Eds.), *Tasks, errors and mental models* (pp. 128–148). London: Taylor and Francis.

Woods, D. D., & Cook, R. I. (1998). *Characteristics of patient safety: Five principles that underlie productive work.* Chicago: CtL.

Woods, D. D., Johannesen, L. J., Cook, R. I., & Sarter, N. B. (1940). *Behind human error: Cognitive systems, computers, and hindsight.* Dayton, OH: Human Systems Ergonomic Information and Analysis Center, WPAFB.

Zimmerman, B., Lindberg, C., & Plsek, P. (1998). *Edgeware: Insights from complexity science for health care leaders.* Irving TX: VHA Inc.

Delivering
Care to Clients

14

Individual as Client

Janet S. Fulton
Carol Baird

Care of the individual client begins with a careful assessment. For clinical nurse specialists (CNSs), care begins with an advanced nursing assessment. What constitutes an advanced nursing assessment? In many care settings, the information collected for an advanced nursing assessment overlaps considerably with a medical history and physical examination. Anecdotally, when nurses are asked to explain the difference between a nursing and medical assessment they often identify the nursing assessment as more holistic. A search of the Cumulative Index to Nursing and Allied Health Literature (CINAHL) was conducted for English articles between the years 1995–2008. The terms *holism* and *holistic nursing* yielded 1,283 articles. The term *nursing assessment* yielded 7,871 articles. Combining these two searches—*holism/holistic nursing* and *nursing assessment*—found only 36 articles. These 36 articles generally focused on nonphysical aspects of assessment, such as spirituality, sexuality, family, culture, and quality of life, suggesting that adding these perspectives or dimensions to a physical assessment, either individually or in combination, created a holistic assessment. Only one article described a theoretical basis for holistic assessment (Sappington & Kelley, 1996). Using modeling and role-modeling theory, Sappington and Kelley assert that nursing care should be grounded in individual uniqueness because clients have knowledge and ability to understand what made them sick and what will make them well.

A CINAHL search of the term *advanced nursing practice* for the same time period (1995–2008) identified 5,756 articles. A combined search of *nursing assessment* and *advanced nursing practice* found 130 articles. Physical assessment of specific symptoms, such as chest pain, shortness of breath, and depressed mood, dominated this group of articles, as well as disease-specific assessment including asthma, diabetes, heart failure, and chronic obstructive pulmonary disease. Articles specific to nurse anesthetists covered topics such as anesthesia risk assessment and preoperative cardiac assessment, whereas articles specific to midwifery discussed fertility assessment and antepartum/postpartum assessment. Several articles addressed specific problems such as domestic violence, sexual assault, and wounds.

Two empiric articles explored the content of advanced nursing assessment (Davidson, Bennet, Hamera, & Raines, 2004; Kelley & Kopac, 2001). Kelley and Kopac surveyed schools of nursing about advanced health assessment courses for nurse practitioner programs and found the major content areas to be: (1) obtaining history and interviewing (99%), (2) physical assessment (99%), (3) ethnic and cultural considerations (90%), (4) developmental assessment (77%), and (5) functional assessment (74%). The least often reported content areas were health promotion and disease prevention. Respondents reported that students were expected to perform head-to-toe physical examinations including eye (fundoscopic) and pelvic examination. In a related study, Davidson and colleagues asked nurse practitioner preceptors to rate the importance of 87 specific assessment competencies for primary care practice. Assessment competencies rated highest were in the cardiovascular, musculoskeletal, and gynecological systems and included the ability to detect and interpret abnormalities in heart rate and rhythm; determine status of circulatory, motor, and neurological systems; and conduct pelvic examinations, including collecting cervical specimens and performing and interpreting speculum and bimanual examinations.

Asked about conceptualizations and theoretical models used to guide assessment, faculty noted challenges in conceptualizing assessment content within nursing theory when using the medical model to establish differential diagnosis of disease conditions (Kelley & Kopac). Among respondents indicating a theoretical basis for assessment, holistic approach was most often reported, followed by systems theory (9%) and functional health (5%).

Findings from the literature search support the observation that advanced nursing assessment is heavily disease-focused and follows the general framework of medical history and physical examination. When the purpose of a health assessment is differential diagnosis of disease, a medical framework is appropriate and necessary. However, little evidence is available describing advanced assessment consistent with a nursing perspective (such as was described in chapter 3). This chapter explores the importance of articulating a theoretical perspective for health assessment, offers a unique purpose of advanced nursing assessment, and suggests an assessment strategy for identifying etiologies amenable to nursing interventions consistent with a theoretical perspective.

ARTICULATING A THEORETICAL PERSPECTIVE FOR ADVANCED ASSESSMENT

The question *What is an advanced nursing assessment?* is part of a larger unknown dealing with the nature of nursing practiced at an advanced level. What is advanced practice in nursing? What are the characteristics? What are the behaviors and outcomes? The ideas offered in this chapter about advanced assessment are *not* intended to provide *the* answer to these questions. Rather, these ideas are offered for consideration in an ongoing dialogue addressing a quest discovering and defining nursing practiced at an advanced level.

Purpose of Health Assessment

The purpose of health assessment is to collect, document, and analyze client information and to draw conclusions supported by data/information. These assessment-based conclusions direct interventions for the purpose of influencing health status. Conclusions require judgment, and conclusions made by nurses about problems amenable to nursing interventions have been called nursing diagnoses. While many judgments are made by nurses in practice, Gordon has long pointed out that the term *nursing diagnosis* is reserved for client conditions that nurses, by virtue of their education and experience, are capable and licensed to treat (Gordon, 2007).

Identifying as nursing diagnosis those conclusions made by nurses based on nursing assessment was introduced into the language of nursing in the 1970s, in part, because of legislative initiatives to recognize the independent practice of nursing as distinct from medicine and to remove statutory requirements for physician supervision of nursing practice. In introducing revisions to the nurse practice act, the New York State Nurses Association included the term *nursing diagnosis* in reference to the distinctive areas in which the nurse exercised, and was expected to exercise, independent judgment (Driscoll, 1976/2007; Fulton, 2007). Scholarly work to develop nursing diagnosis can be traced to the first meeting in 1973 of the National Group for the Classification of Nursing Diagnosis, which later became North American Nursing Diagnosis Association (NANDA). Over the years, integration of nursing diagnosis into practice has been challenging. Carpenito (1995) outlined some of the difficulties resulting from a priori application of labels to all situations in which nurses intervene, including using diagnostic terms without validation and renaming medical diagnoses. Validation problems occur when nurses "change the data to fit the label," for example, using the label *altered nutrition* as a diagnosis for all patients being medically restricted from taking food or fluids by mouth. Renaming medical diagnoses occurs when a nurse uses a label such as *impaired gas exchange* as a diagnosis for patients with chronic obstructive pulmonary disease, asthma, and adult respiratory distress syndrome (Carpenito, 1995). These problems aside, the need to develop nursing diagnosis is of utmost importance for communicating about our nursing conclusions, interventions, and outcomes. For purposes of this discussion, it needs to be underscored that any statement of conclusion made by a CNS or any nurse about a patient problem, whether specified as a nursing diagnosis or not, must be logically consistent with and supported by data that was systematically collected and analyzed. Further, the conclusion should reflect a client health problem amenable to independent nursing interventions. To illustrate: The conclusion may be lower back pain related to positioning, specifically lying supine flat. Interventions are related to repositioning, such as elevating hips or moving to lateral position with knees bent. The etiology of pain, in this example, is body position supine flat. The problem is amenable to independent nursing intervention—repositioning. The specific repositioning intervention will be determined by a more in-depth assessment and understanding of the etiology of the pain problem and contextual limitations. It may be appropriate to administer prescribed medications to alleviate the pain; however, medication is a medical intervention administered based on nursing judgment within the parameters of the medical prescription and intended to alter a different etiology. Etiologies related to position are amenable to independent nursing interventions involving repositioning.

The purpose of an advanced nursing assessment is to support an advanced judgment about a client health problem amenable to independent nursing intervention. While the complexity of possible interventions varies, advanced practice is characterized by the depth and breadth of nursing judgment needed to pinpoint problems and their etiologies, not solely by the complexity of the intervention.

Theoretical Frameworks for Assessment

Assessment concentrates heavily on collection of data about the client (Broom, 2007). The most common framework used for health assessment is the body system framework, which includes a health history and physical examination. Long used in practice, it was more formally organized in a textbook by Bates and Hoekelman (1974). It remains the dominant framework for comprehensive health assessment and is used in teaching physician and nursing students as well as students of other health professions.

The body systems framework includes a health history and a physical examination. The health history focuses on subjective data, including the client's description of symptoms and health problems and other information about the client's social background and lifestyle. Physical examination focuses on objective data determined by an examiner. The physical exam establishes a baseline, identifies normal from abnormal, and validates information obtained during the health history (Barkauskas, Baumann, & Darling-Fisher, 2002). Physical examination requires specific techniques, including inspection, palpitation, percussion, and auscultation, in addition to some special positions and manipulations.

Nursing theoretical frameworks for comprehensive health assessment include Gordon's Functional Health Patterns, Unitary Person Framework, and North American Nursing Diagnosis Association (NANDA) taxonomy (Barkauskas et al., 2002). These frameworks are ways to organize information into categories and under diagnostic labels as opposed to methods for systematically collecting the data. Among the nursing frameworks, Gordon's Functional Health Patterns is the most developed.

Gordon's Functional Health Patterns framework for assessment is based on 11 areas of possible functional health problems. Health problems are determined by assessing functional patterns believed to be influenced by biological, developmental, cultural, social, and spiritual factors. The functional patterns are the following:

1. Health perception—health management
2. Nutrition—metabolic
3. Elimination
4. Activity—exercise
5. Sleep—reset
6. Cognitive—perceptual
7. Self-perception—self-concept
8. Role—relationship
9. Sexuality—reproductive
10. Coping—stress—tolerance
11. Value—belief (Gordon, 2007)

For each functional area, a judgment of whether or not a pattern is functional or dysfunctional is made by comparing assessment data to one or more of the following: (1) individual baselines; (2) established norms for age-groups; or (3) cultural, social, or other norms. Dysfunctional patterns may occur with disease or may lead to disease. A particular pattern has to be evaluated in the context of other patterns and its contribution to optimal function of the client (Gordon, 2007). Unlike the well-established body systems assessment framework, there is no common order for collecting data, no standard questions, and no special techniques of physical examination.

PHILOSOPHICAL VIEW OF ASSESSMENT

Assessment involves combining general knowledge from theory and research with particular knowledge about a client for the purpose of clinical decision making. To explain the paradox of knowledge that is both general (from theory and research) and specific (to a client), Gadow (1995) used a dialectic framework (a method of inquiry in philosophy) to explore the process by which clinical assessment in nursing resolves the opposite positions of general and particular knowledge. The dialectic method was selected because it supports arriving at the most complete understanding of a process. Understanding the overall process, not the outcome, is the goal of this method. Knowledge generated by the dialectic method is considered complete when it incorporates, not eliminates, the opposing elements into the process (Gadow, 1995).

Gadow's (1995) inquiry identified five levels to the assessment process—vulnerability, disengagement, reduction, holism, and engagement. The vulnerable level is focused on the patient's immediate experience and is marked by the patient's vulnerability. The patient is experiencing an urgent and distressing symptom, such as pain or dyspnea. At this level, the focus of assessment is entirely on the patient's subjective report. The patient's experience is the reason for beginning the assessment. No attention is given to exploring the etiology of the problem at this time. At the second level, disengagement, the symptom becomes objectified. The patient's experience of the symptom is reframed in more general terms for the purpose of finding an explanation or etiology. Individual patient distress or suffering associated with the symptom is ignored, and the objectified symptom is moved to an abstract category. At the third level, reduction, the objectified symptom becomes the basis for determining an etiology—the "thing" that explains the symptom. Pain may be explained by orthopedic fracture or local tissue inflammation or many other causes. For some symptoms there may be more than one "thing" that explains the symptom. For example, psychosocial problems may have multiple competing etiologies, such as loss, grief, and anger related to situations of childhood or recent events. Orthopedic fracture may cause pain; however, posture, movement, and other etiologies may also explain pain in the presence of fracture. At the fourth level, holism, multiple competing elements or explanations are viewed simultaneously as the focus shifts back to the individual. The various elements create context. No one data type is more important. Creating a holistic perspective allows the "tangled web" of cause and effect to emerge (Maher & Hemming, 2005). However, while the holistic level provides a comprehensive view of patient experience, the patient is still viewed as an object assembled by the nurse's data analysis, not as a person encountered by another person.

At the last level of assessment, engagement, the patient is engaged as the author of the experience rather than the object of assessment. Internal coherence is created when the patient interprets the data and assigns meaning. Engagement is complete when intersubjectivity is established between the nurse and the patient. The nurse and patient become coauthors of the narrative and reconstruct the situation as meaning. The narrative is no longer objective; it becomes existential as a lived situation. Table 14.1 summarizes the findings of Gadow's (1995) nursing assessment dialectic.

A UNIQUE PURPOSE FOR ADVANCED NURSING ASSESSMENT

A variety of theoretical perspectives and theories are used in nursing practice to explain phenomenon and provide supportive scientific evidence for interventions. Gordon (2007) noted that there is no consensus around a single conceptual focus of nursing and, thus, no consensus on the focus of nursing diagnosis. Depending on the theoretical perspective used to guide practice, nursing diagnoses may be viewed as, for example, self-care agency needs or dysfunctional health patterns.

14.1 | Levels of Nursing Assessment Derived from Dialectic Inquiry

LEVEL OF ASSESSMENT	CHARACTERISTICS
1. Vulnerability	Level of greatest immediacy. Focus on subjectivity (experience) of symptoms. Urgent symptoms receive attention, etiology not addressed.
2. Disengagement	Symptoms are objectified. Experience is framed in general terms; no longer personal. Objectified experiences move to abstract categories for explanation.
3. Reduction	Objectively identifiable elements are the basis for diagnostic certainty. Search for etiology underlying the symptom. Identify a wealth of possible etiologies. Multiple competing etiologies generate greater complexity.
4. Holism	Knowledge about all competing elements is incorporated. Comprehensive view of patient experience in context with no single type of data being more important. Patient viewed as an object assembled by data analysis, not as a person encountered by another person.
5. Engagement	Patient engaged as "author" of experience rather than object of assessment. Patient interprets the data to create internal coherence. Patient and nurse become coauthors of a relational narrative, reconstructing the situation as meaning. Situation becomes unified, existentially, as a lived situation.

From "Clinical Epistemology: A Dialectic of Nursing Assessment," by S. Gadow, 1995, *Canadian Journal of Nursing Research, 27*(2), 25–34.

Nursing's definition of health and health-related problems has evolved to reflect more than body system pathology and biological function. However, labeling nursing as *holistic* does not provide clarity for assessment purposes. Holism as a theoretical perspective has many interpretations, including *adding together different parts to construct a whole* and a more Gestalt notion of *the whole is greater than the sum of parts*. Looking at the nursing assessment literature, it appears that holistic assessment means adding one or more focused assessments, such as a focused assessment on sexuality or spirituality. Focused assessments, individually or in addition to physical assessment of body systems, provide additional information, but conclusions based in a focused assessment are no more holistic than the traditional physical examination of body systems—the conclusions reflect a circumscribed area of interest.

Gadow's finding that the theoretical perspective of the nurse, holistic or otherwise, helps shape a patient's experience suggests that nursing should actively address the theoretical underpinnings of assessment. No one theoretical perspective is absolute or best; however, it is important to have a defined theoretical perspective (or theory) underpinning the assessment process. Defining a theoretical perspective is important for several reasons. First, a theoretical perspective defines data, including necessary data to be collected, what "counts" as data, and boundaries around a complete data set. Second, a theoretical perspective guides data analysis and interpretation by logically aligning data with conclusions. Third, a theoretical perspective aligns conclusions with interventions and outcomes. This logical flow from data collection, analysis, conclusions, interventions, and outcomes is evident when the traditional body systems medical examination framework is used. Using a medical framework to assess body systems for pathological states leads to conclusions about disease, interventions focused on disease treatment, and goals for disease cure or stability. In nursing practice, this logical flow often breaks down as nursing's espoused beliefs about holistic perspective and the conclusions nurses draw about patient problems are often disconnected. Greater attention is needed to clarify the theoretical perspective of holism in particular, and to the theoretical basis of advanced nursing in general.

In a complex multidisciplinary health care environment where team collaboration is paramount, our challenge is to identify a theoretical perspective supporting nursing's unique contributions to patient/ client health outcomes. Self-care, a theoretical perspective that views patients and families engaging in purposeful actions directed at maintaining or improving their health, has been proposed as a theoretical perspective underlying nursing and distinguishing it from other disciplines. Sidani (2003) noted that self-care is a framework that underpins the design of health-promotion interventions and guides nursing practice across the continuum of care. Table 14.2 summarizes Sidani's arguments supporting self-care as a philosophical orientation underlying and distinguishing nursing as a discipline. Considering assessment is a process composed of levels that culminate in a patient–nurse narrative, the self-care perspective would be influential in shaping the intersubjective patient–nurse narrative. A self-care perspective would provide a directed purpose for the nurse–patient relationship and would guide assessment (data collection,

14.2 | Summary of Arguments Supporting Self-Care as a Philosophical Orientation That Underlies and Distinguishes Nursing as a Discipline

ARGUMENTS

1. Self-care serves as a framework that underpins health promotion interventions.

2. Self-care guides practice across the continuum of care in multiple care settings

3. Self-care provides theoretical foundation for psychoeducational, cognitive, behavioral, and symptom management interventions that focuses on:
   a. Self-monitoring, perceiving, and identifying changes in functioning
   b. Judging the meaning and severity of these changes
   c. Assessing options for actions to manage these changes
   d. Selecting and performing appropriate actions

4. Self-care is viewed as an outcome of nursing care where patients are expected to select and perform actions to maintain life, healthy functioning, and well-being.

From "Self-Care," pp. 65–113, by S. Sidani, 2003, in D. M. Doran (Ed.), *Nursing-Sensitive Outcomes*. Boston: Jones and Bartlett.

analysis, and conclusion), drive nursing interventions, and frame outcomes.

The remainder of this chapter describes a self-care perspective for advanced nursing assessment and a foundation for articulating and achieving unique nursing contributions to patient health. Self-care is consistent with nursing's ontology and enjoys considerable empiric evidence.

Self-care is defined as decisions and actions taken by individuals to cope with a health problem and to improve or maintain health status. The notion of self-care has also been referred to as self-management, self-care agency, self-efficacy, and other related terms. While similar in meaning, nuances are present as individual authors use different definitions of similar concepts. For the purpose of the perspective presented here, self-care is considered a broad umbrella term for a philosophical orientation that views patients and families engaging in purposeful actions directed at maintaining or improving their health. The self-care perspective assumes: (1) the purpose of nurse–patient engagement is to support the patient in managing his/her own health; (2) engagement is intersubjective whereby patient and nurse become coauthors of a relational narrative, reconstructing the situation as meaning; and (3) self-care is central to meaning in the nurse–patient narrative.

SELF-CARE PERSPECTIVE FOR ADVANCED NURSING ASSESSMENT

The goal of self-care is an individual's experience of wellness, which is manifest and measured as perceived satisfaction with functional status and quality of life (QOL). Individual wellness is derived from ongoing interaction of life processes—the combination of biological and psychosocial processes of an individual. The processes are ever-present and together are reflected in the total functioning of a human being (Carrieri-Kohlman, Lindsey, & West, 2003). Changes in biological or psychosocial processes are threats to wellness. The purpose of the nursing assessment is to identify threats to wellness (functional status and QOL) and determine etiologies of those threats. Nursing interventions are actions to facilitate self-care and to alter etiologies, thereby alleviating or minimizing threats. Self-care actions initiated by patients/clients at the direction of the nurse alter problem etiologies, thus, alleviating or minimizing threats and improving perceived functioning and quality of life. Threats to wellness and desired self-care outcomes are coconstructed between patient and nurse in the relational narrative of assessment. Figure 14.1 depicts the elements of a self-care theoretical perspective.

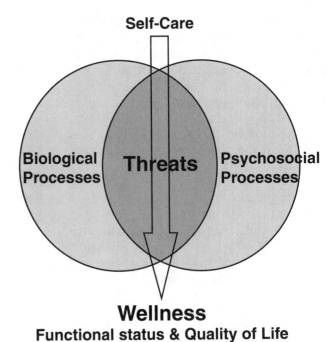

Figure 14.1   Model describing relationships of concepts in a self-care theoretical perspective.

Overview of Self-Care Perspective

Self-Care

Self-care is purposeful actions by patients or their family members directed at maintaining or improving health. Self-care is a complex construct, and definitions may vary based on the *purpose* of the actions and on the *ability* of the individual or family/caregivers. Self-care is different if the purpose is maintenance of current health status by preventive measures or if the purpose is maintenance of chronic disease state. For example, self-care of older adults may have the purpose of maintaining or improving functionality, responsibility, integrity, and/or growth (Hoy, Wagner, & Hall, 2007). Self-care of adults newly diagnosed with epilepsy may have the purposes of management of medications and treatments, safety, seizures, and life issues (Unger & Buelow, 2009). These purposes, however, are dependent upon *abilities*, the patient's emotional status, and physical comfort and functioning. A debate that surrounds the discussion about self-care is whether the concept is appropriate if the individual is unable to perform, that is, paralyzed or comatose.

Orem (as cited in Sidani, 2003, p. 67) considered self-care to be both self-care agency and self-care behavior, although her perspective was rather medical (Redpenning & Taylor, 2003). Self-care agency is the capability of the individual to carryout necessary tasks to maintain, improve, or manage health. This agency comprises multiple domains, including: cognitive (knowledge of health status and behaviors needed), physical (ability to perform needed task), emotional and psychosocial (motivation, desire, environmental, and family support), and performance (the ability to carry out the self-care tasks; Sidani). Self-care behaviors are the processes that individuals or caregivers take in order to maintain or improve health status or manage a health problem. Self-care capability and self-care processes are mutually reinforcing concepts, not separate entities (Hoy et al., 2007). Examples of behaviors are self-monitoring of health, communicating with health care providers and caregivers, coping with and preventing stress, taking medication or following other treatment regimens, changing ways of doing in order to maintain independence, preventing injury, maintaining safety in maneuvering about home and community (including transportation), and learning about health and illness.

Wellness

Wellness is experience; consistent with the nature of experience, wellness is subjective. Wellness is often characterized by pleasant sensations and a perception of comfort (Fakouri & Lyon, 2005; National Association of Clinical Nurse Specialists [NACNS], 2004). As an experience, wellness imbeds individual values, culture, past experiences, and future expectations (DiLalla, Hull, & Dorsey, 2004). Wellness represents balance between the biological strengths and needs and the psychosocial strengths and needs. Wellness can exist in the presence of disease (Moch, 2001). From a nursing perspective, wellness can exist in the presence of disease because wellness is an experience through which individuals, with support as necessary, maximize potential for satisfactory functional status and QOL (Uno & Ruthman, 2004).

Functional Status

Functional status is the perceived ability to perform necessary and valued behaviors for the purpose of meeting basic physiologic needs, fulfilling social roles, and maintaining psychosocial well-being (Leidy, 1994). The adequacy of functional status is determined by an individual based on whatever the individual thinks is adequate or satisfactory for desired activities.

Current function may be distinguished from functional capacity and functional reserve (Doran, 2003). Current functioning is defined as performance dependent on functional *capability*. For example, walking in the community depends on an individual having muscular strength, adequate range of motion of lower extremities, balance, and cardiopulmonary stamina, as well as the motivation to walk that far. Biological processes may limit strength through muscle wasting. Psychosocial processes, such as fear of falling, may limit motivation to walk. An individual with chronic problems of biological processes may have less functional capability. Capability may be improved through interventions, such as exercise. *Functional capacity* is the maximum potential to perform activities. *Functional reserve* is the difference between the current performance and the capacity to perform. Most people have a large reserve that is not tapped in usual or basic needs performance.

Perceived function is associated with well-being (Downe-Wambold & Melanson, 1995); effective coping (Ostwald, Swank, & Khan, 2008); adaptation to changes in health status, environment, or work status (Sandqvist, Scheja, & Eklund, 2008); further disablement (Harrison & Stuifbergen, 2001); self-efficacy for learning new skills (Swor et al., 2003); and perceived cognitive function and neuropsychological performance (Miller, Greene, Montalvo, Ravindran, & Nichols, 1996; Vardy et al., 2008). In addition to the association with well-being, low levels of functioning may predict increased dependency in activities of daily living, increased use of health care services, increased admission to nursing homes, and increased mortality (de Rekeneire et al., 2003).

Perceived functional status may or may not be the same as objective or viewed functioning. Perceived functional status is assessed as a verbal report from the individual. However, verbally reported data may be augmented by physical exam assessment. For example, subjective and objective cognitive status in neurological disorders may be poorly correlated (Schultze-Lutter et al., 2007). Subjective visual effect from cataracts may not be strongly associated with actual objective measure of cataract (Hakim-Banan, n.d.). Younger dialysis patients with high levels of physical performance reported significantly higher strength, mobility, and balance than could be demonstrated using objective measures, suggesting that early impaired sensory nerve function disability may not be realized by patients (Blake & O'Meara, 2004). Safety may become a consideration when perceived function is not well supported by objective measures, as patients over- or underestimate abilities to engage in functional tasks.

Quality of Life

Functional status is closely associated with QOL; however, QOL is not the same as functional status. QOL is the perception of being able to enjoy life and is influenced by but independent of functional status. QOL is also associated with, but not the same as, wellness. An individual may report having satisfactory QOL with poor levels of wellness.

QOL is a broad and complex concept that includes an array of physical and psychosocial characteristics that, if limited or threatened, may affect the individual's ability to derive satisfaction in/from life (Kroenke, Kubzansky, Adler, & Kawachi, 2008). QOL can be influenced by biologic and physiological factors such as symptoms and functional status (Wilson & Cleary, 1995), attachments, and perceived role value, security, and personal control (Grewal & Porter, 2007). Importantly for this discussion, enhanced self-care is associated with greater QOL (Bounthavong & Law, 2008). QOL is independent of physical and social functioning (Lau & McKenna, 2002). In fact, medical therapies to stabilize disease and improve physical function, including pharmacologic agents, have been associated with poorer QOL (Smith, Olin, & Madsen, 2006).

Life Processes

Biological Processes

Biological processes are the micro- (chemical, hormonal, cellular) and macro- (movement, digestion, respiration, etc.) mechanisms that support life, physiologic functioning, and adaptation. These biological processes may be normal and abnormal variations, or they may be pathological. Pathophysiological phenomena may cause alterations in naturally occurring life processes (Carrieri-Kohlman et al., 2003), as can compensatory physiological mechanisms.

Biological processes may be affected by psychosocial processes. Carrieri-Kohlman et al. (2003) divide life processes into five broad areas: regulation, cognition, sensation, protection, and motion. Disruptions to life processes in any of these five areas can threaten an individual's functioning. Disruption in any one area of life processes will cause disruption in others, thus interaction of the areas are mutual and may be additive and/or synergistic, involving one or more of the broad areas. The resulting disruption in functioning results in threats to wellness.

The typical pattern of disruption of life processes tends to vary between specialty populations more greatly than within populations. For example, the pattern of symptoms experienced by persons with head and neck cancer treated with radiation therapy are similar and different from the pattern of symptoms experienced by persons with heart failure. Persons with heart failure share a similar within-group pattern of symptoms that are different from the pattern of symptoms experienced by persons with Alzheimer's disease. Patients with multiple health problems change the symptom pattern even more.

As specialists, CNSs focus on self-care around life processes alterations common within the specialty population; therefore, a comprehensive body system assessment is not often useful. The challenge for CNSs is to develop assessment guidelines for common disruptions in life processes for specialty populations.

Psychosocial Processes

Psychosocial processes are the other half of the life processes and are intimately associated with health and wellness. Disruptions in psychosocial processes may be both etiologic factors associated with a health disruption or consequences of dealing with a health disruption. Psychosocial processes include all of the mental processes necessary for protection, interaction, learning, creation, aesthetics, and valuing. Because health and wellness are not simply a biological phenomenon but the interaction of the individual's perception within a social constructed environment, there are many examples of the interaction of psychosocial processes and health.

Psychosocial processes encompass cognition and emotions. Cognitive processes include orientation, learning ability, perception, beliefs, and negative thinking and may mediate health status through beliefs such as control, learned helplessness, attribution, locus of control, optimism/pessimism, problem solving, and emotion (Cassidy, 1999). Research on learning ability indicates that ability, even controlling for age and education level, has a major role in inadequate health literacy; inadequate health literacy is associated with health outcomes (Levinthal, Morrow, Wanzhu, Jingwei, & Murray, 2008). *Emotions* are responses to events determined by cognition and perception, causing physiological changes, and usually behavior. Pleasure and self-realization are also psychosocial processes; threats to both may lead to threats to wellness. Another psychosocial process often associated with self-care is motivation (Gore-Felton & Koopman, 2008).

Individuals should be considered in context of a social environment. Interpersonal relationship may be considered a psychosocial process; however, relationships are often identified as a social factor necessity for health and wellness. The social part of psychosocial processes of health and wellness include interpersonal and intergroup relationships. Other social factors that are associated with health and wellness are income, employment, education and literacy, gender and gender issues, culture, and environment. For example, increased real and perceived social support is related to improved outcomes after hip fracture (Mortimore et al., 2008). Psychosocial relationships maintain functioning, wellness, and QOL.

Emotions are responses to events determined by cognition and perception, causing physiological changes and usually altered behavior. There are multiple examples of the interaction between emotion and health. For example, evidence suggests that depression is associated with heart disease (Lichtman et al., 2008), negative feelings are related to sleep disturbances (Steptoe, O'Donnell, Marmot, & Wardle, 2008), and anxiety may predict decreased functional status (Harkapaa, 1992).

QOL is defined by psychosocial and social aspects as well as physical aspects. Therefore, psychosocial processes directly affect the perception of wellness (Blane, Netuveli, & Montgomery, 2008; Buenaver, Edwards, Smith, Gramling, & Haythornthwaite, 2008; Davis, 2007; Muslimovic, Post, Speelman, Schmand, & de Haan, 2008). Social factors associated with wellness are often affected by geopolitical issues. Income inequalities, environmental safety, and discrimination certainly affect health, but also QOL. For example, racial/ethnicity disparities in total knee replacement are evident, particularly in black men with no supplemental insurance to Medicare (Hanchate et al., 2008).

Threats to Wellness

Threats to wellness arise from changes in biological and psychosocial processes. Changes in biological processes may lead to physiologic compensatory mechanisms, such as inflammatory processes resulting in pain or pathophysiological alterations resulting in organ-focused disease. Changes in psychosocial processes may result in decreased sensation or perception, decreases in cognition and changes in affect, difficulty with activities of daily living, and alterations in role performance, social relationships, and social support networks (Lindqvist, Widmark, & Rasmussen, 2006).

Threats to function have multiple etiologies that may overlap both biological and psychosocial processes. For example, the ability to provide for personal hygiene requires perception (touch, vision, and hearing), cognition, motivation, and central and peripheral neurophysiologic mechanisms (strength, range of motion). In addition, a suitable environment to allow for hygiene, adaptive equipment, or support from others may also be necessary. Threats to personal hygiene may include interruption in any or part of any of these biological or psychosocial processes.

Threats to QOL are biological and psychosocial. Biological threats to QOL include developmental issues (aging, pregnancy), acute illnesses or injuries, and poorly controlled chronic diseases (Bounthavong & Law, 2008; Chen, Chen, Lee, Cho, & Weng, 2008). Psychosocial threats to QOL include education (Bounthavong & Law), socioeconomic status, employment/occupation (Mountain, Mozley, Craig, & Ball, 2008), and environment (Collier & Truman, 2008). The multidimensional nature of QOL requires skilled assessment to identify complex etiologies. For example, a patient may report limited enjoyment in life. An advanced assessment with relational narrative discovers that the Asian refugee patient is worrying about breast cancer recurrence, compounded by fatigue with difficulty sleeping and lack of appetite plus minimal social network and limited social support from family and friends. The complexity of etiologies requires ongoing, in-depth assessment.

CONDUCTING A SPECIALTY HEALTH ASSESSMENT

This chapter opened by asking, *What constitutes an advanced health assessment?* Thus far, in consideration of the question, we explored a philosophical view of assessment, discussed the importance of articulating a purpose, considered the need for a theoretical perspective, and proposed self-care as a theoretical perspective directed at supporting nursing's unique contribution to patient/client outcomes. Now we need to bring some of these discussion points forward and consider the conduct of assessment.

From the philosophical view, we learned that assessment is a process of the nurse and patient coauthoring a relational narrative. Through narrative a situation becomes unified, not objectively, but as a lived situation. An assessment should include generous opportunity for inclusion of a patient's experience and interpretation of health-related situations or problems along with the CNS's expertise, which also becomes part of the relational narrative.

The purpose of assessment should be stated. CNSs specialize in a delimited area of practice, which may be focused on population (e.g., pediatrics, geriatrics, women's health), problem (e.g., pain, wound management), setting (e.g., critical care unit, operating room, community clinic), or disease/pathology (e.g., diabetes, oncology; American Nurses Association, 2004; NACNS, 2004). CNSs in specialty practice have mastery in the application of science to nursing practice in the specialty. Assessment, for a specialist, is consistent with the specialty area of the purpose of altering the patient's experience though self-care within in the specialty domain. For example, a CNS specializing in diabetes would engage in patient assessment for the purpose of altering the patient's experience of having diabetes.

A theoretical perspective is necessary for guiding the selection and interpretation of assessment data. Contemporary nursing literature and observation suggest that advanced nursing assessment is holistic; however, holism as a theoretical perspective is poorly articulated. Adding focused assessments in domains such as sexuality or spirituality does not make an assessment holistic. Further, every focused narrow assessment should be supported by a theoretical perspective.

Self-care was discussed as a theoretical perspective for advanced nursing assessment by a specialty focused CNS. Self-care is well supported in the nursing literature as a philosophical orientation unique to nursing. Sidani (2003) noted that self-care underpins health promotion interventions; guides practice across the continuum of care in multiple care settings; provides theoretical foundation for psychoeducational, cognitive, behavioral, and symptom management interventions; and is viewed as an outcome of nursing care where patients are expected to select and perform actions to maintain life, healthy functioning, and well-being.

A theoretical perspective of self-care was described. Wellness is experience (subjective) characterized by pleasant sensations and a perception of comfort, and it imbeds individual values, culture, past experiences, and future expectations. Wellness represents balance between the biological life process and psychosocial life processes and is manifest as functional status and quality of life. Self-care is directed at eliminating or minimizing biological and psychosocial threats to wellness, thereby maximizing functional status and quality of life. Advanced nursing assessment involves understanding a patient's meaning of wellness, identifying the gap between a patient's perceived and desired wellness and ability to achieve desired wellness, and drawing conclusions about etiologies of problems preventing closure of the gap. Using a traditional body systems framework, advanced practice nurses have concentrated on gathering a comprehensive medical and surgical history along with a complete system review and physical examination for the purpose of determining a differential disease diagnosis, useful in the practice of primary care. Within a self-care perspective, the purpose of assessment is to determine gaps between perceived wellness (functional status and quality of life), desired wellness, and patient self-care abilities (knowledge, skills, and resources) for achieving desired wellness. Nursing interventions are designed to address the causes (etiologies) of the gaps and assist patients in self-care to achieve desired wellness. Nursing assessment should include data about patient perceptions of wellness adequate for the nurse to engage in an interpretative narrative about the meaning of the wellness experience. Assessment shifts to greater focus on the patient's perspective. Patient perspective of wellness is foreground, with traditional elements of medical and surgical history, habits, lifestyle and physical examination of the nurse/provider-focused assessment as background. CNS practice expertise in a specialty practice drives nursing interventions to address gaps between perceived and desired wellness. Nursing interventions minimize threats and maximize self-care. The outcome of CNS interventions can be measured as improved perception of wellness (functional status and quality of life). Figure 14.2 is a graphic depiction of wellness balanced between threats and self-care.

CNSs in specialty practice areas can use a self-care theoretical perspective to design assessment guidelines for determining gaps and self-care interventions for specialty patient populations. A growing body of scientific evidence is shedding light on the dimensions of the wellness experience for specialty populations. For example, older women with multiple chronic diseases described a core of similar problems (Roberto, Gigliotti, & Husser, 2005). For these women, disease faded into the background, while problems related to functional status and quality of life (pain, falls, sleep

Figure 14.2   Schematic depicting wellness as a balance of life processes and the role of self-care in eliminating or minimizing threats to wellness.

disturbances, reduced energy, worrying, financial strain, medication side effects, and functional limitations) became foreground concerns for daily living. The women in this study described self-care strategies for managing the problems. Here is the place for advanced nursing assessment—to see common problems as threats to wellness, to assess the patient's perception of their experience, and to use a CNS's expertise to cocreate interventions that will reduce threats and improve functional status and quality of life. Thorne, Patterson, and Russell (2003) noted that individuals with chronic disease are experts in self-care with priorities and principles different from textbook recommendations and provider prescriptions.

A SELF-CARE ASSESSMENT FORMAT

What follows is a suggested guide for incorporating the patient's perspective of wellness into advanced health assessment. CNSs are encouraged to develop assessment templates for specialty populations addressing common threats and gaps across specialty and among niche populations, to consider the patient the expert in determining wellness, and to become coauthor in eliminating or minimizing biological and psychosocial threats.

Wellness (Experiential) Data

- Describe your general state of health.
- Describe any health-related problems or concerns.
- What does it mean to you to have these problems or concerns?
- How does any one problem or concern aggravate or cause other problems?

- How do you think nurses or other health care providers can help with any problems or concerns that interfere with your functioning and enjoying life?

Functional Status

- Do you function at the level you think you should?
- Are there any problems or concerns that interfere with your ability to function at your maximum level?
- How much and in what way do problems or concerns interfere with your ability to take care of your personal needs such as bathing and dressing?
- How much and in what way do problems or concerns interfere with your ability to do necessary things such as shopping, cooking, or paying bills?

Quality of Life

- Do you enjoy life as much as you want?
- Any there are there any problems or concerns that interfere with your satisfaction with life or enjoying life as much as you think you can?
- How much and in what way does the symptom or problem affect your feelings, such as feeling sad, worried, or nervous?
- How much and in what way does this symptom or problem interfere with relationships with family and friends?

Psychosocial Processes

Patient's Understanding of Problem or Disease and Cause

- What is your understanding of the problem/ disease?
- What caused the problem?

History of Present Problem or Disease

- Describe the history of your current problem from the time it first started until present. Include how it interfered with things you wanted to do, how it has made you feel, and how it has caused you to change the way you live your life.

Past History of Problem or Disease

- Have you ever had the same or similar problems at another time? If so, when?
- What caused the problem?
- Do you think that past problems are related to current problems? If so, how?
- How did you manage the problem in the past? What did you do?

Patient's Suggestions for Relieving Problem or Disease

- What do you think would help the current problem?
- What do you see as obstacles to getting the help you need?

Family Diseases

- Describe any health problems that family members have had that are similar to your problem.
- How did they manage their problem?
- What happened to these family members?

Family Support

- Who helps you with problems?
- Are you satisfied with the help you get?
- Who could help you but is not? Why not?
- Do you think you can tell this person you need more or different help?

Biologic Processes

Review of Preventative Health Practices/Risk Factors (Data Obtained from Medical Record/Patient Interview)

- Immunizations
- Screenings (hearing, vision)
- Disease: cancer, cardiovascular, etc.
- Allergies: medicine, food, plants, other
- Caffeine/tobacco/alcohol/recreational drug use
- Dental health
  - Do you have a dentist?
  - When was your last dental check-up?
- Exercise
  - Do you exercise regularly? If yes, describe regular exercise routine.
  - What interferes with your exercise routine?
- Nutrition
  - How would you describe your daily diet/foods you eat?
  - What foods do you like?
  - What foods do you not like or avoid?

Patient's Perception of the Relationship Between Lifestyle and Health

- What do you think is or could be the relationship between your lifestyle and your general state of health?

Medications and Medical Therapies

- Current prescribed medications
  - What medications are you taking?

- What are the effects of taking these medications?
- If you skip the medications, do you feel better, worse, or no difference?
- What kinds of concerns do you have about obtaining the medications, such as cost, delivery, or problems getting refills?
- What medications have you taken that were not prescribed for you, such as medications prescribed for a family member with a similar problem?
- What, if any, medications do you think might help that you are not taking, or would help if you stopped taking?
- Over-the-counter medications or supplements
  - What over-the-counter medications or are you taking?
  - What are the effects of taking these medications?
  - What vitamin, mineral, or other nutritional supplements are you taking?
  - What are the effects of taking these supplements?
  - Where did you learn about these over-the-counter medications and supplements?

Physical Alterations

- The extent of a physical examination for advanced nursing assessment varies and should be specific to the specialty patient population and/or health-related problem. For example, where risk of falling is identified, the physical examination should be tailored to include assessment of parameters involving gait, balance, and muscle strength. Physical examination techniques including inspection, palpitation, percussion and auscultation in addition to special tests should be used.

From the assessment data, a CNS draws conclusions about the patient's desired wellness and threats to wellness, both biological and psychosocial; identifies as problems those gaps between desired wellness and patient abilities (knowledge, abilities, and resources); determines the etiologies of problems; and identifies and implements nursing interventions to alter etiologies and promote self-care. A self-care theoretical perspective and proposed model is suggested in this discussion, other theories may be used to support assessment.

DISCUSSION QUESTIONS

1. What constitutes an advanced nursing assessment? Discuss the importance of addressing this question.
2. How does theory guide an advanced nursing assessment? Give an example of how the purpose of an advanced nursing assessment would shift based on the theory guiding the assessment.

3. Discuss the concepts in the self-care perspective presented in this chapter. How would you apply these concepts to your specialty population?

ANALYSIS AND SYNTHESIS EXERCISES

1. Advanced nursing assessment involves coauthoring a narrative with the patient. An emerging body of scientific work is providing insight into the patient's perspective. Consider the following readings and identify meaning that patients may bring to the narrative.
   a. Thorne, S., Paterson, B., & Russell, C. (2003). The structure of everyday self-care decision making in chronic illness. *Qualitative Health Research, 13*(10), 1337–1352.
   b. Thorne, S., Con, A., McGuinness, L., McPherson, G., & Harris, S. R. (2004). Health care communication issues in multiple sclerosis: An interpretive description. *Qualitative Health Research, 14*(1), 5–22.
   c. Paterson, B., & Thorne, S. (2000). Expert decision making in relation to unanticipated blood glucose levels. *Research in Nursing & Health, 23*(2), 147–157.

CLINICAL APPLICATION CONSIDERATIONS

1. Consider the information on the suggested assessment guide and use it to help develop a specialty-focused advanced nursing assessment that targets a selected specialty patient population. Focus on information that will lead to conclusions about problems that are amenable to nursing interventions. The final assessment format may be in a design or configuration of your choosing (e.g., order of information, questions asked, etc.) that best facilitates a coauthored narrative in the context of common threats to wellness, involving biological and psychosocial processes evidenced in the specialty population.
2. Conduct a health assessment of a patient using your specialty assessment format. Revise the format as needed after piloting.

REFERENCES

American Nurses Association. (2004). *Nursing: Scope and standards of practice.* Washington, DC: Author.

Barkauskas, V. H., Baumann, L. C., & Darling-Fisher, C. S. (2002). *Health and physical assessment.* St. Louis: Mosby.

Bates, B., & Hoekelman, R. A. (1974). *A guide to physical examination.* Philadelphia: Lippincott.

Blake, C., & O'Meara, Y. M. (2004). Subjective and objective physical limitations in high-functioning renal dialysis patients. *Nephrology Dialysis Transplantation, 19,* 3124–3129.

Blane, D., Netuveli, G., & Montgomery, S. M. (2008). Quality of life, health and physiological status and change at older ages. *Social Science & Medicine, 66*(7), 1579–1587.

Bounthavong, M., & Law, A. V. (2008). Identifying health-related quality of life (HRQL) domains for multiple chronic conditions (diabetes, hypertension and dyslipidemia): Patient and provider perspectives. *Journal of Evaluation in Clinical Practice, 14*(6), 1002–1011.

Broom, M. (2007). Exploring the assessment process. *Paediatric Nursing, 19*(4), 22–25.

Buenaver, L. F., Edwards, R. R., Smith, M. T., Gramling, S. E., & Haythornthwaite, J. A. (2008). Catastrophizing and pain-coping in young adults: Associations with depressive symptoms and headache pain. *Journal of Pain, 9*(4), 311–319.

Carpenito, L. J. (1995). *Nursing care plans and documentation: Nursing diagnosis and collaborative problems.* Philadelphia: Lippincott.

Carrieri-Kohlman, V., Lindsey, A. M., & West, C. (2003). The conceptual approach. In V. Carrieri-Kohlman, A. M. Lindsey, and C. West (Eds.), *Pathophysiological phenomena in nursing: Human responses to illness* (pp. 1–12). St. Louis: Saunders.

Cassidy, T. (1999). *Stress, cognition and health.* London: Routledge.

Chen, K., Chen, M., Lee, S., Cho., H., & Weng, L. (2008). Self-management behaviours for patients with chronic obstructive pulmonary disease: A qualitative study. *Journal of Advanced Nursing, 64*(6), 595–604.

Collier, L., & Truman, J. (2008). Exploring the multi-sensory environment as a leisure resource for people with complex neurological disabilities. *NeuroRehabilitation, 23*(4), 361–367.

Davidson, L. J., Bennett, S. E., Hamera, E. K., & Raines, B. K. (2004). What constitutes advanced assessment? *Journal of Nursing Education, 43*(9), 421–425.

Davis, L. A. (2007). Quality of life issues related to dysphagia. *Topics in Geriatric Rehabilitation, 23*(4), 352–365.

de Rekeneire, N., Visser, M., Peila, R., Nevitt, M. C., Cauley, J. A., Tylavsky, F. A., et al. (2003). Is a fall just a fall: Correlates of falling in healthy older persons. The Health, Aging and Body Composition Study. *Journal of the American Geriatrics Society, 51*(6), 841–846.

DiLalla, L. F., Hull, S. K., & Dorsey, J. K. (2004). Effect of gender, age, and relevant course work on attitudes toward empathy, patient spirituality, and physician wellness. *Teaching and Learning in Medicine, 16*(2), 165–170.

Doran, D. M. (2003). Functional status. In D. M. Doran (Ed.), *Nursing sensitive outcomes* (pp. 27–64). Boston: Jones and Bartlett.

Downe-Wambold, B. L., & Melanson, P. M. (1995). A causal model of coping and well being in elderly people with arthritis. *Journal of Advanced Nursing, 27,* 1109–1116.

Driscoll, V. M. (1976/2007). The movement to secure statutory definition of the unique and independent practice of nursing. *Clinical Nurse Specialist, 21*(1), 7–12.

Fakouri, C., & Lyon, B. (2005). Perceived health and life satisfaction among older adults. The effects of worry and personal variables. *Journal of Gerontological Nursing, 31*(10), 17–24.

Fulton, J. S. (2007). The unique and independent practice of nursing. *Clinical Nurse Specialist, 21*(1), 5–6.

Gadow, S. (1995). Clinical epistemology: A dialectic of nursing assessment. *Canadian Journal of Nursing Research, 27*(2), 25–34.

Gordon, M. (2007). *Manual of nursing diagnosis.* Boston: Jones and Bartlett.

Gore-Felton, C., & Koopman, C. (2008). Behavioral mediation of the relationship between psychosocial factors and HIV disease progression. *Psychosomatic Medicine, 70,* 569–574.

Grewal, P. K., & Porter, J. E. (2007). Hope theory: A framework for understanding suicidal action. *Death Studies, 31*(2), 131–154.

Hakim-Banan, N. (n.d.). *Association between subjective visual function and both low contrast visual acuity and contrast sensitivity in cataract.* City University London. Retrieved January 21, 2009, from http://www.city.ac.uk/optometry/research/eyenet/projects/cataract.html

Hanchate, A. D., Zhang, Y., Felson, D. T., Ash, A. S., Hanchate, A. D., Zhang, Y., et al. (2008). Exploring the determinants of racial and ethnic disparities in total knee arthroplasty: Health insurance, income, and assets. *Medical Care, 46*(5), 481–488.

Harkapaa, K. (1992). Psychosocial factors as predictors for early retirement in patients with chronic low back pain. *Journal of Psychosomatic Research, 36*(6), 553–559.

Harrison, T., & Stuifbergen, A. (2001). Barriers that further disablement: A study of survivors of polio. *Journal of Neuroscience Nursing, 33*(3), 160–166.

Hoy, B., Wagner, L., & Hall, E.O.C. (2007). Self-care as a health resource of elders: An integrative review of the concept. *Journal of Caring Sciences, 21*(4), 456–466.

Kelley, F. J., & Kopac, C. A. (2001). Advanced health assessment in nurse practitioner programs. *Journal of Professional Nursing, 17*(5), 218–225.

Kroenke, C. H., Kubzansky, L. D., Adler, N., & Kawachi, I. (2008). Prospective change in health-related quality of life and subsequent mortality among middle-aged and older women. *American Journal of Public Health, 98*(11), 2085–2091.

Lau, A., & McKenna, K. (2002). Perception of quality of life by Chinese elderly persons with stroke. *Disability and Rehabilitation, 24*(4), 203–218.

Leidy, N. K. (1994). Functional status and the forward progress of merry-go-rounds: Toward a coherent analytic framework. *Nursing Research, 43,* 196–202.

Levinthal, B. R., Morrow, D. G., Wanzhu, T., Jingwei, W., & Murray, M. D. (2008). Cognition and health literacy in patients with hypertension. *Journal of General Internal Medicine, 23*(8). Retrieved January 21, 2009, from http://www.springerlink.com/content/yg110886517k6863/

Lichtman, J. H., Bigger, J. T., Jr., Blumenthal, J. A., Frasure-Smith, N., Kaufmann, P. G., Lespérance, F., et al. (2008). Depression and coronary heart disease: Recommendations for screening, referral, and treatment: A science advisory from the American Heart Association Prevention Committee of the Council on Cardiovascular Nursing, Council on Clinical Cardiology, Council on Epidemiology and Prevention, and Interdisciplinary Council on Quality of Care and Outcomes Research: Endorsed by the American Psychiatric Association. *Circulation, 118*(17), 1768–1775.

Lindqvist, O., Widmark, A., & Rasmussen, B. H. (2006). Reclaiming wellness-living with bodily problems, as narrated by men with advanced prostate cancer. *Cancer Nursing, 29*(4), 327–333.

Maher, D., & Hemming, L. (2005). Understanding patient and family: Holistic assessment in palliative care. *British Journal of Community Nursing, 10*(7), 318–322.

Miller, R. B., Greene, B. A., Montalvo, G. P., Ravindran, B., & Nichols, J. D. (1996). Engagement in academic work: The role of learning goals, future consequences, pleasing others, and perceived ability. *Contemporary Educational Psychology, 21*(4), 388–422.

Moch, S. D. (2001). Health-within-illness: Concept development through research and practice. *Journal of Advanced Nursing, 28*(2), 305–310.

Mortimore, E., Haselow, D., Dolan, M., Hawkes, W. G., Langenberg, P., Zimmerman, S., et al. (2008). Amount of social contact and hip fracture mortality. *Journal of the American Geriatrics Society, 56*(6), 1069–1074.

Mountain, G., Mozley, C., Craig, C., & Ball, L. (2008). Occupational therapy led health promotion for older people: Feasibility of the Lifestyle Matters programme. *British Journal of Occupational Therapy, 71*(10), 406–413.

Muslimovic, D., Post, B., Speelman, J. D., Schmand, B., & de Haan, R. J. (2008). Determinants of disability and quality of life in mild to moderate Parkinson disease. *Neurology, 70*(23), 2241–2247.

National Association of Clinical Nurse Specialists. (2004). *Statement on clinical nurse specialist practice and education* (2nd ed.). Harrisburg, PA: Author.

Ostwald, S. K., Swank, P. R., & Khan, M. M. (2008). Predictors of functional independence and stress level of stroke survivors at discharge from inpatient rehabilitation. *Journal of Cardiovascular Nursing, 23*(4), 371–377.

Paterson, B., & Thorne, S. (2000). Expert decision making in relation to unanticipated blood glucose levels. *Research in Nursing & Health, 23*(2), 147–157.

Redpenning, K., & Taylor, S. (Eds.). (2003). *Self-care theory in nursing: Selected papers of Dorothea Orem.* New York: Springer.

Roberto, K. A., Gigliotti, C. M., & Husser, E. K. (2005). Older women's experiences with multiple health conditions: Daily challenges and care practices. *Health Care for Women International, 26*, 672–692.

Sandqvist, G., Scheja, A., & Eklund, M. (2008). Working ability in relation to disease severity, everyday occupations and well-being in women with limited systemic sclerosis. *Rheumatology, 47*, 1708–1711.

Sappington, J., & Kelley, J. H. (1996). Modeling and role-modeling theory. *Journal of Holistic Nursing, 14*(2), 130–141.

Schultze-Lutter, F., Ruhrmann, S., Picker, H., Von Reventlow, H. G., Daumann, B., Brockhaus-Dumke, A., et al. (2007). Relationship between subjective and objective cognitive function in the early and late prodrome. *British Journal of Psychiatry, 191*(suppl. 51), s43–s51.

Sidani, S. (2003). Self-care. In D. M. Doran (Ed.), *Nursing-sensitive outcomes* (pp. 65–113). Boston: Jones and Bartlett.

Smith, R. E., Olin, B. R., & Madsen, J. W. (2006). Spitting into the wind: The irony of treating chronic disease. *Journal of the American Pharmaceutical Association, 46*(3), 379–400.

Steptoe, A., O'Donnell, K., Marmot, M., & Wardle, J. (2008). Positive affect, psychological well-being, and good sleep. *Journal of Psychosomatic Research, 64*(4), 409–415.

Swor, R., Compton, S., Farr, L., Kokko, S., Vining, F., Pascual, R., et al. (2003). Perceived self-efficacy in performing and willingness to learn cardiopulmonary resuscitation in an elderly population in a suburban community. *American Journal of Critical Care, 12*(1), 65–70.

Thorne, S., Con, A., McGuinness, L., McPherson, G., & Harris, S. R. (2004). Health care communication issues in multiple sclerosis: An interpretive description. *Qualitative Health Research, 14*(1), 5–22.

Thorne, S., Paterson, B., & Russell, C. (2003). The structure of everyday self-care decision making in chronic illness. *Qualitative Health Research, 13*(10), 1337–1352.

Unger, W. R., & Buelow, J. M. (2009). Hybrid concept analysis of self-management in adults newly diagnosed with epilepsy. *Epilepsy & Behavior, 14*, 89–95.

Uno, K., & Ruthman, J. L. (2004). Wellness as a self-care philosophy for nurses and their leaders. *Holistic Nursing Practice, 20*(1), 3–4.

Vardy, J. L., Zu, W., Booth, C. M., Park, A., Dodd, A., Rourke, S., et al. (2008). Relation between perceived cognitive function and neuropsychological performance in survivors of breast and colorectal cancer. *Journal of Clinical Oncology, 261*(ASCO Annual Meeting Proceedings, Post-Meeting Edition, 15S), 6016.

Wilson, I. B., & Cleary, P. D. (1995). Linking clinical variables with health-related quality of life. A conceptual model of patient outcomes. *Journal of the American Medical Association, 273*, 59–65.

15

Family as Client

Barbara S. O'Brien
Ginette G. Ferszt

Advocating for family inclusion in patient care has been a hallmark of modern nursing practice since its inception. Nightingale facilitated family communication with injured soldiers to boost morale and motivate recovery. More recently, nurses have underscored the importance of family-centered care for every patient/client entering the health care system. Family-centered care is an approach to health care that incorporates active participation of families in the planning, delivery, and evaluation of health care. The family is recognized as a partner with health care providers and included in decision making based on their level of comfort and ability. In some clinical nurse specialist (CNS) practices, the entire family becomes the "client" or the unit of care. In this type of practice, all members of the identified family are considered as a whole when interventions are designed. Pediatric or psychiatric CNSs are frequently compelled to incorporate care designs that foster effective adjustment and adaptation of the entire family unit in achieving desired outcomes. When working with the family as a unit, assessment and interventions strategies are highly complex. Regardless of the nature of family interventions designed by the CNS, family inclusion in nursing care and patient decision making is increasingly recognized as an essential component of care.

Dynamic shifts in health care today reflect continued efforts to effectively involve families in patient care. Challenges created by a fast-paced delivery system—including shortened length of hospital stay, technologically driven diagnostics that yield rapid results, and the need for prompt decision making—increasingly press nurses to develop trust with family members in abbreviated periods of time. At the forefront of this movement, family-centered care and family as client have emerged as essential nursing care

concepts and philosophies. Families are an integral part of the continuum of care, and their effective involvement with the patient and providers can profoundly influence patient outcomes. As informed consumers, families are no longer content to take back-seat positions to professionals. They are demanding more information and greater participation in issues related to the care of a loved one. Recently, the Institute of Medicine (IOM) supported patient-centered health care systems where treatment recommendations and decision making included patients' (and family) preferences (IOM, 2001). In addition, today's focus on cost-containment has generated a resurgence of home care provisions so that inclusion and support of families becomes increasingly salient in accomplishing safe, optimal recovery for the vast majority of patients.

Families vary greatly in their capacity to respond to health-related stressors. In many cases, staff nurses adeptly manage the family education, support, and resource needs required to facilitate continuing care. However, it is important to recognize that the specific nature of the challenge and the abilities of the family will impact adjustment and adaptation. For families with established, functional systems who are experiencing alterations that fall within their capacity to respond, the staff nurse is generally able to provide the support that sufficiently responds to family needs. However, staff nurses may not have the time, knowledge and/ or skills to respond to complex family needs, especially in light of the increasing nursing workloads combined with high patient acuity and shortened lengths of hospital stays. Consequently, home care issues may surface that escalate the risk of poor patient outcomes or increase recidivism rates, all contributing to the escalating cost of health care. Additionally, the risk of resulting low patient satisfaction ratings and conflict situations escalate when family needs are neglected.

The CNS is the ideal resource to respond to the increasing needs of today's complex families. This chapter addresses CNS interventions for the family unit, focusing on the family as client and the family as the context of care. Strategic interventions in advocating for and role modeling family-centered care are discussed. Within the CNS spheres of practice framework described by the National Association of Clinical Nurse Specialists (NACNS; 2004), CNSs must be competent in addressing family needs. This practice includes assessing family needs and designing interventions for families experiencing the stress of illness/injury as well as providing support and education to staff while establishing system changes that address family needs and focus on positive patient care outcomes.

BACKGROUND

The literature is rich in descriptions of CNS practice involving families. CNSs intervene to help families in acute care, outpatient, private practice, and community-based settings and in numerous specialties, including but not limited to community health, critical care, gerontology, medical-surgical, neurology, pediatrics, maternal child health, psychiatric mental health, and rehabilitation. The following discussion provides a few examples that illustrate the scope of CNS practice.

In critical care, CNSs have made significant contributions, intervening to promote communication between the patient, family, and health care staff in these stressful care settings. Notable success has been reported in decreasing length of stay in intensive care units (ICUs) as a result of improved communication between patients, families, and staff facilitated by CNSs teamed with the medical director (Ahrens, Yancey, & Kollef, 2003; Coyle, 2000). Coyle described the benefit of the CNS in assuming a primary supportive role for families by providing information and answering very difficult questions related to health care decisions about a family member with suspected brain-stem death.

Gerontological CNSs continue to be in high demand because the current population of Americans over the age of 65 is 36 million, or 12% of the population. By 2030, the number is expected to rise to 20%, or 71.5 million (Burbank, 2007). Despite this growing need, attracting enough CNSs to serve the health care requirements of this rapidly growing population is a persistent challenge (Thornlow, Auerhahn, & Stanley, 2006). Gerontological CNSs practice in a wide variety of settings, including acute care, long-term care facilities, outpatient practices, senior housing facilities, and in the community. A positive impact on a number of patient outcomes resulted from the use of advanced practice

registered nurses (APRNs) in long-term care facilities (Ryer et al., 2000). Decreased hospital readmissions along with prolonged stabilization of the patient's mental status resulted in decreased family distress. Austrom et al. (2006) described the benefits of providing care to Alzheimer's patients and their families in the primary care setting by multidisciplinary teams coordinated by a geriatric advanced practice nurse. Furthermore, positive patient outcomes for elders receiving institutional or home care may depend on successful integration of family resources and coping abilities. The CNS is uniquely positioned to provide this support.

In pediatric care, CNSs have provided support and education for families of children in acute care and home care settings. Davis (2006) described her role as the primary point person for families who have a child with ear, nose, and throat (ENT) problems. She provided expert support and education from the beginning of the child's hospitalization through discharge. In home care, CNSs have provided essential follow-up for low birth weight babies in the transition from hospital to home (Brooten et al., 2002). In-home and telephone support for 4 months for these infants and their families resulted in an increase in the mothers' confidence in providing care for her infant and a decreased use of emergency departments and pediatrician offices (Lasby, Newton, & von Platen, 2004). Canam (2005) described a qualitative study with 16 CNSs who organized and provided health care for children with complex needs and their families across the continuum of care. In addition to focusing on individual children and their families, the CNSs described the potential for contributing to high-quality and cost-effective care at the population level.

Oncology CNSs have provided psychosocial support and education for families in diverse settings. CNSs in community oncology programs have enhanced communication across the continuum of care and improved patients' and families' abilities to successfully navigate complex systems (Vooght & Richardson, 1996). Oncology CNSs in a perioperative nurse liaison program intervened with a designated family point person for families experiencing high degrees of distress and were able to demonstrate decreased patient and family anxiety while improving communication (Cunningham, Hanson-Heath, & Agre, 2003). CNSs have also been identified as having an important role in providing support and education for patients receiving chemotherapy for colorectal cancer and their families (Wright & Myint, 2003).

The practice of psychiatric mental health CNSs is diverse. In hospital acute care settings, the psychiatric consultation liaison nurse (PCLN) has flourished, particularly as the complexity and acuity of health care has grown exponentially. PCLNs conduct psychiatric mental health assessments and provide crisis and brief counseling to patients and families and consultation and education to nursing staff. Psychiatric CNSs have also assumed primary provider responsibilities for mental health services to burn patients and their families (Summers, 1991) and counseled families whose family member was dying (Skilbeck & Payne, 2003). Within the last decade, critical incident stress debriefing has also come under the purview of the psychiatric mental health CNS practice. Ragaisis (1994) noted that intervention at the family level decreased their anxiety by providing education regarding the posttrauma response.

Psychiatric CNS practice has also expanded into the community setting. Combining psychiatric mental health nursing and case management skills, CNSs have provided holistic nursing care to clients and families in the home following discharge from psychiatric hospitals (Ward-Miller, 1996). Elder (1986) described the benefit of the CNS working in the home with families who have a child with developmental disabilities. By educating families on how to manage problematic behaviors, family stress was significantly decreased. Psychiatric mental health CNSs have also made significant contributions in intensive home-based crisis intervention and family education programs (Amundson, 1989). By teaching families new problem-solving skills and providing in-home family support, crises that could have resulted in needing to place a child in foster, group, or institutional care have been averted.

These selective examples illustrate the importance of CNS practice focusing on family involvement. A long and rich history of the beneficial impact of CNS intervention with family is documented in the literature.

CARING FOR FAMILIES: CNS FOCUS

Important challenges confront families when a member develops an acute or chronic health problem. The response of the family to this altered state will depend on many variables and warrants a systematic analysis. Nurses expect families to be responsive to their suggestions and teaching. Typically, busy bedside nurses expect that families will be amenable to their suggestions, instructions, and any limitations imposed by the health care system. Although the majority of families acquiesce to these system conditions, such as limited visiting hours, a dilemma arises for the family whose response fails to conform to expectations. For these families, significant conflict can arise between family members and health care providers. When conflict with family members occurs, staff nurses frequently consult a CNS. While a CNS may be able to negotiate a resolution to the conflict, future crises may be averted by mentoring and coaching staff nurses in providing early attention to family issues and building on family strengths.

CNSs work with families in multiple care settings. Family management issues may present different challenges depending on the setting and CNS specialty practice area. For the CNS educated in management of psychiatric/psychological phenomena, engagement in family therapy approaches aimed at assessing and altering family behaviors and interactions may be indicated. Nonpsychiatric CNSs are commonly involved with management of family responses specific to identified health care issues. In these circumstances, the goal of family assessment is evaluation of the effectiveness of family activities and coping strategies needed for immediate and/or ongoing management of an impaired member. While the two functions are not mutually exclusive, the distinction is important. These varying goals of care require a different and distinct skill set to encourage the achievement of adaptive family outcomes. Because educational programs preparing psychiatric CNSs include specialized techniques for emotional responses that may include family therapy approaches, these methods will not be addressed in this chapter. When available, it is recommended that CNSs working in other health care areas take advantage of consultation from psychiatric CNS colleagues to assist with families exhibiting behavioral pattern challenges or a history of psychiatric problems. In most instances, the CNS can have tremendous impact on family adaptation when armed with a systematic approach for assessment and intervention.

Positive patient outcomes often require a team approach when addressing family concerns and needs. Internalized personal attitudes, biases about families, and what constitutes an appropriate response to the needs and care of an ill member can affect the actions of health care providers. Premature judgment of family reactions can be devastating to therapeutic relationships. Therefore, the CNS needs to recognize and examine personal values as well as those of collaborating staff to avoid compromising care outcomes. Actions and responses that are appropriate for one family may be completely unrealistic or unacceptable for another. Family composition and coping strategies are dependent on many factors. Therefore, it is important for the CNS to obtain a comprehensive understanding of the family system, family members' perceptions of the situation, and response patterns.

SPHERES OF INFLUENCE

Nurses often make valiant efforts to work with families experiencing illness stressors. Unfortunately, absence of a systematic approach to assessment coupled with time constraints may result in ineffective actions. When the situation is compounded by direct conflicts between staff and family, the task is even more daunting and neglected. Early attention to family issues and the use of family strengths to avert the development of a crisis are important strategies that the CNS can incorporate into clinical practice. Operating in the three spheres of influence, the CNS can make great strides to improve patient and family outcomes, educate staff to work effectively with families, and effect organizational and policy-level changes to advocate for family care across all settings. Effective management of family issues necessitates the use of all three spheres of influence of the CNS (NACNS, 2004):

1. Patient/client: use of specific knowledge of assessment of family stress and adaptation as well as the use of therapeutic family intervention strategies.
2. Nurses and nursing practice: focus on prevention strategies targeting implementation of staff education programs as well as role modeling of appropriate interventions needed to work effectively with families in crisis.
3. Organization/system: apply research and leadership skills designed to create a hospitable environment of care that will incorporate family needs.

Sphere I: Family Focus

Family Assessment and Intervention

CNSs prepared in the specialties of pediatrics, psych–mental health, or family therapy have typically incorporated practice competencies for assessing and intervening with family units. Because a family is a dynamic system, intervention requires specialized practice competencies. All CNSs can benefit by improved understanding of the family as an integrated unit.

Use of a model can provide a framework to organize thinking, focus assessment, and facilitate interpretation of data (Meleis, 1991). Confronted with the same health care problem, it is difficult to predict how different families will respond. While numerous family theories have been formulated, the Resiliency Model of Family Stress, Adjustment, and Adaptation has been selected as a useful approach for the CNS working with families in acute, chronic, and community settings (McCubbin & McCubbin, 1987; McCubbin & Thompson, 1991; McCubbin, Thompson, & McCubbin, 1996, 2003). Since its inception, this model has continued to evolve and to be used by nursing and other disciplines from the social sciences.

Application of this model is consistent with the first sphere of influence related to the practice of CNSs: patient/client. The model relates important variables specific to the assessment of family stress and adaptation and provides a guide for developing therapeutic family intervention strategies.

The Resiliency Model describes a framework for working with families throughout the illness trajectory. It has been applied to a variety of health care challenges for families in various stages of development and across socioeconomic boundaries (Danielson, Hamel-Bissell, & Winstead-Fry, 1993). The model identifies interacting factors that influence family adaptation. Numerous valid and reliable assessment instruments are available to obtain systematic, objective data useful in designing effective interventions for each unique situation. Use of the model can serve as a foundation to guide the CNS to a greater understanding of issues involved in providing family care. The Resiliency Model is an expansion and compilation of the work of Hill (1949), the Double ABCX Model of Family Stress (McCubbin & Patterson, 1981), and the Typology Model of Family Adjustment and Adaptation (McCubbin & McCubbin, 1987). These theories take into consideration available family resources, family perception of the stressor, and established family coping patterns and problem-solving skills. The Resiliency Model reframes these multiple factors and expands the model for the purpose of explaining family adaptation (Danielson et al., 1993).

The Resiliency Model has practical application for CNSs working in inpatient settings as well as in community care areas. Because health issues may precipitate family stress/crisis, having a model to guide understanding of a family's response patterns can facilitate designing effective, individualized nursing interventions. The Resiliency Model focuses on identifying and building on family strengths. Families may be in either the initial (adjustment) or long-term (adaptation) phases of response to illness.

The *adjustment phase* of the model is initiated when a new illness stressor places a demand on the family system. The adjustment phase begins when the family becomes aware of an illness or injury that provokes more than a limited and contained response. Such stressors include accidents, traumatic injuries, or any illness diagnosis. Health concerns evoke a cascade of effects that influence family actions, reactions, and functions. Severity of illness will impact family response: The more severe the illness (stressor), the greater the impact on the family system. For example, a planned elective surgery for hip replacement for an older adult member is unlikely to demand major, long-term changes for the family and could be expected to be far less distressing than an unanticipated accident resulting in a spinal cord injury for a young adult.

Family vulnerability highlights the importance of other factors that may impact the stress experience. The existence of concurrent, multiple stressors increases a family's vulnerability to effective management of a new demand. If the illness represents the single stressor requiring adjustment, it will be easier to focus on needed activities required to meet the illness demands. Conversely, a family grappling with multiple changes will be highly vulnerable. Events such as the recent death of a family member, relocation of a family member (e.g., sending a child to college), financial difficulties (e.g., loss of wages), and marital friction may all increase family vulnerability. The additional stressors often tax the family's capacity to manage the illness situation and may be enough to adversely affect the ability to respond to the transitions and strains produced by the illness. The model uses the term *pile-up* to label this phenomenon. Multiple stressors compound in a synergistic manner and can alter interpersonal relationships and threaten stability of the family system. In these circumstances, members may become overwhelmed, have difficulty coping, or be plummeted into a crisis mode if buffering factors are inadequate to manage the situation.

To appropriately evaluate the impact of vulnerability, one must consider other factors that may influence family adjustment. Family types, the existing established patterns of functioning for a family, provides information about the ability of the family to deal with the illness event. It is important to determine how the family usually operates and behaves. The range of family types and established behavior patterns can be extensive. In general, the most resilient families are described as cohesive but flexible. A cohesive family remains emotionally, if not physically, close and supportive despite changes in circumstances. A flexible family is able to realign priorities and relationships in order to accomplish mutual goals. These families are highly adaptive and have clear open communication patterns. Family roles can change to accommodate the needs of the ill family member. Families with characteristics of cohesion and flexibility are better able to effectively problem solve and manage stressors. Families that are disorganized, loosely bonded, and inflexible should be considered at-risk. For example, a disorganized family may have difficulty communicating among themselves and, subsequently, bombard the nurses with questions and complaints. Ineffective communication often leads to confusion for both the family and the health care team. These families often have difficulty collaborating, problem solving, and making health care decisions. Chaotic activity is evidenced in the care setting where disagreements, control issues, hostility, and displaced priorities are commonly exhibited.

Family resistance resources is a variable in the model that considers the strengths and capabilities of the family system that are useful in managing the stressful situation. Resistance factors serve to provide the family with the ability to avert a crisis or major family disruption. For example, in a flexible family system, the ability and willingness of members to assume roles previously held by the ill member provides a smooth transition for recovery within the family system. Assessing resistance factors facilitates identifying interventions to support those strengths that are useful in promoting effective adjustment. Appropriate assessments might include evaluation of economic stability, cohesiveness, flexibility, hardiness, shared spiritual beliefs, traditions, celebrations, routines, and organization (McCubbin & McCubbin, 1993).

Though extremely significant, the family's view of their situation is often ignored. If perception is everything, then family appraisal of the stressor demands priority attention. Problems may be created when health care providers inadvertently act on their own beliefs regarding the meaning of the illness and its expected impact on the family system. It is most important to acknowledge that individual appraisal of any event is personal and, therefore, variable and subjective. Avoidance of imposing external beliefs in the situation is imperative. In order to help a family adjust to a member's illness, nurses need to understand the family's perspective of the situation. If viewed as a catastrophic, uncontrollable event, adjustment will require interventions aimed at providing education and realistic expectations to avert further deterioration. On the other hand, a family viewing the situation as a challenge will benefit from support in their efforts to rally an effective defense.

The last factor, problem solving and coping, takes into account the abilities that exist within a family to confront new or distressing situations. Problem-solving skills require the family to identify the problem, break it into manageable parts, and take action to resolve it. Some families do not communicate openly, directly, and effectively, therefore, communication within the family must be assessed. Distressed communication between family members frequently evokes difficulties and creates conflicts among the family members and in the health care environment. For example, a family member may infer that nursing care is inadequate when the real issue is anxiety about the family's ability to manage the affected individual at home.

Techniques to reinforce problem-solving skills include support of previously effective strategies and keeping the focus on the problem and not the family members. Clarifying decisions and strategies may avert competitive or even hostile reactions over power and control issues. Undoubtedly, most nurses have confronted difficulties in this area when decisions related to life-support measures, comfort measures, or nursing home placement were being considered.

These elements of typology, appraisal, problem-solving skills, and availability of resources interact as the family strives to manage the illness-related stressor. Eventually, the response culminates in some level of adjustment for the family. The model predicts that if all factors are in balance and function to reduce the level of tension in the family, there will be a *bonadjustment*, an optimistic and constructive ability to manage the situation. Illness places a major strain on the family system because there are often burdensome demands that occur in all of the components of the model. Yet, many families are capable of making this adjustment with little or no assistance. When demands are too high, *mal-adaptation* may result. Demands can include shifting roles within the family, changing goals (or even values), new rules or priorities, boundary changes, and alterations in patterns of functioning (McCubbin & McCubbin, 1993). When demands exceed mediating factors, maladjustment occurs and a resulting crisis may loom. Too frequently, it is only at this juncture that the CNS is consulted. Problems in the health care setting escalate as families in crisis exhibit disorganization and disruptive behaviors. Nurses and other care providers describe the situation as out-of-control and express fear of negative patient and family outcomes. McCubbin and McCubbin caution against labeling these families as dysfunctional. It is the experience of crisis that initiates the adaptation phase. When things are very painful, humans tend to seek assistance in reducing suffering. Therefore, the CNS should approach these situations armed with the knowledge that with supportive care these families are likely to be amenable to interventions and strategies that enable them to better manage their situation.

When illness recovery has a distinct resolution, interventions targeting adjustment may be enough. Once the illness resolves, the family is likely to reestablish itself at a previous or higher level of functioning. Conversely, if the family has maladjusted to the stressor or the changing situation adversely impacts adjustment, a crisis may occur. If emotional stability is at risk, additional assistance may be indicated, such as a referral for family counseling. However, the CNS should anticipate entry into the next phase of the model when working with families dealing with chronic illness. Chronic conditions will create periodic additional or ongoing demands for the family.

The adaptation phase of the Resiliency Model explains the interacting factors that affect family response in this stage. While the factors are similarly labeled, the duration of the stressor requires major and enduring change within the family—adaptation as opposed to adjustment. *Adjustment* involves immediate and often temporary changes in managing an illness, whereas *adaptation* infers acceptance of more durable and long-lasting alterations. Family survival may depend on the acceptability of these changes within the family group. Successful adaptation is defined as the existence of a balance between meeting individual member needs and the well-being of the family as a whole (Danielson et al., 1993). No single strategy can be prescribed in any of the components, and as in the adjustment phase, the interactions between the variables will change the approach. Also, effective adaptation to chronic illness will require integration with the larger community, including the health care system. This mutual relationship facilitates identification of appropriate care, support, and essential education provided to families, while the families reciprocate by following through on the plan of care.

As a family strives to manage a chronic illness, challenges to their prior adjustment will be inevitable. The CNS should anticipate and monitor the occurrence of pile-up over time. Families will become increasingly vulnerable to crisis when demands related to the chronic illness mount or when factors required in managing the situation are compounded by other stressors, strains, and transitions of family life. When pile-up of stressors is suspected, the CNS needs to identify impending or actual stressors impacting the family. Assessment of life changes, hardships, concurrent competing demands, prior strains, situational demands, efforts to cope, ambiguities, and normal life-cycle transitions experienced by the family need to be explored. A clinical interview and assessment is important in identifying issues in this area and in affirming rapport with the family. Additionally, the CNS might elect to use a structured assessment instrument designed to measure family stress (see Table 15.1). When stressors are overwhelming, a family crisis situation may ensue. Again, family strengths and resources are rallied in an attempt to manage the situation. Many components of family response need to be reassessed in an effort to obtain currently valid data to guide future interventions to assist with adaptation. It is important for the CNS to identify the family types and newly instituted patterns of functioning as multiple family types exist. In general, families with greater breadth and depth in their patterns of functioning will be better equipped to support family integrity, unity, flexibility, and predictability when struggling to manage an illness and its long-term impact. To supplement the clinical interview, instruments are available to the CNS to assist in determining family types; two of these are provided in Table 15.1.

Additionally, it is important to reassess the adaptive strategies being used by the family. Historically established patterns may be inadequate in the face of new demands imposed by the illness. However, the adoption of new methods may be problematic as well. For example, a mother may seek employment outside the home to decrease the burden of financial stress resulting from the illness, or a family may move closer to health services for the ill member. Such changes may evoke a chain reaction because needs, desires, and roles of other family members can be dramatically impacted. In assessing this component, the clinical interview should focus on the family's values, priorities, expectations, goals, and rules over time as well as on any change in patterns of family functioning and their impact on the system. Effective patterns will be congruent with family functioning and positively correlated with the ease and level of adaptation to the illness. Assessment of family patterns provides insight into functioning and elucidates important family strengths and valued resources.

15.1 | Assessment Instruments for Family Assessment/Functioning

INSTRUMENT	PRIMARY REFERENCE	FOCUS OF MEASURE
Family Inventory of Life Event and Changes (FILE)	McCubbin & Thompson, 1991	Evaluates stressors present in family at one point in time
Family Hardiness Index	McCubbin & Thompson, 1991	Identifies stress resistance and adaptation resources, mitigating stressors and demands
Family Time and Routines Scale	McCubbin, & Thompson, 1991	Family integration and stability
Family Inventory of Resources for Management (FIRM)	McCubbin & Thompson, 1991	Measures family social, psychological, community, and family income resources
Social Support Index	McCubbin, Patterson, & Glynn, 1996	Measures type and availability of social support for family
Family Problem Solving & Communication	McCubbin, Thompson, & McCubbin, 1996	Explores type of problem-solving methods used by family and primary communication patterns existing within the system
Coping Health Inventory for Parents (CHIP)	McCubbin & Thompson, 1991	Measures coping skills of families where a child has a health condition; greater repertoire of coping skills predicts improved family management
Family Crisis-Oriented Personal Evaluation Scale	McCubbin & Thompson, 1991	Identifies problem-solving and behavioral strategies used in difficult or problem situations
Family's Sense of Coherence Index (FSOC)	McCubbin, Thompson, & McCubbin, 1996	Evaluates degree of connection and loyalty within family unit
Family Index of Resiliency and Adaptation (FIRA-G)	McCubbin & Thompson, 1991	Evaluates flexibility for use of various problem-solving strategies

From *Family Measures: Stress, Coping and Resiliency* (CD-ROM), by H. I. McCubbin, A. Thompson, and M. A. McCubbin, 2003, Madison: University of Wisconsin.

Efforts to adapt will be affected by available family resources. Effective assessment in this area should include review of resources of the individual family members, the family working as a unit, and the community. Resources may be tangible (having a handicapped accessible home) or intangible (such as personality attributes of family members). Desirable and abundant resources facilitate adaptation. The CNS needs to assess existing resources while planning interventions for the acquisition and maintenance of ongoing support needs. Case managers and social workers can be valuable in identifying and procuring resources, such as assistive devices, financial relief, and community support systems. Intangible resources are more difficult to identify but may have significant influence on the level of adaptation. For example, a caregiver who is depressed is likely to have a diminished capacity to meet the demands of the situation regardless of past performance. There are myriad family resource considerations, and the unique constellation of these factors can affect family hardiness and the ability to adapt at any point in time. Family interviews often reveal resources that are operational and those that are lacking in a specific situation. To assist in this process, the Family Inventory of Resources for Management (FIRM) can be useful (see Table 15.1).

Social support is an important and powerful interpersonal resource for family adaptation. Broadly defined, it includes all persons and agencies that may assist the family in coping with the illness. Extended family, personal friends, health care providers, and even government policies can serve as affirming sources of support to families coping with illness conditions. Recent attention and policy statements at the national and international level have legitimized attention to effective pain management for many. A broad network of effective social support promotes family adaptation by enhancing a sense of respect and efficacy on the part of the family as well a sense of being valued in the larger community. Families may openly share social support resources with providers on interview, but additional assessment can be accomplished through administration of specific assessment instruments (see Table 15.1).

The Resiliency Model describes three levels of family appraisal that impact family adaptation. *Level 1* occurs in the adjustment phase and refers to the family's definition of the stressor and it's impact—how they view the illness. *Level 2*, the situational level, requires an assessment of the family's appraisal of their capacity to cope with the challenge—their ability to balance the demands with the strengths and capabilities of the family. These appraisals must be re-evaluated over time and can vacillate from positive to negative depending on the circumstances at the time. Many factors affect the family's assessment of the situation and are capable of altering perceptions. For example, when a family member is initially diagnosed with a myocardial infarction, families may panic, fearing the worst. With successful treatment, family fears may be substantially allayed and optimism (realistic or not) may result. If treatment fails or the member develops heart failure, this appraisal will shift again as the family must adjust to new circumstances and arrive at a revised interpretation of the meaning, demands, and suspected outcomes of the situation. It must be noted that the family's appraisal of the situation may differ significantly among the members and from that of health care providers. Evaluation should focus on the impact of the perception on effective adaptation and what strategies need to be employed to reduce adverse outcomes. Positive appraisals of an illness and the family's ability to manage it will support effective problem solving, coping, and use of resources directed at adaptation. The CNS needs to encourage families to share their thoughts and feelings about the illness and its impact on the family, thus, obtaining data useful in designing interventions to support realistic and constructive appraisals. Even for families dealing with terminal illness, a positive outlook is possible by focusing on interventions such as spending quality time with the member or facilitating a "good death."

Level 3, family schema appraisal—family meaning, requires insight into the meaning the family attaches to the illness and the subsequent family changes. Arriving at a shared family meaning of the illness and its impact on the family system is a complex endeavor requiring time and effort on the part of the family. Most providers have heard families report that the presence of an unexpected stressful event, such as the birth of a handicapped child, "brought the family together." It may even be stated that such cohesiveness would not have otherwise occurred. Accomplishments in this area involve a reappraisal of family values, goals, priorities, rules, and expectations and a realignment of the

perception of the family, its meaning to the members, and even its patterns of functioning resulting from the illness situation. The family's ethnic, religious, and sociocultural background will influence how the family appraises and makes meaning of the situation that they are confronting. The new meaning involves the intense work of altering expectations, reframing previously held views, and arriving at a family schema that is accepted by all members. The CNS is challenged to elicit data from the family that reveals their shared meaning and understanding of their situation. Cultural factors must be accounted for in this process. Data about the family's meaning and understanding of the situation can be used to support development of a positive and constructive view that is congruent with the changed family situation.

The last variable of the model that interacts to influence family adaptation is problem solving and coping. Coping behaviors are defined as efforts of a family member or the family as a whole to reduce or manage a demand on the system. While problem solving is frequently viewed on the individual level, it can operate as a coordinated effort across the family system. A plan can be established so that various members assume complementary functions to accomplish a desired outcome. In a family with a handicapped child, older siblings may assume more household tasks to enable the parents to have quality time with each other and other children in the family. Danielson et al. (1993) noted that coping and problem solving may be directed at: (1) reducing or eliminating stresses and hardships, (2) acquiring additional resources, (3) managing family system tension, and (4) shaping the appraisal at both the situational and the schema level. Having a broad array of problem-solving and coping strategies combined with an open, honest, and effective communication style establishes a positive environment for adaptation. As an adjunct to the clinical interview, the CNS may select an instrument developed to measure family problem-solving and coping skills (see Table 15.1).

The components of the model interact to predict the effect on adaptation outcomes for families managing an illness situation. In *bonadaptation*, family coherence is demonstrated through alignment of family schema and patterns of functioning, appropriate growth and development of members, maintenance of family integrity, and the existence of mutually supportive relationships with the community. For families dealing with chronic illness, this process is ongoing and requires revision as the illness or family situation undergo change. The continuing nature of the adjustment requires the CNS to be vigilant in systematically re-evaluating and addressing emergent family needs. Assessment of the family related to all factors that influence adaptation is imperative. Again, instruments specifically designed to assess family adaptation can be useful (see Table 15.1).

The Resiliency Model integrates a multitude of factors that influence family response to illness events. This explanation is useful in assessing family adjustment and/or adaptation and in designing effective interventions needed to provide assistance to families in their struggle to manage stress and garner appropriate support. Left unaddressed, illness stressors can result in harmful outcomes for patients and their families.

Sphere II: Nursing and Nursing Practice

Formal and informal educational programs for nurses and other health care professionals must be built into the fabric of our health care systems in order to meet the needs of today's diverse families. Formal, ongoing educational programs must include topics such as cultural and religious influences on family responses to a patient's illness, cultural and spiritual needs or concerns of families, family coping styles, the family developmental life cycle, preparing children for visiting their loved one, the prevention and management of crisis, and assessing families for anxiety, depression, and posttraumatic stress disorder (Hughes, Bryan, & Robbins, 2005; Jones et al., 2004). CNSs can provide updates and ongoing attention to these issues for nursing care personnel and students.

CNSs can facilitate staff participation in the development of informational materials for patients and families in hospital or community settings. Print and video materials can assist families with understanding the dimensions of an illness or treatment and provide a realistic perspective upon which to shape their response. In one hospital, a video illustrating a realistic portrayal of a code was made available to families struggling with a resuscitation decision. The CNS viewed the video with family members and facilitated a question-and-answer discussion. This intervention often paved the way for families to engage in decisions with an improved understanding of the implications for the patient.

Children are curious, and in many families it is appropriate for children to visit members in the acute care setting. It is important to prepare children for what they will see and hear in an effort to avoid misinterpretations that may result in enduring traumatic experiences. In preparing children for visiting their loved one, particularly in a critical or intensive care unit, the CNS can provide age-appropriate educational programs. These programs, designed to reduce the fear and anxiety experienced by children, may be one-on-one, pretaped videos, storybooks, or other formats familiar to children. Staff may need to be reminded of the importance of child visitation and also supported with strategies to assist in making it a satisfactory experience for all.

Attitudes toward health, illness, and health care providers are strongly influenced by ethnic factors (Campinha-Bacote, 2003; Friedman, 1992; Herz, 1987;

McGoldrick, 1982). When individuals respond to an illness in a manner that is similar to a member of the health care subculture, they are most often labeled *normal* (Herz). Given the changing demographics in our country, nurses are caring for individuals and families from a broad spectrum of ethnic backgrounds who often respond differently than the expected norm. It has long been known that emotional expressiveness in minority cultures is less valued by the dominant culture (McGoldrick), and families who respond with a great deal of emotion may be judged in a negative way or misunderstood by health care providers. The judgment of health care personnel influences the health care agency's attitude. CNSs can facilitate effective response to families in stressful situations by encouraging an attitude of respect for diversity.

CNSs can assume a pivotal role in interacting with families and educating nursing staff. Ethnic bias can blind one to another's reaction to illness (Friedman, 1992). Because our cultural values and assumptions are usually outside of our awareness and we see the world through our own "cultural filters" (McGoldrick, 1982), assisting the staff, in a gentle way, to explore their own values, beliefs, and assumptions is often a first step. Providing consultation to nurses and educating them about different cultures must be a priority in today's health care systems.

Given the high level of stress that nurses experience at various times during their career, support services for staff must also be an integral part of health care systems today. Staff support is needed to decompress and confront feelings about family members, their reactions and behaviors, or patient care outcomes. In the past, support groups for nurses have often come under the purview of psychiatric CNSs, mainly, the PCLN. However, CNSs in other specialties can also provide support for nurses in a variety of ways. For instance, one of the authors developed a creative approach for supporting and empowering nurses in clinical situations where they had provided care for a patient who was hospitalized for a long period of time. In one situation, the patient's pain and related distress were unable to be totally relieved. Often, the nurses felt inadequate in their inability to provide comfort for this patient. When the patient died, nurses, residents, unit secretaries, family members, nursing assistants, and clergy were brought together around the patient's bed. The purpose of this ritual was to remember the patient but also to provide the opportunity for health care professionals and other staff members to acknowledge each other and all of their efforts. Gathered together over the patient, the surgical resident recalled a time when he had chastised one young nurse for intrusion on his time by calling him in the middle of the night. However, in reflection, the resident was able to acknowledge the importance of the nurse advocating for the patient. This intervention facilitated the grieving process of staff and enabled them to reflect positively on their efforts to provide appropriate care. Perhaps more importantly, this intervention made it possible for the team to reframe the staffs' efforts by acknowledging and validating their actions despite the outcome of death of the patient.

Another avenue for role modeling and educating nursing staff about family needs as well as designing family interventions is regular interdisciplinary patient care conferences. These conferences provide an opportunity for establishing honest, accurate, and understandable information to be communicated to families. Questions and concerns raised by family members can also be addressed individually and collectively. An intervention study conducted in a neonatal ICU reported that using a shared decision-making model in scheduled meetings between health care professionals and patients resulted in less conflict, more accurate knowledge, more realistic parent expectations, and improved provider relationships with families (Penticuff & Arheart, 2005).

The CNS can play an integral role in working with staff to provide knowledge, competence, and confidence for integrating families in patient care to promote quality outcomes. CNSs can also serve the nursing staff by providing expert knowledge and skills for managing difficult and challenging family situations, whether through role modeling, education, or personal support. Clearly, this resource function serves to promote job satisfaction and staff retention. These factors further highlight the value-added service of the CNS in the practice setting.

Sphere III: Organization/System

The CNS must work to advocate for inclusion of the family as a partner in multidisciplinary decision making and care. To accomplish this goal, attention must be focused on broader organizational and societal policies that appropriately incorporate a family focus in health care. Research and leadership skills of the CNS are useful in promoting an environment of care that fosters family involvement and emphasizes family-centered care.

Improving the environment of care for families may necessitate challenges to existing practices. The CNS must become actively involved in evaluating the needs of families and the practices of nurses and other health care providers in working with families. The conduct and dissemination of nursing research on family care is needed to substantiate best practices. Long-standing disputes over access to patients in the institutional setting is a classic exemplar. Notably, restrictive policies related to flexibility in visiting hours, visitation by young children, and even pet visitation policies are being reviewed in many facilities. These practices need to be challenged and revised based on the best

evidence to ensure care that promotes quality patient/family outcomes.

Institutional environments need to consider the needs of families as well. Becoming involved in the creation or redesign of a facility affords the CNS an opportunity to promote areas where families feel welcome and not external to the care setting. While attractive lounge areas are important, providing a private, quiet, and safe space for visitors; ensuring comfortable sitting or sleep accommodations; and access to staff care providers represent more enduring needs. For the most part, these needs have not been adequately addressed and may create artificial barriers to family involvement in care procedures. The CNS is prepared to explore family environmental needs and to implement cost analysis profiles measuring the impact on patient response.

Challenging long-established policies and embedded beliefs may lead to dramatic changes in health care practice. For example, while many health care providers may resist the movement, evidence is mounting that family presence at resuscitation procedures is beneficial. Not only are patients and families expressing a desire to be present (Bassler, 1999), but studies have indicated that with appropriate preparation and support during the event, families reported that witnesses felt comforted that everything was done to save the loved one and that they experienced no greater stress than a control group (Kidby, 2003; Meyers et al., 2000; Robinson, MacKenzie-Ross, Campbell, Egleston, & Prevost, 1998). As families are invited to observe care processes, a reduction in legal actions may be an additional benefit. The CNS needs to be active in pursuing evidence to advocate for best practice agency policy changes that will increase responsiveness to family needs and outcomes and that are supported by financial efficacy.

As the population continues to age, provisions for palliative care are an increasingly relevant concern. Recently, Clinical Practice Guidelines for Quality Care were developed (National Consensus Project for Quality Palliative Care, 2004). Families need to know that their loved one is being treated with respect and that suffering is kept at a minimum. Additionally, families need emotional support and timely, honest information about what to expect in the dying process (Teno et al., 2004). The growing need and evidence guiding the provision of palliative care will impel greater CNS involvement in this important area of practice. Organizations need to be presented with accurate facts that support implementation of conscientious, cost-effective decisions regarding palliative care services.

Finally, nurses can and should influence the development of health policy on the local, state, and federal levels (Reinhard, 2002; White, 2002). CNSs need to advocate for improved agency-to-agency communication.

Policies affecting timely patient/family information that protects confidentiality when moving across the system, such as transfer to another facility or discharge to the home setting, must be established, monitored, and evaluated to ensure continuity of quality care. Public policy impinging on the access to care or stigmatization of patients returning to communities needs attention. HIV/AIDS, escalating antibiotic resistant infections, attention to effective pain management, and potential public health crises, such as the threat of an avian flu epidemic or a bioterriorism attack, are examples of contemporary issues where public education, assistance, and policy decisions have been impacted by the actions of nurses. Additionally, CNSs need to be involved in the development of comprehensive, evidence-based standards of care. Nurses are capable of viewing practice from a variety of perspectives. The CNS can take the lead in representing family inclusion in standards wherever relevant.

To accomplish outcomes in this area, CNSs may choose to serve on hospital committees, community boards, and local, state, or national committees. The ability to conduct or support research studies and to analyze and logically apply research findings to practice is a process where CNSs must use their expertise to advocate for patient/family care. Exercising leadership skills, expert interpersonal communications, and advanced knowledge are essential in influencing policies directed at meeting the needs of patients and families in the face of dynamic changes in the health care system.

SUMMARY

The integration of family care into nursing practice continues to evolve. While other models and theories of family may be equally relevant, the Resiliency Model was selected to provide the CNS with a systematic approach for assessment and development of intervention strategies for families confronting a health care challenge. Examples of methods and instruments useful in obtaining comprehensive assessment leading to effective therapeutic interventions were presented. Provisions for family care across the three spheres of influence of CNS practice were highlighted. The need for CNS leadership in family care requires a continued focus on the development of this practice component.

DISCUSSION QUESTIONS

1. In your professional life, how would the elements of the Resiliency Model have been helpful in preventing personal bias about family responses that might impact nursing care?

2. How would you incorporate the issues related to power and family structure into the Resiliency Model?
3. What family stressors have you confronted in your own practice?
4. What interventions have you employed when working with a challenging family situation? How might a theoretical model help you to design effective new methods?
5. How can the CNS promote collaboration with the total health care team in meeting the challenge of family care in your setting?
6. What evidence-based practice project would be relevant to the enhancement of family care in your nursing specialty?
7. What policy changes can you identify that would promote family involvement and bonadaptation?

DISCUSSION

1. Reflect on your past clinical experiences with a challenging family that stands out in your mind. Identify possible reasons for the difficulty you experienced in delivering family-centered care. Refer to the Resiliency Model, and consider other interventions that you might use in the future with this type of family that might be more successful.
2. Reflect on a current challenge in a family clinical situation. Apply the three levels of influence to analyze how you might have been effective in all three spheres of influence.

SUGGESTED ACTIVITY

Select a movie: for example, *My Big Fat Greek Wedding, Away from Her*

Points to Consider: Observe your responses to different family members as you watch this movie. Identify which family member(s) you would have the most difficulty communicating with and discuss possible reasons for your responses. Discuss methods or interventions you could employ to improve the situation.

REFERENCES

Ahrens, T., Yancey, V., & Kollef, M. (2003). Improving family communication at the end of life: Implications for length of stay in the intensive care unit and resource use. *American Journal of Critical Care, 12*(4), 317–323.

Amundson, M. J. (1989). Family crisis care: A home-based program for child abuse in Hawaii. *Issues in Mental Health Nursing, 10*(3/4), 285–296.

Austrom, M. G., Hartwell, C., Moore, P., Perkins, A., Damush, T., Unverzgagt, F. W., et al. (2006). An integrated model of comprehensive care for people with Alzheimer's disease and their caregivers in a primary setting. *Dementia: The*

International Journal of Social Research and Practice, 5(3), 339–352.

Bassler, P. C. (1999). The impact of education on nurses' beliefs regarding family presence in a resuscitation room. *Journal for Nurses in Staff Development, 15*(3), 126–131.

Brooten, D., Genaro, S., Knapp, H., Jovene, N., Brown, L., & York, R. (2002). Classic article: Functions of the CNS in early discharge and home follow up of very low birthweight infants. *Clinical Nurse Specialist: The Journal for Advanced Practice Nursing Practice, 16*(2), 85–90.

Burbank, P. (2007). Introduction. In P. Burbank (Ed.), *Vulnerable older adults. Health care needs and interventions* (pp. xviii–xxiv). New York: Springer.

Canam, C. (2005). Illuminating the clinical nurse specialist role of advanced practice nursing: A qualitative study. *Canadian Journal of Nursing Leadership, 18*(4), 70–89.

Campinha-Bacote, J. (2003). Guest editorial: Cultural desire: The key to unlocking cultural competence. *Journal of Nursing Education, 42*(6), 239–240.

Coyle, M. A. (2000). Meeting the needs of the family: The role of the specialist nurse in the management of brain death. *Intensive and Critical Care Nursing, 16*(1), 45–50.

Cunningham, M. F., Hanson-Health, C., & Agre, P. (2003). A perioperative nurse liaison program: CNS interventions for cancer patients and their families. *Journal of Nursing Care Quality, 18*(1), 16–21.

Danielson, C. B., Hamel-Bissell, B., & Winstead-Fry, P. (1993). *Families, health, and illness.* St. Louis: Mosby.

Davis, C. (2006). Lending an ear. *Nursing Standard, 20*(22), 20–22.

Elder, J. H. (1986). Behavioral management for families of emotionally handicapped and/or developmentally delayed children. *Issues in Mental Health Nursing, 8*(1), 37–49.

Friedman, M. (1992). *Family nursing. Theory and practice.* Norwalk: Appleton and Lange.

Herz, F. B. (1987). Ethnicity, families and life-threatening illness. In M. Leahey & L. Wright (Eds.), *Families and life-threatening illness* (pp. 232–233). Springhouse, PA: Springhouse Corporation.

Hill, R. (1949). *Families under stress.* New York: Harper & Row.

Hughes, F., Bryan, K., & Robbins, I. (2005). Relatives' experiences of critical care. *Nursing in Critical Care, 10*(1), 23–30.

Institute of Medicine. (2001). *Crossing the quality chasm: A new health system for the 21st century.* Washington, DC: National Academies Press.

Jones, C., Skirrow, P., Griffiths, R. D., Humphris, G., Ingleby, S., Eddleston, J., et al. (2004). Post-traumatic stress disorder-related symptoms in relatives of patients following intensive care. *Intensive Care Medicine, 30*, 456–460.

Kidby, J. (2003). Family witnesses cardiopulmonary resuscitation. *Nursing Standard, 17*, 33–36.

Lasby, K., Newton, S., & Von Platen, A. (2004). Neonatal transitional care. *Canadian Nurse, 100*(8), 18–23.

Lewis, A., & Levy, J. S. (1982). *Psychiatric liaison nursing.* Reston, VA: Reston Publishing Co.

McCubbin, H. I., & Patterson, J. M. (Eds.). (1981). *Systematic assessment of family stress, resources and coping: Tools for research, education and clinical intervention.* St. Paul, MN: Family Social Stress.

McCubbin, H. I., Patterson, J. M., & Glynn, A. (1996). Social support index. In H. McCubbin, A. Thompson, & M. McCubbin (Eds.), *Family assessment: Resiliency, coping, and adaptation—Inventories for research and practice.* Madison: University of Wisconsin.

McCubbin, H. I., & Thompson, A. (1991) *Family assessment inventories for research and practice* (2nd ed.). Madison: University of Wisconsin.

McCubbin, H. I., Thompson, A., & McCubbin, M. (Eds.). (1996). *Family assessment: resiliency, coping and adaptation—Inventories for research and practice.* Madison: University of Wisconsin.

McCubbin, H. I., Thompson, A., & McCubbin, M. (2003). *Family measures: Stress, coping and resiliency* (CD-ROM). Madison: University of Wisconsin.

McCubbin, M., & McCubbin, H. I. (1987). Families coping with illness: The resiliency model of family stress, adjustment and adaptation. In H. McCubbin & A. Thompson (Eds.), *Family assessment inventories for research and practice* (2nd ed., pp. 3–232). Madison: University of Wisconsin.

McCubbin, M., & McCubbin, H. I. (1993). Family coping with illness: The resiliency model of family stress, adjustment and adaptation. In C. Danielson, B. Hamel-Bissell, & P. Windstead-Fry (Eds.), *Families, health, and illness* (pp. 21–63). St. Louis: Mosby.

McGoldrick, M. (1982). Ethnicity and family therapy: An overview. *Ethnicity and family therapy* (pp. 3–30). New York: The Guilford Press.

Meleis, A. (1991). *Theoretical nursing: Development and progress.* Philadelphia: J. B. Lippincott.

Meyers, T. A., Eichhorn, D. J., Guzzette, C. E., Clark, A. P., Klein, J. D., Taliaferro, E., et al. (2000). Family presence during invasive procedures and resuscitation: The experience of family members, nurses, and physicians. *American Journal of Nursing, 100*(2), 32–43.

Mohit, D. (2002). Psychiatric home care and family therapy: A window of opportunity for the psychiatric clinical nurse specialist. *Archives of Psychiatric Nursing, 14*(3), 127–133.

National Association of Clinical Nurse Specialists. (2004). *Statement on clinical nurse specialist practice and education* (2nd ed.). Harrisburg, PA: Author.

National Consensus Project for Quality Palliative Care. (2004). Clinical Practice Guidelines for Quality Palliative Care, Executive Summary. *Journal of Palliative Medicine, 7*(5), 611–627.

Penticuff, J. H., & Arheart, K. L. (2005). Effectiveness of an intervention to improve parent-professional collaboration in neonatal intensive care. *Journal of Perinatal Neonatal Nursing, 19*, 187–202.

Ragaisis, K. M. (1994). Critical incident stress: A family nursing intervention. *Archives of Psychiatric Nursing, 8*(1), 38–43.

Reinhard, S. (2002). State government: 50 paths to policy. In D. Mason, J. Leavitt, & M. Chaffee (Eds.), *Policy and politics in nursing and health care* (pp. 481–513). St. Louis: Saunders.

Robinson, S., MacKenzie-Ross, S., Campbell, H., Egleston, C., & Prevost, A. (1998). Psychological effects of witnessing resuscitation on bereaved relatives. *The Lancet, 3*(52), 614–617.

Ryer, M. B., Snyder, M., Gross, C. R., Savik, K., Perason, V., Krichbaum, K., et al. (2000). Value outcomes: The use of APRN's in long term care facilities. *The Gerontologist, 40*, 654–662.

Skilbeck, F., & Payne, S. (2003). Emotional support and the role of clinical nurse specialists in palliative care. *Journal of Advanced Nursing, 43*(5), 521–530.

Summers, T. M. (1991). Psychosocial support of the burned patient. *Clinical Care Nursing Clinics of North America, 3*(2), 237–244.

Teno, J. M., Clarridge, B. R., Casey, V., Welch, L. C., Wetle, T., Shield, R., et al. (2004). Family perspectives on end-of-life care at the last place of care. *Journal of the American Medical Association, 291*(1), 88–93.

Thornlow, D. K., Auerhahn, C., & Stanley, J. (2006). A necessity not a luxury: Preparing advanced practice nurses to care for older adults. *Journal of Professional Nursing, 22*(2), 116–122.

Vooght, S., & Richardson, A. (1996). Community oncology. A study to explore the role of a community oncology nurse specialist. *European Journal of Cancer Care, 5*(4), 217–224.

Ward-Miller, S. (1996). The psychiatric clinical nurse specialist in the home care setting. *Nursing Clinics of North America, 31*(3), 519–525.

White, K. (2002). The federal government. In D. Mason, J. Leavitt, & M. Chaffee (Eds.), *Policy and politics in nursing and health care* (pp. 515–542). St. Louis: Saunders.

Wright, K., & Myint, A. S. (2003). The colorectal cancer clinical nurse specialist in chemotherapy. *Hospital Medicine, 64*(6), 333–336.

16

Community as Client: Clinical Nurse Specialist Role

Naomi E. Ervin

The specialty of *community health nursing* was titled *public health nursing* until the late 1960s (Freeman, 1970; Sullivan, 1984). Recently, members of the specialty are encouraging a return to this original title to better reflect the focus of the specialty on the community or population. Defined as a synthesis of knowledge from nursing and social and public health sciences (American Public Health Association, 1996), public health nursing may be practiced in any setting. The hallmark of the practice is prevention of illness and injury toward improvement of the health of communities or populations.

In early public health nursing textbooks, the emphasis was on the community (Freeman, 1950). In a later book, Freeman (1970) stated: "The purpose of community health nursing is to further community health through the selective application of nursing and public health measures within the framework of the total community health effort" (p. 31). The focus on the community has been expanded and refined over the decades but remains essentially true to the original focus. This chapter provides an overview of the historical, theoretical, conceptual, and ethical background and foundations of advanced public/community health nursing practice.

HISTORICAL BACKGROUND

In 1948, Esther Lucile Brown issued a report calling for the incorporation of public health nursing and related sciences into collegiate undergraduate curriculums. This recommendation was implemented in 1965, making public health nursing a required component of all undergraduate baccalaureate nursing programs. The implementation of this requirement provided one basis for the development of graduate programs. An additional basis for graduate public/community health nursing programs resulted from the 1967 publication of a Western Interstate Council on Higher Education in Nursing (WICHEN) monograph series, one of which was about community health nursing. These documents provided a theoretical basis for practice through a conceptual framework based on key concepts from theories and practice (Sullivan, 1984).

Early in the development of the specialist level of public health nursing, master's programs were housed in schools of public health long before 1967. The trend to offer master's programs in schools of nursing began in the 1970s with phasing out of public health nursing master's level study in most schools of public health (Ervin, 2007). Because the first programs to prepare clinical nurse specialists (CNSs) began in the 1950s in schools of nursing (National League for Nursing, 1958), public health nursing differed from the larger nursing profession at the inception of the specialty.

During the late 1970s and early 1980s, when public health nurse leaders were concerned about the focus of the specialty, a conference was planned to address the definition and title of the specialty. The Consensus Conference on the Essentials of Public Health Nursing Practice and Education was held in 1984 to define public health nursing and community health nursing and to identify education needed for generalist and specialist practice. The term *community health nurse* was referred to in the consensus document as an umbrella term for any nurse working in the community. A *community health nurse specialist* was defined as "a nurse with at least a master's degree in any area of nursing, such as maternal-child health, psychiatric-mental health or medical-surgical nursing or some sub-specialty of any clinical area" (Consensus Conference, 1985, p. 4). A *public health nurse specialist* is prepared at the graduate level with a focus in the public health sciences. One recommendation from the Consensus Conference was that a certification examination be developed.

The differentiation between community health nursing and public health nursing has not been clearly identified by the profession. The title of the specialty continues to be in flux, as indicated in the introduction. A useful rubric for differentiating the specialty from practice in the community is to use the term *community-based nursing* as nursing in the community and *public/community health nursing* to refer to the specialty. In this chapter, the author uses the term *public/community health nursing* as the title of the specialty that focuses on care of the community or population.

Another step toward realization of a certification examination came with the development of standards of practice. The 1986 American Nurses Association's (ANA) *Standards of Community Health Nursing Practice* delineated differences between the generalist and the specialist. These standards identified the specialist's practice as care of the community. The certification examination for the clinical specialist in public/community health nursing was developed by a committee with representatives from both the ANA and the Public Health Nursing Section of the American Public Health Association. The examination was offered for the first time in October 1990. The original content areas of the certification examination closely approximated the essential content areas identified in the authoritative documents at that time, for example, epidemiology, biostatistics, community assessment and diagnosis, nursing theory, management theory, and research (ANA, 1986; Consensus Conference, 1985; Selby, Riportella-Muller, Quade, Legault, & Salmon, 1990). The committee that developed the original certification examination was chaired by the author of this chapter.

The original standards of practice were revised by representatives of the Quad Council of Public Health Nursing Organizations, which is composed of the ANA, the Association of Community Health Nursing Educators, the Association of State and Territorial Directors of Nursing, and the Public Health Nursing Section of the American Public Health Association (Quad Council, 1999). The 1999 document was deliberately titled public health nursing to more accurately reflect the definition of the specialty that was widely accepted at that time. Review of the 1999 scope and standards document was begun in 2004 with representation from the four member

organizations of the Quad Council. The revised standards were published in 2007 (ANA, 2007). The revised scope and standards statement contains measurement criteria, which are indicators of competent practice, for both generalist and specialist roles.

Public/community health nursing has almost always been defined as care of individuals, families, and communities (ANA, 1986; Freeman, 1950; Gardner, 1926). Care at the population level is paramount in advanced practice. Direct care of individuals and families is included in the scope of practice of the public/community health nurse generalist and specialist (American Nurses Credentialing Center, 2006; Quad Council, 1999).

THEORETICAL AND CONCEPTUAL BACKGROUND

The foundations of advanced practice are in the categories of philosophical, conceptual, and knowledge. A major philosophical framework for practice of the public/community health nurse specialist is social justice (Ervin, 2002a). Complementary to social justice is the field of environmental justice, which focuses on fair treatment of populations under laws, policies, and regulations about the environment (Institute of Medicine [IOM], 1999). Among the major concepts included in advanced community health nursing practice are nursing, public health, primary prevention, health promotion, population focus, community, autonomy, and interdisciplinary practice (Ervin, 2002a). The public health sciences particularly include biostatistics, epidemiology, and environmental health. Theoretical foundations are found in the areas of, but not limited to, health behavior, health promotion, disease and injury prevention, health education, demography, and ecology.

Several models of practice at the advanced level have been developed and are described in the literature. The most prevalent models are community as client (Anderson & McFarlane, 1988), community as partner (Anderson & McFarlane, 2004), Helvie's energy theory (1998), and the Integrative Model for Holistic Community Health Nursing (Laffrey & Kulbok, 1999).

The focus of care is the community or population for the clinical specialist in public/community health nursing. The core processes used at the advanced practice level are community assessment, program planning, program implementation, and program evaluation (Ervin, 2002a). The Public Health Nursing Competencies (Quad Council, 2004), based on the public health competencies developed by the Council on Linkages (Council on Linkages between Academia and Public Health Practice, 2001), provided added clarification for the specialist role. The public health competencies are general and apply to all categories of public health workers. A task group of representatives of the Quad Council, including the author, used the public health competencies to delineate competencies at the levels of staff nurse, specialist, and administrator. The resulting document spells out the level of competencies expected of the CNS in public/community health nursing.

The title *clinical specialist* in public/community health nursing has not been widely adopted by practice settings. An informal review of local health department Web sites revealed little use of the title. Position titles listed were director, consultant, supervisor, coordinator, and public health nurse. More striking is that the term *community health nurse* is used instead of *public health nurse* in some state and local health departments (Ervin, 2007).

Whatever model is employed by advanced practice public/community health nurses, the paradigm of multiple determinants of health remains a constant. Health and disease are outcomes of complex factors referred to as multiple determinants of health (Evans, Barer, & Marmor, 1994). This paradigm is becoming more accepted as scientists discover causes of health and disease previously unknown or understood differently. New knowledge has helped us to understand how the physical environment has a much greater effect on health and disease than we believed in previous centuries. The evidence about the physical environment and its relationship to the human condition is also becoming more accepted (IOM, 1995, 1999).

APPLICATION TO CNS PRACTICE

The National Association of Clinical Nurse Specialists' (NACNS) *Statement on CNS Practice and Education* (2004) is not a natural fit with all aspects of advanced public/community health nursing practice. On one hand, the competencies are worded to be directed primarily at care of individuals, but this section provides interpretation of the patient/client sphere of influence that fits with the community as client. On the other hand, the statement on CNS practice does not contain all aspects of CNS practice that are key to competent advanced public/community health nursing practice. Broad areas that have been omitted are included in this section. Components related to systems and staff education are universally compatible with all specialties of CNS practice.

Patient/Client Sphere of Influence

The major goals of public/community health nursing are to prevent disease and injury and to promote health of communities and populations. These goals contrast with the goal of CNSs in other specialties: "to decrease or prevent symptoms/suffering and improve functioning" (NACNS, 2004, p. 18). CNS services may also be sought by patients or clients to maintain or improve health by modifying risk behaviors and increasing health-promoting lifestyles. One major difference between the goals of community health clinical nurse specialists (CHCNSs) and CNSs in other specialties is the client: the community versus the individual or family.

As emphasized elsewhere in this chapter, the patient/client of the CHCNS is the community or population under the jurisdiction of a CHCNS's responsibility. For example, in a local health department, the CHCNS may be responsible for the residents of a specific county, which could contain a few thousand to a few million residents. The ability to "take care" of thousands of individuals has been questioned. The CHCNS does not take care of each individual but organizes programs, services, collaboratives, and/or partnerships to meet protection, prevention, and health promotion gaps in services not provided by other sectors of the community (IOM, 1988).

Services made available to a community through an agency with CHCNSs are not just in a community but are part of a community. This means that the CHCNS develops outreach activities to take services to people and does not wait until people come to a facility. For example, a community nursing center may hold an immunization day at a local elementary school or Women, Infants, and Children (WIC) program site. WIC is a federal program that provides grants to states for supplemental foods, health care, referrals, and nutrition education for low-income pregnant, breast feeding, and non-breastfeeding postpartum women and to infants and children up to age 5 who are at nutritional risk (Food & Nutrition Service, USDA, n.d.).

The first core competency listed in the NACNS statement is: "Use knowledge of differential illness diagnoses and treatments in comprehensive, holistic assessments of patients within the context of disease, diagnoses, and treatments" (NACNS, 2004, p. 25). The language of disease and treatments is not a good match with the words used to define competencies of CHCNSs. For competent community practice, advanced practice nurses need knowledge of community diagnoses and interventions, which may equate to treatments, at the community and/or population levels, but treatments convey more of a connotation to care of ill individuals.

The basis for developing programs and services is a community assessment. The outcome of such an activity is comparable to the assessment done on an individual patient: a diagnosis. In public/community health nursing, the diagnosis is at the community or population level and is labeled community diagnosis or community health diagnosis (Ervin, 2002a; Muecke, 1984; Neufeld & Harrison, 1990). Diagnoses serve the same purpose at the individual or community level: to provide the focus for identifying the intervention or potential interventions to address the diagnosis or problem.

As with a diagnosis about an individual, identifying the cause of the community diagnosis is a necessary step in order for an appropriate intervention to be determined or developed. Evidence-based interventions are a necessary component of the CHCNS's practice for effectiveness and desired outcomes. Causes of problems or conditions at the community level are numerous. The evidence to determine what is the cause or causes of a specific diagnosis must be obtained after the community assessment process is completed, if not collected during the process. Infant mortality is one example of a problem that has multiple causes, for example, SIDS, low birth weight, birth injury, and congenital anomalies. With the details about the factors related to infant mortality in a specific community, the CHCNS can explore the research about specific interventions to decrease infant mortality. For example, if the leading cause of infant mortality in a specific community is low birth weight, then the risk factors for low birth weight need to be explored. Low birth weight due to poor maternal nutrition may require a much different intervention than low birth weight related to young maternal age.

For CHCNS practice, interventions are embedded in programs or services delivered to an aggregate or community in need of such actions (Ervin, 2002a). For example, if statistics demonstrate a low rate of immunization among specific members of a population or community, the intervention of immunizations must be delivered in a program designed to reach children and adults in need of immunizations. The outreach program must be tailored to reach such members of a community in order to protect not only the specific individuals but also the total community to prevent outbreaks of preventable diseases. Immunizations for adults also decrease costs to society and prevent deaths from preventable illnesses such as pneumonia among adults over the age of 65 years.

Interventions applied to ameliorate community diagnoses may be policy development and enforcement (Public Health Nursing Section, 2001). CHCNSs practice in an interdisciplinary mode in many practice settings, but they may also work with professional organizations to bring about policy changes. Policy development may be at local, state, or national level. One example in which public health nurses have been involved for many years is legislation to prohibit smoking in public places. Other policy areas that require continued attention are access to health care, safety in the community, and surveillance.

Public/community health nursing practice is based on evidence (NACNS, 2004), but evidence-based interventions are not abundant. In a survey of local health departments, a large majority of agencies reported using evidence in practice, but most guidelines were from other public health agencies and not specific to nursing (Ervin, Bell, & Bickes, 2009). The most frequently used model for implementing evidence-based practice in public/community health nursing is the Minnesota model (Public Health Nursing Section, 2001). The model, informally titled the "intervention wheel," integrates three components: the population basis of interventions, three levels of practice (community, systems, individual/family), and 17 public health interventions. *Interventions* are defined as "actions taken by public health nurses on behalf of individuals, families, systems, and communities to improve or protect health status" (Public Health Nursing Section, 2001, p. 1). Each intervention is described, and documentation is provided for the evidence base in the publication.

One example of an intervention employed by advanced practice public/community health nurses is coalition building. The intervention is aimed at promoting and developing alliances among organizations for a common purpose. Through this intervention, linkages are built, problems are solved, and local leadership is enhanced to address health concerns. Steps for coalition building include recruiting members, developing preliminary objectives and activities, convening the coalition, estimating needed resources, selecting a coalition structure, maintaining the coalition, and conducting continuous process and outcome evaluation (Public Health Nursing Section, 2001).

Nurses and Nursing Practice Sphere of Influence

Although the title of clinical specialist is not often used in public/community health nursing practice, the role of nurses with advanced preparation is often directed toward the sphere of influence of nurses and nursing practice. The titles *supervisor, director, coordinator,* and *inservice educator* have position descriptions with components related to this sphere of influence. Assisting public/community health nurses to become more effective is a major part of any public/community health nurse in an advanced role.

A preferred approach to developing the competencies of staff nurses is through the process of coaching (Ervin, 2005). Building on baccalaureate education, the CHCNS provides regular guidance for each nurse to emphasize strengths and focus on improving areas of less strength. The first activity for implementing a clinical coaching process is an assessment of the nurse's strengths and weaknesses. This assessment may be conducted in several ways, but a self-assessment should be part of the process. The CHCNS then schedules regular appointments with the nurse to discuss the assessment and develop objectives and a plan for achieving the objectives.

In public/community health nursing practice, most staff nurses have some preparation in the care of the community, but the CHCNS can make great strides for team strength by working with each nurse individually as well as in group activities. For example, the basis of program planning is a community assessment. Most advanced practice public/community health nurses do not conduct community assessments by themselves; a group effort is generally needed in order to accomplish this task in a timely manner. Furthermore, most staff nurses do not have time in their assignments to gather data and information unless they are given some direction about how to do this efficiently. The CHCNS plans the community assessment with the knowledge of team assignments, strengths, and time constraints for team members.

The evidence base for public/community health nursing comes from a variety of fields, for example, epidemiology, health behavior, and health promotion. Many studies have identified effective interventions for various aggregates of the population. Agencies that base practice on evidence generally have policies, procedures, protocols, and guidelines for nurses' use (Ervin et al., 2009). The organizational approach to evidence-based practice is appropriate because each nurse could not possibly review research and other evidence and develop interventions to meet community needs (Ervin, 2002b).

Several resources are available for nurses to use in practicing from an evidence base. Among those already mentioned is the "intervention wheel" (Public Health Nursing Section, 2001). Also available for nurses' use are books on evidence-based practice (e.g., Brownson, Baker, Leet, & Gillespie, 2003; Melnyk & Fineout-Overholt, 2005), data-based articles about research findings, and research syntheses (e.g., Rice & Stead, 2004). Over 20 years of research supports the effectiveness of home visiting to pregnant, low-income women and their children (Olds, Henderson, Tatelbaum, & Chamberlin, 1986; Olds & Kitzman, 1990; Olds et al., 1997). CHCNSs locate resources about evidence-based practice so that the evidence base for practice is readily available in each agency.

In addition to the evidence base for practice in specific agencies, CHCNSs engage in life-long learning to maintain and enhance competence (NACNS, 2004). Membership in professional organizations is one approach for accomplishing this goal. Several organizations provide opportunities for learning as well as leadership involvement. In addition to the NACNS and the ANA, associations specific to public/community health nursing are the Public Health Nursing Section of the American Public Health Association, the Association of Community Health Nursing Educators (ACHNE), and the Association of State and Territorial Directors of Nursing (ASTDN).

Organization/System Sphere of Influence

Advanced practice public/community health nurses often hold positions that require them to have influence and control of organization or system activities, such as director of a community nursing center or director of public health nursing. Such positions of authority permit nurses to have more control over practice as well as the development of policies that support quality community care. However, many official agencies, such as local and state health departments, function within structures and policies determined outside the influence of the nursing department or service area (Turnock, 2004). For example, state regulations may dictate the perimeters of health department functions as well as the qualifications of directors of public/community health nursing at the local level. Some states require that local health departments meet accreditation criteria that may have been developed without nursing representation. In public health, advanced practice nurses may gain more influence in the organization/system sphere by serving on state boards of health, holding policy positions in the offices of state legislators and national congresspersons, and gaining appointment to state regulatory agencies.

One of the greatest constraints for practice in public official agencies often is the lack of funding for activities to benefit the community-at-large. Because most funding for official public health agencies comes from taxes, local voters often decide the fate of funding. Funding for local official agencies is also derived from state and federal funding, both of which are, in turn, derived from taxes. Advanced public/community health nurses are also involved in writing grants to generate funding.

For community nursing centers, the issue of sustainability is paramount as a focus for the CHCNS who establishes and practices in such a center (Glick & Kulbok, 2002; Krothe, 2002; Murphy, 1995). Revenue generated from third-party reimbursement is the second largest stream of revenue for CHCNS services. Because much of the focus for these services is prevention, reimbursement may not be abundantly available. Often, too, the population who needs prevention services is not insured or is underinsured.

EVALUATION

The basis for evaluation of the effectiveness of interventions by the CHCNS is the evaluation plan, which is developed as part of the program planning process. The evaluation plan puts forth explicit measurable outcomes. Some of the outcomes may be at the individual, family, group, aggregate, or community level. At times, outcomes may be identified at more than one level because of the type of intervention. For example, a smoking cessation program for pregnant women may track the smoking cessation level in specific sessions attended by the women but also track the percentage of women who reported smoking during pregnancy by reviewing birth certificates. Each outcome measure is important to monitor the success of a long-term community program.

In evaluating the impact of interventions of the CNS in public/community health nursing, the ideal measures are those at the community or population level. Some common measures of population health include mortality, morbidity, infant mortality, and immunization levels (Valanis, 1999). However, these indicators of health at the community level are difficult to attribute to the actions of CHCNSs or to any one organization in the community, such as the local health department.

Program planning by the CHCNS provides a mechanism for the specialist to develop realistic measures of success for specific programs. The programs may be provided through local health departments or any other community-focused organization, such as a community nursing center, visiting nurse association, or community health center. Rather than measure outcomes for the total community, the CHCNS must develop outcome measures for the target population or community segment identified as in need of the service or intervention.

In order to determine if an intervention had an effect, the CHCNS must gather baseline data about the target population before the intervention is implemented. For example, the immunization level of 2 year olds in a specific targeted geographical community was identified at 29% by the local health department. The CHCNS identified that the immunization level of 2-year-old children attending the community nursing center was also 29%. If resources allow for a program to reach all 2-year-old children in the community, the follow-up evaluation would need to survey all children in that community. The resources to conduct this type of intervention and evaluation are rarely available to community nursing centers. However, through chart audits, the nursing staff could identify the immunization levels of children who attended the nursing center. If children did not return to complete an immunization series, the CHCNS would need to include a portion of the intervention that called for follow-up by phone, e-mail, mailed reminder notices, home visits, or a combination of these methods for reaching parents.

One example of a project to improve outcomes was coordinated by the author working with a home health care agency. The program focused on improving outcomes for patients with heart failure. Patients who had home visits after the inservice education program for the nursing staff improved in several outcomes, including fewer hospitalizations, improved medication adherence, and more exercise (Ervin, Scrivener, & Simons, 2004).

Working with low-income communities is often the focus of CHCNSs. Examples of the outcomes focused upon in these communities are increasing the immunization levels of targeted groups such as homeless children, prevention and early detection and treatment of lead poisoning, and preventing low birth weight infants (Ervin, Nelson, & Sheaff, 1999). Other examples of improvements in a community's health can be seen in the work done by community nursing centers to provide care in low-income communities in various parts of the country. Numerous examples demonstrate that advanced practice nurses are among the vanguards in recognizing that barriers to health care create inequities that will not be solved by the government anytime soon (IOM, 2003; Murphy, 1995).

ADVANCED NURSING PRACTICE

Focus on the population or community for public/community health nursing practice is applicable at both the generalist and specialist levels. However, the specialist level encompasses the total spectrum of practice activities in providing leadership to nurses who practice at the generalist level. Knowledge and skills required to fulfill the specialist role are acquired at the master's or doctoral level. Baccalaureate nursing education provides the foundation for graduate study.

Interventions to address community or population issues are based on a broad array of knowledge about biostatistics, epidemiology, demography, health behavior, environmental health, and health policy, as well as advanced nursing knowledge. The CHCNS is qualified to develop or adapt interventions and plan programs needed to implement the interventions. Generalist public/community health nurses are members of teams to implement the interventions. The scope and standards of practice delineate the criteria for both the generalist and specialist levels of practice (ANA, 2007).

Although the scope of practice for the generalist and specialist is a continuum, the public/community health nursing generalist in some agencies may provide care to individuals and families more than to total communities and populations. In order to maintain or enhance the health of a community, often interventions are carried out at the individual level, such as immunizations. Care at the individual level is not a negation of the community focus but part of the total scope of practice needed to achieve healthy communities.

ETHICAL CONSIDERATIONS

Advanced practice public/community health nurses embrace the code of ethics that applies to all nurses. The code of ethics makes reference to individuals as patients and specifically lists the community as a patient in the second edition (ANA, 2001). As outlined earlier, a major philosophical foundation and ethical orientation for advanced public/community health nursing practice is social justice. The original focus of public health nursing was care of indigent families, especially in the major cities of the United States (Sullivan, 1984). Even though public health nursing services were expanded to the total population in the early 20th century, the ethical ideals of the specialty have persisted.

Social justice calls for equal entitlement of all persons to basic aspects of a healthy life, such as health protection and minimum standards of income. This approach requires that the total society protects the public's health versus the idea that the individual's lifestyle needs remediation (Beauchamp, 1999; Fry, 1985). Societal protection of health is mandatory if societies are to prosper because individuals cannot provide the infrastructure to support small and large communities for items such as clean air and water.

The greatest advancements in health have been made through public health measures such as control of communicable diseases and regulation of air, water, sewage treatment, and food quality. These and other public health measures have contributed greatly to the 30-year increase in the life span in the 20th century (Brownson et al., 2003). Without an investment in the public health approach that the public's right to safe water, air, food, and environment is greater than the market approach (Shi & Singh, 2003), the United States would not have as high a standard of living as it now enjoys. If individuals purchased what each could afford, millions of individuals and families would live in squalor. The U.S. society is not without inequities (Ervin & Bell, 2004), but society has made strides toward improving the environment and standard of living for millions of citizens and residents.

Advanced public/community health nurses are committed to achieving the *Healthy People 2010* objectives, which are focused on eliminating health disparities and increasing the quality and years of healthy life for Americans (U.S. Department of Health and Human Services, 2000). Achieving the objectives is in part dependent upon access to health services. CHCNSs work toward improving access to services through various interventions, for example, developing community nursing centers, promoting equity in access to services, and improving health care coverage through legislation. Assessing access to health services includes ethical questions about who has access and why (Bambas & Casas, 2003). Note that access to medical care is not the total answer to eliminating disparities. Health services include a broad range of care that encompasses mental health, nutrition, and nursing. Because most health insurance coverage is for medical care, communities and individuals are often without preventive and early

detection services that could decrease the burden of disease and injury in low-income populations.

DISCUSSION QUESTIONS

1. What advanced public/community health nursing practice conceptual frameworks are commonly found in the literature? Describe one of them.
2. How has society influenced the development of advanced public/community health nursing practice?
3. How do public/community health nursing and community-based nursing differ?
4. What place does social justice have in advanced public/community health nursing practice?
5. How does the code of ethics for nurses compare with the social justice orientation?

ANALYSIS AND SYNTHESIS EXERCISES

1. For a specific geographical community, locate vital statistics about the population and compare and contrast with the state and national vital statistics for the same time period.
2. Gather data about the leading causes of death for a specific geographical community, and formulate one community diagnosis. Use comparisons with the state and U.S. statistics.
3. Locate environmental standards for air and water quality. Analyze the data about air and water quality for a specific community using the standards.
4. Identify the location of toxic sites in a specific geographical community. Compare morbidity and mortality data for the populations who live near these sites with state and national morbidity and mortality data for selected conditions, for example, asthma, cancer, or premature births.

CLINICAL APPLICATIONS

1. Interview three key leaders of a specific community to gain their perspectives of the leading community problems.
2. Identify the three leading health problems or potential problems in a given community.
3. Compare the three leading health problems identified for a specific community with the focus of the major health care providers in the community.

REFERENCES

American Nurses Association. (2001). *Code of ethics for nurses with interpretive statements*. Washington, DC: American Nurses Publishing.

American Nurses Association, Council of Community Health Nurses. (1986). *Standards of community health nursing practice*. Kansas City, MO: Author.

American Nurses Association. (2007). *Public health nursing: Scope and standards of practice*. Silver Spring, MD: Author.

American Nurses Credentialing Center. (2006). *Clinical nurse specialist in public/community health nursing certification*. Retrieved January 22, 2007, from http://www.nursingworld. org/ancc/cert/eligibility/CNS_CommHealth.html

American Public Health Association, Public Health Nursing Section. (1996). *Definition and role of public health nursing*. Washington, DC: Author.

Anderson, E. T., & McFarlane, J. M. (1988). *Community as client: Application of the nursing process*. Philadelphia: Lippincott.

Anderson, E. T., & McFarlane, J. M. (2004). *Community as partner: Theory and practice in nursing* (4th ed.). Philadelphia: Lippincott.

Bambas, A., & Casas, J. A. (2003). Assessing equity in health: Conceptual criteria. In R. Hofrichter (Ed.), *Health and social justice: Politics, ideology, and inequity in the distribution of disease* (pp. 321–334). San Francisco, CA: Jossey-Bass.

Beauchamp, D. E. (1999). Public health as social justice. In D. E. Beauchamp & B. Steinbock (Eds.), *New ethics for the public's health* (pp. 101–109). New York: Oxford University Press.

Brown, E. L. (1948). *Nursing for the future*. New York: Russell Sage Foundation.

Brownson, R. C., Baker, E. A., Leet, T. L., & Gillespie, K. N. (2003). *Evidence-based public health*. New York: Oxford University Press.

Council on Linkages Between Academia and Public Health Practice. (2001). *Core competencies for public health professionals*. Washington, DC: Public Health Foundation/Health Resources and Services Administration.

Ervin, N. E. (2002a). *Advanced community health nursing practice: Population-focused care*. Upper Saddle River, NJ: Prentice Hall.

Ervin, N. E. (2002b). Evidence-based nursing practice: Are we there yet? *Journal of the New York State Nurses Association, 33*(2), 11–16.

Ervin, N. E. (2005). Clinical coaching: A strategy for enhancing evidence-based nursing practice. *Clinical Nurse Specialist, 19*(6), 296–301.

Ervin, N. E. (2007). Clinical specialist in community health nursing: Advanced practice fit or misfit? *Public Health Nursing, 24*(5), 458–464.

Ervin, N. E., & Bell, S. E. (2004). Social justice issues related to uneven distribution of resources. *Journal of the New York State Nurses Association, 35*(1), 8–13.

Ervin, N. E., Bell, S. E., & Bickes, J. T. (2009). Evidence-based nursing practice in local public health. *Michigan Journal of Public Health, 3*(1), 33–46.

Ervin, N. E., Nelson, L. L., & Sheaff, L. (1999). Preventing adverse outcomes: A population focus. *Journal of Nursing Care Quality, 13*(6), 25–31.

Ervin, N. E., Scrivener, K., & Simons, T. (2004). Using the linkage model for integrating evidence into nursing practice. *Home Healthcare Nurse, 22*(9), 606–611.

Evans, R. G., Barer, M. L., & Marmor, T. R. (Eds.). (1994). *Why are some people healthy and others not?* New York: Aldine de Gruyter.

Food & Nutrition Service, U.S. Department of Agriculture. (n.d.). *Woman, infants, and children*. Retrieved September 10, 2007, from http://www.fns.usda.gov/wic/

Freeman, R. B. (1950). *Public health nursing*. Philadelphia: Saunders.

Freeman, R. B. (1970). *Community health nursing practice*. Philadelphia: Saunders.

Fry, S. T. (1985). Individual vs. aggregate good: Ethical tension in nursing practice. *International Journal of Nursing Studies, 22*(4), 303–310.

Gardner, M. S. (1926). *Public health nursing* (2nd ed.). New York: Macmillan.

Glick, D. F., & Kulbok, P. A. (2002). Revising programs. In N. E. Ervin, *Advanced community health nursing practice: Population-focused care* (pp. 451–462). Upper Saddle River, NJ: Prentice Hall.

Helvie, C. O. (1998). *Advanced practice nursing in the community*. Thousand Oaks, CA: Sage.

Institute of Medicine. (1988). *The future of public health*. Washington, DC: National Academies Press.

Institute of Medicine. (1995). *Nursing, health, & the environment*. Washington, DC: National Academies Press.

Institute of Medicine. (1999). *Toward environmental justice*. Washington, DC: National Academies Press.

Institute of Medicine. (2003). *Unequal treatment: Confronting racial and ethnic disparities in healthcare*. Washington, DC: National Academies Press.

Krothe, J. S. (2002). Monitoring program implementation. In N. E. Ervin, *Advanced community health nursing practice: Population-focused care* (pp. 349–369). Upper Saddle River, NJ: Prentice Hall.

Laffrey, S. C., & Kulbok, P. A. (1999). An integrative model for holistic community health nursing. *Journal of Holistic Nursing, 17*(1), 88–103.

Melnyk, B. M., & Fineout-Overholt, E. (2005). *Evidence-based practice in nursing & healthcare: A guide to best practice*. Philadelphia: Lippincott.

Muecke, M. A. (1984). Community health diagnoses in nursing. *Public Health Nursing, 1*(1), 23–25.

Murphy, M. (Ed.). (1995). *Nursing centers: The time is now*. New York: National League for Nursing Press.

National Association of Clinical Nurse Specialists. (2004). *Statement on clinical nurse specialist practice and education* (2nd ed.). Harrisburg, PA: Author.

National League for Nursing. (1958). *The educational preparation of the clinical nurse specialist in psychiatric nursing*. New York: Author.

Neufeld, A., & Harrison, M. J. (1990). The development of nursing diagnoses for aggregates and groups. *Public Health Nursing, 7*, 251–255.

Olds, D. L., Eckenrode, J., Henderson, C. R., Jr., Kitzman, H., Powers, J., Cole, R., et al. (1997). Long-term effects of home visitation on maternal life course and child abuse and neglect. Fifteen-year follow-up of a randomized trial. *Journal of the American Medical Association, 278*(8), 637–643.

Olds, D. L., Henderson, C. R., Jr., Tatelbaum, R., & Chamberlin, R. (1986). Improving the delivery of prenatal care and outcomes of pregnancy: A randomized trial of nurse home visitation. *Pediatrics, 77*(1), 16–28.

Olds, D. L., & Kitzman, H. (1990). Can home visitation improve the health of women and children at environmental risk? *Pediatrics, 86*(1), 108–116.

Public Health Nursing Section. (2001). *Public health interventions: Applications for public health nursing practice*. St. Paul: Minnesota Department of Health.

Quad Council of Public Health Nursing Organizations. (1999). *Scope and standards of public health nursing practice*. Washington, DC: American Nurses Publishing.

Quad Council of Public Health Nursing Organizations. (2004). Public health nursing competencies. *Public Health Nursing, 21*(5), 443–452.

Rice, V. H., & Stead, L. F. (2004). Nursing interventions for smoking cessation. *Cochrane Database Systematic Reviews, 1,* CD001188.

Selby, M. L., Riportella-Muller, R., Quade, D., Legault, C., & Salmon, M. E. (1990). Core curriculum for master's community health nursing education: A comparison of the views of leaders in service and education. *Public Health Nursing, 7*(3), 150–160.

Shi, L., & Singh, D. A. (2003). *Delivering health care in America* (3rd ed.). Gaithersburg, MD: Aspen.

Sullivan, J. A. (Ed.). (1984). *Directions in community health nursing.* Boston: Blackwell.

Turnock, B. J. (2004). *Public health: What it is and how it works* (3rd ed.). Boston: Jones and Bartlett.

U.S. Department of Health and Human Services. (1985). *Consensus conference on essentials of public health and nursing practice and education.* Rockville, MD: U.S. Department of Health and Human Services, Bureau of Health Professions, Division of Nursing.

U.S. Department of Health and Human Services. (2000). *Healthy people 2010.* Washington, DC: U.S. Government Printing Office.

Valanis, B. (1999). *Epidemiology in health care* (3rd ed.). Stamford, CT: Appleton & Lange.

Population-Based Data Analysis

Ann L. Cupp Curley

There is increasing awareness among health care professionals of the importance of population-based care. Problems are defined (diagnoses) and solutions proposed (interventions) for defined populations or subpopulations. While clinical decision making related to individual patients is important, it has little impact on overall health outcomes for populations. Population strategies have the potential to change norms. Clinical nurse specialists (CNSs) are in the unique position of being educated to provide evidence-based care to specialty populations (Nelson, Holland, Derscheid, & Tucker, 2007). These populations may be defined by the demographic characteristics of the population, the setting or environment, the type of care required, or the diagnosis (National Association of Clinical Nurse Specialists [NACNS], 2004). Evidence-based practice (EBP) as it relates to public health seeks to bring clinical practice and public health together through the use of population health sciences in clinical practice (Heller & Page, 2002). The focus of population-based care is on populations at risk, comparison groups, and demographic factors. It is concerned with the patterns of delivery of care and outcomes measurement at the population or subpopulation level.

How can we improve the quality of care for our patients by taking a population-based care approach? If we altered how we define our population, how would the care we provide differ, and who would benefit from this difference? What would be the cost benefit of changing how we provide individual care based on a deeper understanding of population health needs? These are questions that the CNS encounters in everyday practice. Successful CNS practice depends on the ability to recognize the difference between the individual and population approaches to the collection and use of data

and the ability to assess needs and evaluate outcomes at the population level. This chapter provides the CNS with the tools to be able to follow a critical chain of evidence and avoid the pitfalls of faulty inference in population analysis.

BACKGROUND

The historical evolution of epidemiology and public health provides a background for an understanding of the population approach to patient care. The publication of Farr's "Vital statistics" in J. R. McCullach's *A Statistical Account of the British Empire* in 1837 laid the foundation for the use of vital statistics in public health. Up until the 19th century, appeals for public health reform were based on subjective observations and were dependent on emotional appeal. Vital statistics supplied public health reformers with objective data and the ability to support their requests for reform with facts and figures. For example, using information that he gathered on cholera victims, Snow compared the incidence rates for cholera in one water district with those in another to support his hypothesis that cholera resulted from the contamination of water supplies. Perhaps one of the earliest documented examples of EBP occurred in 1854 when the handle of the contaminated well in London was removed, resulting in a sharp decrease in the incidence rate for cholera and the end of an epidemic.

Florence Nightingale was educated in arithmetic, geometry, and algebra. During the Crimean War, she used statistical analysis to plot the incidence of preventable deaths among British soldiers. She created a diagram to dramatize the unnecessary deaths caused by unsanitary conditions and the need for reform. After the Crimean War, Nightingale worked with Farr to standardize data collection and classification in hospitals. This work led to the development of her Model Hospital Forms. She used the standardized data to support her crusade for hospital reform, especially improvements in sanitation (Dossey, 2000). With her analysis, Florence Nightingale revolutionized the idea that social phenomena could be objectively measured and subjected to mathematical analysis. She was one of the earliest health care practitioners to collect and analyze data in order to persuade people of the need for change. Her work in medical statistics led to her election in 1858 to the Statistical Society of England (Dossey, 2000; Lipsey, 2006).

Since Farr and Nightingale, the use of statistics in public health has expanded and become more sophisticated. Statistics are now used to explain the linkages between many different variables and health and disease. The Framingham Heart Study is one of the most important population studies ever carried out in the United States and provides an example of how the methods pioneered by early practitioners such as Farr and Nightingale can be effectively employed. Established in 1948 and still in operation, it has generated over 1,000 scientific papers to date. Before Framingham, most health care providers believed that atherosclerosis was an inevitable part of the aging process and that blood pressure was supposed to increase with age. The idea that individuals could modify risk factors (a term coined by the study) tied to heart disease, stroke, and other diseases did not exist until then, and this is one of the key findings of this study (National Heart, Lung and Blood Institute [NHLBI] & Boston University, 2007).

The Nurses Health Study was established in 1976 with funding from the National Institutes of Health (NHI). The primary goal was to investigate the potential long-term consequences of the use of oral contraceptives, but the goal has since expanded to include the investigation of other diseases and conditions. Every 2 years cohort members receive a questionnaire about diseases and health-related topics, including smoking, hormone use, and menopausal status. It has also expanded to include investigations into the risk factors for major chronic diseases in women. The Nurses Health Study has made many contributions to the understanding of women's health. It was through this study that it was discovered that women who used estrogen plus testosterone to reduce postmenopausal symptoms were about twice as likely to develop breast cancer as women who had never used postmenopausal hormones.

A point of interest is that nurses were originally chosen for the study because investigators believed that nurses would be highly likely to respond to the surveys and not drop out of the study. This has proven true, as response rates have been consistently high and the mortality rate due to participant drop out is low (Department of Health and Human Services, NHI, & NHLBI, 2007).

The work of Farr, Snow, Nightingale, and others laid the foundation of today's studies; however, statistics must be used with caution. Health is a multidimensional variable—factors that affect health, and that interact to affect health, are numerous. Many relationships are possible. There are problems inherent in the use of statistics to explain differences between groups. Although statistics can *describe* disparities, they cannot *explain* them. It is left to the researchers to explain the *differences*. In addition to the problem of using statistics to explain differences, one must also be aware of the validity and reliability of the data. There are problems associated with the categorizing and gathering of statistics during the research process that can have an effect on how the data should be interpreted. In order to formulate change, one must do more than just collect data—one must look at the theoretical issues associated with explaining the relationship between the variables. Practice must clearly indicate a commitment to high standards for research with an emphasis placed on adherence to careful and thorough procedure and ethical practice.

ISSUES IN POPULATION-BASED ANALYSIS

Population strategies are used to identify populations at risk and to evaluate interventions at the population level that have a far-reaching effect. When evaluating data at the population level, it is important to avoid ecologic fallacy. An ecologic fallacy occurs when an observed association in a population is assumed to exist on an individual level. For example, higher rates of falls are seen in elderly populations than in younger populations. Polypharmacy also occurs at higher rates in elderly populations, and we might be tempted to believe that polypharmacy is responsible for the higher rates of falls. However, we cannot conclude that whenever an elderly individual falls it is due to polypharmacy. Population-based evaluation and planning depend on understanding the many and varied factors that influence health and disease. Statistics alone cannot explain relationships between variables or differences among groups. The CNS should emphasize the use of sound investigative principles and a broad theoretical perspective to interpret the results. When a clinical problem is identified, one of the next steps is a systematic review of the literature to discover what is already known about the issue.

Another potential difficulty in population research is that indirect associations can appear causal. An indirect relationship occurs when a factor and an attribute seem to be related only because of some underlying common condition. A classic example occurred when Farr detected an inverse relationship between cholera and altitude. This finding seemed to support the then commonly held belief that cholera was caused by bad air or *miasmas*. In fact, cholera deaths occurred more frequently at low-lying altitudes because the water was less pure in these areas. When a factor appears to be causally linked to a health problem, additional studies and further scrutiny are warranted in order to rule out alternative explanations.

PRINCIPLES OF POPULATION-BASED ANALYSIS

The five basic principles of the population approach to care described by Ibrahim, Savitz, Carey, and Wagner (2001) provide a framework for the CNS in the area of population-based evaluation. These principles include the following: a community perspective, a clinical epidemiology perspective, EBP, an emphasis on prevention, and an emphasis on outcomes.

The *community perspective* refers to the collection of data related to the frequency of disease, disability, and death in a population and the number of people in the population of interest. This information allows the CNS to calculate rates. The evaluation of outcome measures in populations begins with an identification of the totality of health problems, the needs of defined populations, and the differences among groups. The rates calculated from these numbers can help the CNS target populations at risk and supply the evidence for changes in clinical practice.

The *clinical epidemiology perspective* refers to the need to manage all patients with similar needs or problems—congestive heart failure patients, for example, or dependent elderly people being cared for at home. The care of specialized groups is the core of CNS practice.

Evidence-based practice (EBP) is a principle of population-based health care and one of the core competencies of CNS and basic nursing practice (American Nurses Association [ANA], 2004; NACNS, 2004). EBP is defined as the conscientious integration of best research evidence with clinical expertise and patient values and needs in the delivery of quality, cost-effective health care (Burns & Grove, 2005). The basic sciences of public health (particularly epidemiology and biostatistics) provide tools for the CNS working with specialized populations to provide evidence for effective interventions.

Prevention can also best be carried out at the population level. For example, a falls prevention program within a hospital can lead to decreased injuries and related costs. Interventions that are appropriate at the

individual level and applied at the population level can result in a far-reaching effect.

Outcomes measurement refers to collecting and analyzing data using predetermined outcomes indicators for the purposes of making decisions about health care (ANA, 2007). Outcomes research in CNS practice is research that focuses on the effectiveness of nursing interventions. Outcomes measurement in population-based care begins with the identification of the population and the problem, followed by the generation of a clinical question related to outcomes. An outcomes measure should be clearly quantifiable, should be relatively easy to define and diagnose, and should lend itself to standardization.

In outcomes measurement, the CNS is ultimately concerned with whether or not a population benefits from an intervention (care). The CNS also needs to be concerned with the question of efficacy (does the intervention work under ideal conditions?) and effectiveness (does it work under real life situations?). Other important considerations are efficiency (cost-benefit), affordability, accessibility, and acceptability.

Four general types of outcomes provide a comprehensive model for outcomes measurement. They are: functional outcomes (such as the ability to perform ADLs), cost outcomes (cost of care), clinical outcomes (such as pain management) and satisfaction outcomes (such as family satisfaction with patient care), according to Oermann and Floyd (2002).

POPULATION-BASED ANALYSIS FOR CNS PRACTICE

Methods derived from epidemiology can be used to: identify the etiology or the cause of a disease and the risk factors, identify the impact of risk factors in a population, determine the extent of a disease and/or adverse events found in a population, evaluate both existing and new preventative and therapeutic measures and modes of health care delivery, and provide the foundation for developing public policy and making regulatory decisions.

Descriptive Epidemiology

Descriptive epidemiology is used to describe the distribution of disease and other health-related states and events in terms of personal characteristics, geographical distribution, and time. There are four types of descriptive studies: case reports, case series, correlation studies, and cross-sectional surveys. This chapter will focus on the use of correlation studies and cross-sectional surveys in population analyses. The data used in descriptive studies is often readily available—from hospital records, census data, or vital statistics records.

Correlation Studies

Correlation studies are also referred to as ecologic studies. Ecologic studies are used to conduct studies of group or population characteristics. In ecologic studies, rates are calculated for characteristics that describe populations and used to compare frequencies between different groups at the same time or the same group at different times. They are useful for identifying long-term trends, seasonal patterns, and event-related clusters. Because data are collected on populations instead of individuals, an event cannot be linked to an exposure in individuals, and the investigator cannot control for the effect of other variables (confounders). A confounder is a variable that is linked to both a causative factor and the outcome. A good example of the effect that a confounder can have is provided in Gordis (2004). He describes a study that seemed to link coffee consumption with pancreatic cancer. Later investigation revealed that coffee consumption is closely related to cigarette smoking. In this particular case, coffee consumption served as a confounder.

A study by Babones (2008) provides an illustration of a correlational study. The author used data from the *World Institute for Development Economics Research* to investigate the relationship between inequality and three population health outcomes (life expectancy, infant mortality, and murder rate) in more than 100 countries. The results of these analyses indicate that income inequality correlates negatively with population health. That is, populations in poorer countries experience poorer health, and populations in wealthier countries experience better health. The author points out that, "the existence of a correlation between income inequality and population health does not, in itself, imply a causal relationship between the two variables" (p. 1623). These data indicate a relationship between the variables—but not a causal one. There are many possible explanations for the relationship, including (but not exclusively) cultural and social differences among the countries.

Cross-Sectional Studies

In cross-sectional studies, both exposure to a factor and an outcome are determined simultaneously. They provide a "snap shot" at one point in time. One problem with cross-sectional studies is that the investigator is studying prevalent cases only—not new cases—and the cases may not be representative. They exclude people who have died, and temporal relationships are difficult to determine. Cross-sectional studies can be used to suggest possible risk factors and to identify prevalence rates, but they are not useful for evaluating interventions.

Mosack and Shore (2006) conducted a cross-sectional study to examine the screening of depression among pregnant and postpartum participants in a community-based program. They used archival data from 98 women participating in a community-based visiting nurse program. Depression screening was conducted using two instruments, the Center for Epidemiologic Studies Depression scale (CES-D) and the Edinburgh Postnatal Depression scale. Based on available prevalence rates, both screening instruments identified more women as depressed than anticipated. The authors point out that the two instruments that were used are both screening tools—not diagnostic instruments—therefore, "the results were not entirely unexpected." However, the findings still led the authors to conclude that it is important to screen pregnant and postpartum women.

This study serves to illustrate both the advantages and the disadvantages of cross-sectional studies. Because the women were screened just once, the study missed any women who were previously depressed but not depressed at the time of the study and any women who became depressed after the data were collected. On the other hand, a cross-sectional study is fairly quick and can be used to identify prevalence rates for specified populations—as this one did.

Rates

Knowledge of the distribution of illness and injury within a population can provide valuable information on etiology and can lay the foundation for the introduction of new interventions. Rates are a useful method of measuring attributes, illness, and injury in a specific population, and they can also be used to evaluate outcomes. Both low and high rates can provide useful information for the CNS.

The *Data and Trends Reports* published by the Centers for Disease Control (CDC) provide an example of how rates can be used to identify trends and provide policy makers with information for designating resources. The CDC surveys the incidence and prevalence of many diseases and conditions. These figures provide health care workers and policy makers with information on the risks and burden of various diseases and conditions. For example, the *Diabetes Data & Trends* report (CDC, 2007) reveals that the rate of newly diagnosed cases of diabetes in people ages 18 to 44 in the United States has increased from 1.7 per thousand in 1980, to 2.0 per thousand in 1990, to 2.7 per thousand in 2000, and to 3.4 per thousand in 2005.

In rates, the numerator is the number of events that occur during a specified period of time, and the denominator is the average population of interest during that time period. The numerator is divided by the denominator, then this number is multiplied by a constant—either 100, 1,000, 10,000, or 100,000—and is expressed as per that number. Simply put, the rate is calculated as follows:

Rate = Numerator/Denominator x Constant Multiplier

In order to calculate rates, the CNS must first have a clear and explicit definition of the patient population and of the event. For a rate to make sense, anyone represented in the denominator must have the potential to enter the group in the numerator.

Rates can be either crude or specific. Crude rates apply to an entire population without any reference to any characteristics of the individuals in it. Crude mortality rate is an example. To calculate crude mortality, the numerator is all deaths during a specific period of time. The denominator is the number of people in the population of interest. Typically, the population number that is used is the population at midyear.

Specific rates can also be calculated. Specific rates are calculated after a population has been categorized into groups. Let us suppose that a CNS wants to calculate the yearly fall rate for patients 65 years of age and older who are on a particular unit. The formula would be as follows:

Total number of falls of patients 65 years of age and older during the specified year (numerator) divided by total number of patient days of patients 65 years of age and older for that unit during the year (denominator) X 100 = rate per 100.

In order to compare rates in two or more groups, the events in the numerator must be defined in the same way, the time intervals must be the same, and the constant multiplier must be the same. Rates can be used to compare two different groups or one group during two different time periods. Returning to the example about falls, the fall rates could be compared on the same floor but at two different times, for instance, before and after implementation of a planned intervention.

Formulas for the rates discussed in this chapter as well as many other useful examples can be found in Table 17.1.

Incidence rates describe the occurrence of new events in a population over a period of time relative to the size of the population at risk. Prevalence rates are the number of all cases of a specific disease or attribute in a population at a given point in time relative to the size of the population at risk. Incidence provides information about the rate at which new cases occur—it is a measure of risk. The formula for the incidence rate for Type II diabetes in a community is as follows:

Total number of people diagnosed with Type II diabetes in a population during the year (numerator) divided by population at midyear (denominator) X 1,000 = rate per 1,000.

Prevalence measures the amount of an existing problem during a specific time and is a measure of burden.

The formula for the prevalence rate for Type II diabetes during 1 year in a community is as follows:

Total number of people with Type II diabetes in a population during the year (numerator) divided by population at midyear (denominator) X 1,000 = rate per 1,000.

In the previous formula, all newly diagnosed cases for the year plus existing cases are included. It is important to note that undiagnosed cases are not captured in either prevalence rates or incidence rates.

The *Diabetes Data & Trends* report (CDC, 2007) shows that the incidence rate of diabetes in adults aged 18 to 79 has increased from 493 per 100,000 in 1980 to 1,440 per 100,000 in 2005. These data show a four-fold increase in new cases in the United States during a 25-year period. The prevalence of diabetes in the same population during the same period increased from 5,600 per 100,000 to 15,800 per 100,000 (CDC, 2007). Information on the rising incidence and prevalence of diabetes in the United States has led to increased attention to factors that cause diabetes (especially lifestyles) and programs targeted at primary prevention.

Incidence rates provide us with a direct measure of how often new cases occur within a particular population and provide some basis on which to assess risk. By comparing incidence rates among population groups who vary in one or more factor, the CNS can begin to get some idea of the association between a factor and risk. For example, taking the example on falls one step further, if the CNS compares the fall rates on two different floors and discovers that they are significantly different, the characteristics of the two floors can be compared and the etiology can be hypothesized.

The case fatality rate is often used to determine when to use a screening test and for evaluating acute, infectious diseases. It is a measure of the probability of death among diagnosed cases. Its usefulness for chronic diseases is limited because the length of time from diagnosis to death can be a long one. The formula is as follows:

The number of deaths due to the disease in a specified period of time divided by the number of cases of the disease in the same period of time X 100.

The case fatality rate can provide health care professionals with information on how deadly a disease is.

Standardization of crude rates is an important consideration in ecologic studies. Standardization is used to control for the effects of age and other characteristics in order to make valid comparisons of rates. Age adjustment is an example of rate standardization and perhaps the most important one. No other factor has a bigger effect on health outcomes than age. Consider the problem of comparing two communities with very different age distributions. One community has a much higher mortality rate for cancer than the other one, leading investigators to consider a possible environmental hazard in that community—when in fact that community's aging population is the factor most responsible for the higher rate. Age adjustment allows a researcher to eliminate the problem of age differential and, thus, compare rates for health events across population groups or to assess changes in rates over time.

There are two methods of age adjustment: direct and indirect. The direct method applies observed age-specific rates to a standard population. The indirect method

 | Calculating Rates

TYPE	DESCRIPTION	
Incidence rates	Describe the occurrence of *new* disease cases in a community over a period of time relative to the size of the population at risk. *RISK*	
	Incidence rate = $\dfrac{\text{Number of new cases during a specified period}}{\text{Population at risk during the same period}}$	X constant multiplier
Prevalence rates	Are the number of *all* cases of a specific disease in a population *at a given point in time* relative to the population at risk. *BURDEN*	
	Prevalence rate = $\dfrac{\text{Number of existing cases at a specified time}}{\text{Population at risk at the same specific time}}$	X constant multiplier
Crude rates	Summarize the occurrence of births (crude birth rate) or deaths (crude death rate); the numerator is the number of events, and the denominator is the average population size.	
	Crude death rate = $\dfrac{\text{Number of deaths in a population during a specified time}}{\text{Average population estimate during the specified time}}$	X constant multiplier
Specific rates	Are used to overcome some of the biases seen with crude rates; they are used to control for variables such as age, race, gender, and disease.	
	Age-specific death rate = $\dfrac{\text{Number of deaths for a specified age group during a specified time}}{\text{Population estimate for the specified age group}}$	X constant multiplier
Case fatality rates	Used to measure the percentage of people who die after diagnosis with a certain disease and within a certain time after diagnosis.	
	$\dfrac{\text{Number of individuals dying during a specified period of time after disease onset or dx}}{\text{Number of individuals with the specified disease}}$	X constant multiplier
Proportionate mortality ratio	Useful for determining the leading cases of death	
	$\dfrac{\text{Number of deaths from a specified cause in the United States during specified time period}}{\text{Total deaths in the United States during the specified time}}$	X 100
Years of potential life lost (YPLL)	Used for setting health priorities; predetermined standard age at death in United States is 65 years.	
	$\dfrac{\text{65 – age at death from a specific cause = X}}{\text{Add the years of life lost for each individual for specific cause of death = YPLL}}$	
Sensitivity	The ability of a screening test to identify accurately those persons with the disease = TP / (TP + FN)	
Specificity	Reflects the extent to which it excludes the persons who do not have the disease = TN / (TN + FP)	
Positive predictive value	= TP / (TP + FP)	
Negative predictive value	= TN / (TN + FN)	

TP = True positives   TN = True negatives
FN = False negatives   FP = False positives

applies the age-specific rates of a standard population to the age distribution of an observed population.

As mentioned previously, rates can be used to describe the distribution of disease and other health-related states and events, but sometimes the CNS may be more concerned with knowing how data can be used to describe the relevancy of clinical practice. Health impact assessment is the assessment of the potential health effects, positive or negative, of a particular intervention on a population. The number needed to treat (NNT) statistic, the disease impact number (DIN), and the population impact number (PIN) are formulas that are used in health impact assessment. NNT is the number of patients needed to receive a treatment to prevent one bad outcome. DIN is the number of those with the disease in question among whom one event will be prevented by the intervention. PIN is the number of those in the whole population among whom one event will be prevented by the intervention. Years of potential life lost (YPLL) measures premature mortality, the productive years that are lost related to early death (Gordis, 2004).

More extensive information on health impact assessment formulas and standardization can be found in most advanced epidemiology texts. It is important for the CNS involved in population-based evaluation to be aware of these concepts.

Analytic Epidemiology

Analytic epidemiology looks at the origins and causal factors of diseases and other health-related events. They are often carried out to test hypotheses formulated from a descriptive study. The goal of analytic epidemiology is to identify factors that increase or decrease risk. *Risk* is the probability that an event will occur. For example, a patient who smokes might ask the CNS, "What is the likelihood that I will get lung cancer if I continue to smoke?"

Although descriptive studies allow a basis for comparison and can provide the CNS with data to identify etiology and differences among groups, further studies need to be carried out in order to determine the significance of a factor. To do this, the CNS can use comparison of exposed and nonexposed groups; comparison is an essential component of population studies. One design is the case–control study.

Case–Control Studies

In a case–control study the CNS must first identify a group of individuals with the attribute of interest (cases). A second group is identified without the attribute of interest (controls). The proportion of those *cases* who were exposed to the suspected causal factor are then compared to the proportion of the cases who were not exposed, and the proportion of the *controls* who were

exposed are compared to the proportion of the controls who were not exposed. The measure of the effect of exposure is expressed as an odds ratio (OR), which is the ratio of the odds of having been exposed if you are a case to the odds of having been exposed if you are a noncase. If the exposure is not related to the attribute, the odds ratio will equal 1. If the exposure is related to the attribute, the odds ratio will be less than 1.

In a case–control study, if there is an association of an exposure with an attribute, the prevalence of history of exposure should be higher in persons who have the attribute in cases than in controls. It is important to keep in mind that only a subset of the population will be at risk from a particular exposure—in other words, only a proportion of those exposed will become a case as a result of their exposure. The calculation of the odds ratio can tell the CNS something about the risk of exposure in becoming a case—it does not calculate certainty. The fact that an elderly individual is overmedicated may put that person at risk for a fall, but it does not mean that that person *will* fall.

There are some problems with case–control studies that the investigator must keep in mind. People in the groups are not randomly assigned—association may be the result of exposure to another, unknown, variable. The problem with randomization in case–control studies is that the investigator cannot always assign exposure to a variable randomly for ethical reasons.

Case-control studies can be used to study the effects of an intervention. A case-control design was used to evaluate the impact of an advanced practice nurse (APN) intervention to reduce restraint use in hospitalized nursing home patients (Bourbonniere, Strumpf, Evans, & Maislin, 2003). Three different odds ratios were computed for three different staffing models. The results are displayed here:

Model #1 P .001, OR 0.23, 95% CI 0.10–0.55

Model #2 P .001, OR 0.23, 95% CI 0.10–0.51

Model #3 P .001, OR 0.23, 95% CI 0.10–0.55

Note that the OR is less than 1 in each model—signifying a negative relationship between the APN intervention and restraint use. Selection of the sample is an important step in case–control studies. Definite criteria should be used so that there is no ambiguity about how to distinguish between a case and a control. Exposure is not always all or nothing. Controls should resemble the cases as closely as possible except for exposure to the factor under study. If the cases are drawn from a particular clinic, then ideally the controls should be drawn from the same clinic population. Matching is one method that can be used to select a sample so that potential confounders are distributed equally between the cases and controls. A good example would be if a CNS planned to evaluate an intervention to reduce burden among caregivers of dependent elderly in the home. It is known that men and women have characteristics that affect the caregiver role (in general, for example, women find the physical demands of caregiving more burdensome than do men). By matching gender in the study, the CNS can eliminate this potentially confounding factor (gender). The problem with matching is that the investigator is not always aware of all of the potentially confounding factors, and it can be expensive and time consuming to match each subject in a study.

Recall bias is also an important consideration in case–control studies. This can happen when people who experience an adverse outcome think over and remember the events leading up to the outcome. It makes it more likely that they will recall details that people who did not experience the adverse outcome will not. A woman who gives birth to a child with birth defects is more likely to remember every event leading up to and including birth than a woman who gives birth to a normal baby. This can lead to a false association between an event (such as a fall) and a birth defect.

Cohort Studies

Cohort designs can be either prospective or retrospective. In a *prospective* cohort design, the investigator selects a group of individuals who were exposed to a factor and a group of nonexposed individuals and follows both groups to compare the incidence of an attribute (more than two groups can be compared in this design). In a *retrospective* cohort design, exposure is ascertained from past records and outcome is ascertained at the time the study begins. If an association exists between the exposure and the outcome, then the proportion of the incidence rate of the exposed group will be greater than the incidence in the nonexposed group. The ratio of these is the relative risk (RR), which is the incidence rate in the exposed divided by the incidence rate in the nonexposed. RR is the measure of the strength of an association between an exposure and a disease.

If the relative risk is equal to 1 (numerator equals the denominator), then the risk to the two groups is equal. If the relative risk is greater than 1 (numerator is greater than the denominator), the risk in the exposed groups is greater than the risk in the nonexposed group. If the relative risk is less than 1 (denominator is greater than the numerator), the risk in the exposed group is less than the risk in the nonexposed group.

Cohort studies are carried out when the investigator has good evidence that links an attribute to an outcome, when the time interval between exposure and the attribute is short, and when the outcome occurs relatively often.

A cohort study was carried out to ascertain characteristics that would predict cessation or continuation of antiretroviral therapy (ART) postpartum (Tedaldi et al., 2002). The health care team of the women in the study included a CNS, a nurse practitioner, and a physician. Two groups of women were divided between those who discontinued ART postpartum and those who continued ART. Relative risk was carried out for several demographic characteristics. A significant factor for continuation of ART in this study included Latina ethnicity (risk ratio = 0.24, confidence interval = 0.06–0.87). The RR of .24 indicates that women of Latina ethnicity in this study were likely to continue ART postpartum, that is, the number of women of Latina ethnicity who discontinued ART (numerator) was less than the number of women of Latina ethnicity who continued ART (denominator).

One of the major problems with cohort studies is that they can be time consuming and expensive if the sample needs to be followed for any length of time. The longer the time period, the more likely that participants will be lost for follow-up. This can lead to problems with calculating incidence rates. Recall that in the Nurses Health Study one reason for choosing nurses was because of the belief that they would have a low drop out rate. Cohort studies are not feasible if there is difficulty involved in identifying exposed versus nonexposed populations or when data for the subjects is incomplete or lacking.

Case–Control and Cohort Studies

It is important to understand that the difference between case–control and cohort studies is not a function of calendar time. In case–control studies the investigator begins with people who have the attribute of interest and those who do not. In cohort studies the investigator begins with exposed and nonexposed individuals. Case–control and cohort studies are used to establish etiologic relationships. If associations are found, further studies are necessary to determine causal links and to prevent ecologic fallacy. When examining the results of case–control and cohort studies it is important for the CNS to consider whether or not all other explanations for an identified association have been eliminated. No single epidemiological study can satisfy all criteria for causality. The CNS needs to look at the accumulation of evidence as well as the strength of individual studies.

Risk

Relative risk and the odds ratio are measures of the association between a factor and an outcome. They can be used to derive causal inference, but they do not provide any information regarding the actual change in magnitude of a risk related to a factor. *Risk* is the probability of an event occurring. *Attributable risk* (AR) is an estimate of the amount of risk that is attributable to a risk factor and is calculated in cohort studies. The formula for the AR is as follows:

$$AR = (\text{risk in exposed}) - (\text{risk in nonexposed})$$

If an exposure is harmful, the AR will be greater than 0. If an exposure is protective, the AR will be less than 0. If a study determines that the likelihood of dying in middle age is .2 for someone who is normal weight and .4 for someone who is morbidly obese, then the AR for being obese is .4 – .2 = .2.

Population attributable risk is important to policy makers. For the previous example the question becomes, "Among the general population, how much of the total risk for death in middle age is due to morbid obesity?" This decade, the question about how much risk is accrued to people who are overweight has become a concern for health care professionals and policy makers alike.

Randomized Trials

Randomized trials are useful for evaluating treatments (including technology) and for assessing new ways of organizing and delivering health services. In population-based studies, the issue is often health promotion and disease prevention, rather than treatment of an existing disease. The intervention is undertaken on a large scale—with the target involving defined populations rather than individuals—and often involves educational, program, or policy interventions. When carefully designed, randomized trials can provide the strongest evidence for a cause-and-effect relationship.

The basic design of a clinical trial is to assign the sample randomly to either receive the new treatment or not to receive the new treatment. The difference between a randomized trial and a cohort study is that in a randomized trial, the subjects are randomly selected to be exposed or not be exposed. Inclusion and exclusion criteria for the participants must be precise and spelled out in advance. As with cohort studies, more than two groups can be compared in this design. Analysis is carried out to determine how many people in the new treatment group (or groups) improve and how many people in the current treatment group improve.

A clinical trial design was used to evaluate the effects of a pedometer-intervention for low-active adolescent girls (Schofield, Mummery, & Schofield, 2005). The purpose of the study was to compare the effectiveness of daily step count targets with time-based prescription (the more traditional method) for increasing the health-related physical activity of low-active adolescent girls. The study was carried out over a 12-week period. The participants were assigned to a control group, a pedometer group, or a minutes group. The pedometer

group set daily step count targets, while the time group set time-based goals for physical activity. The authors used ANOVA to analyze the differences among the groups. There was a significant difference in activity between the pedometer group and the time group, suggesting that this piece of technology has the potential to change the activity behavior of low-active adolescent girls in the short term. The investigators state that more research is needed. This study illustrates how useful the clinical trial design is for testing a new intervention on a specialized population.

Sample Size

Sample selection and sample size determination is a critical step in the research process. Determining the sample size is an important factor in determining whether or not the investigator has ample resources to carry out the study and what size sample is required in order to identify true differences and associations. Power analysis is used to determine sample size. There are several factors that influence the size of the sample that is needed—power, effect size, and significance.

Significance is the probability that an observed difference or relationship exists. Power is the capacity of the study to detect differences or relationships that actually exist in the population–the capacity to correctly reject a null hypothesis, that is, prevent a Type II error. The larger the power required, the larger the necessary sample size. The smaller the sample size, the smaller the power of the study. Effect size is the actual differences between groups and treatments. It can be determined by reviewing previous studies and pilot studies. The smaller the effect size, the larger the necessary sample size. The more stringent the significance level, the greater the necessary sample size.

Power analysis can be conducted using computer programs. There are many free software programs available on the Internet to assist with power analysis. Typing sample size calculation in a search engine such as Yahoo! or Google will lead the investigator to many sites. Power analysis allows the CNS to use resources efficiently and to provide data that are meaningful (Burns, 2000; Duffy, 2006).

Screening

Screening is used to describe programs that deliver a testing mechanism to detect disease in groups of asymptomatic individuals. It is a method used in secondary prevention for early detection in order to improve prognosis. There are several concepts that are important to understand about screening.

Screening is neither available nor appropriate for all diseases. In order for a screening program to be effective, certain criteria should be met: (1) the target population needs to be identifiable and accessible, (2) the disease should affect a sufficient number of people to make screening cost-effective, (3) the disease should be relatively serious, (4) an effective treatment is available for the disease, and (5) the preclinical period should be sufficient to allow treatment before symptoms appear so that early diagnosis and treatment make a difference in terms of outcome. To be effective, it is necessary for the screening test to be sensitive enough to detect most cases of the disease and to be specific enough to exclude most other causes of positive results. Screening tests should also be relatively inexpensive, easy to administer, and have minimal side effects (Gordis, 2004).

The validity of a screening test refers to its ability to accurately identify those who have the disease. Sensitivity and specificity are measures of a screening test's validity. *Sensitivity* is a measure of a screening test's ability to accurately identify disease when it is present. *Specificity* is the probability of a negative test when the disease is absent. The *positive predictive value* is a measure of the probability of a positive test result when the disease is present. The *negative predictive value* of a test is a measure of the probability that the disease is absent when there is a negative test. The higher the prevalence of a condition in a population the higher the predictive value. The formulas can be found in Table 17.1.

The CNS can evaluate the success of screening programs by determining whether or not there is a reduction in overall mortality, a reduction of the case fatality rate in screened individuals, an increase in the percentage of cases detected at earlier stages, a reduction in complications, and improvement of quality of life in screened individuals.

ETHICAL CONSIDERATIONS IN POPULATION-BASED EVALUATION

Population-based evaluation provides the CNS with information for EBP. There is no reason to assume that a new intervention or therapy will have only positive effects; research can detect evidence of harm as well as benefit. The question is not whether or not studies should be conducted, it is *how*. Ethics is as important as a sound methodology in population research. Population-based interventions should relate to a well-understood disease etiology, be feasible, and entail an appropriate trade-off of rights of the individual against benefit that is accrued to the population. Population-based research can have direct and often immediate societal relevance, and although this research involves human subjects, they may derive no personal benefits from the results of a study.

One of the best examples of population research that violated the principle of "do no harm" was the Tuskegee Study. The U.S. Public Health Service, working with the Tuskegee Institute, began the study in 1932. Nearly 400 low-income Black men with syphilis were enrolled in the study. They were never told they had syphilis, and they were never treated. At the start of the study, there was no proven treatment for syphilis. After penicillin became a standard cure in 1947, the medicine was withheld from the men. The Tuskegee scientists wanted to continue to study how the disease spreads and kills. The experiment lasted four decades, until public health workers leaked the story to the media. Many family members also became infected—and died—as a result. The *New York Times* exposed the study in 1972—40 years after the study began and after many articles on the study had been printed in professional journals (National Public Radio, 2002).

In 1978, the National Commission for the Protection of Human Subjects of Biomedical and Behavioral Research created *The Belmont Report: Ethical Principles and Guidelines for the Protection of Human Subjects of Research*. *The Belmont Report* sets forth the basic ethical principles required for research involving human subjects. Autonomy (the right of self-governance), beneficence (prevent evil or harm to others), and justice (balance between the benefits of participating in a study and the burden) are the three core principles of *The Belmont Report*.

The CNS should be aware of some special considerations in population-based research. A randomized trial can provide strong evidence for adopting a new intervention, but not all interventions are appropriate for study. A randomized trial is considered unethical if the current intervention is believed to be the best available whether or not that fact has been established scientifically by well-designed studies. A good example would be a study to determine whether or not legislation to prevent people from talking on hand-held cell phones while driving decreases motor vehicle accidents. It would be unethical to undertake a clinical trial where some people would be randomly selected to talk on a cell phone while driving.

Group comparison is a basic method in population-based research, and a related issue is the use of race and ethnicity as a grouping variable. Genetic research has been unable to find a clear genetic break between races, and biological differences are poorly understood. Using race to identify subgroups is of questionable validity. Ethnicity may be a better category, but if it is used the researcher should have a justifiable reason for the use of ethnicity as a variable, and it should be clearly defined. No variable should be used routinely, and there should be a clear and justifiable reason for the use of every variable.

There are also special ethical concerns related to screening programs. Individuals in a well population take part in screening programs, and health care professionals need to show that the benefits of screening outweigh the costs. Screening programs should be safe and free of side effects. Errors in results can cause concerns. False positive results create both extra costs for diagnostic procedures and anxiety for the individual. False negative results are equally problematic because they can place an individual at ease and make them less likely to seek help when they have early symptoms of a disease.

The CNS who is involved with population-based research has an obligation to protect and consider the interests of the populations they study. Population-based research must be concerned with the larger systemic effects that research in that population will have. Consider again the issue of race. Using ethnicity as a subgroup allows researchers to identify health disparities and to direct health resources appropriately. On the other hand, using ethnicity as a variable may serve to stigmatize certain subgroups by relating undesirable lifestyles (such as drug use) to a particular subgroup. When a CNS is making decisions related to population-based evaluation, the decisions need to be based on a sound methodological framework that includes ethical considerations of the effect of the research on the population as a whole.

CONCLUSION

Two nurse practitioners enrolled in a doctorate in nursing practice program investigated the fall rate in a long-term care/subacute rehabilitation setting (LTC/SAR; Rosner & Sirkin, 2007). They found that the facility was near the 50th percentile for falls when compared to similar institutions and that there was a need for an improved fall prevention program particularly in the SAR. Following an in-depth literature review to gain a better understanding of the known contributors to falls and a careful evaluation of the existing fall prevention program, a comprehensive, interdisciplinary fall prevention program was initiated in the SAR. The program was evaluated using a cohort design, with fall rates calculated for the SAR population before and after the intervention. The fall rate decreased from 19 falls per 1,000 patient days before the intervention to 9 falls per 1,000 patient days after the intervention with a relative risk (RR) of 0.4, demonstrating a decreased risk of falling after the intervention.

This project provides an example of how population methods can be used to identify a problem, design and implement an intervention, and evaluate the intervention to improve patient care.

SUMMARY

Population-based analysis is a complex practice area, and the challenges for the CNS are diverse. Interventions

at the population level can have a more far-reaching effect than interventions at the individual level. A falls intervention program based on carefully researched evidence will have a bigger impact on fall rates in a hospital than an uncoordinated, individual approach. The CNS requires skills in EPB, comprehensive assessment, and evaluation of interventions at the population level. Population-based data can assist the CNS to target at-risk populations, identify risk factors, evaluate interventions, and make decisions to improve the health of populations. This chapter outlined the basic principles and processes of population-based analysis. The CNS can use this information in practice and also to explore the issues further.

DISCUSSION QUESTIONS

1. During 1996, 215 new cases of AIDS were reported in Williamson, a city of 500,000. This brought the total number of active cases of AIDS to 2,280. During this time there were 105 deaths attributable to the disease.
   a. What was the incidence rate per 100,000 for AIDS during 1996?
   b. What was the prevalence rate of AIDS per 100,000?
   c. What is the cause-specific death rate of AIDS?
2. Let us hypothesize that body mass index (BMI) is associated with Type II diabetes. Using health records, ascertain the BMIs of adolescents at your clinic who have not been diagnosed with diabetes. Classify every individual as either obese or not obese, and then follow each one over time. Classify each adolescent who is diagnosed with diabetes as a case and each one who is not as a control. Match cases and controls in your study for age and gender. Out of 20 adolescents who are obese, 17 are diagnosed with diabetes. Four out of 20 adolescents who are not obese are diagnosed with diabetes. (See Exhibit 17.1.)
   a. What is the study design?
   b. What is the appropriate statistic for testing the hypothesis?
   c. Carry out the calculations.
   d. Why use other clinic patients for the control group?
3. Use Exhibit 17.2 to answer the following questions:
   a. What is the sensitivity of the test?
   b. What is the specificity of the test?
   c. What is the positive predictive value?
   d. What is the negative predictive value?
   e. What effect do you get from lowering the screening cut-off point in terms of false positives and false negatives?
4. Go to: http://www.cdc.gov/nccdphp/burdenbook 2004/toc.htm; research the state that you live in or work in.

EXHIBIT 17.1 SUMMARY OF CLINIC INFORMATION

	Cases	Controls
Obese	17	4
Not obese	3	16
Total	20	20

EXHIBIT 17.2 SCREENING INFORMATION

Screening Test Results	Population		Total
	Disease	No Disease	
Positive	TP 66	FP 98	164
Negative	FN 84	TN 9,752	9,836
Total	150	9,850	10,000

a. What is the burden of chronic diseases in this state?

b. How do the leading causes of death in the state compare to U.S. figures?

c. Identify five important risk factors that need to be targeted in the state.

d. Identify vulnerable groups. Who do targeted services need to be provided to?

ANSWERS TO DISCUSSION QUESTIONS

1. Answer
   a. 215/500,000 x 100,000 = 43 cases per 100,000
   b. 2,280/500,000 x 100,000 = 456 cases per 100,000
   c. 105/500,000 x 100,000 = 21 deaths per 100,000
2. Answer
   a. This is a cohort design.
   b. Relative risk
   c. $RR = \dfrac{17/17 + 4}{3/3 + 16} = .81/.16$

   RR = 5.06 Risk is > in exposed than
   　　　　　　　　 nonexposed group

   d. Matching is one method that can be used to select a sample so that potential confounders are distributed equally between the cases and controls. Controls should resemble the cases as closely as possible except for exposure to the factor under study.
3. Answer
   a. TP/ (TP + FN) 66/ (66 + 84) = .44 or 44%
   b. TN/ (TN + FP) 9,752/ (9752 + 98) = .99 or 99%

c. TP/ (TP + FP) 66/ (66 + 98) = .402 or 40%

d. TN/ (TN + FN) 9,752/ (9,752 + 84) = .991 or 99%

e. Lowering the screening cut-off level that distinguishes between diseased and nondiseased populations will increase the false positives and decrease false negatives. Sensitivity will be increased, and specificity will be decreased.

REFERENCES

American Nurses Association. (2004). *Nursing: Scope and standards of practice.* Washington, DC: Author.

American Nurses Association. (2007). *NDNQI national database of nursing quality indicators.* Retrieved January 21, 2009, from https://www.nursingquality.org/FAQPage.aspx#1

Babones, S. J. (2008). Income inequality and population health: Correlation and causality. *Social Science & Medicine, 66,* 1614–1626.

Bourbonniere, M., Strumpf, N., Evans, L., & Maislin, G. (2003). Organizational characteristics and restraint use for hospitalized nursing home residents. *Journal of the American Geriatrics Society, 51,* 1079–1084.

Burns, K. (2000). Power and effect size: Research considerations for the clinical nurse specialist. *Clinical Nurse Specialist, 14*(2), 61–68.

Burns, N., & Grove, S. (2005). *The practice of nursing research: Conduct, critique, and utilization* (5th ed.). St. Louis: Elsevier Saunders.

Centers for Disease Control. (2007). *Diabetes data and trends.* Retrieved January 9, 2009, from http://www.cdc.gov/diabetes/statistics/incidence/fig1.htm

Department of Health and Human Services, National Institutes of Health, National Heart Lung and Blood Institute. (2007). *Women's health initiative.* Retrieved January 9, 2009, from http://www.nhlbi.nih.gov/whi/index.html

Dossey, B. (2000). *Florence Nightingale: Mystic, visionary, healer.* Springhouse, PA: Springhouse Corporation.

Duffy, M. (2006). Resources for determining or evaluating sample size in quantitative research reports. *Clinical Nurse Specialist, 20*(1), 9–12.

Gordis, L. (2004). *Epidemiology* (3rd ed.). Philadelphia: Elsevier Saunders.

Heller, R., & Page J. (2002). A population perspective to evidence based medicine: "Evidence for Population Health." *Journal of Epidemiology and Community Health, 56,* 45–47.

Ibrahim, M., Savitz, L., Carey, T., & Wagner, E. (2001). Population-based health principles in medical and public health practice. *Journal of Public Health Management Practice, 7*(3), 75–81.

Lipsey, S. (2006). *Mathematical education in the life of Florence Nightingale.* Retrieved January 9, 2009, from http://www.agnesscott.edu/lriddle/women/night_educ.htm

Mosack, V., & Shore, E. (2006). Screening for depression among pregnant and postpartum women. *Journal of Community Health Nursing, 23*(1), 37–47.

National Association of Clinical Nurse Specialists. (2004). *Statement on clinical nurse specialist practice and education* (2nd ed.). Harrisburg, PA: Author.

National Heart, Lung and Blood Institute & Boston University. (2007). *The Framingham Study.* Retrieved January 9, 2009, from http://www.framinghamheart study.org/

National Public Radio, Inc. (2002). *Remembering Tuskegee*. Retrieved January 9, 2009, from http://www.npr.org/programs/morning/features/2002/jul/tuskegee/

Nelson, P., Holland, D., Derscheid, D., & Tucker, S. (2007). Clinical nurse specialist influence in the conduct of research in a clinical agency. *Clinical Nurse Specialist, 21*(2), 95–100.

Oermann, M., & Floyd, J. (2002). Outcomes research: An essential component of the advanced practice nurse role. *Clinical Nurse Specialist, 16*(3), 140–144.

Rosner, N., & Sirkin, A. (2007). *A multifaceted falls reduction strategy in a sub-acute rehabilitation setting.* Unpublished doctoral capstone project, University of Medicine and Dentistry of New Jersey, School of Nursing, Newark.

Schofield, L., Mummery, W., & Schofield, G. (2005). Effects of a controlled pedometer-intervention trial for low-active adolescent girls. *Medicine & Science in Sports and Exercise, 37*(8), 1414–1420.

Tedaldi, E., Willard, S., Gilmore, J., Holdsworth, C., Dix-Lassiter, S., & Axelrod, P. (2002). Continuation of postpartum antiretroviral therapy in a cohort of women infected with human immunodeficiency virus. *Journal of the Association of Nurses in AIDS Care, 13*(1), 60–65.

Client-Focused Teaching: The Role of the Clinical Nurse Specialist

Kelly A. Goudreau

CLIENT-FOCUSED TEACHING: THE ROLE OF THE CLINICAL NURSE SPECIALIST

Client-focused teaching has undergone many name changes over the years. Names for the process are varied and include patient education, patient-centered teaching, and client-focused education. Each of these variations reflects a need to clearly define the process of providing needed information to the individual who is experiencing a health challenge of either short- or long-term impact. Today, the focus from many organizations, such as The Joint Commission (2008) and the Institute for Healthcare Improvement (IHI) in collaboration with the Institute of Medicine (IOM; 2004), is on empowering or activating the patient to manage their own care more effectively. Issues around providing education to patients and focusing on the needs of the patients as they seek specific information are many. One of the issues is frustration of both the patient/client and the health care provider due to the plethora of conflicting information now available to patients/clients. Additional frustrations on the part of the health care provider include whether or not the patient/client is ready to listen and use the information presented (readiness to learn), how best to get the information to the patient/client in an understandable manner (health literacy), and finally, how best to assess whether or not the information has had a positive effect on the patient/client (assessment of learning outcomes).

What role does the clinical nurse specialist (CNS) play in this ongoing dance between the patient/client and the health care provider working to inform the patient/client? A concentration on client-focused teaching/patient education is specifically reflected in the outcomes of CNS practice articulated by the National Association of Clinical Nurse Specialists (NACNS) *Statement on Practice and Education* (2004). In the statement, NACNS identifies that two of the expected outcomes of CNS care and function are: (1) development of innovative educational programs for patients, families, and groups that are then implemented and evaluated; and (2) expertise in diagnosis and treatment to prevent and remediate, or alleviate illness and promote health with a defined specialty population (2004, pp. 25–26). This chapter relates patient education concepts and offers evidence-based interventions to support critical elements of CNS practice.

Client-focused teaching is an important function of nursing practice and critical to the role of the CNS. This chapter addresses:

1. The current practice of client-focused teaching/patient education in the clinical environment,
2. The changing role of client-focused teaching/patient education in health care delivery, and
3. Evidence-based strategies that the CNS can use to support nursing staff and other health care providers to effectively educate patients/clients.

BACKGROUND

Staff nurses within a hospital system, home care, or long-term care environment must demonstrate how their practice meets certain standards of care established by The Joint Commission (2008), the major accrediting agency for most health care facilities. A focus on patient education is a component of the delivery, design, and testing of nursing interventions related to preventing, lessening, or alleviating the illness experience. Educating patients in the management of their own care is integral across the health care continuum, health promotion and disease prevention, and in the diagnosis, treatment, and self-management of acute and chronic diseases. The CNS provides support for both the staff nurse and the patients as they attempt to meet the educational needs of the patients/clients regardless of the setting (home, inpatient, rehabilitation, or long-term care).

In addition to the role in CNS practice and outcomes (NACNS, 2004), patient education is also mandated by The Joint Commission (2008). CNSs typically play a key role in ensuring that strategies are put in place to meet or exceed The Joint Commission standards. In the past there was a separate section in The Joint Commission standards that addressed patient education. With the recent revisions, however, now the expectations for patient education are dispersed across almost all of the standards. Specific Joint Commission standards that refer to patient education include the following: assessment of patients' learning needs, infection control, national patient safety goals, medication management and reconciliation, transfer and follow-up care, participation in decisions about care, receiving information in an understandable manner, how to seek assistance if the patient's condition changes, and informed consent (The Joint Commission, 2008).

The role of the CNS expands beyond meeting the needs of nursing staff and accrediting agencies and addresses the needs of patient care directly. CNSs care for patients with both acute and chronic disease within a specialty population (NACNS, 2004). Of note is the fact that the chronic disease burden in the United States will continue to increase as the population ages (Rothman & Wagner, 2003). The CNS's role in this area needs to be especially evident. To effectively self-manage chronic disease, patients must understand their condition(s) and the disease process. They must also be able to self-monitor, record, and track self-monitoring data; know what, when, and how to report changes in their condition; problem solve; modify their medications, diet, and physical activity as appropriate; enlist the support and involvement of family members and their social support systems; and cope on a day-to-day basis (Lorig, 2001; Rothman & Wagner, 2003; Wagner et al., 2005). The CNS educates patients with chronic disease regarding the information and skills needed to accomplish these critical tasks. As an advanced practice nurse, the CNS may also be the patient's point of contact regarding the self-monitoring data and offer guidance about

needed changes in the treatment plan. The CNS also offers advice and suggestions to help patients solve self-management problems.

The CNS also plays a key role in the development and use of evidence-based interventions to provide in-depth education and counseling to patients and family members. The challenge is to select effective patient education and counseling interventions for use in time-limited clinical encounters.

Like health care delivery and the role of the CNS, patient education has evolved. In the 1970s, patient education was frequently viewed as offering patients print materials or audiovisuals to provide information about their conditions and the diagnostic or surgical procedures they were about to undergo. The educational content frequently focused solely on anatomy and pathophysiology emulating the medical model of teaching. Clinicians truly believed that providing information in this way would motivate patients to comply with the treatment plan and make the recommended health behavior changes. This approach was frequently unsuccessful in accomplishing either education or compliance with treatment plans.

There are several reasons for this lack of success. The first reason for this failure was the misconception that information alone, especially about anatomy and pathophysiology, was sufficient to cause people to change health behaviors. Another reason for lack of success was the common use of fear messages. Clinicians believed that if they informed patients about the negative consequences of noncompliance, patients would certainly follow the treatment plan and make the recommended lifestyle changes. There is ample evidence to suggest that fear messages are ineffective (Wagner et al., 2005). Fear elicits anxiety. Most people who experience anxiety try to avoid the situation that is making them anxious, which in turn makes it very difficult to positively influence a patient's willingness to adhere to treatment plans and make the desired health behavior changes (Nolte, Elsworth, Sinclair, & Osborne, 2007). The patient education materials of this era were designed to foster compliance. Patients who appeared in these materials and audiovisuals were usually depicted as Caucasian. Little, if any, attempt was made to tailor and personalize patient education materials to age, race, gender, or ethnicity of the specific target audience for whom they were intended.

The field of patient education has evolved both conceptually and as a field of practice since the 1970s. An ample body of research currently exists on evidence-based interventions drawing from the health education, nursing, clinical psychology, and health care communications literature (Wagner et al., 2005). The evolution of patient education parallels changes in society, health care delivery, and the patient's role. In the 1970s, the relationship between patients, physicians, and health care team members was significantly different than it is today. Physicians were considered to be solely responsible for designing treatment plans and the subsequent regimens, and there was little opportunity for other members of the health care team, much less the patient, to contribute to the design of the treatment plan. The patient was held responsible and accountable for carrying out the treatment plan as designed by the physician, but there were few attempts to solicit patient input in order to create a tailored, individualized treatment plan that accommodated the patient's goals and lifestyle. We now know that the better a treatment plan is tailored to accommodate the patient's goals and lifestyle, the more likely it will be followed (Bruce, Lorig, & Laurent, 2007).

THE CURRENT PRACTICE OF CLIENT-FOCUSED TEACHING/ PATIENT EDUCATION IN THE CLINICAL ENVIRONMENT

Two key differences between the 1970s and the clinical practice of client-focused education today are: (1) the client is expected to be a full partner and the key decision maker in how their health will be managed (Turner, Thomas, Wagner, & Moseley, 2008), and (2) in order to be key decision makers, the client must clearly understand the health care issues, and health literacy is key to that understanding (U.S. Department of Health and Human Services [USDHHS], 2000a, 2000b). Patients are now recognized as key active participants in the process of health care. An informed and empowered patient is active and participatory in his or her own care and also takes greater responsibility for his or her own health care outcomes. This active participation is necessary to achieve the desired clinical outcomes. Their activated and empowered participation also impacts the economics of health care delivery (Ament, 2008; Goudreau et al., 2008; Kennedy et al., 2007; Mayer & Villaire, 2004). Patients need information and skills in order to:

1. Access health care services. Patients must not only be able to access the needed health care services in a timely manner, they must also have the skills needed to navigate complex health care delivery systems and interface with insurers.
2. Adopt a healthy lifestyle to promote health, prevent disease, and enhance their quality of life.
3. Prepare for diagnostic tests and procedures.
4. Participate as active partners in all aspects of their care.
5. Self-manage acute and chronic diseases and conditions.
6. Obtain optimal benefits from rehabilitation.
7. Engage the needed support from family members and friends.
8. Employ the needed coping skills.
9. Communicate effectively with their providers and members of the health care team.

The kind of communication needed to do this is fostered by a true partnership between patients and their providers and health care team members (Schwartzenberg, Cowett, Van Geest, & Wolf, 2007).

CNSs are able to lay a foundation for this therapeutic relationship and, depending on the clinical practice environment and the population they work with, they can maintain it over time. This is especially important for patients with chronic diseases. The role of the CNS in inpatient care allows for standardization, assessment of appropriate materials, and the introduction of patient education through a variety of methods and techniques. Methods include such processes as print media, verbal instruction, computer-based instruction, and return demonstration (London, 1997). The CNS role in outpatient environments ensures that the initial work done by the inpatient nursing staff can be maintained or modified to better meet the patient/client needs. Patients/clients are seen more than just in the hospital or in a clinic visit and can now be maintained on an ongoing basis.

In order to be a full partner in their own health care, the patient/client must be able to communicate effectively with their provider. Communication must be reciprocal and must include ways to contact the provider or team when questions arise and answers are needed. The changing era of the information age has seen increased expectations for communication between patients and their providers. As patients become more technology savvy and increasingly competent, they are seeking greater amounts of information from both their provider and other sources such as the Internet. They are also demanding immediate opportunities to communicate with their providers. As a result, use of secure e-mail between patients and members of the health care team is now possible and increasingly being used (personal communication, David Douglas, Director of Technology Information Management Systems, Portland VA Medical Center, December 21, 2008; Lorig, Ritter, Laurent, & Plant, 2006). In order to make this an effective environment for learning and support of client-focused education, patients need to be comfortable with and understand the process and the "business" rules for both how and what is appropriate for this method of communication. Just as there is an expectation of behavior in a personal interaction, there are also behavioral expectations in an online environment.

When a patient is admitted to an inpatient area, a rehabilitation unit, or is simply seeing their provider in a time-limited clinic interaction, there is a need to clearly and effectively communicate and understand. A health partnership cannot be established if there is a lack of understanding of the topics at hand. Health literacy is a key element in ensuring that patients/clients understand the content being presented or discussed.

Health care providers are not always good at creating materials or presenting content that truly meets the needs of the patients/clients they are intended to serve. Content is not clear or simply is too complex to assist comprehension (Schwartzenberg et al., 2007; Seligman et al., 2007). These poor efforts at provision of health information that is inappropriate to the patient/client needs only serve as bad examples of how to accommodate low health literacy.

Health literacy was identified as a major issue in the U.S. Department of Health document *Healthy People 2010* (USDHHS, 2000a) and continues to be an issue on the rise today (Toofany, 2007). In *Healthy People 2010* (USDHHS, 2000b), health literacy is defined as "the degree to which individuals have the capacity to obtain, process, and understand basic health information and services needed to make appropriate health decisions" (p. vi). All people need health literacy skills to find their way to the right place in a hospital, self-monitor and self-manage chronic and acute conditions, safely take prescribed medications, fill out medical and insurance forms, and communicate with members of the health care team.

A national survey of adults in the United States found a significant number of Americans have low-level general literacy skills that hamper their participation in the economy and society (Kirsch, Jungeblut, Jenkins, & Kolstad, 1993; National Center for Education Statistics, 2003). Upwards of 90 million Americans "were much less likely to respond correctly to the more challenging literacy tasks in the assessment—those requiring higher level reading and problem-solving skills. In particular, they were apt to experience considerable difficulty in performing tasks that required them to integrate or synthesize information from complex or lengthy texts" (p. xvii). These difficulties with general literacy are only compounded when one considers the complexity of health care information and the added stressors of learning about a health condition not previously known.

People from all ages, races, incomes, and education levels are challenged by health literacy. Individuals with limited health literacy incur medical expenses that are up to four times greater than patients with adequate literacy skills, costing the health care system billions of dollars every year in unnecessary doctor visits and hospital stays (IHI & IOM, 2004). The health literacy problem is compounded by the fact that most patients hide their confusion because they are too ashamed and intimidated to ask for help.

Effective communication between health care providers and their patients is hindered when patients or family members have limited health literacy. Difficulties in communication can cause medical errors, delay in care, treatment mishaps, and other costly, unwanted consequences that are sometimes fatal (IHI & IOM, 2004). Issues surrounding health literacy are recognized by The Joint Commission, as well (2008). The Joint Commission mandates patients' right to receive information in a manner that they can understand. Elements of this standard deal with information specifically tailored to the patient's age, language, and ability to understand and accommodation of physical and cognitive impairments.

Patient and environmental health literacy relate to the CNS's core competencies in the client direct care, nursing practice, and organizations and systems spheres of practice. The CNS impacts the patient/client directly by ensuring that he/she understands the content presented to them by the provider or other health care staff. The CNS impacts the care provided by the nurse through defining the issues surrounding patient/client-focused education and providing support and education to the nursing staff. Specifically, the CNS educates the nursing and support staff about how to empower patients/clients and how to create materials that are within the boundaries of health literacy guidelines. The CNS impacts the health care system by putting in place policies and programs that allow for and encourage an active and participatory patient/client. Additionally, the fact that these policies and programs are based on the best available evidence adds to the value the CNS brings to the clinical environment. The final system-level impact of the CNS is the standardization of patient/client educational materials and processes at an appropriate grade level and with a culturally appropriate focus. Each of these influences at the patient/client level, the nursing staff level, and the systems level will lead to improved patient/client outcomes.

Most health education materials should be written at the sixth-grade reading level to accommodate current health literacy levels in the United States (McLaughlin, 1996). Using materials that incorporate the appropriate reading level and a clear graphical layout can make a big difference in promoting patients' comprehension because appropriate graphics and pictures reinforce the written text. Many options are available for evaluating the reading level of written materials. Most focus on sentence length, complexity of words used, numbers of words in a phrase, and number of syllables in the words. The Fleisch-Kincaid test is often built into current software programs readability indices and can be used to assess a document's reading level.

CNSs can also decrease the demands on patient literacy through effective patient–clinician communication. Most patients want and need to have effective relationships with their physicians and health care team members. Providing patients with pamphlets, directing patients to a Web site, or having patients watch a video can supplement but never replace face-to-face interactions. Successful discussions with patients about health behavior change and self-management are founded on trust and a therapeutic relationship. Effective relationships help patients take a more active role in their health care. The CNS can extend the invitation for patients to participate in different ways at different times. The goal is to keep the dialogue flowing.

Two issues must be taken into consideration when looking at any health education and client-focused interventions related to acute or chronic illnesses: (1) the client is expected to be a full participant in the health care process, and (2) health literacy is potentially compromised. The CNS is an essential element in the assessment of the client/patient and their ability to fully participate. Methods to approach clients/patients must be based in evidence-based practice and firmly founded in theoretical constructs that provide strength to the interventions and provide methods to evaluate the outcomes. There are many theories and processes that have been proposed, and many of those are being currently researched. The impact of the patient participation and ability to understand the content is key to whichever method/theoretical model that is used.

CONCEPTUAL AND/OR THEORETICAL SUPPORT: EVIDENCE-BASED PATIENT EDUCATION INTERVENTIONS

There are many different theoretical constructs for patient/client-focused educational interventions. The Joint Commission (2008), *Healthy People 2010* (USDHHS, 2000a), and the Institute of Medicine (2004) have all pointed to the need for activated, empowered, and informed patients/clients, therefore, research is underway to find the best methods to achieve improved patient outcomes. Evidence-based patient education can be integrated into all aspects of CNS practice through a variety of methods and techniques. Due to the current time constraints in health care (Ament, 2008; London, 1995), many of the evidence-based methodologies discussed in this section are those that can be easily accomplished in time-limited clinical encounters. Others are longer term but are supportive of the overall concepts of empowerment and activation of the patient/client in their own care.

The Joint Commission (2008) mandates that patient education must be based on each patient's needs and ability to understand. This requires assessing the preferred learning modality of the patient and documenting the stated educational needs, including any physical, cognitive, and social barriers that may impact the patient's ability to learn the needed information and skills. Identification of the patient's needs and concerns facilitates the integration of the clinical and patient priorities. These patient-centered or client-focused needs assessment techniques use active involvement of the patient because they focus on the patient's ownership of the problem, identification of the issues, and problem solving.

Some of the theories that can be used to provide a foundation for the educational intervention that follows the assessment include the Salient Belief Model (Miller, 1957), the Health Belief Model (Rosenstock, Strecher, & Becker, 1994), and the Stages of Change Model (Prochaska & DiClemente, 1983). A more recent midlevel theory and application focuses on how to address and empower patients/clients who have chronic diseases and assists in long-term management of the chronic disease. The Chronic Disease Self-Management Program (CDSMP; Lorig, 2001) offers some hope for positive long-term outcomes of care.

Salient Belief Model

One of the quickest and most effective strategies to elicit patient concerns is based on the work of Miller (1957). Miller's "Salient Belief Model" is based on research that demonstrates that people have a limited number of strong beliefs about any topic. Miller identified that the number of strong beliefs an individual can have can be as many as seven (plus or minus two). If you can determine what those beliefs are, you can design your teaching to address those beliefs and concerns.

The term *salient* is derived from the Latin word *salire,* to leap or jump. Synonyms for salient include: apparent, obvious, self-evident, first, or significant. A clinician can use the Salient Belief Model as an assessment strategy in a one-on-one situation with a patient. To identify the patient's salient beliefs, ask, "When you think of _____, what do you think of?" Here's an example that's not related to health, "When you think of Thanksgiving, what do you think of?" People may respond with family gatherings, turkey, football, or the beginning of the holiday shopping season. Although asked the same question, the responses demonstrate the diversity of strong beliefs on Thanksgiving. If a CNS needed to effectively educate an individual about Thanksgiving, the topic would be framed around its relationship to the person's response to the salient belief question. A CNS questioning two patients who are not taking their antihypertensive medications might discover that one worked swing shifts and found it difficult to follow the regimen due to differences in work schedule. Another might express concern regarding loss of sexual function. The CNS can then approach these two patients with very different counseling strategies.

CNSs can use the Salient Belief Model to identify patient concerns and then to frame their education to those specific needs and concerns. These are tools that the CNS can use with difficult situations where the staff nurse and other clinicians have not had success.

The Health Belief Model

The Health Belief Model (Rosenstock et al., 1994) was first described by U.S. Public Health officials in the 1950s in an effort to define the process of change and how best to motivate an individual to change existing health behaviors. The model defines that in order for a change to occur in an individual's health behaviors there must be some motivating factors. These factors initiate the change in behavior and assist in sustaining the change until it becomes a habit. The model contains perceived threat: There must be a perceived threat to the individual in order for a change to be initiated. The threat consists of two parts: (a) perceived susceptibility and (b) perceived severity of a health condition. Perceived susceptibility is the individual's subjective perception of the risk of contracting a health condition. If they do not perceive that they are susceptible, then there will be no change made to the health behaviors that are likely to lead to the health condition. Perceived severity is feelings concerning the seriousness of contracting an illness or of leaving it untreated and is based on the evaluations of both medical and possible social consequences. This particular belief falls clearly into the 1970s perspective of health education and could be used to generate fear in the individual in order to motivate action on their part. Although the Health Belief Model can still be used today, the provider needs to be aware of the tendency toward potential use of scare tactics. In an environment that is attempting to empower a new generation of learners, this tendency needs to be taken into consideration and used carefully.

The second part of the Health Belief Model relates to perceived benefits to participating in the prescribed treatment plans. The empowered and activated patient will likely see this as the most palatable component of the model, and it includes the individual belief about the effectiveness of strategies designed to reduce the threat of illness. There are, however, also perceived barriers that would prevent the individual from participating. These barriers include the potential negative consequences that may result from taking particular health actions, including physical, psychological, and financial demands. In the health care environment of today, where many individuals do not have sufficient health care plans to provide support for long-term maintenance of chronic illnesses, this can be a defining factor in the success of the planned change.

Cues to action, the final element in the Health Belief Model, includes events, either bodily (e.g., physical symptoms of a health condition) or environmental (e.g., media publicity), that motivate people to take action. It remains, however, an area of the Health Belief Model that has not been systematically studied.

Other variables also articulated in the model include the impact of: (1) indirect, diverse demographic, psychosocial, and structural variables that affect an individual's perceptions of their ability to change; and (2) the belief of the individual that they are able to be successful, or self-efficacy (Bandura, 1977).

Stages of Change Model

An additional perspective on how an individual can be approached regarding health behaviors and how they are impacting activities of daily living is the Stages of Change Model, first articulated by Prochaska and DiClemente (1983). The stages of change are experienced by each individual and can be used to assess whether an individual is ready to make changes in their lives and whether or not those changes are likely to be maintained over time. Stage 1 is *precontemplation.* When in this stage the individual has the health problem (whether he/she recognizes it or not) and has no intention of changing. Stage 2 is *contemplation.* In contemplation the individual recognizes that there is a health problem and is seriously thinking about changing. They have not yet made any plans to change at this time. The third stage of change is *preparation for action.* When preparing for action the individual recognizes the problem and intends to change the behavior within the next month. At this time some behavior change efforts may be reported, but whatever has been defined as the successful behavior change criterion has not yet been reached. The fourth stage of change is *action.* In this stage the individual has enacted consistent behavior change for less than 6 months. Without positive reinforcement of the change they may revert to the contemplative or precontemplative stage. Use of both overt and covert reinforcements is appropriate at this stage, in addition to social support and avoiding high-risk cues. The final stage is *maintenance.* In order to reach this stage the individual must maintain the new behavior for at least 6 months.

Another theory or model of care that is increasing in use and has shown successful outcomes is the midlevel theory of chronic disease self-management (Lorig, 2001). The CDSMP is clearly evidence based with more than 20 years of research supporting the findings that patients feel empowered and activated and make changes in their lives that are manageable and maintained over time (Kennedy et al., 2007; Lorig, 2001). The program consists of a combination of self-directed change that is supported by a peer group that is sustained over a period of 6 weeks. Although this is not a program that can be managed quickly in a short interaction with a client, it is one that can be managed by the CNS with his or her client/patient population. The CDSMP model brings the best of patient empowerment, peer support, health literacy, and ongoing positive interaction with the health care system together into a single program.

APPLICATION TO CNS PRACTICE

There are several evidence-based strategies to help patients change their health behaviors. In the process of learning how to improve delivery of patient education services, it is important to understand the factors that help a person gain control over specific health behaviors.

Each of the theories identified has specific elements that can be applied directly to CNS practice. Although conceptual, each of the models previously identified can be used by the CNS as he or she addresses specific patient/client education needs.

The first action by the CNS as he/she addresses the individual patient/client is to assess the educational needs. Next is to identify how best to address the needs in collaboration with the patient/client and the health care team. Each of the models previously identified indicates a need to assess the patient/client, their preferred method of learning, and whether or not they are ready to make the subsequent behavioral changes required to attain improved health outcomes.

Self-efficacy theory (Bandura, 1977), a component of both the Stages of Change (Prochaska & DiClemente, 1983) and the CDSMP (Lorig, 2001), can be used in two ways: first with the health care providers as they are releasing control of the management of the patient's/client's health plan and again when assisting the patient to feel more self-assured as they assume the management of their own care. It is important to remember self-efficacy relates to a person's belief about his or her ability to do some future activity. It is predictable and related to a specific activity. It is not a personality trait.

Self-efficacy involves:

1. Behavior choices—Which activities people will choose to attempt and which they will avoid. People will not attempt behaviors they believe are impossible even if they have the needed skills to complete the task.
2. Effort—How much effort people will expend and how long they will persist in the face of obstacles. Some people will persevere longer trying to complete a task despite obstacles and failures.
3. Amount of anxiety tolerated—How much anxiety or distress people experience during their efforts.

A CNS can use self-efficacy theory to help patients change health behaviors. When suggesting a change in the treatment that requires a new health behavior, ask the patient, "On a scale from 1 being totally unsure and 10 being totally sure, how certain are you that you will be able to (identify the behavior)?" The numerical score is important. People who give themselves scores of 7 or higher are much more likely to be able to perform the behavior. Scores of less than 7 indicate the need to go back and problem solve. People have very different reasons regarding why they feel they cannot perform a behavior. By working with a patient to identify his/her specific concerns, you can effectively problem solve with the patient to facilitate the needed health behavior change (Lorig, 2001).

In dealing with patients/clients it is important to discuss options and specifically ask the patient/client what behavior they want to change. Assist the patient/client to select one behavior that they feel they can realistically change within the period of time that they identify. Typically small increments of time are more achievable and realistic. Assist the patient to make a plan that will help them to achieve the goal. It is important that the patient/client identify previous activity related to this behavior that will help them to be successful in this attempt.

The CNS can do this by asking what problems the patient/client is expecting to encounter. Once difficulties have been identified, the CNS can ask them to identify strategies that could overcome the issues, then re-ask the self-efficacy question. Plan to follow-up with the patient as needed or appropriate. At the point of follow-up, congratulate the patient if he/she was successful; problem solve if the patient experienced difficulty or was not successful.

There are several ways to enhance patients' self-efficacy. Modeling is one technique. Modeling is also called imitation learning. This technique is effective for learning new behaviors and strengthening previously learned behaviors that are slipping. When dealing with any patient/client, offer them models or examples of others similar to the patient/client (i.e., condition, age, educational background, job, social support system) who have successfully dealt with similar problems related to self-management or coping strategies. Your patient may develop a stronger belief in his/her own capabilities if the person is similar in age, sex, social status, situation and type of problem. By using multiple events or models, the patient will be more likely to identify with one of the subjects or situations. It is also important to offer an example of a person who had to cope with problems and work out solutions in order to attain mastery.

The modeling technique can also be used in patient education classes or groups. In a group teaching session, when one participant poses a problem, an effective group leader will not offer the solution. The CNS should facilitate group problem solving by asking,

"Does anyone have a suggestion for solving this problem?" The CNS can write down the ideas on a flip chart or dry erase board and probe the group for additional suggestions. After several suggestions have been made, turn to the person who posed the problem or question and ask, "Does this offer you a few hints you can use?" After group members have offered suggestions, the CNS may contribute a few more. In using this process, the group members become models for the group. The process generates creative solutions and, because group members have helped each other, enhances their self-efficacy.

Motivational interviewing is another technique that the CNS can use to assist patients/clients in the process of change (Hall & Finegood, 2006; Miller & Rollnick, 2002; Rollnick, Miller, & Butler, 2008). Often described in collaboration with Prochaska and DiClemente's (1983) Stages of Change, motivational interviewing is a process of assisting the client to more clearly define reasons why change has not been successful in the past. Of utmost importance is recognition that the patient/client is in complete control of the decision to make a change. The health care provider must always remember the patient's/client's right to refuse to change.

The first component of motivational interviewing is to establish rapport. Rapport is an essential element if the relationship is to develop into the therapeutic discussion that will assist patients/clients to change. As an advanced practice nurse, the CNS is in the best position to assist patients/clients to change. There are four core motivational interviewing skills:

1. Express empathy—acknowledge that there are issues that must be addressed.
2. Roll with resistance—resistance is normal and must be acknowledged as a component of the change process.
3. Develop discrepancy—create "cognitive dissonance" or the acknowledgement of the difference between where the individual is at the present and where they would like to be once their goal is accomplished.
4. Promote self-efficacy and change—encourage successful outcomes and assist the patient/client with reaffirmation of their success. (Hall & Finegood, 2006)

Use of motivational interviewing permits the CNS to demonstrate respect for the patient's values, preferences, and needs, while at the same time encouraging the change that the patient/client is seeking. Motivational interviewing helps identify patients' concerns and needs via asking open questions, for example, "What's concerning you most right now?" CNSs can use patients' responses to tailor treatment plans to their specific concerns, goals, and lifestyles. Open questions also help identify behaviors that patients would like to change by

focusing on the patient's motivation, willingness, and ability to change specific behaviors.

Conversations about behavior change optimally occur when patients and CNSs view each other as partners, an important component of the spirit of motivational interviewing. Patient–CNS partnership also maintains the relationship even if the patient is not ready to take action. The CNS can ask, "As your clinical nurse specialist, I am concerned about you and your health. I recognize (Reflective Listening) that you have said that, for now, you are not interested in *(insert health behavior change)*, but out of my concern for you, may I have your permission to ask about it in the future?"

Motivational interviewing also encourages CNSs to express empathy. When patients share their concerns or fears, CNSs can offer emotional support, another dimension of patient-centered care. Understanding the patient's feelings and perspectives without judging or blaming does not need to imply acceptance. Acceptance is possible without agreement or endorsement. The CNS may differ with a patient's views and respectfully express the divergence. However, it is extremely important to listen to patients to understand their perspectives. Listening, accepting, and respecting patients' perspectives builds the therapeutic, patient-centered relationship.

Setting the agenda is the next component of motivational interviewing. Setting the agenda permits the CNS to identify and respect the patient's values, preferences, and expressed needs, the first component of patient-centered care. CNSs can effectively use this information to create a treatment plan specifically tailored to each patient, increase adherence, and engage the patient in health behavior change. It also opens the door to discussion about possible health behavior changes. Permitting patients to identify behaviors they would like to change immediately increases buy-in with the change process. Patient engagement is another attribute of patient-centered care.

CNSs can assess importance to patients by affirming patients' past successful behavior changes or coping strategies. This enhances patient confidence to make new health behavior changes. For example, "Remember when you started walking more, and you started by just walking to the mailbox, then worked your way up gradually to walking for 30 minutes a day?" or "Remember when we added two new medicines to the ones you were already taking? You did a great job juggling times you take your medicines, even though one of the new ones could not be taken close to mealtimes."

Motivational interviewing also includes assessing readiness. It can be done using the self-efficacy needs assessment technique ("People can differ a lot when it comes to how ready they are to *[insert health behavior change]*. How ready do you think you are?") or using numerical scale ("If 0 was totally unprepared and 10 was absolutely sure you will be able to *[insert health behavior change]*, what number would you give yourself?"). If the patient responds less than 7, it alerts the CNS to the likelihood that the patient will not be able to succeed with the behavior change.

Additional probing may identify specific barriers that the patient would need to overcome, and the CNS may be able to help the patient find ways to resolve those problems. The CNS can also ask the patient what it would take to achieve a higher number. Then, the CNS can specifically deal with the issues the patient identifies.

Negotiation is a critical component of the partnership, the therapeutic relationship, and patient-centeredness. It permits clinicians to use their clinical expertise, and it allows patients to use their knowledge of their goals and lifestyle experiences to achieve the desired clinical outcomes while keeping patients in control. Asking open questions, affirming, reflective listening, and summarizing help clinicians and patients discuss possibilities for behavior change. These core skills help patients make changes that are important to them and lead to enhanced health outcomes.

Motivational interviewing is an effective way to enhance patient–clinician communication and facilitate health behavior change. Its effects are more powerful than active listening or simple reflection used alone. Motivational interviewing also helps clinicians build therapeutic relationships. It creates rapport and engages patients in discussions about their needs, priorities, and health behavior change. To counsel patients most effectively, it is important for clinicians to use a variety of approaches (Miller & Rollnick, 2002), self-efficacy, and modeling, along with motivational interviewing. These strategies compliment motivational interviewing. They permit clinicians to work with each patient as an individual and use evidence-based counseling techniques to gain important information to create the most effective treatment plan, engage the patient, and support health behavior change.

Health literacy is an issue that cannot be forgotten as you deal with the issue of change and informing the patient/client of their options. Keeping in mind that health literacy is an issue for approximately two-thirds of the American population, Chew, Bradley, and Boyko (2004) identified a series of questions that allow for a fast screening of patients who may have low health literacy. These questions focus on how often an individual must ask for assistance, confidence levels, and admitting difficulty with understanding written materials. Unfortunately, they rely on the individual being able to admit they have difficulty understanding information. CNSs can easily and quickly assess health literacy by asking the patient to repeat information that has been shared with them in their own words (London, 1997).

It is important to remember that print materials are most effectively used as an adjunct to support, complement, augment, and remind patients of what is important for maintaining or improving their health. They can also use print materials to share information about their condition and treatment plan with family members. By using the following communication techniques, CNSs can effectively counsel patients and family members who have limited health literacy skills:

1. Ask open-ended questions to ascertain patients' comprehension.
2. Use everyday language to explain terms.
3. Build on what the patient knows.
4. Be alert for nonverbal behavior that indicates misunderstanding.
5. Provide opportunities for patients to report on what they have understood.
6. Provide names and numbers for staff that can be called for questions.

The "teach-back" technique is recommended to nonjudgmentally permit patients to report what they have learned in a patient education session. The CNS can use questions such as:

1. "So I can make sure that I was clear, please tell me what you think we have discussed during this visit," or
2. "Please tell me what you will tell your wife/husband about the changes we have made in your treatment plan at today's visit."

The emphasis is a check on the clarity of the CNS, not a test of the patient.

Each of the methods described in this section are active ways in which a CNS can implement elements of the models described in the previous section. By using these tools the CNS can have a significant impact on the patients/clients and the health care team. Ultimately, the goal is to provide examples, models, and behaviors that will increase the likelihood of success in patient health outcomes. The CNS also has a role to play in the system.

SYSTEMS LEVEL HEALTH LITERACY

Because of the leadership role of CNSs, they can also impact the health literacy of the care environment. Patients must navigate the physical grounds and buildings of health care facilities, read signs and informational postings, complete forms, find the correct departments, and correctly check-in for services. CNSs can assume a leadership role in assessing their health care environments and clinical settings. In addition to information on health literacy and strategies to effectively educate patients and families with limited health literacy, the Harvard School of Public Health's Health Literacy Program provides information on how to conduct an environmental health literacy assessment. One of the valuable resources on the Harvard Health Literacy Program's Web site is the text of the seminal work on health literacy written by Doak, Doak, and Root (1985). Upon their retirement, the team of Doak, Doak, and Root offered the text of their book to the Harvard School of Public Health Literacy Program with permission to make it freely available to all disciplines to promote health literacy in hospitals and other health care organizations. This book provides CNSs with very specific strategies to educate patients and family members with low health literacy.

EVALUATION OF PATIENT/ CLIENT-CENTERED TEACHING

Patient/client-centered teaching focuses on the use of interpersonal relations skills as well as the use of print materials that are tailored to the needs of the patients/clients. Evaluation of the interpersonal relationship is not easily measured. Assessment of clinical outcomes resulting from the interaction and adherence to the treatment plan agreed to by the patient/client in collaboration with the health care provider are perhaps the best measure. These must be measured on a one-to-one basis, however, and are difficult to quantify. Measurements of established criterion, such as ability to stay within evidence-based boundaries of care (i.e., performance measures for hemoglobin A1C for diabetic patients), may be an indirect measure of the success of patient/client-centered teaching. To use these measures as a potential direct measurement of success is difficult and biased at best.

Evaluation of materials is much easier to accomplish. The use of the Simple Measure of Gobbledygook (SMOG) scale provides a process to evaluate printed materials (McLaughlin, 1996). The SMOG scale in collaboration with the Fleish-Kincaid analysis of grade level also provides a means to measure the health literacy levels of various educational materials provided to the patient/client as a supplement to any other educational process. As mentioned previously, it is important to maintain reading levels between the sixth and eighth grade in order to reach the majority of the U.S. population.

ETHICAL CONSIDERATIONS

There is a potential for breach of ethics in any circumstance where a health care provider has access to a patient/client's personal feelings related to their

self-efficacy to make change. Each and every CNS should be vigilant to the potential abuses of patients/clients in their vulnerable state.

CONCLUSION

The roles and responsibilities of CNSs offer important opportunities at the direct client care through the health system level to impact patients' quality of life and clinical outcomes. They can also serve as role models and mentors to nurses and other clinical disciplines in promoting use of evidence-based patient education and counseling techniques. Their role in effectively educating patients and family members and positively impacting the health care environment promotes care that is patient-centered.

Through the use of techniques and tools that support the patient/client as they make changes in their lifestyle and health, the CNS can impact the patient, the nursing staff, and the system. Through these actions on the three spheres of influence the care of patients/clients will be improved.

A focus on empowerment, activation, and inclusion of the patient in a manner that they can understand can only result in improved cost-effectiveness and increased access for patients/clients everywhere. The time has come for patient/client-focused education that increases the ability of the individual to make decisions regarding his/her care. The CNS can and does play a significant role in making it possible.

DISCUSSION QUESTIONS

1. If you were to ask a group of CNSs (barring unforeseen events) to rate on a scale from 10 being absolutely certain to 1 being absolutely uncertain how likely it is that they will successfully get dressed tomorrow morning, most will respond "10." Ask the same group of CNSs how likely it is that they could successfully scale Mount Everest tomorrow, and their responses may be very different. Discuss how you have seen this same kind of situation play out with patients in the clinical area. How would you apply self-efficacy theory to assist the patient to perhaps see themselves doing something that they may consider impossible?

2. According to Hall and Finegood (2006), 40% of the population is in precontemplative stage of change, 40% are in contemplative, and only 20% of the population is engaged in active change processes. Does this number surprise you? Why or why not?

3. What types of patient education material does your facility have? Are there any gaps in the information available and the information that your patients

need? Are there standardized patient/client education materials available, or does each unit use something different?

ANALYSIS AND SYNTHESIS EXERCISES

1. Think of an individual that you have worked with or who may be a part of your circle of family or friends who has successfully managed to change their health behaviors and has sustained the change over a year or more. What was it that assisted them to make the change? If you do not know of anyone who has successfully changed health behaviors, think of someone who has attempted change. Why do you think they were not successful?

2. Interview a leader of a CDSMP (you can often find one by doing a search online for leaders in your area). Ask them about their background. Are they a health care provider or a lay person? Ask them about the program and why they chose to become a leader. What role do you see the CNS having in support of a CDSMP group?

3. Look at the patient/client education materials in your facility. Do a SMOG analysis and a Fleish-Kincaid analysis of the grade level of the materials. Do your materials meet the standard? What would need to be done to make them meet the standard?

REFERENCES

Ament, L. (2008). Getting patients to follow treatment plans is challenging, costly. *Hospitals and Health Networks*, April. Retrieved February 11, 2009, from http://www.hhnmag.com/hhnmag_app/jsp/articledisplay.jsp?dcrpath=HHNMAG/Article/data/04APR2008/0804HHN_InBox_DisMgt&domain=HHNMAG

Bandura A. (1977). Self-efficacy: Toward a unifying theory of behavior change. *Psychology Review, 84*, 191–215.

Bruce, B., Lorig, K., & Laurent, D. (2007). Participation in patient self-management programs. *Arthritis and Rheumatism, 57*(5), 851–854.

Chew, L. D., Bradley, K. A., & Boyko, E. J. (2004). Brief questions to identify patients with inadequate health literacy. *Family Medicine, 36*(8), 588–594.

Doak, C. C., Doak, L. G., & Root, J. H. (1985). *Teaching patients with low literacy skills*. Philadelphia: J. B. Lippincott.

Goudreau, K. A, Geiselman, J., Sutterer, W., Tarvin, L., Toothaker, A., Pincock, L., et al. (2008). Economics of standardized patient education materials with veteran patients. *Nursing Economic$, 2*(26), 111–115, 121.

Hall, D., & Finegood, K. (2006). *Motivational interviewing: Enhancing readiness to change*. Retrieved December 29, 2008, from http://www.nadcp.org/preconference/Pre-Conf_Motivational_Interviewing.pdf

Institute for Healthcare Improvement & Institute of Medicine. (2004). Health literacy: A prescription to end confusion. In L. Nielsen-Bohlman, A. M. Panzer, & D. A. Kindig (Eds.), *Institute of Medicine Committee on Health Literacy*. Washington, DC: National Academies Press.

Kennedy, A., Reeves, D., Bower, P., Lee, V., Middleton, E., Richardson, G., et al. (2007). The effectiveness and cost effectiveness of a national lay-led self care support programme for patients with long-term conditions: A pragmatic randomised controlled trial. *Journal of Epidemiology and Community Health, 61*(3), 254–261.

Kirsch, I., Jungeblut, A., Jenkins, L., & Kolstad, A. (1993). *Adult literacy in America: A first look at the findings of the National Adult Literacy Survey. Publication #9375*. Washington, DC: National Center for Education Statistics, U.S. Department of Education.

London, F. (1995). Teach your patients faster and better. *Nursing, 95*(August), 68, 70.

London, F. (1997). Return demonstrations: How to validate patient education. *Nursing, 97*(February), 32j.

Lorig, K. R. (2001). *Patient education: A practical approach* (3rd ed.). Thousand Oaks: Sage.

Lorig, K. R., Ritter, P. L., Laurent, D. D., & Plant, K. (2006). Internet-based chronic disease self-management: A randomized trial. *Medical Care, 44*(11), 964–971.

Mayer, G., & Villaire, M. (2004). Low health literacy and its effectives on patient care. *Journal of Nursing Administration, 34*(10), 440–442.

McLaughlin, G. (1996). SMOG grading—A new readability formula. *Journal of Reading, 12*(8), 639–646.

Miller, G. (1957). The magical number seven, plus or minus two, some limits on our capacity for processing information. *Psychological Review, 63*, 81–97.

Miller, W. R., & Rollnick, S. (2002). *Motivational interviewing: Preparing people for change* (pp. 201–216). New York: Guilford Press.

National Association of Clinical Nurse Specialists. (2004). *Statement on clinical nurse specialist practice and education* (2nd ed.). Harrisburg, PA: Author.

National Center for Education Statistics. (2003). *National survey of adult literacy*. Retrieved February 11, 2009, from http://nces.ed.gov/pubsearch/pubsinfo.asp?pubid=2007469

Nolte, S., Elsworth, G. R., Sinclair, A. J., & Osborne, R. H. (2007). The extent and breadth of benefits from participating in chronic disease self-management courses: A national patient-reported outcomes survey. *Patient Education and Counseling, 65*(3), 351–360.

Prochaska, J. O., & DiClemente, C. C. (1983). Stages and processes of self-change of smoking: Toward an integrative model of change. *Journal of Consulting and Clinical Psychology, 51*(3), 390–395.

Rollnick, S. R., Miller, W. R., & Butler, C. C. (2008). *Motivational interviewing in health care: Helping patients change behavior*. New York: Guilford Press.

Rosenstock I., Strecher, V., & Becker, M. (1994). The Health Belief Model and HIV risk behavior change. In R. J. DiClemente & J. L. Peterson (Eds.), *Preventing AIDS: Theories and methods of behavioral interventions* (pp. 5–24). New York: Plenum Press.

Rothman, A. A., & Wagner, E. H. (2003). Chronic illness management: What is the role of primary care? *Annals of Internal Medicine, 138*, 256–261.

Schwartzenberg, J. G., Cowett, A., Van Geest, J., & Wolf, M. S. (2007). Communication techniques for patients with low health literacy: A survey of physicians, nurses and pharmacists. *American Journal of Health Behavior, 31*(Suppl.1), S96–S104.

Seligman, H. K., Wallace, A. S., DeWalt, D. A., Schillinger, D., Arnold, C. L., Shilliday, B. B., et al. (2007). Facilitating behavior change with low literacy patient education materials. *American Journal of Health Behavior, 31*(Suppl. 1), S69–S78.

The Joint Commission Standards. (2008). Retrieved December 3, 2008, from http://www.jointcommission.org/NR/rdon lyres/F53D5057–5349–4391–9DB9-E7F086873D46/0/health_ literacy_exec_summary.pdf (p. 6).

Toofany, S. (2007). Learning the language of health. *Nursing Management, 14*(6), 10–14.

Turner, S. L., Thomas, A. M., Wagner, P. J., & Moseley, G. C. (2008). A collaborative approach to wellness: Diet, exercise and education to impact behavior change. *Journal of the American Academy of Nurse Practitioners, 20,* 339–344.

U.S. Department of Health and Human Services. (2000a). *Healthy People 2010: Understanding and improving health.* Retrieved December 3, 2008, from http://www.healthypeople.gov/document/pdf/uih/2010uih.pdf

U.S. Department of Health and Human Services. (2000b). *Health literacy, January 1990 through 1999.* NLM Pub. No. CBM 2000–1. Bethesda, MD: NLM. Retrieved December 29, 2008, from http://www.healthypeople.gov/document/HTML/Volume1/11HealthCom.htm#_Toc490471350

Wagner, E. H., Bennett, S. M., Austin, B. T., Greene, S. M., Schaefer, J. K., & Vonkorff, M. (2005). Finding common ground: Patient centeredness and evidence based chronic illness care. *The Journal of Alternative and Complimentary Medicine, 11*(Suppl. 1), S7–S15.

The Business of Clinical Nurse Specialist Practice

Consultation in the Clinical Nurse Specialist Role

Geraldine S. Pearson

Consultation has been a central component of the clinical nurse specialist (CNS) role since the role was first identified in the 1950s and implemented as part of specialty role designation. It is prominently identified in the newest competencies proposed for CNSs by the National Association of Clinical Nurse Specialists (NACNS; 2004). Historically, nurses prepared at the master's level as specialists in clinical nursing were seen as part of a movement to improve care. Peplau (1965), Reiter (1966), and Smoyak (1976) all wrote about specialized clinical preparation as an additional educational component of traditional nursing education. Consultation was an integral part of this expanded nursing role and remains one of the core competencies of the CNS role. Defined as the indirect provision of care through helping others implement change, the process of CNS consultation has reflected the tumultuous fiscal and professional pressures that nursing in general has faced. These pressures include managed care and reimbursement issues, funding streams, erosion of the value placed on the CNS role, and the inherent difficulty capturing the essence of the CNS role, especially with regard to consultative activities and outcome measures. For CNSs the purpose of consultation is to implement a unit of change that will result, either directly or indirectly, in improved health care. The CNS consultant may deal with various systems, including educational, health care, and corporate environments. Consultation may be case specific to an individual, group specific to staff or patients, or system specific. Consultation is often integrated into direct care roles and occurs in all specialties of advanced practice nursing. Some aspect of consultation is usually central to the functioning of a CNS regardless of the nursing practice specialty.

Many theorists, both in nursing and in other disciplines, have identified the structure and process of consultation with distinct boundaries and rules. In reality, consultation activities, like much of the CNS role, have evolved and changed, often to fit the CNS practice situation. Berragan (1998) noted that consultation in nursing appears to follow two trends: "external or independent consultancy where the incumbents focus purely upon this role as their 'job,' and internal consultation where consultancy is seen as an integral part of their role and is a subrole of the advanced practitioner" (p. 139). These two trends are applicable to the consultation roles taken by CNSs in the current health care system. Barron and White (2009) advocate differentiating clinical consultation from other CNS roles involving comanagement, referral, and supervision. Their algorithmic model carefully details the process of consultation from request to consultative intervention and assessment.

It is impossible to underestimate the influence of third-party reimbursement and fiscal restraints on the CNS consultation role, at least as it was originally conceptualized. The fiscal constraints on the CNS role, including the need for direct third-party reimbursement, have had a significant impact on role continuation and development. Many CNSs have compromised with the fiscal pressures or the systems where they practice and incorporate the consultative process into other aspects of their work that are more likely to result in third-party reimbursement.

In spite of the financial complexities of continuing to do consultation as the predominant part of a CNS's job, most nurses in a CNS role would cite consultation as the arena where they have the most impact on a changing health care system. It is the area of work where all the skills possessed by a CNS are called into play and actively used as part of a consultation process.

The CNS role requires knowledge, expertise, and experience in an area of specialty practice. Consultation evolves out of the evidenced expert knowledge base of a CNS who knows how to practice and how to improve situations through indirect application of expertise. This chapter reviews the historical development of consultation in CNS practice, conceptual models of consultation, and outcome measures pertaining to efficacy of the consultative role.

HISTORICAL PERSPECTIVE

The role of consultant is rooted in specialty practice, which, in turn, has been the hallmark of the CNS role. The 1960s saw an increase in graduate nursing programs that trained nurses in specialty fields. This trend continued into the 1970s and was influenced dramatically by the federal funding available to nurses who went on to graduate study (Hoeffer & Murphy, 1984). By 1980, the American Nurses Association (ANA) had issued a social policy statement that defined specialization in nursing for its nursing members and community constituents. From here developed the Council of Clinical Nurse Specialists, which first met in 1983 and became a forum for CNSs, their developing role, and their evolution within specialty practice. The entry level for CNS practice is a graduate nursing degree originally defined with key components of educational content in theory, clinical practice, and research (Field, 1983). Course content around the consultation role was generally embedded in the clinical practice aspect of educational preparation.

Barron (1989) noted that consultation has historically been an essential part of the CNS role. The key types of consultation are divided into expert, resource, and process consultation. The expert is seen as having unique skills necessary to prescribe specific solutions to problems in specific situations. In contrast is the resource consultant, who provides relevant information allowing the consultee to choose alternative solutions (Sparacino & Cooper, 1990). The third type of consultation, involving process, initiates changes in situations that allow the consultee to make decisions applicable to this situation and ones in the future (Kohnke, 1978).

Historically, Berragan (1998) suggested that nurses, in the early years of the CNS role, were reluctant to take on the role of consultant. She suggested that this was rooted in a lack of suitable role models and nurses questionable need for consultation. Chinn and Wheeler

(1985) suggested that consultation models in nursing were impeded because of the perceived inferiority of nursing when compared to medicine. It was also suggested that the consultation role development was rooted in the development of nursing knowledge within the framework of womens' positions within a largely patriarchal medical system (Hagell, 1989).

In the 1970s and 1980s, the consultation role in nursing was promoted in the United States, specifically for advanced practice nurses and CNSs (Blake, 1977; Lareau, 1980). In Britain, Wright and Pearson (in Marr, 1993) began the nurse consultant role in the 1980s in nursing development units. Wright (1991) and Marr (1993) began the work in Britain at the same time that Braddock and Sawyer (1985) were defining nurse consultation in the United States, and Keane (1989) was describing similar role development in Australia.

Fenton (1985, p. 33) further developed Benner's model of expert nursing practice (1984) by defining the consulting role as a specific domain of CNS practice. She noted that this aspect of the CNS role included:

■ Providing patient care consultation to the nursing staff through direct patient intervention and follow-up;
■ Interpreting the role of nursing in specific clinical patient care situations to nursing and other professional staff; and
■ Providing patient advocacy by sensitizing staff to the dilemmas faced by patients and families seeking health care.

Fenton's early descriptors of the consultation aspect of the CNS role are one of the few that directly identify advocacy as an important component to consultation. As such, the provision of improved patient care is the goal of a consultative process whether through direct or indirect means.

Currently, consultation is one of the core competencies for CNSs (NACNS, 2004) and is prominently noted to be part of revised competencies. Consultation is accomplished within three spheres of influence, including patient/family, nursing personnel, and organizational systems (NACNS, 2004). The CNS is both a resource and a process consultant (Klein, 2007).

As a resource consultant, CNSs provide relevant information that enables the staff nurse and others to make decisions based on alternatives. As a process consultant, the CNS facilitates change so that decisions can be made in specific and future situations. "CNS consultation can be measured by outcome achievement and documentation of specific process activities" (Klein, 2007, p. 13).

Klein notes that consultation can be both internal (within the institution) or external (outside the institution). External consultation can involve specialty organizations, other health care providers, or other health care systems (Klein, 2007).

In current practice, the consultation provided by a CNS of any specialty is complex, complicated, elegant, astute, and powerfully effective in transitioning systems of care. Most often integrated into a broader CNS role, consultation continues to be a hallmark of CNS practice with the ultimate aim of improving patient care.

CONCEPTUAL MODELS OF CONSULTATION

Hamric and Spross (1989) defined *consultation* as an interactional process occurring between two professionals trying to solve a problem. Most consultation is based on a problem-solving approach. Lippitt and Lippitt (1978) note that "the ultimate goal of consultation is learning, change, and growth" (p. 130).

Certainly one of the first nursing theorists to touch on the consultative practice of the CNS, at least indirectly, was Patricia Benner (1984). Her research on clinical expertise identified seven domains of practice defining the process of clinical judgment. These include: the helping role, administering and monitoring therapeutic interventions and regimens, effective management of rapidly changing situations, the diagnostic and monitoring functions, the teaching–coaching function, monitoring and ensuring the quality of health care practices, and organizational and work role competencies. The process of consultation is embedded in each domain. Inherent in a consultation practice is clinically expert knowledge about a particular disease entity or population of people (Spross & Baggerly, 1989). Benner would likely view nurses at the expert level of practice as embodying the characteristics necessary to be a nurse consultant.

Barron and White (2009; in the newest edition of Hamric, Spross, and Hanson [Eds.], *Advanced Practice Nursing: An Integrative Approach*) defined the distinct differences between the processes of consultation, collaboration, comanagement, and referral. Consultation is distinguished by the degree to which the nurse assumes direct responsibility for clinical management. Consultants are generally not responsible for the direct management of the clinical dilemma for which they are consulting. If they become responsible for the direct clinical intervention, then the process moves away from consultation and into comanagement or supervision. The consultee assumes responsibility for the clinical outcomes and is free to use or not use the advice offered by the consultant.

Approaches to consultation are varied and may be based on specific or multiple theoretical structures. Also, in the current practice arena for CNSs, consultation is less likely to be bounded to strict rules and structures and more apt to ebb and flow with the clinical work inherent in the CNS role. This is influenced by utilization of resources, reimbursement for services, and workforce needs. Few health care systems have the luxury of employing a CNS who does only consultation. Most CNSs integrate consultation into other core competencies of the role.

Gerald Caplan is best known for his model of mental health consultation rooted in his work in Israel in 1949 when, as a child psychiatrist, he was faced with the mental health needs of 16,000 immigrant children. He believed that a traditional model of referral, diagnosis, and psychotherapy of individual children was not possible. As a response he developed an indirect service model of consultation with colleagues caring for groups of children. Eventually his model was used by nurses and clergy, and it has become the framework for mental health consultation used by many disciplines (Caplan, Caplan, & Erchul, 1995).

Caplan (1970) defined consultation as a process in which a specialist's help is sought to identify ways of system or work problems. He advocated for the following principles:

- Guide the development of consultation by understanding its ecological field.
- Explicate all consultation contracts.
- Keep the consultant relationship noncoercive.
- Promote consultee-centered consultation.
- Avoid uncovering types of psychotherapy.
- Use the displacement object.
- Foster orderly reflection.
- Widen frames of reference.
- Train those who consult to be consultants. (Caplan et al., 1995, pp. 25–26)

Caplan and Caplan (1993) also conceptualized four models for consultation. These included client-centered case consultation, consultee-centered case consultation, program-centered administrative consultation, and consultee-centered administrative approach. Differences in individual or system define the specific consultation model.

While Caplan's model has been used widely in school environments, many CNSs, especially those working in psychiatric settings, use his principles to guide their consultation work. Caplan et al. (1995) emphasized that consultation is only one part of a "larger conceptual framework designed to prevent mental illness and promote mental health in the population at large" (p. 30). His model also tends to be more structured in terms of consultative role and behavior than the roles taken by CNSs. Caplan's major premise has great applicability to nursing practice. He maintains that consultation is only one piece of a larger conceptual framework aimed at preventing mental illness and promoting mental health. Similarly, CNSs involved with nonpsychiatric specialty areas are likely to see consultation as one part of their role.

In the early decades of the CNS role, there was much debate about the consultative role being a primary or subrole for CNSs. It was argued that consultation was the foundation for the educator, researcher, and clinician roles that make up the CNS components of functioning (Noll, 1987). Currently, most would agree that the process and function of consultation is integrated into all aspects of the CNS role.

Alvarez (1990) described developmental stages of consultative relationships of psychiatric CNSs in non-acute settings. They were seen as testing via crisis referrals, referrals by a few psychologically minded staff, widening islands of staff support, regular inservices and increasing visibility, regular referrals and active working relationships, and skilled staff using the consultant as a source of education and support for staff-generated interventions.

Blake and Mouton (1983) proposed an organizational consultative model used by many nurses. It involved a definition of four focal issues (power/authority, morale/cohesion, norms/standards, and goals/objectives) and their interdependence. Defining change in one focal issue influences functioning in the other issues. Interventions were planned accordingly and included the following categories: acceptant, catalytic, confrontation, prescription, and theories and principles.

The most evolved descriptions of the CNS consultation role have come from Barron (1989) and Barron and White (2009). They wrote about the CNS as consultant and outlined the steps needed to facilitate this process. Modeled along the nursing assessment, they included assessment, planning the intervention, the intervention, and evaluation/closure. Barron advocated for an organizational assessment whenever a CNS consultant entered a system. She also identified establishing relationships and negotiating roles with administrators, physicians, and other professionals as essential to the process. Establishment of credibility involves fostering effective mutual relationships with consultees that ultimately allows the CNS "to offer practical, theoretically sound, successful problem-solving strategies and clinical expertise" (p. 137). Barron and White (2009) defined an ecological model of CNS consultation that considered characteristics of the nurse consultant, characteristics of the consultee, patient and family factors, and situational factors. Formal and informal consultation and various consultation situations can include CNS to CNS, CNS to physician, and CNS to staff nurse consultations.

SPECIALTY DIFFERENCES IN CNS CONSULTATION

Many specialty areas of nursing have developed strong CNS components and role development. These include pediatrics, oncology, cardiology, internal medicine, community health, and psychiatry.

The specialty of psychiatric nursing has been cited as the first to develop curriculum-specific education around the consultation role. In 1946, with the passage of the National Mental Health Act, research and training funds were given to the core mental health disciplines (Hamric, 1989). The designation of psychiatric nursing as one of these core disciplines furthered the scope of psychiatric nursing education and practice and likely fostered the early development of the CNS role specifically aimed at psychiatric consultation liaison nursing.

Psychiatric consultation liaison nurses (PCLNs) often serve as systems' consultants in their work settings, using systems theory to assess feelings, motivations, and interactions with others. The goals are often to resolve interpersonal difficulties and conflicts among staff and to facilitate change. The ultimate goals are improved outcomes and better patient care (Robinette, 1996).

The PCLN role is well-defined in the literature as a role taken by nurses who have both psychiatric/mental health and medical-surgical experience. They practice mostly in medical-surgical inpatient or outpatient settings and long-term care facilities (Happell & Sharrock, 2001; Minarik & Neese, 2002).

OUTCOME EVALUATION OF CNS CONSULTATION

Because the consultation role of the CNS is often integrated into other work tasks and is sometimes difficult to quantify, many have struggled with measuring outcome. In spite of these difficulties, it is essential that the aspects of CNS practice that result in change be measurable and quantifiable to illustrate their value to the individuals and organizations that fund the practice. Prevost (2002) noted that CNSs can demonstrate cost-effectiveness by understanding the data elements that define changes. These can include admission rates, average lengths of stay, rates of complication, numbers of educational consultation requests, employee turnover rates, and rates of infection. Measuring the outcome means understanding exactly what is to be measured to gauge change or improvement.

Oermann and Floyd (2002) identified a comprehensive outcome model that included clinical, functional, costs, and satisfaction. They see outcome studies as complimentary to evidence-based practice. Findings are integrated into practice and subsequent outcome studies "validate the effectiveness of those interventions and confirm whether they continue to work over time" (p. 142). Prevost (2002) emphasized the need to quantify clinical expertise and to justify the CNS role by measuring, communicating, and marketing effectiveness, impact, or outcome.

The concept of outcome has become increasingly important in this fiscally driven health care environment. Consultation activities of the CNS are especially subject to scrutiny because many of these clinical activities are difficult to quantify or measure. Consultation is a specialized nursing intervention with focus on various systems. Yakimo (2006) has written about measuring outcomes in psychiatric consultation liaison nursing, noting that little attention has been paid to outcomes in this area of specialization. This is likely true in other subspecialties of CNS.

Yakimo, Kurlowicz, and Murray (2004) reviewed PCLN studies that illustrated effective interventions by CNSs acting in a consultative role. These included reduction of demanding patients' requests of staff nurses' time (Mallory, Lyons, Scherubel, & Reichelt, 1993), decreasing length of stay associated with untreated mental health issues (Ragaisis, 1996), and identifying and treating delirium and depression in the elderly (Kurlowicz, 2001).

Yakimo (2006) has advocated for a broader emphasis on comprehensive outcome dimensions relating to the patient and family, the provider, and the institution. The Donabedian model of health care delivery suggests that there are three sources of evidence from which quality can be determined: structure, process, and outcome (Donabedian, 1966, 1980). Yakimo and others (2004) advocate using a systematic model to evaluate the outcome of consultative activities. Types of outcome include clinical, psychosocial, functional, fiscal, and satisfaction. Oermann and Floyd (2002) note that advanced practice nurses are in the best position to conduct the outcome studies demonstrating the effectiveness of their practice.

Brooten and Naylor (1995) have questioned whether or not traditionally measured outcomes are sensitive enough to evaluate nursing actions. This has particular implications for nurse consultation activities, often integrated into other aspects of nursing practice, difficult to quantify and measure.

This issue is applicable to more recent literature. Fairley and Closs (2006), in their study evaluating a nurse consultant's clinical activities and the effect on patient outcomes, note that clinical activities were complex processes involving clinical judgment and decision making. They found it difficult to pinpoint the exact activities that resulted in their definition of patient care success: "a state free from risk or harm that optimizes rehabilitation" (p. 1113).

SUMMARY

The consultation aspect of the CNS role has evolved and grown into a well-accepted, essential part of advanced nursing practice. The nursing literature is filled with descriptive papers and anecdotes about successful nursing consultations at all subspecialties of CNS practice. It is more difficult to find research-based evidence about the efficacy of the role, probably because it is very difficult to measure the outcome of consultation.

Nearly all CNSs engage in some process of consultation as part of their nursing role. The groups and individuals who have benefited from the process of consultation do not question the utility of CNS consultation. The complexity of the consultation role assumed by CNSs has evolved in direct proportion to the development of the total role. CNSs in a variety of specialty practice arenas use consultation as part of their daily work. Most engage in consultation as part of their more multidimensional CNS role.

There is increasing pressure on nurses who provide consultation to identify and measure the direct impact of the intervention, especially as it relates to reducing health care costs. It is essential that nurses engaged in consultation begin systematically measuring the effect of this intervention. At no other time in the history of the consultative role has this been more essential. By illustrating the value of the activity in measurable terms, nurses will ensure that they can continue offering the creative, dynamic, thoughtful consultative activities that directly and indirectly improve and enhance patient care.

DISCUSSION QUESTIONS

1. What role does consultation have in current CNS practice?
2. Can a CNS practice without incorporating consultation in their role?
3. How does consultation differ across specialties of CNS roles?
4. What is the advantage of adhering strictly to a theoretical model of consultation versus developing a version that fits the practice, situation, and needs of the consultee?
5. When, after receiving nursing education, is a CNS able to provide effective consultation? What factors influence this?
6. What are the pitfalls of offering consultation?
7. How does a CNS integrate the other aspects of functioning, such as direct care or teaching, with a consultation role? Identify the positives and negatives of this when all parts of the role are integrated in the same setting.
8. How does the CNS build in the research component to their consultative practice that builds an evidence-based practice and justifies the consultation?
9. What administrative and clinical supports are required by a CNS in order to offer consultation?

ANALYSIS AND SYNTHESIS

1. Choose one description of a CNS consultation in literature from the past 3 years. Evaluate the paper from the perspective of use of a theoretical model, role description, and incorporation of evaluation that is measurable and determines effectiveness.
2. Evaluate the clinical practices of five CNSs. Query them about the role of consultation in their work and the ways they measure their effectiveness.

CLINICAL APPLICATIONS

1. Observe a consultation conducted by a CNS. Note the following:

   ■ How did the consultation begin? Did it have a discreet beginning, or was it integrated into the CNS role?
   ■ What was the predominant question from the consultee?
   ■ What theoretical model did the CNS use while conducting the consultation?
   ■ How did the consultation fit into the CNS role and the setting?

2. Develop a consultation project in a clinical setting where you are practicing. Include the following:

   ■ Identify the individuals requesting the consultation (consultees).
   ■ Listen to the request for consultation. Is it related to an educational need, a clinical problem, a staffing problem, or another issue influencing care?
   ■ Develop a plan for providing the consultation, including the consultee in the process.
   ■ Ascertain the evaluation of the consultation, identifying measurable goals and objectives while quantifying whether or not the consultation accomplished original goals of the process.

STEPS TO CNS CONSULTATION

1. Request for consultation is received.
   a. Define the type of consultation requested (consultee-centered, patient-centered, program-centered).
   b. Define the role of the individuals requesting the consultation.
   c. Assess the issues involved.
   d. Decide whether or not consultation can be provided.
2. CNS agrees to conduct the consultation.
   a. Define the question and the issues.
   b. Define the recipients of the consultation.

   c. Define the intervention that could potentially come from the consultation.
3. Consultation is provided.
   a. Document process and progress.
   b. Determine need for follow-up.
4. Evaluate outcome of consultation.

Adapted from Barron and White (2009)

CASE STUDY OF CONSULTATION PROCESS FOR CHILD AND ADOLESCENT PSYCHIATRIC CNS

Jane is a CNS working on an inpatient child unit in a large metropolitan hospital. The average length of stay on the unit is 7 days, and the average age of the child patients is 10 years. The head nurse for the unit, Tim, requests a consultation about a particular staff person with whom he is "struggling." Jane determines that this is a consultation to the head nurse about a program- (staff-) centered issue. The head nurse will be using Jane's consultation to better provide supervision to the staff nurse. Jane will have no role in any formal intervention with the staff person.

After establishing the process of the consultation and their roles, the consultation begins. Tim begins to define his difficulties with the staff nurse and the way this individual interacts with very young children on the unit. As he talks about his observations, he also shares his self-doubts, and his concerns that he is overreacting to what he is observing.

Jane asked Tim to define the role expectations for the staff nurse and to think about the ways this staff person was meeting these expectations. She also asked Tim to think about why he was hesitant to confront this particular staff. He shared that the individual's age and long experience was in direct contrast to his relative newness to the head nurse role. Jane and Tim looked at what he brought to the role and discussed ways of supervising the staff so she would have more positive interactions with the younger patients on the unit.

One week later, when Jane and Tim spoke again, he indicated that the supervision process had gone "much better" with this person and that the consultation helped him. Jane documented the consultation and filed it. She made sure Tim knew he could use her consultative expertise in the future with other unit issues.

REFERENCES

Alvarez, C. A. (1990). The psychiatric clinical nurse specialist in the non-acute setting. In P. S. A. Sparacino, D. M. Cooper, & P. A. Minarik (Eds.), *The clinical nurse specialist: Implementation and impact* (pp. 145–162). East Norwalk, CT: Appleton & Lange.

American Nurses Association. (1980). *Nursing: A social policy statement.* Kansas City, MO: Author.

Benner, P. (1984). *From novice to expert: Excellence and power in clinical nursing practice.* Upper Saddle River, NJ: Prentice Hall.

Barron, A. M. (1989). The CNS as consultant. In A. B. Hamric & J. A. Spross (Eds.), *The clinical nurse specialist in theory and practice* (2nd ed., pp. 125–146). Philadelphia: W. B. Saunders.

Barron, A. M., & White, P. A. (2009). Consultation. In A. B. Hamric, J. A. Spross, & C. M. Hanson, (Eds.), *Advanced practice nursing: An integrative approach* (4th ed., pp. 191–216). St. Louis: Elsevier.

Berragan, L. (1998). Nursing practice draws upon several different ways of knowing. *Journal of Clinical Nursing, 7*(3), 209–217.

Blake, P. (1977). The clinical specialist as nurse consultant. *Journal of Nursing Administration, 7*(10), 33–36.

Blake, R. R., & Mouton, J. S. (1983). *Consultation: A handbook for individual and organizational development* (2nd ed.). Reading, MA: Addison Wesley.

Braddock, B., & Sawyer, D. (1985). Becoming an independent consultant. *Nursing Economics, 3*(6), 332–335.

Brooten, D., & Naylor, M. (1995). Nurses' effect on changing patient outcomes. *Image, 27,* 95–99.

Caplan, G. (1970). *The theory and practice of mental health consultation.* New York: Basic.

Caplan, G., & Caplan, R. B. (1993). *Mental health consultation and collaboration.* San Francisco: Jossey-Bass.

Caplan, G., Caplan, R. B., & Erchul, W. P. (1995). A contemporary view of mental health consultation: Comments on "Types of Mental Health Consultation" by Gerald Caplan (1963). *Journal of Educational and Psychological Consultation, 6,* 23–30.

Chinn, P. L., & Wheeler, C. E. (1985). Feminism and nursing. *Nursing Outlook, 33*(2), 74–77.

Donabedian, A. (1966). Evaluating the quality of medical care. *Milbank Member Fund Quarterly, 44*(3, Suppl.), 166–206.

Donabedian, A. (1980). Methods for deriving criteria for assessing the quality of medical care. *Medical Care Research and Review, 37*(7), 653–698.

Fairley, D., & Closs, S. J. (2006). Evaluation of a nurse consultant's clinical activities and the search for patient outcomes in critical care. *Journal of Clinical Nursing, 15,* 1106–1114.

Fenton, M. V. (1985). Identifying competencies of clinical nurse specialists. *Journal of Nursing Administration, 15,* 31–37.

Field, L. (1983). Current trends in education and implications for the future. In A. B. Hamric & J. Spross (Eds.), *The clinical nurse specialist in theory and practice.* New York: Grune & Stratton.

Hagell, E. I. (1989). Nursing knowledge: Women's knowledge. A sociological perspective. *Journal of Advanced Nursing, 14*(3), 226–233.

Hamric, A. (1989). History and overview of the CNS role. In A. Hamric & J. Spross (Eds.), *The clinical specialist in theory and practice* (pp. 3–18). Orlando, FL: Grune & Stratton.

Hamric, A. B., & Spross, J. A. (1989). *The clinical nurse specialist in theory and practice* (2nd ed.). Philadelphia: W. B. Saunders.

Happell, B., & Sharrock, J. (2001). The psychiatric consultation-liaison nurse: Towards articulating a model for practice. *Journal of Psychiatric and Mental Health Nursing, 8,* 411–417.

Hoeffer, B., & Murphy, S. A. (1984). *Specialization in nursing practice.* Kansas City, MO: American Nurses Association.

Klein, D. G. (2007). From novice to expert. In M. G. McKinley, (Ed.), *Acute and critical care clinical nurse specialists: Synergy for best practices* (pp. 11–28). St. Louis: Saunders.

Kohnke, M. (1978). *Case for consultation in nursing: Designs for professional practice.* New York: Wiley.

Kurlowicz, L. H. (2001). Benefits of psychiatric consultation-liaison nurse interventions for older hospitalized patients and their nurses. *Archives of Psychiatric Nursing, 15*(2), 53–61.

Lareau, S. C. (1980). The nurse as clinical consultant. *Topics in Clinical Nursing, 2*(3), 79–84.

Lippitt, G., & Lippitt, R. (1978). *The consulting process in action.* San Diego: University Associates.

Mallory, G. A., Lyons, J. S., Scherubel, J. C., & Reichelt, P. A. (1993). Nursing care hours of patients receiving varying amounts and types of consultation/liaison services. *Archives of Psychiatric Nursing, 7*(6), 353–360.

Marr, J. F. (1993). Consultant nurse. *Surgical Nurse, 6,* 25–26.

Minarik, P. A., & Neese, J. B. (2002). Essential educational content for advanced practice in psychiatric consultation liaison nursing. *Archives of Psychiatric Nursing, 16*(1), 3–15.

National Association of Clinical Nurse Specialists. (2004). *Statement on clinical nurse specialist practice and education* (2nd ed.). Harrisburg, PA: Author.

Noll, M. (1987). Internal consultation as a framework for clinical nurse specialist practice. *Clinical Nurse Specialist, 1,* 46–50.

Oermann, M. H., & Floyd, J. A. (2002). Outcomes research: An essential component of the advanced practice nurse role. *Clinical Nurse Specialist, 16*(3), 140–144.

Peplau, H. E. (1965). The nurse in the community mental health program. *Nursing Outlook, 13*(11), 68–70.

Prevost, S. S. (2002). Clinical nurse specialist outcomes: Vision, voice, and value. *Clinical Nurse Specialist, 16*(3), 119–124.

Ragaisis, K. M. (1996). The psychiatric consultation-liaison nurse and medical family therapy. *Clinical Nurse Specialist, 10*(1), 50–56.

Reiter, F. (1966). The nurse-clinician. *American Journal of Nursing, 66*(2), 274–280.

Robinette, A. L. (1996). PCLN's: Who are they? How can they help you? *American Journal of Nursing, 96*(7), 48–50.

Smoyak, S. A. (1976). Specialization in nursing: From then to now. *Nursing Outlook, 24*(11), 676–681.

Sparacino, P.S.A., & Cooper, D. M. (1990). The role components. In P.S.A. Sparacino, D. M. Coooper, & P. A. Minarik (Eds.), *The clinical nurse specialist: Implementation and impact* (pp. 11–40). East Norwalk, CT: Appleton & Lange.

Spross, J. A., & Baggerly, J. (1989). Models of advanced nursing practice. In A. B. Hamric & J. A. Spross (Eds.). *The clinical nurse specialist in theory and practice* (2nd ed., pp. 19–40). Philadelphia: W. B. Saunders.

Wright, S. (1991). The nurse as consultant. *Nursing Standard, 5,* 31–34.

Yakimo, R. (2006). Outcomes in psychiatric consultation-liaison nursing. *Perspectives in Psychiatric Care, 42*(1), 59–62.

Yakimo, R., Kurlowicz, L. H., & Murray, R. B. (2004). Evaluation of outcomes in psychiatric consultation-liaison nursing practice. *Archives of Psychiatric Nursing, 18*(6), 215–227.

Mentoring

Kelly A. Goudreau

It is the supreme art of the mentor to awaken joy in creative expression and knowledge.

—*Albert Einstein*

The art of mentoring is a complex interchange of give, take, readiness to learn, sensing of readiness to learn, and integration of the learners needs as perceived by both the learner and the mentor. This dynamic dance typically takes place within the context of a one-on-one relationship established between two people: a mentor and his or her protégé. There are other models of mentorship that are described in the literature (Goran, 2001; Grossman, 2007), but the key concept is one of sharing of knowledge and information from one who is more experienced or expert with one who seeks to learn from the expert (Busen & Engebretson, 1999; Yoder, 1990). The definition of mentoring or mentorship is more than just teaching skills, however. It also includes career counseling, guidance, advice, and enhanced opportunities for career advancement as a result of the networks that the mentor has established that assist the protégé. The role of the clinical nurse specialist (CNS) as the expert clinician, guide, and mentor to the experienced and inexperienced nursing staff embodies the best of the concept of mentorship.

Although the concept of mentoring has been in existence for centuries, there is little research-based literature on the topic. The enculturation of the concept as an expectation, however, has occurred in relatively recent history. Over the past 30 years, mentoring was integrated into the stream of consciousness in the business world and has become a construct of the CNS's world. Mentoring is both provided and received by the CNS as he or she develops and grows. The expectation is to return the gift that was provided by a mentor through mentoring the next generation of staff nurses and CNSs as they grow and develop.

The intent of this chapter is to provide an overview of the current state of the literature on mentoring and mentorship, define conceptual models of mentoring and mentorship currently in use, apply these models to CNS practice in a variety of settings, and discuss the current cultural expectation for mentoring and mentorship. Examples of how and why to implement the concept in practical terms is provided.

MENTORSHIP: WHERE DID IT COME FROM?

The concept of mentoring and mentorship is actually derived from Ancient Greek mythology. In the Odyssey, the story purportedly written by Homer (Fitzgerald, 1961), Odysseus (Ulysses) left his young son, Telemachus, in the hands of Mentor, who guided him into becoming a loved and trusted leader in his father's absence. The story brings in elements of Greek mythology through the introduction of the concept that it was not actually a man named Mentor who guided and taught young Telemachus but was in fact the goddess Athena in disguise. The principle is that a more experienced person can provide counsel and guidance to the less experienced person who is learning and growing under the watchful eye of their mentor. According to Peddy (2001), although it has not changed significantly, a more contemporary description of a mentor is "a friend and role model, an able advisor, a person who lends support in many different ways to one pursuing specific goals" (p. 28).

The Roman Catholic Church saw mentoring as an important means of succession planning. The church leaders identified that in order for the church to ensure its continued success, not only did they have to draw in new members but there also needed to be a sense of community. In an effort to achieve that sense of community they established formal mentoring relationships between clergy and community youth. Mentoring was identified as a professional responsibility of all the members of the church. Mentoring young members of the church to become devout practitioners and take the place of the aging clergy provided continued growth and development of the church. Not only was growth achieved but an increased diversification in the ranks of parishioners was attracted to the church as the young of the various populations became church leaders. The church increased its ability to reach out to the widening array of cultures they were attempting to convert.

The concept of mentoring became embedded in the business world for the same reasons articulated by the church. Success of any business rests on planning and growth of the potential pool of candidates for leadership. Succession planning in the face of a shrinking pool of employable personnel is a strong driver of the rationale for mentoring. The same reasons exist currently in nursing.

Current statistics in nursing indicate that by the year 2020 there will be a shortfall of 340,000 available nurses (Hart, 2007; Health Resources and Services Administration, 2006). These statistics are well-known in nursing, and it is not surprising that mentoring and mentorship are key concepts that can play a major role in both recruiting and retaining nurses. Mentoring and mentorship is a primary component in keeping nursing a viable profession for the same key reasons that the church identified:

- Succession planning in a time of shortage,
- Increasing diversity in both culture and age variation in the workplace, and
- The need for a sense of community and professional responsibility.

A variety of so-called mentoring programs have become prevalent in the current age. A number of facilities that hire nurses have developed residency or internship programs with the focused goal of both attracting and retaining new nurses graduating from schools of nursing (Bally, 2007; Hayes & Scott, 2007; Hunnerkopf, 2007; Poynton, Madden, Bowers, & Keefe, 2007). Key to these programs is the relationship that is established between the new graduate and their preceptor/mentor. Expectations for these preceptors do not often extend beyond the relationship with the new graduate and assessment of their competence to provide minimally safe patient care. These skills do not often move beyond the skills of a staff nurse. The preceptors are not mentors in the truest sense of the meaning found in the literature (Grossman, 2007; Yoder, 1990). According to Dracup and Bryan-Brown (2004), "mentors do more than teach

skills; they facilitate new learning experiences, help new nurses make career decisions, and introduce them to networks of colleagues who can provide new professional challenges and opportunities" (p. 450). The overall intent of the residency is to decrease the numbers leaving the profession through development of current registered nurses (RNs) as preceptors or mentors, provision of support to new RNs, and increasing overall satisfaction with the profession through opportunities for growth, development, and collegial relationships for both the mentor and the protégée. The role of the CNS clearly fulfills all of these expectations.

LITERATURE REVIEW

A clear definition of *mentorship* versus *preceptorship* has been the primary confusion within the literature. The concept of mentoring and mentorship as described in this chapter has been clearly defined and articulated by only a few authors (Angelini, 1995; Grossman, 2007; Murray, 2001; Shea, 2001; Stewart & Kreuger, 1996; Yoder, 1990; Yonge, Billay, Myric, & Luhanga, 2007). Most authors on the topic assume that the reader has the same understanding of the concept, and they proceed to describe the relationship as one that is focused on skills attainment. Typically, in U.S. and Canadian literature the relationship focused on skills attainment is called preceptorship rather than mentorship (Grossman, 2007; Yonge et al., 2007). Mentoring and mentorship is most accurately defined as follows:

> Mentoring in nursing encompasses a guided experience, formally or informally assigned, over a mutually agreed-on period, that empowers the mentor and mentee to develop personally and professionally within the auspices of a caring, collaborative, culturally competent, and respectful environment. (Grossman, 2007, p. 28)

There has been tremendous international interest in mentoring recently. This interest, however, has only served to perpetuate the confusion and lack of clarity surrounding the terms *preceptorship* and *mentorship*. The work surrounding the initiation of Project 2000 in the United Kingdom has generated tremendous interest in the process and outcomes of what is being called mentoring and mentorship (Andrews & Wallis, 1999; Hyatt et al., 2008; Moseley & Davies, 2008; Nettleton & Bray, 2008; Webb & Shakespeare, 2008). An additional international discussion on mentoring and mentorship is the Leonardo da Vinci project undertaken in the European Union (Fulton et al., 2007). On closer examination of the articles, however, it is clearly evident that in both instances the articles describe support of the nursing students who are entering the workplace in greater numbers now that the educational institutions are responding to the call for increased enrollment. The articles describe mentorship as a supportive educational environment that links the student with a particular individual who will assess their clinical competency. In the United States, these relationships are more often called preceptorships rather than mentoring relationships.

Although the concept of mentoring and mentorship has existed for literally generations, there has been very little actual research on the topic. Perhaps this is due to the current state of confusion regarding the extent to which the support is provided and the duration of the support. Articles in both the business and nursing literature are most likely to be anecdotal in nature and discuss the "how to" of mentoring rather than assessing research-driven benefits of mentoring (Cahill & Payne, 2006; Tuohig, 2007). In many research-focused articles the concept of mentoring has not been defined clearly, so it is difficult to determine if the research was conducted on mentoring or preceptoring as the concept; there continues to be confusion about the terms (Dyer, 2008; Fulton et al., 2007; Hyatt, Brown, & Lipp, 2008; Moseley & Davies, 2008; Myall, Levett-Jones, & Lathlean, 2008; Nettleton & Bray, 2008; Webb & Shakespeare, 2008; Yoder, 1990).

For purposes of the research review, and application within the advanced practice role, mentoring is defined much as Yoder (1990) and later Grossman (2007) and Yonge and colleagues (2007) defined it and includes a component whereby the mentor specifically works with the protégée to develop a long-term plan for specific personal development in addition to skills development. Areas that need growth are collaboratively identified by both the mentor and the protégée and, in turn, are developed, explored, and expanded. Unfortunately, there is little research that examines this definition and the outcomes of same.

The research that has been done with the broader definition in mind has been structured around the implications of the relationship between the mentor and the protégée and, subsequently, the behaviors that are most conducive to establishing and maintaining the mentoring relationship (Allen, Eby, & Lentz, 2006; Nedd, Nash, Galindo-Ciocon, & Belgrave, 2006; Nickle, 2007). The focus on individual development has been identified as a means to increase personal and professional satisfaction for both the mentor and the protégée (Finley, Ivanitskaya, & Kennedy, 2007). By clearly identifying opportunities for improvement and opportunities for personal development, the mentor and the protégée are collaborative partners, and both have stated they experience personal satisfaction with both the growth and the relationship that develops (Shea, 2001). Although not research-based, Shea blends the concepts of preceptoring and mentoring but distinctly separates them in terms of time and structure. He describes various

stages of the relationship on a continuum ranging from highly structured, short-term relationships (preceptorships) to informal, long-term friendships that are intermittent in nature but are sustained relationships that last from 3 years to a lifetime (mentorships).

Research conducted includes both qualitative and quantitative work (Angelini, 1995; Benner, 1984; Dyer, 2008; Dracup & Bryan-Brown, 2004; Nedd et al., 2006; Nickle, 2007; Schweibert, 2000; Stewart & Kreuger, 1996). Unfortunately, most of the work is survey or self-report in nature and has little academic or scientific rigor. Additionally, there is little that has been done in terms of evaluation of the outcomes of a mentoring relationship (Grossman, 2007).

The work done to date supports the anecdotal perceptions that there is value in the relationship that is largely of an intangible nature but is reported as positive for both the mentor and the protégée (Allen et al., 2006; McKinley, 2004; McWeeny, 2002; Morse, 2006; Robert Wood Johnson Foundation, 2004; Zucker et al., 2006). Further, the relationship that holds the most promise of sustained and positive outcomes are the informal long-term friendships described by Shea (2001; Allen et al., 2006).

CONCEPTUAL AND/OR THEORETICAL SUPPORT FOR MENTORING

The rigorous research that has been conducted has been based on one of three conceptual frameworks or theories. Within nursing, Benner (1984) is the most frequently cited work that supports the perception that an individual can move from being a novice to being an expert under the watchful eye of a guide, or through self-reflection and experiential growth (Nedd et al., 2006). Although this theory provides some strength to the concept of mentoring, it is not specifically focused on the relationships of the novice with the experts in their environment and provides tangential support for the premise that mentoring will strengthen and ensure overall satisfaction with the new role.

The issue of a lack of strong theoretical constructs to support research and researchable outcomes of mentoring and mentorship are also found outside of nursing. Strong theory development was undertaken in the field of psychology, however, and theoretical constructs around mentoring relationships by Kram (1985) suggest that mutual interpersonal appreciation is key to being able to initiate and maintain a mentoring relationship. Kanter's (1977) work on organizational development and individual development also provides theoretical structure to mentoring relationships in the workplace similar to that posited by Kram. These theories are rarely seen within nursing, however.

Finally, the strongest theoretical construct that directly relates to mentoring is that presented by Collins, Brown, and Holum (1991) in their discussion of the theories of a Russian educator, Lev Vygotsky (Nickle, 2007). Collins et al. describe the theory of constructivism as defined by Vygotsky. Vygotsky was a contemporary of Piaget's, but neither man knew of each other due to the fact that the iron curtain separated their research during their lifetimes. What Vygotsky, and later Collins et al. (1991), described is a process where a mentor/teacher/guide assesses the learner's abilities with lower and upper thresholds of comfort. That comfort zone is called the zone of proximal development, and it is the job of the guide and mentor to push the learner to move along the continuum of learning and establish new upper and lower boundaries of comfort and understanding. The guide and mentor sets up a "scaffolding" of support that protects the learner as they initially begin to learn a new process or are placed in a new environment. Gradually, the scaffolding is removed as the mentor assesses that the learner is comfortable and able to perform the duties or interactions without support. This dynamic assessment and release of the learner as they move across the continuum of learning and through the zone of proximal development describes the process of mentoring. The theory of social constructivism emphasizes the interaction of the environment and the social structures that support learning. It truly brings the theories of Benner (1984), Kram (1985), and Kanter (1977) into a dynamic whole that provides a strong foundation for continued research and evaluation of outcomes. It, too, however, has not been strongly introduced into the nursing literature at this time (Nickle, 2007).

APPLICATION TO CNS PRACTICE: HOW TO USE MENTORING IN YOUR ENVIRONMENT

Through the mentoring relationships established in residency programs and orientation, the CNS can have direct influence on welcoming, assessment of strengths, identification of areas needing improvement, and ongoing support that ultimately results in retention of the nursing staff. The theories of Lev Vygotsky and his successors are lived on a daily basis in the role of the CNS in the clinical environment. By welcoming, assessing strengths and areas for improvement, and then supporting the neophyte in the clinical environment, the CNS is a mentor. It is the CNS who constructs the scaffolding around the new nurse and creates the environment in which the learner feels safe to learn. This protection extends not

only to the learner but also to the patients for whom the learner is caring. The expert nurse, in the form of the CNS, is able to not only monitor the learning of the new nurse but also provide the safety net for the patient as the CNS assesses the efficacy of the care provided by the neophyte.

Evidence of the strength of this relationship can be indirectly assessed through the role of the CNS in the magnet movement. CNSs play two pivotal roles in the recent surge of hospitals seeking magnet status: (1) They are the advanced practice nurses (APNs) that are most visible to the staff and provide the support to new nurses as expert clinicians, and (2) they are most often the individuals who manage and coordinate the magnet journey (American Nurses Credentialing Center, 2005; personal communication, Jane Walker, August 28, 2008).

The key elements of magnet where CNSs have the greatest impact or influence are in 5 of the 14 forces: (1) Force 1: Quality of Nursing Leadership; (2) Force 3: Management Style; (3) Force 6: Quality of Care; (4) Force 11: Nurses as Teachers; and (5) Force 14: Professional Development. As a leader on the unit or within the facility, the CNS role models the behaviors of leadership and management. As the expert clinician on the unit or in the specialty area, the CNS has a direct influence on the quality of the nursing care, exemplifies the role of nurses as teachers, and provides a role model for the less experienced nurses. Finally, it is in the professional development force that the CNS has the greatest influence as a mentor.

The three spheres of influence that a CNS functions within are the patient/client sphere, the nursing/nurses sphere, and the systems sphere (National Association of Clinical Nurse Specialists [NACNS], 2004). The one that the CNS has the greatest role as a mentor is within the nursing/nurses sphere of influence. Within the mentor role that the CNS plays, he or she is able to provide the greatest strength to the establishment of clearly defined competencies and evaluation processes to assess whether or not the neophyte has attained these competencies. Regardless of whether or not the initial orientation is called a preceptorship, residency, or internship, the CNS plays a pivotal role. Direct one-on-one interaction in support of both the new and experienced nurses means that the CNS provides a coaching role at the very least and, in many instances, a mentoring relationship with many of the staff over time. This relationship extends not only to the direct relationship with each nurse but also to the creation of a culture of mentoring by all staff. Grossman (2007) noted that in her vision of a mentoring culture in nursing, "clinical nurse specialists . . . may allow a mentoring staff to expand the nursing science base in everyday work with patients" (p. 27). The use of evidence-based practice principles and sharing of the evidence with staff creates a culture of excellence and quality that can only be attributed to the presence of an APN in the clinical environment (LaSala, Connors, Pedro, & Phipps, 2007).

Additional provisions of mentoring in the CNS influence on the nursing/nurses sphere is the mentoring of masters or doctoral students who are becoming CNSs. A component of the CNS role is the expectation that those who are expert in being the expert clinician will share their lessons learned with the neophyte CNS. Mentoring the next generation of APNs is paramount to the continuation of the role and the direct influence on the quality and safety of the patient care.

In either the mentoring of new staff nurses or the mentoring of new CNSs, the role of the experienced CNS is to assess the learning needs of the nurses/ nursing staff and then assist them to move along the continuum of learning within their comfort level and beyond. By stretching the zone of proximal development (Nickle, 2007), the learner moves beyond their current capability under the watchful, supportive eye of the CNS.

According to Lakasing and Francis (2005), the characteristics of the most successful mentors include the following: knowledge of how societal systems, processes, or things work; strong values that are parallel to the institution and the profession; technical competence; strong character that allows and encourages growth in the mentee; knowledge of how to behave in a social situation; understanding of how to get things done in or through the organization; strong moral standards that encourage the development of same in the mentee; and understanding of other people and their viewpoints. Each of these is an essential competency for the successful CNS. These themes have been reiterated in recent work done in the European Union through the MAITRE project (Miller & Storey, 2007). The MAITRE Project (which is an acronym that stands for *M*entoring tr*AI*ning ma*T*erials and *RE*sources) is a research collaborative that is looking at what mentor competencies are and how they can be standardized then measured across multiple disciplines and countries. *Maitre* is a French word that means "master" and is intended to convey that there is a way to master the art of mentoring as well as to be a master of the protégé.

Within the systems sphere of influence and in relation to mentoring, the CNS works collaboratively with the education and/or nursing professional services department to provide system-wide, consistent programs that will encourage and develop nurses and assist them in feeling supported and mentored by their peers and/or by the CNS. Through a thorough needs assessment and day-to-day interaction with the nursing staff, the CNS is often able to identify the broad learning needs for learners and demonstrate to the systems-level education department what the specific learning needs may be across the facility.

EVALUATION OF MENTORING AND MENTORSHIP

Within the NACNS *Statement on Practice and Education* (2004), the one clear outcome that is addressed in relation to mentoring is within the nursing/nurses sphere of influence. Identification of the necessary knowledge and skill development in nurses is a key outcome of CNS practice (NACNS, 2004). It is unfortunate, however, that very few research studies have been conducted to assess this particular outcome for CNSs, or any other discipline for that matter. Most of the information related to mentoring is anecdotal and not research-based at all.

Buddeberg-Fischer and Herta (2006) conducted a literature review within the medical literature in relation to evaluation of formal mentoring programs for medical students and doctors. They identified that only 16 articles met their criteria for inclusion in the study, and none of them discussed evaluation of the programs. Nursing literature is, as previously stated, confused on the definition of mentoring. This confusion creates a situation where some formal evaluations may have been done in relation to preceptor relationships rather than mentoring relationships, which then focus on the short-term attainment of competencies and skills versus the lasting, guiding relationship of a mentorship (Webb & Shakespeare, 2008).

Outside of nursing and health care literature the situation is similar, whereby authors continue to have anecdotal information rather than research-based outcomes assessment. Boldra, Landin, Repta, Westphal, and Winistorfer (2008) identify that the benefits of mentoring include improved retention, leadership development, succession planning, and a sense of increased organizational commitment on the part of the mentees. This has not, however, been substantiated through research.

When evaluation has been research-based, data that has been collected on the evaluation of mentor programs has been descriptive in nature. Most often, when evaluation of a mentor relationship is discussed, regardless of the perception of it being a true mentorship or preceptorship, the data defines the level of satisfaction with the relationship or the program itself (Weiss et al., 2008).

This lack of research data to support the mentor relationship is problematic and needs to be addressed. It is the realm of the CNS to address issues related to the mentoring, coaching, and precepting of new nurses or experienced nurses who have moved into new clinical areas. Perhaps the CNS should lead the way in creation of a sound research process to fully evaluate the outcomes of mentoring, precepting, or coaching and the relative value of each to the organization in which they practice.

ADVANCED NURSING PRACTICE: WHY IS MENTORING AN ADVANCED SKILL?

Regardless of the research base or the anecdotal nature of the perceptions, it is clear that most, both internal or external to the profession, consider mentoring an essential component of current needs to retain and develop personnel. The role of the advanced practice CNS has been defined as an essential element. By being the clinical expert who oversees the quality and safety of the care being provided by the nursing staff and by guiding, coaching, role modeling, and mentoring the staff, the CNS is an element that must be present.

Staff nurses in general do not have the time to mentor other staff nurses. Their role is correctly focused on provision of care to the patient population. They will sometimes assist student nurses or peers who are new to the environment, but typically, if there is something that needs attention beyond the basic assessments, they will refer it to the CNS.

The nurse manager, although they carry advanced skills in leadership and management, is not always the clinical expert. They refer issues of clinical competence to the CNS to address. Through this assessment and referral the CNS can be both the coach/guide and potentially address issues of mentorship with promising new nurses. They work in partnership with both the nurse manager and the staff nurse to assist the further development of staff. Working within the nurses/nursing sphere of influence is an essential component of the CNS role and is clearly an advanced skill.

ETHICAL CONSIDERATIONS

The ethics of mentoring are not often discussed in the literature, yet, there are many instances of the establishment of a code of ethics associated with mentoring. The code of ethics in most instances outlines the need for mutual respect, confidentiality, and boundaries. It is clear that from the outset there is a power differential in the relationship, with the mentor having more power than the protégé. The power differential can be a cause of concern if it is not used appropriately.

Most often the power differential can cause nothing more than blurring of the lines between being a casual friend versus mentor as the relationship is established and maintained over a long period of time. Unfortunately, the power differential can also lead to a

misuse of the relationship for personal gain on the part of the mentor and potentially may even result in the outcome being an inappropriate sexual relationship.

The competence of the mentor is utmost when a mentor/protégé relationship is being considered in either a formal mentoring program or an informal mentored relationship. The mentor has a responsibility to ensure that the protégé has the best opportunity to learn, and that can only be accomplished if the mentor is knowledgeable and can share their expertise and network of connections with the protégé. If the mentor knows that they are not the correct person who can assist and advance the protégé, they need to acknowledge that and step away.

The CNS is in the unique position of being a clinical expert and guide/coach and mentor to many nurses and nursing staff on the unit. He or she can clearly see the current relationships and the dynamics of those relationships. As a clinical expert and guide, the CNS has the responsibility to ensure that any mentor relationships are healthy and bound by ethical precepts. If they are not, the CNS has a moral and ethical responsibility to bring them to the attention of those who can best address the issues. As a guide and role model on the unit, the CNS is expected to have the highest moral and ethical standards and uphold those expectations in the staff on the unit. As such, he or she represents the best of what professional nursing is and can be.

SUMMARY

It is clear from the literature that mentoring is perceived to have many benefits. Benefits that are expressed are that mentoring allows organizations to grow and flourish by: (1) developing, satisfying, and retaining employees; (2) advancing the development of experienced staff by encouraging them to become mentors; (3) improving organizational climate, performance, and image; (4) allowing for the creation of clinical expert networks; and (5) increasing diversity within the discipline.

Although these benefits are not clearly established through research outcomes, the anecdotal benefits have been discussed thoroughly in the literature. The expectation that every professional nurse will guide and mentor another has been firmly implanted in the social fabric of the discipline. The benefits are personal and typically include the sense that the knowledge gained through years of experience will not be lost as one generation transitions and passes responsibility to the next.

The role of the CNS in this process is clear. As an APN working directly in the influence of staff, the CNS has a significant role to play as mentor, guide, and role model. How do we bring this all together? The expectation of being a mentor needs to be incorporated into the education of the CNS as he or she masters the role. The

CNS needs to focus on individual development for the staff and themselves. Through the perpetual process of assessing the needs of the staff and then seeking or building the resources needed to further develop the clinical skills, personal attributes, or professional comportment, the CNS plays a key role in the development of nurses and nursing as a profession.

REFERENCES

Allen, T. D., Eby, L. T., & Lentz, E. (2006). Mentorship behaviors and mentorship quality associated with formal mentoring programs: Closing the gap between research and practice. *Journal of Applied Psychology, 91*(3), 567–578.

American Nurses Credentialing Center. (2005). *ANCC Magnet recognition program—recognizing excellence in nursing services.* Retrieved January 12, 2009, from http://www.nursecredentialing.org/Magnet.aspx

Andrews, M., & Wallis, M. (1999). Mentorship in nursing: A literature review. *Journal of Advanced Nursing, 29*(1), 201–207.

Angelini, D. (1995). Mentoring in the career development of hospital staff nurses: Models and strategies. *Journal of Professional Nursing, 11,* 89–97.

Bally, J.M.G. (2007). The role of nursing leadership in creating a mentoring culture in acute care environments. *Nursing Economics, 25*(3), 143–148.

Benner, P. (1984). *From novice to expert: Excellence and power in clinical nursing practice.* Menlo Park, CA: Addison-Wesley.

Boldra, J., Landin, C., Repta, K., Westphal, J., & Winistorfer, W. (2008). The value of leadership development through mentoring. *Health Progress, 89*(4), 33–36.

Buddeberg-Fischer, B., & Herta, K. D. (2006). Formal mentoring programmes for medical students and doctors: A review of the Medline literature. *Medical Teacher, 28*(3), 248–257.

Busen, N. H., & Engebretson, J. (1999) Mentoring in advanced practice nursing: The use of metaphor in concept exploration. *The Internet Journal of Advanced Nursing Practice, 2*(2). Retrieved January 12, 2009, from http://www.ispub.com/ostia/index.php?xmlFilePath = journals/ijanp/vol2n2/mentoring.xml

Cahill, M., & Payne, G. (2006). Online mentoring: ANNA connections. *Nephrology Nursing Journal, 33*(6), 695–697.

Collins, A., Brown, J. S., & Holum, A. (1991). Cognitive apprenticeship: Making thinking visible. *American Educator, 15*(3), 6–46.

Dracup, K., & Bryan-Brown, C. (2004). From novice to expert to mentor: Shaping the future. *American Journal of Critical Care, 13*(6), 448–450.

Dyer, L. (2008). The continuing need for mentors in nursing. *Journal for Nurses in Staff Development, 24*(2), 86–90.

Finley, F. R., Ivanitskaya, L. V., & Kennedy, M. H. (2007). Mentoring junior healthcare administrators: A description of mentoring practices in 127 U.S. hospitals. *Journal of Healthcare Management, 52*(4), 260–269.

Fitzgerald, R. (1961) *Translation of Homer: The Odyssey.* New York: Doubleday.

Fulton, J., Bohler, A., Hansen, G., Kauffeldt, A., Welander, E., Santos, M., et al. (2007). Mentorship: An international perspective. *Nurse Education Practice, 7*(6), 399–406.

Goran, S. F. (2001). Mentorship as a teaching strategy. *Critical Care Nursing Clinics of North America, 13*(1), 119–129.

Grossman, S. C. (2007) *Mentoring in nursing: A dynamic and collaborative process.* New York: Springer.

Hart, K. (2007). The aging workforce: Implications for health care organizations. *Nursing Economics, 25*(2), 101–102.

Hayes, J. M., & Scott, A. S. (2007). Mentoring partnerships as the wave of the future for new graduates. *Nursing Education Perspectives, 28*(1), 27–29.

Health Resources and Services Administration. (2006). *Preliminary findings: 2004 national sample survey of registered nurses.* Washington, DC: U.S. Department of Health and Human Services.

Hyatt, S. A., Brown, L., & Lipp, A. (2008). Supporting mentors as assessors of clinical practice. *Nursing Standard, 22*(25), 35–41.

Hunnerkopf, P. (2007). Clinical learning. *Nursing Standard, 21*(20), 59.

Kanter, R. M. (1977). *Men and women of the corporation.* New York: Basic Books.

Kram, K. E. (1985). *Mentoring at work: Developmental relationships in organizational life.* Glenview, IL: Scott Foresman.

Lakasing, E., & Francis, H. (2005). The crisis in student mentorship. *Primary Health Care, 15*(4), 40–41.

LaSala, C. A., Connors, P. M., Pedro, J. T., & Phipps, M. (2007). The role of the clinical nurse specialist in promoting evidence-based practice and effecting positive patient outcomes. *Journal of Continuing Education in Nursing, 38*(6), 262–270.

Miller, A., & Storey, P. (2007). *MAITRE: Mentoring trAIning maTerials and REsources—Appendix 2—Mentor competencies and rationale.* Retrieved January 12, 2009, from http://www.amitie.it/maitre/training/html/comtab_eng.html

McKinley, M. G. (2004). Mentoring matters: Creating, connecting, empowering. *AACN Clinical Issues Advanced Practice in Acute Critical Care, 15,* 205–214.

McWeeny, M. (2002). The changing mosaic of mentoring. *Creative Nursing Journal, 3,* 3–4.

Morse, J. M. (2006). Deconstructing the mantra of mentorship: In conversation with Phyllis Noerager Stern. *Health Care for Women International, 27,* 548–558.

Moseley, L., & Davies, M. (2008). What do mentors find difficult? *Journal of Clinical Nursing, 17*(12), 1627–1634.

Murray, M. (2001). *Beyond the myths and magic of mentoring: How to facilitate an effective mentoring process* (2nd ed.). San Francisco: Jossey-Bass.

Myall, M., Levett-Jones, T., & Lathlean, J. (2008). Mentorship in contemporary practice: The experiences of nursing students and practice mentors. *Journal of Clinical Nursing, 17,* 1834–1842.

National Association of Clinical Nurse Specialists. (2004). *Statement on clinical nurse specialist practice and education* (2nd ed.). Harrisburg, PA: Author.

Nedd, N., Nash, M., Galindo-Ciocon, D., & Belgrave, G. (2006). Guided growth intervention: From novice to expert through a mentoring program. *Journal of Nursing Care Quality, 21*(1), 20–23.

Nettleton, P., & Bray, L. (2008). Current mentorship schemes may be doing our students a disservice. *Nurse Education in Practice, 8,* 205–12.

Nickle, P. (2007). Cognitive apprenticeship: Laying the groundwork for mentoring registered nurses in the intensive care unit. *Dynamics: Canadian Association of Critical Care Nurses, 18*(4), 19–27.

Peddy, S. (2001). *The art of mentoring: Lead, follow and get out of the way.* Houston TX: Bullion Books.

Poynton, M. R., Madden, C., Bowers, R., & Keefe, M. (2007). Nurse residency program implementation: The Utah experience. *Journal of Healthcare Management, 52*(6), 385–396.

Robert Wood Johnson Foundation. (2004). *Nurse Executives Fellow Program.* Retrieved January 12, 2009, from http://futurehealth.ucsf.edu/Program/rwj/

Shea, G. (2001). *Mentoring: How to develop successful mentor behaviors* (3rd ed.). Boston: Thompson Crisp Learning.

Schweibert, V. (2000). *Mentoring: Creating connected, empowered relationships*. Alexandria, VA: American Counseling Association.

Stewart, B., & Krueger, L. (1996). An evolutionary concept analysis of mentoring in nursing. *Journal of Professional Nursing, 12,* 311–321.

Tuohig, G. (2007). *Nurse mentoring: Creating a professional legacy*. Retrieved January 12, 2009, from https://www.nnsdo.org/dmdocuments/NurseMentoring.pdf

Webb, C., & Shakespeare, P. (2008). Judgements about mentoring relationships in nurse education. *Nurse Education Today, 28,* 563–571.

Weiss, L. M., Williams, C. A., Wetzel, D. E., Drake, A. C., Cumberlander, L. B., & Gordon, C. L. (2008). Veterans Health Administration mentoring model for new nurse executives. *Nursing Administration Quarterly, 32*(3), 226–229.

Yoder, L. (1990). Mentoring: A concept analysis. *Nursing Administration Quarterly, 15*(1), 9–19.

Yonge, O., Billay, D., Myrick, F., & Luhanga, F. (2007). Preceptorship and mentorship: Not merely a matter of semantics. *International Journal of Nursing Education Scholarship*. Retrieved January 12, 2009, from http://www.bepress.com/ijnes/vol4/iss1/art19/

Zucker, B., Goss, C., Williams, D., Bloodworth, L., Lynn, M., Denker, A., et al. (2006). Nursing retention in the era of nursing shortage. *Journal for Nurses in Staff Development, 22*(6), 302–306.

Project Management: A Core Competency for Professional Nurses and Nurse Managers

Robert Loo

Health care in North America has been undergoing dramatic changes marked by increasing health care costs and job demands on nurses and nurse managers (McGillis Hall & Donner, 1997). The size, complexity, and costs of the health care system in North America, arguably the largest service industry in the region and probably the world (Sapienza, 1997), strongly underscore the need for highly effective and efficient nurse management systems (Aroian et al., 1997; Carnevale, 1997; Manion, Sieg, & Watson, 1998; Wilmot, 1998). Nurse managers and educators need to train themselves and staff in project management to help promote efficient and effective management. Although some organizations may want to adopt project management as their main management approach (i.e., management-by-projects), other organizations may simply want to superimpose project management on their current organizational structure and management practices and use a project management approach as projects arise.

The project management approach offers the following strengths:

- It is action and results oriented—it gets the job done.
- It is led. Projects require effective leadership to achieve goals successfully. Effective leadership does not mean "autocratic" leadership but the flexible use of different leadership styles depending upon the type of project, the qualifications and experience of the project staff, and such other factors as time pressures from management.
- It provides a single point of contact, the project leader, with project staff, management, stakeholders, and so on.
- It fosters a synergistic and creative "we" instead of "me" atmosphere because it brings together a multidisciplinary team focused on achieving a common goal within a deadline and budget and to quality standards.
- It promotes effective personal work habits and management skills especially in planning and controlling techniques.

Recognition of the power of project management has resulted in many educational and training organizations offering courses in this field. Also, some organizations offer in-house project management training (Loo, 1991). More generally, project management training ranging from 1-day sessions to 1-week courses are readily available in most urban centers through training organizations or management consulting firms. Those interested in project management training should consult the Project Management Institute (PMI) document, *A Guide to the Project Management Body of Knowledge* (PMI, 1998), to appreciate the scope and depth of the nine major knowledge areas that make up the project management discipline.

PROJECT MANAGEMENT AND HEALTH CARE MANAGEMENT

It should be evident that a project management approach with its strong goal-orientation, detailed planning and controlling, and accountability could help ensure the successful completion of projects, ameliorate the stress levels that many health staff and managers feel, and help solve the "free rider" problem sometimes found in group work fostering cooperative learning and management skills development.

IMPLEMENTATION RECOMMENDATIONS FOR EFFECTIVE PROJECT MANAGEMENT

Any organization or manager considering introducing project management should attend to several key factors that can mean success or failure (Johns, 1999; Meredith & Mantel, 1999; Stuckenbruck, 1988).

Organizational and Staff Commitment

The genuine commitment of senior management to a project management approach is essential; otherwise, staff will soon detect that the exercise is simply a token one, and they will not make the effort to properly use the project planning tools and other techniques. A large body of literature shows that using a project management approach results in more effective and efficient management in a variety of organizational contexts including health care (Johns, 1999; Meredith & Mantel, 1999; Stuckenbruck, 1988); therefore, advocates can convince senior management of the benefits of implementing project management.

Project Leadership

Project managers must be effective leaders because it is people who do the work and often under time pressures and other sources of stress (Zimmerer & Yasin, 1998). Research has found that effective project leaders have strong interpersonal communication skills, can motivate team members and maintain motivation even during frustration periods in the project, and have effective conflict resolution skills for handling conflicts within the project team and with management among other stakeholders. Effective project managers have flexible leadership styles; they are able to use different styles appropriately with different team members and at different stages in the project life cycle. For example, a junior staff member might require a more *directive* leadership style compared to a senior team member who might require only a *delegation* style (Loo, 1994).

Training

At least some basic project management training needs to be provided to managers and staff. Loo (1990) demonstrated that even a 1-day course can be effective in organizations. Many training organizations and universities offer a wide variety of project management training, including custom training for specific organizational needs. A practical approach to initiate project management training would be to first send nurse trainers on a formal project management training course; a 3- to 5-day course should be comprehensive enough for such trainers. Then those nurse trainers could tailor short courses, perhaps 1-day courses, to offer within organizations. One short course should target nurse managers who need to know not only the sorts of basic project management techniques and tools that are discussed in the following section but also the leadership skills required for team building and maintaining high motivation among project staff (Loo, 1994; Meredith & Mantel, 1999). It is appreciated that most nurse managers have these sorts of skills, but leadership skills need to be reviewed because of the high stress in projects based on time pressures and interpersonal conflicts that usually occur among team members, as well as between the project team and senior management. One short course should target staff who would serve on project teams to train them in basic project management techniques and tools.

Training and Learning Methods

The two most commonly used training and learning methods in project management are short lectures and practical exercises. Short lectures are useful in presenting facts to those learning project management. However, project management is an applied management discipline for getting work done so skills are most important; therefore, practical exercises in applying project management techniques are most important. It is recommended that trainers alternate short lectures and practical exercises to facilitate effective learning. For example, a lecture on project planning rationale and methods should be followed by a practical individual or group exercise requiring trainees to apply project planning to a relevant health care scenario, such as planning for the implementation project for a new software program or clinical procedure.

ORGANIZATIONAL LEARNING

Training nurses and managers so they learn project management is important, but organizational learning is also important. The lessons learned, both good and bad, from a specific project must find their way throughout the organization so that other managers and teams can benefit from effective project management techniques and experiences and avoid pitfalls that threaten the success of problem projects (Cavaleri & Fenton, 2000). Nurse trainers should incorporate the lessons learned from past projects to improve future training courses by building on past successes and, most importantly, ensuring that the same mistakes are not repeated.

Project Management Systems

A wide variety of PC software packages (Promisel, 1999) are readily available at reasonable costs, especially for IBM-compatible systems. The PMI publishes an annual software survey in its *PM Network* magazine. These software packages offer a wide range of planning, controlling, resourcing, and reporting capabilities that are useful throughout the project life cycle.

Evaluation

It is important that the introduction and effectiveness of project management be evaluated to determine if, in fact, project management improves the effectiveness and efficiency of projects as well as the skills of participating staff in both the technical (e.g., planning, controlling) and people (e.g., team-building skills, communication skills, conflict management skills) side of management. A discussion of project evaluation and audit approaches and techniques is provided by Loo (1985) and others in a special issue of the *Project Management Journal.* Hormozi, McMinn, and Nzeogwu (2000) recently added to the emphasis on project evaluation in the termination phase with a discussion of costs.

Project management follows a life cycle from a conceptual phase to a termination phase. This life cycle view reflects the influence of the systems approach to the development of project management. A typical life cycle for projects progresses from a conceptualization phase (initiating the project), to the detailed project planning phase, to the execution or implementation phase, and finally, to the project termination or closeout phase.

PROJECT PLANNING

As with all planning, project planning consists of determining in advance what is to be done, starting with an overall plan and then detailed planning in the development phase. One planning tool in the conceptual phase is the project description. Typically, a 1-page project description or project statement evolves over the conceptual phase. This document, as shown in Exhibit 21.1, presents a concise and precise overview of the project's purpose or objective, the terms of reference or mandate under which the project is justified, and a brief description of the methodology (e.g., a patient or employee satisfaction survey; a clinical trial) to be used in the project, as well as key milestones (e.g., project start and finish dates). This document is an important communication tool for the project team, management, and other stakeholders (e.g., client) in the project. It can also be the stimulus for setting up a contract in the case of externally contracted projects.

As the project manager completes the project description with input from management or the client among other stakeholders, the manager should also perform a strengths, weaknesses, opportunities, and threats (SWOT) analysis to determine what strengths and weaknesses the organization and project team

---

EXHIBIT 21.1 FORMAT FOR A PROJECT DESCRIPTION

Project Title: Use a short, unique and meaningful title.

Unit: Identify the organizational unit/team conducting the project.

Purpose: The purpose statement is a concise and clear statement of the overall objective of the project starting with an action verb, "To . . . ." It is sometimes useful to also specify what the project is not addressing if there is any ambiguity; this is part of "scope management."

Terms of Reference: The client/organization and the client's contract position and incumbent are identified. The project manager and any other key personnel already assigned to the project are identified. The reporting structure is specified as well as the estimated budget and budget constraints.

Methodology and Milestones: A brief description of the main methodology is presented; for example, a questionnaire survey of a stratified random sample of 200 employees. Major milestones are specified, especially for the project start and completion dates as well as key intermediate milestones such as an end-of-fiscal year project review.

have with respect to the proposed project, what opportunities the proposed project offers the organization, and what threats the project might present to the manager and organization. A SWOT analysis can help the project manager decide whether or not to pursue the proposed project. The start of a model SWOT analysis for a "Training Needs Assessment" project is shown in Exhibit 21.2.

Many potential problems or issues may be identified during any planning process; therefore, issues analysis is an important part of the planning process (see Exhibit 21.3, for a generic planning chart). The use of issues analysis charts, as shown in Exhibit 21.4, aids project staff in describing all potential issues or

problems and to share these issues with other project members and the client in order to determine the impact on the project and action to be taken. An issues impact assessment (see Exhibit 21.5) complements the issues analysis by addressing two major decision factors: the probability of the issue occurring during the life of the project (a high probability or very likely to occur; medium probability or likely to occur; and a low probability or unlikely to occur) and the potential negative impact on the project (a high impact that could mean project failure; a medium impact causing serious performance problems; and a low impact resulting in an inconvenience or disruption). For example, conducting a training needs assessment project creates

EXHIBIT 21.2 A SWOT WORKSHEET

Strengths
—We have experience conducting
training needs assessment projects.
—We have the trainers with the expertise
to assist in the needs assessment
project and to develop and deliver
training courses.

Opportunities
—Outputs from this training needs
assessment project will be useful for
the organization's and the human resource
department's strategic planning
and the development of future
managers.
—Results from this project will help the
organization identify areas for improvement
in staff recruitment and
placement activities.

Weaknesses
—Unit managers resist giving staff time
off to attend training courses. Unit
managers give staff training a low priority.
—The unions have not been helpful in
the past in helping to provide resources
for the organization's training efforts.

Threats
—There may be cuts to budgets in the
coming year, and the training budget
is vulnerable.
—There will be a major restructuring
of the organization, and the training
function may be eliminated.

EXHIBIT 21.3 A GENERIC PLANNING CHART

Project Title: Training   Needs   Assessment
Project Manager: (name)
Date chart completed: __/__/__

Activity and Output	Accountability	Estimated Time		Required Resources
		Work time	Elapse time	
001				
Conduct a literature search, produce a bibliography and a critical review on "training needs assessment"	(name)			$300 for literature purchase & printing Bibliography
002				

EXHIBIT 21.4 A GENERIC ISSUES ANALYSIS CHART

Project Title: Training   Needs   Assessment
Project Manager: (name)
Date chart completed: __/__/__

Issue/Problem	Impact Assessment	Action to be Taken
001 The training budget might be cut next year	Could be a high-impact and high probability event because we will not have the budget to develop and deliver training courses	Develop a contingency plan with alternative, cost-efficient training delivery (e.g., OJT, self-directed study)
002		

EXHIBIT 21.5 AN ISSUES IMPACT ASSESSMENT WORKSHEET

Issue Statement: Because next year's budget may be reduced, the training budget is most vulnerable to cutting.

	Impact		
	High	Medium	Low
Probability High			
Medium			
Low			

EXHIBIT 21.6 A GENERIC GANTT CHART

Project Title: Training   Needs   Assessment
Project Manager: (name)
Date chart completed: __/__/__

Activity	Week
01: Conduct literature search and review and draft the Bibliography of training needs assessment.	1 2 3 4 5 6 7 8 9 10 11 12
02: Draft the training needs assessment questionnaire.	
03: Pretest questionnaire with 10 staff and do debriefing.	

expectations among staff that the health care organization will follow through with training and development programs and courses; however, as we all know, training budgets are often among the first budgets to be cut when funding becomes tight. Possible actions could be to use a train-the-trainer approach, on-the-job training, and coaching for high-potential staff among other cost-efficient training delivery alternatives. Such contingency planning ensures that the unforeseen is anticipated and appropriate actions are planned so the success of the projects is not jeopardized and unintended negative impacts, such as staff dissatisfaction, are minimized.

Having completed the process of developing the planning charts along with the resource time requirements and the issues analysis, the project team can now develop a Gantt chart to display the activities over the time period for the project (see Exhibit 21.6). The use of Gantt charts, unlike Program Evaluation and Review Technique (PERT) and Critical Path Method (CPM), does not require any special training, and it is quite suitable for small projects (less than $500,0000 and no longer than 1 year). This visual presentation of project activities is easy to communicate to anyone, and it serves to remind project staff at a glance of what activities are supposed to be done at what times.

PROJECT MONITORING AND CONTROL

With planning complete, the project implementation or execution phase can begin. The Gantt chart continues to be used to monitor progress on the project and identify problems, especially activities falling behind schedule. The use of milestones is essential in planning and controlling projects. Milestones are placed at critical points in a project where major decisions must be made. For example, in Exhibit 21.6, a milestone (open triangle) was placed after the pretesting of the survey questionnaire (activity 003) because the team would know whether the questionnaire was working as intended or whether there were serious problems with the questionnaire (e.g., misinterpreted questions). If there were serious problems, then management would have to decide whether to start over with the development of another questionnaire, salvage the current questionnaire, replace the project manager, or some other option.

Besides the use of milestones, another commonly used control tool is the project status report. These reports are typically scheduled monthly or, in very short projects, weekly or every 2 weeks to ensure that the project manager and client can track a project and take timely corrective actions if necessary to modify a project. As seen in Exhibit 21.7, these reports briefly describe three main areas: the current status of the project, any problems or issues that arose since the last report and the actions taken, and any upcoming milestones and approved changes to the work plan. These reports are usually kept to one page; it is not the intent of project management to generate unnecessary paper or create bureaucrats but simply to ensure project success through careful planning, monitoring, and controlling. The project control cycle is illustrated in Exhibit 21.8.

CONCLUSION

The project management approach can be easily and quickly superimposed on existing management approaches in virtually any organization to help managers and staff complete projects successfully, deal

---

EXHIBIT 21.7 A PROGRESS STATUS REPORT

Project Title: Training   Needs   Assessment

Reporting period: __/__/__ To __/__/__

Prepared by: (name)

Project Status	A brief description of activities and outputs completed since the last project status report.
Issues & Actions Taken	What problems or issues have arisen during the reporting period and how they have been resolved.
Upcoming Milestones	Upcoming outputs and milestones covering the coming reporting period as well as changes to the work plan.

EXHIBIT 21.8 THE PROJECT CONTROL CYCLE

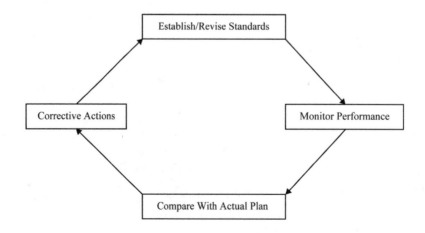

effectively with work load stress, learn better, and develop basic management skills that will serve them well throughout their careers. Benefits accrue to the organization as well with projects and other activities being completed within deadlines, budgets, and expected quality standards. Clearly, a project management approach presents a win–win outcome all around.

EDITORS' NOTE

This article adapted with permission from Loo, R. (2003). Project management: A core competency for professional nurses and nurse managers. *Journal for Nurses in Staff Development, 19*(4), 187–193.

REFERENCES

Aroian, J. F., Horvath, K. J., Secatore, J. A., Alpert, H., Costa, M. J., Powers, E., et al. (1997). Vision for a treasured resource, Part 1: Nurse manager role implementation. *Journal of Nursing Administration, 27*(3), 36–41.

Carnevale, F. A. (1997). The practice of management in nursing: From novice to expert. *Canadian Journal of Nursing Administration, 10*(2), 7–13.

Cavaleri, S. A., & Fenton, D. S. (2000). Integrating organizational learning and business praxis: A case for intelligent project management. *The Learning Organization, 7*, 251–258.

Hormozi, A. M., McMinn, R. D., & Nzeogwu, O. (2000). The project life cycle: The termination phase. *SAM Advanced Management Journal, 65*, 45–51.

Johns, T. G. (1999). On creating organizational support for the project management method. *International Journal of Project Management, 17*(1), 47–53.

Loo, R. (1985, August). Evaluation in the project management environment. *Project Management Journal, XVI*(3), 36–41.

Loo, R. (1990). One-day project management training: Is it possible? *1990 Proceedings of the Project Management Institute Annual Symposium,* 568–574.

Loo, R. (1991). Project management training in Canadian organizations. *International Journal of Project Management, 9*(4), 250–257.

Loo, R. (1994). Situational project leadership. *1994 Proceedings of the Project Management Institute Annual Symposium,* 574–577.

Manion, J., Sieg, M. J., & Watson, P. (1998). Managerial partnerships: The wave of the future. *Journal of Nursing Administration, 28*(4), 47–55.

McGillis Hall, L., & Donner, G. J. (1997). The changing role of hospital nurse managers: A literature review. *Canadian Journal of Nursing Administration, 10*(2), 14–39.

Meredith, J. R., & Mantel, S. J., Jr. (1999). *Project management: A managerial approach.* New York: Wiley.

Project Management Institute. (1998). *A guide to the project management body of knowledge.* Newton Square, PA: Author.

Promisel, R. (1999). Project management basics. *IIE Solutions, 31*, 39–47.

Sapienza, A. M. (1997). Four challenges for health project managers. *PM Network, 11*(7), 26–29.

Silverman, M. (1888). *Project management: A short course for professionals.* New York: Wiley.

Stuckenbruck, L. C. (Ed.). (1988). *The implementation of project management: The professional's handbook.* Reading, MA: Addison-Wesley.

Wilmot, M. (1998). The new ward manager: An evaluation of the changing role of the charge nurse. *Journal of Advanced Nursing, 28*, 419–427.

Zimmerer, T. W., & Yasin, M. M. (1998). A leadership profile of American project managers. *Project Management Journal, 29*, 31–38.

Economic and Financial Considerations for Clinical Nurse Specialists

Leeann Blue
Mary L. Fisher

Health care economics exerts remarkable control on nursing practice in the United States. The American Association of Colleges of Nursing (AACN, 2007) lists health care economics literacy to be an essential core skill for all advanced practice nurses. The U.S. health care system changes over time, but it has reflected a revenue stream that comes from private payer insurance and government sources. This funding stream for health care does not fund all those who require health care services. The uninsured represent 15.8% of our population, or 47 million Americans. This is a 22% increase since 2000 (U.S. Census Bureau, 2007). Funding for the uninsured may come from charity sources, self payment, or cost shifting (charging more to other groups to cover the costs for this group).

The U.S. health care system has seen consistent increases in costs, which then results in careful and constant government and employer review of the resources expended. This environment requires careful consideration of efforts within the system to deliver cost-effective care to individuals and the community. Understanding the value the clinical nurse specialist (CNS) brings to the efficient delivery of care is essential to addressing these economic concerns.

The objectives for this chapter are to: (1) describe an overview of U.S. health care economics and the financial challenges faced by the health care system,

(2) define key economic terms associated with the U.S. health care economy, and (3) describe how the CNS role can impact or influence the health care economy. The chapter closes with a conclusion and discussion questions.

U.S. HEALTH CARE ECONOMICS

Health care is an important part of the overall economy in the United States and has gained a lot of attention because of the increasing costs and need for resources attributed to our health care delivery. National health care expenditures went from $245.8 billion in 1980 to $1,299.5 billion in 2000 (4.3 times) and are expected to rise to $2,815.8 billion in 2011 (Center for Medicare and Medicaid Services [CMS], 2007a). Those increased costs will most certainly generate pressure for providing the best value of health care and for new solutions to deliver effective, efficient, and safe health care. Questions about how much health care the country can afford continue to surface, and decisions about what types of services are a fundamental right of all citizens is yet to be addressed.

U.S. health care economics stands apart from our normal understanding of the U.S. free enterprise economic system. Our economy is built on a concept of supply and demand in a market where consumers and traders are free to exchange goods and services for currency. A direct exchange and interchange between purchasers and traders in the purchasing process is fundamental for free enterprise to work. Any system that bypasses that direct exchange stands to limit the free market and to undermine our free enterprise system.

One aspect of a purchase decision that is directly undermined by blocks in the direct exchange between purchasers and traders is quality. The extent to which quality is transparent and publicly reported impacts a consumer's ability to make informed decisions. Consumers balance their need for quality with what they plan to pay. In making purchasing decisions based on this balance, consumers serve as a control on the free enterprise system. Their demand for quality at a certain price point drives the market to control costs while still providing a quality product. Without that dynamic, costs can spiral out of control and quality can go unchecked.

There are many consumer advocacy groups who test products and provide data to consumers to assist their decision making. For example, consulting *Consumer Reports* before making a major purchase or calling the Better Business Bureau to check on a contractor are expected aspects of consumerism.

Separation of the Health Care Consumer From Price

Health care stands apart from these normal consumer–product relationships within our free market. We rarely know the costs of health care before we have consumed the product. This creates an in-elastic demand setting where, in health care, demand is insensitive to changes in price (Chang, Price, & Pfoutz, 2001). Consumers, therefore, cannot exert control over quality.

This focus on consumers understanding and seeing the quality outcomes within our health care system is changing. CMS requires all hospitals that receive funding from this source to share in the public realm their patient satisfaction data and quality core measures from several different high-volume diagnoses. This provides the consumer transparency related to patient care outcomes, process measures, and patient satisfaction with services delivered in different provider settings (CMS, 2007b).

This is a very new aspect to our health care environment and is intended to provide the patient/family/community with the information needed to help drive patient care delivery decisions. CMS and private insurers will continue efforts to provide transparency in health care outcomes and satisfaction data as another tool to benchmark best practice and to ensure that the consumer has access to the data to help make decisions (CMS, 2007b).

While health care costs are of increasing concern, the health care consumer is shielded from evaluating quality in relation to cost for health care decisions. Insured consumers are affected because:

1. They do not always know the true costs of care delivered.
2. Health care coverage providers may negotiate discounts for health care products or services, which then leads to inconsistent pricing across the health care system.
3. Health care coverage providers may limit access to certain types of care by withholding coverage for certain transactions (e.g., setting limits for psychiatric care).
4. Health care providers may limit access to care by limiting provider participation (e.g., Preferred Provider Organizations—PPOs reimburse more for in-plan providers than out-of-plan providers; Health Maintenance Organizations—HMOs only pay for in-plan providers and use gatekeepers to limit specialty referrals).
5. Health care providers may limit access to care by instilling large copays and deductibles.
6. Health care providers may deny coverage, period.

Uninsured consumers are affected as well:

1. Providers engage in "cost shifting" by inflating charges to uninsured people to cover losses from care that is not reimbursed in contractual discounts.
2. If the uninsured cannot pay up-front costs, they may not get nonemergency care or very important preventative care.
3. Clinical providers may limit their exposure to uninsured people by closing their practice to new patients.
4. One of the top reasons cited for bankruptcies in the United States is catastrophic health care costs.

The Health Care Price Index

There are many reasons for separation of the consumer from price in our health care system, and those reasons may have helped contribute to a health care price index (HCPI) that has risen faster than other consumer prices for the last 20 years and consumed 16% of the gross domestic product (GDP) in 2006, or $2 trillion annually (Catlin, Cowman, Hartman, Heffler, & The National Health Expenditure Accounts Team, 2009). "As a percentage of GDP, national health spending is projected to reach 17.7 percent by 2012, up from 14.1 percent in 2001" (CMS, 2007a). Because these costs are the highest of any industrialized nation, American products are less competitive on the world market. One example of this is the fact that health care costs add $1,100 to the cost of every car made in the United States (Fisher, 2005).

Other factors that impact the HCPI include labor costs and inflation, technological advances, pharmaceutical development costs and inflation, malpractice costs, inflation of medical-related supplies and equipment, building expansion and competition for customers, insurance company profits, and chronic illness in an aging population.

Health Care Consumers' Need for Agency

Consumers usually inform themselves about products before they make a major purchase. In some highly technical purchases, the consumer still must rely on experts to advise them. In health care, the majority of our transactions as consumers are technically and medically complex, and our reliance on experts is much more complete. This places a burden of agency on providers. *Agency* refers to authority given to a provider with unique knowledge to make decisions about the care of another and to consume health resources in the process (Propp, Krubert, & Sasson, 2003). Agency carries with it a moral obligation to act in the patient's best interest even when not in the provider's best interest. This is a key precept for the transparency of sharing outcomes by hospitals with the public.

Competition Within Health Care

Another concept inherent in the free enterprise system is competition. While we have a lot of competition existing in health care, it is often not the normal competition intended to inform consumers and influence their decision making. Much of the competition in health care is aimed at the true decision makers—providers and insurers. Consumers may be targets of advertising, but much of it is of the "ask your doctor about . . ." type. This type of advertising often does not serve to educate the consumer about a product but to trigger the consumer to ask a provider if they need the medication or treatment. This type of marketing is intended to have consumers pressure providers to provide the medication or treatment, even if not required by the consumer's medical needs. Marketing directly to the consumer is becoming more of a focus and will likely continue.

Providers are competing for insurance contracts, often based on cost alone. Until insurers receive pressure from employers (the majority of nongovernmental insurance is employer-sponsored) to negotiate contracts based not only on costs but also on quality outcomes, there is no incentive on the part of insurers to care about quality. There is a trend for employers to begin looking at quality as a factor in insurance negotiations. Offering quality health care can be seen to be in the employer's best interest in order to attract and retain the best employees and to keep the workforce productive. A long-term perspective is needed for employers to take this view, however.

Access to Care

Access is another important issue within our health care economy. A key issue in access has to do with the growing number of uninsured in the United States. There were 47 million uninsured Americans in 2006 (15.8% of all Americans), according to the most recent available census data. This figure has been steadily rising, in part because of a steady decline in employer-sponsored health insurance and the limiting of eligibility for government-sponsored health care. Medically indigent Americans often seek inappropriate care in emergency room (ER) settings due to lack of access to primary care. By using very costly ER settings inappropriately, overall costs of health care rise, but the individual is shielded from the normal market pressures because there is no intent or capacity to pay for the service.

Regulation Mechanisms

There have been many efforts to curb health care spending for over 30 years. As the major payer of health care bills (government sources accounted for 45% of health care dollars spent in 2001), the federal government has been active in regulating the health care industry. In the 1970s, certificate of need (CON) approval was required before major health care facility building could occur. Prospective payment, a federal program that designed diagnostic related groups (DRGs) as a mode to reimburse for care, was operational in 1983. This system is still in effect today for Medicare and Medicaid reimbursement. The DRG system is consistently reviewed and changes made to reflect practice utilization and costs. CMS has started a process of consistent auditing of clinical providers' documentation to ensure that they meet the criteria for payments. This effort is called Recovery Audit Contractor audits.

In the 1980s, private industry responded by seeking access controls through development of HMO and PPO models. These so-called capitated models share risk for insurance coverage with providers by paying based on covered lives in a variety of negotiated contract forms instead of paying directly for services provided. This type of contracting provides an incentive to providers to ration care unless quality outcome standards are negotiated at the same time (Fisher, 2005).

The Move to Pay for Performance

The effort of CMS in 2008 and beyond is to have hospitals and providers share their actual performance data, to provide transparency of the outcomes of care, and to not pay for events caused by errors within the hospital setting that were not anticipated. This effort is called the Medicare Pay for Performance (P4P) initiative. The foundation for effective pay for performance initiatives is collaboration with providers and other stakeholders to ensure that valid quality measures are used. Through these collaborative efforts, CMS is developing and implementing a set of P4P initiatives to support quality improvement in the care of Medicare beneficiaries. Within a hospital setting, these initiatives focus on an initial set of 10 quality measures by linking the reporting of these measures to the payments that the hospitals receive for each Medicare discharge. Hospitals that participate and submit all of the required data receive their full Medicare DRG payments. As of 2008, nearly all (98.3%) of the hospitals eligible to participate in this program are complying with the requirements of this provision.

There are several other pilot P4P initiatives occurring, and mostly likely these will spread to most health care delivered within the United States. The Physician Group practice Demonstration, Chronic Care Improvement Program, End Stage Renal Disease Management Program, and Care Management for High Cost Beneficiaries are just a few of the demonstration projects occurring at this time (CMS, 2008).

Nursing Labor Supply

There is a world-wide nursing shortage. Donelan, Buerhaus, DesRoches, Dittus, and Dutwin (2008) predict that the shortage will reach 500,000 by 2025. Because of the continually increasing demand for nurses, health care institutions are in competition for scarce nursing resources. What are the salaries and incentives necessary to attract and retain nurses? How must the work environment improve? The success of magnet designated facilities in this area is an example of the extent of competition. One burning question that remains unanswered is: How must nursing practice change if supply continues to be less than demand for nursing services in the future? CNSs are uniquely positioned as experts in the delivery of care to impact this issue.

CNS Impact on Hospital and Nursing Care

The CNS can provide direct care or help to establish best practice for a patient care population or service that adds value to the care delivery model. The CNS role impacts health care within the patient/client sphere, the nurses/nursing sphere, and the system/organizational sphere (National Association of Clinical Nurse Specialists [NACNS], 2004).

The CNS can impact each of these spheres in several ways:

1. Being the expert direct care provider for complex cases.
2. Being the expert for providing evidence-based best practice through:
   a. Educating/mentoring staff nurses on evidence-based practice in bridging the gap between what is known and what is done at the bedside,
   b. Developing and implementing evidence-based best practice guidelines, and
   c. Identifying indicators for and monitoring outcomes of practice within a care setting.
3. Conducting clinical inquiries into future care delivery models.

CNS Role in Limiting CMS Losses

CMS in its P4P initiative will no longer pay for certain events that occur within the hospital setting that were caused by the hospital. This effort for the first phase became effective October 2008. For many of these events, nursing has a major role in identifying and applying best practice interventions to limit the hospital's exposure to loss. These events include (CMS, 2008):

1. Pressure ulcer stages III and IV
2. Falls and trauma
3. Surgical site infection after bariatric surgery for obesity, certain orthopedic procedures, and bypass surgery (mediastinitis)
4. Vascular-catheter–associated infection
5. Catheter-associated urinary tract infection
6. Administration of incompatible blood
7. Air embolism
8. Foreign object unintentionally retained after surgery

Understanding Cost Analysis as an Important Tool

A key skill for the CNS to acquire is a detailed understanding of the financial impact of nursing interventions (equipment, pharmaceuticals, and care delivery) to the costs of providing care for patients or a community. One aspect of that financial analysis is how to calculate labor costs associated with nursing care. Early research on cost analysis of nursing care focused on "costing out" nursing services. These studies often were conducted for the purpose of measuring productivity, comparing costs of nursing delivery models, establishing models to directly charge patients for nursing costs, and relating nursing costs to other cost models, most notably DRG categories. Costing efforts have evolved with economic and practice changes to the health care system. For example, most studies in the 1980s were performed in acute care hospitals, whereas more studies now relate to a variety of settings.

"Today, cost analysis of nursing care focuses on justifying the cost effectiveness of professional practice models, evaluating redesign efforts, and monitoring and controlling nursing costs within an ever-tightening, cost-conscious health care environment" (Fisher, 2006, pp. 112–113). Within the context of rising capitation penetration, cost analysis is essential to accurate capitation bidding and financial viability of the parent organization. As "best practices" benchmarking pushes the envelope of competitive bidding, demonstrating cost-effective nursing practice becomes essential to securing managed care contracts.

Cost and efficiency of nursing procedures or treatments continue to be studied. Capasso and Munro (2003) compared two wound treatments (saline vs. hydrogel). While costs for both treatments were comparable for wound closure rate and treatment supplies, saline was significantly more expensive. The saline treatment required a higher number of home nursing visits, accounting for the difference in cost. This example demonstrates the multifactorial nature of costing research and the need to look beyond the obvious in doing such analyses.

Another fertile area for cost analysis is to evaluate cost differences among professional practice models. However, most of these studies use proprietary practice models that are difficult to duplicate in other settings. Variables are identified in these studies that do impact nursing costs, such as nursing turnover, ratio of productive to nonproductive hours, and nursing satisfaction. Complex issues emerge for this type of analysis. Relative productivity across discipline levels, recruitment, training, and impact on quality must be added to the equation.

Cost-Effectiveness Evaluation

As the U.S. economic picture darkens, with ever-increasing percentages of the GDP being consumed with health care costs, continuing efforts focus on cost containment, quality improvement, and the dynamic between the two. What is the benefit of reducing costs for an episode of care if that care is substandard and results in future health care costs associated with readmission, chronic illness, complications, or death? Analyzing costs, without measuring quality, will not get us where we want to go.

CNS programs and projects designed to improve care must demonstrate cost-effectiveness and be evaluated on the patient/family, personnel, system, and community levels (Welch, Fisher, & Dayhoff, 2002). In cost-effectiveness analysis, we may compare the differences in costs to the differences in outcomes of several

possible program choices. This analysis is appropriate where one specific outcome is clear and is expressed as a health status goal, such as percentage loss of excess body weight compared to ideal weight for bariatric surgery. Where multiple outcomes are relevant and must be evaluated in a weighted manner, then a cost-utility analysis is performed. In cost-benefit analysis, "we replace the health indices with dollar measures of benefits" (Jacobs & Rapoport, 2004, p. 376).

"All cost analysis is based on assumptions that must be examined and made explicit when reporting findings" (Fisher, 2006, p. 112). Be leery of studies that describe cost-analysis but fail to report the underlying assumptions of the model.

What are some quality outcome measures that must be considered in a nursing cost-benefit or cost-effectiveness analysis?

1. Length of stay—This variable correlates highly with nursing work as measured by such variables as acuity indexes, task/procedure complexity, direct nursing care hours, and patient charges.
2. Quality patient outcomes—patient satisfaction, clinical outcomes appropriate to DRG type and comorbidities, reduction of nurse-sensitive complications and failure-to-rescue, liability costs associated with failed care, CMS P4P measures, and National Quality Forum and National Database of Nursing Quality Indicators measures that are nursing sensitive. The CNS can help teach, review, and set up policies and procedures to structure a foundation for best practice. In addition, the CNS needs to monitor and provide ongoing education to help prevent these events from reoccurring.
3. Nurse factors—Adding to cost of care are nurse factors that may be difficult to measure, that is, nurse turnover, ratio of productive to nonproductive hours, training costs, nurse satisfaction, and education level of the nurse.
4. Patient education outcomes—This area of frequent CNS responsibility can be aided by a model to evaluate the cost-effectiveness of patient education programming offered by Welch and colleagues (2002). The growth of capitation and cost analysis of nursing services will need to take new directions. As critical pathways (benchmark performance tools) evolve as care guides, the costs of pathway changes on nursing delivery, patient outcomes, and case costs must be calculated. What are the most efficient *and* effective pathways toward resolution of a given health problem? What practice setting or level of care is appropriate for patients at each step of the pathway? For example, when is it safe to transfer a fresh open heart patient from critical care to a stepdown environment? (Earliest transfer to a least costly delivery mode saves money.) These types of calculations may be critical for institutions to secure managed

care contracts in a cost-competitive environment. Determining what activities can be safely eliminated from a pathway without negatively impacting care outcomes will have cost and resource savings as we move to "best demonstrated practices."

Finally, we must move toward a cost-effectiveness analysis model that incorporates the outcomes of nursing practice. This aspect has been especially elusive given the generic and group nature of nursing practice. With multiple nursing providers impacting a patient's care, how do we separate the relative contributions of each person or each subspecialty of nursing practice that a patient may experience in the course of their care from contributions of other disciplines? Additionally, we need to quantify the costs of increased patient mortality and failure to rescue associated with changes in nurse–patient ratios based on recent landmark studies by Aiken (2002) and Cho (2003).

Understanding the health care current economics and staying on top of trends will help the CNS to be able to effectively contribute to patient care. Further skills in the budgeting and finance area are essential for contemporary CNS practice.

HEALTH CARE BUDGETING 101

Most CNSs will encounter budgets. In many cases, the CNS will have fiscal responsibility for at least a program budget that falls within an operating budget (see Glossary of Budgeting Terms later in this chapter). Specific budgeting practices are unique to organizations and will not be covered here. The framework for budgeting is described.

All health care organizations practice budgeting discipline. Each year, either on a calendar or fiscal year schedule, the organization decides how to spend its money in relation to its overall goals. It is vital that the budget process be tied to strategic planning for the organization so that scarce resources are aligned with strategic goals. Corporate fiscal officers determine the schedule, format, and processes used in budgeting. Most organizations have budget support resources allocated to assist in the budgeting process.

Each organization will have operating, capital, and cash budgets. The time cycles for these three types of budget will differ.

Operating Budgets

The most complex aspect of budgeting is the operating budget. For most service organizations, the major dollar amount in this category is personnel costs. Also included in the operating budget are supplies and equipment, as well as utilities and overhead costs. The operating budget is especially tied to volume and acuity predictions. In addition, inflation factors are often provided by finance based on industry predictions.

Personnel

Health care cannot be provided without an adequate workforce with the right skill mix, experience, and licensure. The organization must be competitive in their salary and benefit structures to ensure a stable workforce. Salary increases must be factored into the personnel budget for the coming year. Salary increases may include cost of living adjustments (COLA) and merit increases that are based on performance indicators. Benefit costs have become a challenge for all employers as health care costs have sky-rocketed and consumed more and more of dollars reserved for salaries. Benefits also include life insurance, retirement, travel, paid time off, disability, and family leave. All must be factored for inflation in the personnel budget.

Productive and Nonproductive Costs

A factor that greatly impacts the personnel budget is the nonproductive hours that are paid out. This category includes vacation, holiday, sick time, or a combined flexible paid time off allotment, as well as bereavement, military, education, and workman's compensation time multiplied by the hourly salary of each employee.

Regulation of Staffing

Who can do what is regulated by state licensing laws in many cases, so the CNS must become knowledgeable about state law. Personnel are further broken down into direct care and indirect care providers.

Direct and Indirect Care

Direct care is exactly what the name implies. Those activities that are directly associated with care to the patient, including the documentation of care, are calculated into the direct care hours. Nurses may also have indirect care hours that include orientation, continuing education and inservices, meetings, and other activities that take them away from the bedside. Personnel who support care indirectly such as unit secretaries and transporters are considered indirect care providers. How these categories are calculated into budgeted nursing hours per unit of service differs widely across institutions.

Units of Service and Acuity

Institutions often track the amount of care patients receive by looking at the direct care hours per unit of service. A unit of service differs based on the clinical setting. For example, in an inpatient setting, the unit of service used is nursing hours per patient day. In a clinic setting, nursing hours per visit or procedure may be used. In the operating room, the unit of service is nursing hours per case. Often an acuity factor is used in addition to units of service to distinguish that patients require varying amounts of care based on their severity of illness or ability to complete activities of daily living.

Volume Projections

A vital role the CNS can play in budgeting is assisting with volume projections. Because the CNS fundamentally understands the business of care, he/she should know when to expect seasonal variations, what the trends in care are that may impact the business practices of the specialty, and if changes in best practices may impact length of stay.

Supply and Equipment

Supplies needed for the operations of the unit are in this category of the operating budget. Again, some supplies are directly linked to care. In those cases, they are considered variable needs because how much is needed depends on patient volume and acuity. Other supplies are fixed in that their use is not dependent on patient volume. Minor equipment that does not meet the definition of a capital expenditure is part of the operating budget. CNSs frequently impact the costs associated with this category by their work related to product comparisons.

Overhead

Each budget center is allocated their share of overhead. This is either done on a prorated cost per square foot of space (if the unit has a physical location) or based on a formula related to volume of service. Overhead often includes administration, utilities, maintenance, housekeeping, and other nonrevenue generating support services.

Capital Budgets

A plan for proposed expenditures for facilities, equipment, or software over $2,000 and with a durable life exceeding 2 years is called the capital budget. Capital budgets are often constructed on a different budget cycle from the operating budget. Funds for capital expenditures are considered separate from operating funds and often come from profits. Even in a nonprofit enterprise, revenue in excess of expenditures is created and that excess profit must be put back into the institution to maintain nonprofit status. There are never enough capital dollars to meet the huge demand for updated equipment or facilities. These requests are often adjudicated by a panel of executive officers and board members. It is often a political process. The approved capital request will be assigned a date for availability of funds as part of the cash budget process.

Cash Budgets

Institutions use the practice of encumbering funds to ensure there will be cash to meet obligations. For example, if employees are accruing sick time, the money to pay for that benefit must be available. Payroll must be met. Other ways institutions control cash flow are to limit their inventory liability (just-in-time supplies), keep their personnel costs in check, schedule their capital purchases, and enhance their debt collection.

Foundation Accounts

Philanthropy assists institutions in serving the public. Donations account for more and more of the program development monies for organizations. An endowment will fund a program off of the income from a principle that is not touched. Generally, foundations allot from 4% to 5% of an endowment's total to be used in a given year. Of course, this is dependent on income, and if the market is down, the income may not be there to give a payout on an account in a given year.

Budget Compliance and Monitoring

It is not enough to prepare and approve a budget. It must be tightly monitored and continuously updated to make sure reality meets expectation. Variance reporting is the mechanism most institutions use to monitor the budget on a monthly basis. In this type of report, the manager analyzes why the actual is different from the budgeted amount in each category. This is called exception reporting.

Often, volume and acuity variances account for much of the problem. Sometimes the variance is due to the fact that the manager failed to budget for an important item, or a new practice has changed the rules. For example, when universal precautions were implemented suddenly in the late 1980s, no one had anticipated their latex glove budgets increasing by $1 million.

CNS Budget Considerations

The main thing for a CNS to know about budgets is accountability. Being accountable to ensure your programming needs are included in the budget process is vital to your success. Being accountable to keep costs within budget is expected.

ETHICAL CONSIDERATIONS

We have to ask ourselves if health care is viewed as a right or a privilege in our society. Such a question is fundamental to whether or not we, in fact, have a health care system for all Americans. Our answer to this question also impacts our actions as providers of care. What are the unmet needs of those we serve? How do we advocate for vulnerable populations? What is our obligation to provide services that lose money? What is our perspective on wellness care versus illness-related services? Understanding the impact of economics for health care clearly can help you to formulate a full picture for your ethical professional practice and your budgeting decisions.

CONCLUSION

The CNS role can impact our health care economy and has been demonstrated in the research as doing so by reducing hospital costs and length of stay, reducing frequency of emergency room visits, improving care practices through critical review and analysis of care and equipment/supplies required for patient care, increasing patient satisfaction with nursing care, and reducing medical complications in hospitalized patients. It is critical for CNSs to stay aware of the current health care environment dynamics and their impact on safe, quality, efficient patient care.

DISCUSSION QUESTIONS

1. Describe how the current U.S. health care economy is shifting to one of transparency related to health care outcomes and how you, as a CNS, can make a difference in this transparency. Identify the sources you can access to identify national benchmarks for costs of care and cost of complications.
2. Why it is so important for the CNS to be aware of the current economic trends within health care?
3. List a care process or technology/equipment implementation where you believe the CNS could add value for its adoption within your care setting, and describe the value in terms of dollars and benefits.
4. How will you, as a CNS, respond to CMS's new P4P initiative?
5. What do you believe to be the major economic priority for your role as a CNS?

GLOSSARY OF BUDGETING TERMS

Capital budget: A plan for proposed expenditures for facilities, equipment, or software over $2,000 and with a durable life exceeding 2 years.

Cash budget: A plan for the cash flow of the organization with special attention to timing the outflow of resources to ensure adequate cash to meet the organization's goals.

Cost benefit analysis: An economic analysis that compares all of the costs associated with a program, service, or project with the anticipated or real benefits.

Debt: Money owed to any creditor.

Depreciation: The annualized loss of value in a durable piece of equipment or structure that is directly related to its anticipated functional life and need for replacement.

Economy of scale: The optimum scale of operation needed to produce the services at the lowest cost per unit basis.

Fiscal year: The unit of time chosen by an organization for its budgeting and reporting cycle.

Internal rate of return: The annualized, compounded return rate, which can be earned on invested capital or the yield on the investment. This figure assists organizations to make business decisions about which services to offer.

Lost opportunity costs: Costs associated with tying up resources in one area when those resources could produce increased revenues in another area. This calculation is used to determine priorities for business choices. It is the value of the path not taken.

Operating budget: The annual budget needed for the operations of a unit. It includes equipment, space, utilities, personnel, depreciation, and supplies.

Product line (service line) budget: An operating budget that includes all service areas associate with a product or service, e.g., cardiac service line budget would include multiple areas associated with the care of cardiac patients.

Return on investment: The time needed to recoup the initial investment and start-up costs of a new venture.

Variance analysis: A monthly analysis of the variations from budgeted allocations. This analysis often compares actual to budgeted costs and relates them to volume and acuity fluctuations.

REFERENCES

Aiken, L. H, Clark, S. P., & Sloan, D. M. (2002). Hospital staffing, organization and quality of care: Cross national findings. *Nursing Outlook, 50*(5), 187–194.

American Association of Colleges of Nursing. (2007). *The essentials of master's education for advanced practice nursing.* Retrieved January 21, 2009, from http://www.aacn.nche.edu/education/mastessn.htm

Capasso, V., & Munro, B. (2003). The cost and efficacy of two wound treatments. *Association of periOperative Registered Nurses Journal, 77*(5), 984, 986, 988–992.

Catlin, A., Cowman, C., Hartman, M., Heffler, S., & The National Health Expenditure Accounts Team. (2008). National health spending in 2006: A year of change for prescription drugs. *Health Affairs, 27*(1), 14–29.

Centers for Medicare and Medicaid Services. (2007a). *Health care spending as part of GDP historical.* Retrieved April 26, 2007, from http://www.karlloren.com/healthinsurance/p1.htm

Centers for Medicare and Medicaid Services. (2007b). *Letter to State Medicaid Directors.* Retrieved July 31, 2008, from http://www.cms.hhs.gov/SMDL/downloads/SMD073108.pdf

Centers for Medicare and Medicaid Services. (2008). *Home page.* Retrieved September 1, 2008, from http://www.cms.hhs.gov

Chang, C., Price, S., & Pfoutz, S. (2001). *Economics and nursing: Critical professional issues.* Philadelphia: F. A. Davis.

Cho, S. H., Ketefian, S., Barkauskas, V. H., & Smith, D. G. (2003). The effects of nurse staffing on adverse events, morbidity, mortality, and medical costs. *Nursing Research, 52*(2), 71–79.

Donelan, K., Buerhaus, P., DesRoches, C., Dittus, R., & Dutwin, D. (2008). Public perceptions of nursing careers: The influence of the media and nursing shortages. *Nursing Economics, 26*(3), 143–150, 165.

Fisher, M. L. (2005). Overview of health care delivery. In J. M. Black & J. H. Hawks (Eds.), *Medical-surgical nursing: Clinical management for positive outcomes* (7th ed., pp. 121–131). Philadelphia: W. B. Saunders Co.

Fisher, M. L. (2006). Cost analysis of nursing care. In J. J. Fitzpatrick (Ed.), *Encyclopedia of nursing research* (2nd ed., pp. 112–114). New York: Springer.

Jacobs, P., & Rapoport, J. (2004). *The economics of health and medical care.* Boston: Jones and Bartlett Publishers.

National Association of Clinical Nurse Specialists. (2004). *Statement on clinical nurse specialist practice and education* (2nd ed.). Harrisburg, PA: Author.

Propp, D. A., Krubert, C., & Sasson, A. (2003). Healthcare economics for the emergency room physician. *Emergency Medicine, 21*(1), 55–60.

U.S. Census Bureau. (2007). *Income, poverty, and health insurance coverage in the United States: 2006.* Washington, DC: U.S. Census Bureau. Retrieved August 23, 2008, from http://www.census.gov/prod/2007pubs/p60–233.pdf

Welch, J. L., Fisher, M. L., & Dayhoff, N. (2002). A cost-effectiveness worksheet for patient-education programs. *Clinical Nurse Specialist Journal, 16*(4), 187–194.

Technology Management in Complex Health Care Settings

Patricia O'Malley

Over the past 100 years, hospitals have become centers of technology for the diagnosis and treatment of disease. Health care environments increasingly depend on nurses to accept new roles and greater responsibilities with emerging technology to ensure success in patient care and outcomes. Despite nursing's continuous emersion in technology, nursing is generally unaware of the meaning, significance, or impact of technology on nursing practice (Barnard, 2001).

Technological dominance has become a priority in health care. Technology has been described as an instrument and a human activity and defines Western culture (Heidegger, 1977). There is no aspect of nursing practice that has not been touched by technology (Locsin, 2001a). How technology has extended roles in medicine and nursing continues to be debated. However, history suggests that nursing has afforded no resistance to assuming the responsibility for the knowledge and tasks associated with technology application in health care. Furthermore, technology application is increasingly delegated to nursing, which requires intense education, competency assessment, and time-consuming repetitive tasks (Barnard, 2001). Technological competency defines contemporary nursing practice (Locsin, 2001a).

While technology brings the nurse closer to the patient by virtue of task performance, technology can also provide a path for the dehumanization of the patient. The clinical nurse specialist (CNS) has a unique role in assisting nurses to embrace the human–technology interface in health care *and* preserving the art and science of caring in an age of ever-accelerating technological advancement (Locsin, 2001a).

This chapter explores the relationship of technology and the CNS role in health care. This chapter provides many tools and resources for the CNS to use in any environment where technology application is an integral part of the plan of care. Before exploring the current state of technology in health care, a brief review of the history of technology in health care is required.

HISTORY OF TECHNOLOGY IN HEALTH CARE

The home was the primary site for medical care in the 1900s. The mean life expectancy was 47 years, and 95% of births occurred at home. Pneumonia, influenza, tuberculosis, and dysentery were the primary causes of death. During this period, medical imaging was introduced. The average time for a head X-ray required 11 minutes of exposure time, and patients generally received large doses of radiation. Electrocardiogram (ECG) was introduced in 1901 using a string galvanometer that used a magnet that weighed nearly 600 pounds (Ridgway, Johnson, & McClain, 2004). Thermometers, anesthesia, blood pressure sphygmomanometers, surgical instruments, and sterilizers were in use in hospitals (Richter, 2004; Welter, 2004).

From 1919 to 1939, increasing work in medical instrumentation was accomplished, and the iron lung and radiation treatment were introduced. The golden years for electronics were 1945–1959, and the application of military and university research and development technologies combined with the Hill-Burton Act of 1947 provided the foundation for the transformation of hospitals. Emerging technology for this period included prototypes of heart valves, dialysis, the first pacemaker, oscilloscope, cardiopulmonary bypass, and respirators. Radionuclide technology—the precursor to nuclear medicine as well as ultrasound—was introduced (Ridgway et al., 2004).

The technology "arms race" began in the 1960s. Hospitals raced to purchase emerging technology developed through increased funding by the National Institutes of Health (NIH) to universities for biomedical engineering training. The average battery life for a pacemaker was extended to 12 to 18 months, and the first DC defibrillator replaced the 1950s AC defibrillator. Lasers, hyperbaric oxygen therapy, silicone implants, fiber optic endoscopes, fetal heart monitors, and computers were introduced during this period. Multichannel laboratory analyzers were introduced, which provided hospitals a path for profit in laboratory testing. The first heart bypass surgery was performed in 1964, followed by the heart transplant in 1967 and the artificial heart in 1968. The birth of the World Wide Web occurred in 1969, when the U.S. Department of Defense merged four university computer networks and named the network the Advanced Research Projects Area Net (ARPANET), which would expand and eventually become the Internet (Ridgway et al., 2004).

The boom of community hospitals in the 1970s increased the number of hospitals in the United States to 5,875. With the expansion of clinical engineering programs, high-tech digital computer-controlled medical devices emerged. Computed tomography (CT) scan was introduced during this time, as well as anesthesia machines and nuclear batteries (Richter, 2004; Ridgway et al., 2004).

The emergence of fixed price health care reimbursement in the 1980s, coupled with the *Medical Waste Tracking Act of 1988* and expensive maintenance contracts for technology maintenance and repairs, slowed technology acquisition as an increasing number of hospitals closed. Magnetic resonance imaging was introduced in 1984 (Ridgway et al., 2004).

Tight budgets and control of labor expenses resulted in erosion of working conditions in hospitals in the 1990s. During this decade, information technology (IT) began to emerge in the health care environment along with positron emission tomography (PET) and single photon emission computed tomography (SPECT) scanners and gamma knives (Ridgway et al., 2004).

The recent technology explosion of medical informatics may result in the greatest transformation of health care. The electronic medical record and integration with increasingly complex clinical systems and nanotechnology promises to make the environment of care paperless and immediately accessible by every care provider anytime and anywhere (Ridgway et al., 2004). Hidden in the promises of medical informatics are the realities associated with implementation (Shekelle, Morton, & Keeler, 2006). Difficult workflow alterations, culture change, role redesign, programming and design flaws, and new medical errors are just a small sample of the obstacles that the CNS faces in the current health care setting (O'Malley, 2007).

Technology has increased the complexity and cost of health care. The merging of science, technology, and engineering have changed hospitals into technology centers with associated medical specialties rather than a place for the sick (Welter, 2004). Balancing cost with return on investment has become an increasingly difficult issue because technology is refined and modified as soon as it is released (Clancy, 2006a).

Rising labor costs, declining reimbursement, data-driven patient outcomes, and keeping pace with technology development is the current environment of care. The CNS role in health care is well-positioned to discern technological rhetoric from science and determine the risks, benefits, alternatives, and limits of technology for organizations, nursing practice, and patients (Lanzafame, 2006).

NURSING AND TECHNOLOGY

While appearing as no more than a footnote in the history of medical technology, nursing was indispensable for the technological transformation of health care during the 20th century (Barnard & Cushing, 2001). Since the 1930s, nurses have been increasingly linked with technology. Matching equipment to procedures, supervision of use, improvisation, sterilization, troubleshooting, and maintenance continue to contribute to the functional redundancy of many aspects of practice (Sandelowski, 2000). While technology has extended the science around the nursing process, it has also blurred the distinctions between nursing, medicine, and other health professions (Sandelowski, 2000).

Nurses remain the primary users of technology in health care. Medical devices include a variety of tools, instruments, and machines that are used to assess, treat, sustain, and comfort patients. Responsible for the application, operation, and troubleshooting of a variety of medical devices, nurses also interpret technology and reduce fears for patients and families (Sandelowski, 2000).

As more and more technology enters the environment of health care, the boundaries between patient and machine and technical versus professional nursing have become increasingly blurred. Implicit in the mechanization of health care is that technology can be substituted for a nurse. However, experience suggests that *without* a nurse, the technology–patient interface is wrought with safety issues and significant adverse events (Sandelowski, 2000).

While *purposes* of technology can be clearly articulated in complex health care systems, the *consequences* of technology implementation are rarely adequately factored for the organization (David, Judd, & Zambuto, 2004). Whether *instrument* or a *product*, technology organizes human activity, labor, and choices. Technology is defined by structure, purpose, and use. Exhibit 23.1 describes the varied purposes of technology in health care today (David et al., 2004). Exhibit 23.2 describes some of the primary technologies purchased by the health care organizations in the United States (Gaev, 2004). All technology has a predictable life cycle that should be the basis of CNS assessment, planning, and evaluation. Figure 23.1 describes the life cycle of technology for any health care organization (David et al., 2004). Exhibit 23.3 describes important elements the CNS may consider when evaluating the interface of medical devices during the life cycle (Gaev, 2004; Haselkorn, Rosenstein, Rao, VanZuiden, & Coye, 2007).

TECHNOLOGY PROCUREMENT

Hospitals adopt technology out of clinical necessity, to support operations, or because of market forces, as described in Exhibit 23.4 (David et al., 2004). In 1999, hospitals worldwide spent $155.5 billion on medical devices and $66.5 billion was spent in the United States alone. Devices included capital equipment, computer-based systems, disposables, reusables, and other supplies. Increasingly, hospitals face balancing cost and quality with rapidly emerging advances in technology and limited capital to enable staff to become familiar with the device.

Successful hospitals link technology acquisition and management with the mission and strategic plan of the

EXHIBIT 23.1 PURPOSES OF TECHNOLOGY IN HEALTH CARE

Purposes of Technology
1. Diagnostic
2. Therapeutic
3. Rehabilitation
4. Increase efficiency
5. Increase cost-effectiveness
6. Increase reimbursement
7. Decrease risk
8. Decrease error
9. Decrease exposure risk
10. Recruitment of staff

EXHIBIT 23.2 UNITED STATES—MAJOR CATEGORIES OF MEDICAL DEVICE SALES

Major Categories
1. Incontinence supplies
2. Blood glucose monitoring
3. Wound closure products
4. Implantable defibrillators
5. Soft contact lenses
6. X-ray equipment
7. Orthopedic fixation devices
8. Pacemakers
9. Examination gloves
10. Coronary stents
11. Ultrasound equipment
12. Arthroscopic accessory instruments
13. Magnetic resonance imaging
14. Computed tomography
15. Monitoring systems
16. Medical information technology
17. PACS (picture archiving and retrieval systems)

EXHIBIT 23.3 INTERFACES OF MEDICAL DEVICES

Dyad	Interface Elements
Device–User	Nursing is usually the greatest user of technology; majority of errors with application are user errors; training, competency, and surveillance requirements
Device–Patient	Does the device accommodate the physiological variance of human beings?; degree of activity/movement restriction
Device–Environment	Conditions necessary for storage and use: temperature, humidity, electrical power, shielding from electromagnetic fields, and connections to special gases
Device–Accessories	Accessories: cost, strength, average shelf and use life, cleaning requirements compared to disposables

organization. A dedicated multidisciplinary committee armed with a *consistent plan* for technology assessment, evaluation, implementation, and monitoring can forge this important link (Haselkorn et al., 2007, White, 2007).

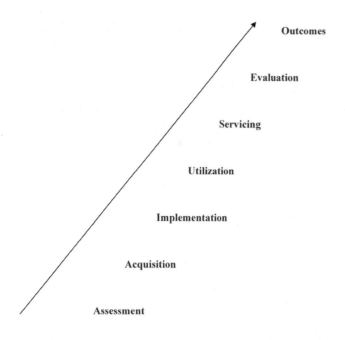

Figure 23.1 Life cycle of technology.

From "Introduction to Medical Technology Management Practices" (pp. 101–107), by Y. David, T. Judd, and R. Zambuto, 2004, in J. Dyro (Ed.), *Clinical Engineering Handbook*. Boston: Elsevier Academic Press.

EXHIBIT 23.4 RATIONALE FOR TECHNOLOGY ADOPTION

Rationale	Indices
Clinical Necessity	Meet standards of care
	Increase quality of care
	Improve quality of life
	Enhance safety
	Treat disease
	Reduce length of stay
	Support care protocols
Operations Support	Increase efficiency
	Expand or develop services
	Reduce errors
	Regulatory compliance
	Reduce dependence on user skill levels
	Integrate departments
	Reduce maintenance loads
Market Preference	Increase access to care
	Improved customer satisfaction
	Increase return on investment
	Improve revenue stream
	Impact market share

Members from all disciplines should know purposes and objectives of the committee. A proactive approach in seeking emerging technology should underlie the objective of completing a comprehensive impact analysis. Beginning with a formal request for information, the CNS should obtain references from the vendor early. Beware of relying solely on vendor information. More often, vendor summaries are biased and designed to attract prospective buyers rather than presenting a balanced and realistic presentation of the benefits and limits of the device (Keller, 2004). Exhibit 23.5 describes the elements required for a comprehensive analysis necessary for the CNS to make an informed decision about medical devices (Harding & Epstein, 2004; Haselkorn et al., 2007; Rosenstein, O'Daniel, & Geoghan, 2003; Wilson, Kumor, & Bar, 2007). Sources of evidence for informed decision making are described in Exhibit 23.6a and 23.6b (Baretich, 2004; Matuszewski, 1997). The outcome of any technology assessment is a function of how relevant information is at the time the decision is made (Rosen & Gabbay, 1999).

The CNS must plan for problems associated with technology assessment. Once there is broad acceptance of a medical device based on insufficient evidence, there is little incentive to complete a critical evaluation. However, critical evaluation is necessary for an informed decision and to reduce the emergence of unseen problems in the clinical setting later. Exercise great caution when evaluating clinical trials, which often have small samples, inconsistent procedures across trials, lack of randomization, and focus on *intermediate* rather than *final* outcomes. Then the CNS can bring to the table all the evidence to promote a rational and cost-effective decision for the acquisition and use of new and existing technology (Matuszewski, 1997).

Hospitals who are part of a group purchasing organization (GPO) avoid many problems associated with technology acquisition. The ability to negotiate group rate discounts for medical devices helps control cost but limits choice. Products are usually *not* selected for clinical utility, effectiveness, or safety. More often, products are selected based solely on the lowest negotiated price. Even more problems can occur when the contract requires a sustained commitment to purchase a set volume of medical devices to secure a negotiated price (Keller, 2004). Furthermore, individual GPO member hospitals usually do not have direct input in device selection, and products are often chosen without consideration of the unique needs of each GPO member. Technology assessment committees and the CNS can provide invaluable direction to the GPO for appropriate medical device selection. Finally, common problems associated with technology assessment that can be avoided by careful planning are described in Exhibit 23.7 (David et al., 2004).

Clinical trials are an important part of technology procurement, and the CNS often facilitates medical device

EXHIBIT 23.5 REQUIRED ELEMENTS FOR COMPREHENSIVE TECHNOLOGY ASSESSMENT

Factor	Elements
Technology type	Therapeutic, diagnostic, or supportive Alternative products
Return on investment—Costs	Life cycle of the medical device Purchase versus lease Plan for upgrades Maintenance Replacement Accessories Disposables Reimbursement
Quality	Comparison with like technologies Other user experiences and outcomes Shelf life of associated disposables Parts availability
Safety	Potential adverse events Redundancy Back-up systems Competency requirements
Safety *(continued)*	Biomedical training Monitoring requirements Outcomes of device failure Availability of loaner equipment
Staffing	Surveillance requirements Transport requirements Credentialing
Service line	Acceptance Clinical justification Expected utilization Integration in existing services Communication requirements Market impact and penetration Support of strategic plan and organizational mission
Vendor control	Ability to pace the rate of device introduction Inventory control Shipping, freight, installation costs Duration of price guarantees
Vendor control *(continued)*	Vendor support during introduction Staff training support Post–device introduction support Resources after implementation
Regulatory	Labeling Liability Insurance Consent issues Maintenance requirements Current Food and Drug Administration (FDA) status History of vendor clearance to market the device Local, state, and federal codes

(Continued)

EXHIBIT 23.5   REQUIRED ELEMENTS FOR COMPREHENSIVE TECHNOLOGY ASSESSMENT (*CONTINUED*)

Users	Competency requirements
	Training requirements
	Ease of use
	Human factors
	Ability to maintain proficiency
	Associated clinical procedures
Users *(continued)*	Available written materials or manuals
	Staff evaluations
Contract considerations	Warranty details
	Payment schedules
	Grounds for cancellation
	Price protection
	How future versions of the device will be made available
	Time table for implementation

EXHIBIT 23.6A   SELECTED SOURCES OF EVIDENCE FOR TECHNOLOGY ASSESSMENT

Sources

Manufacturer guidelines
Evaluation/experience of other users
Focused literature reviews
Government patent review
Clinical trials
Expert opinion
News media
Specialty organization guidelines/standards

trials in clinical areas. Before beginning any trial, obtain relevant department and vendor support. After arranging time with manufacturers for use of the medical device, offer in-service training for all staffs impacted by the trial. User and service manuals should be part of the education process and readily available once the device is in use. Schedule any classes in areas with easy access and low distractions. Provide notebooks in trial areas for staff to write questions and concerns when the CNS is not available. To obtain staff evaluation regarding the device (e.g., ease of use), the CNS should consider preparing and administering a short written survey (Canlas, Hall, & Shuck-Holmes, 2004; Harding & Epstein, 2004; Haselkorn et al., 2007).

Training super users to serve as resources on individual units to extend the expertise of the CNS is a wise intervention for complex medical devices. In-house maintenance from the vendor or manufacturer is critical during the trial. After approval, in-house clinical engineers must also be as well-trained as the manufacturer service providers to ensure safety and to complete required preventative maintenance (Canlas et al., 2004; Harding & Epstein, 2004; Haselkorn et al., 2007).

In summary, successful technology procurement is based on prepurchase evaluation, expected life cycle, and cost-benefit analysis of maintenance, depreciation, and obsolescence. This knowledge, combined with outcomes from clinical trials and staff feedback, can help the CNS and the organization make the best decision required for technology procurement (Canlas et al., 2004). Every decision must include consideration for the reality of limited resources and increasing demands. The CNS should balance the choice of any technology with the possible loss of choice in the future of more cost-effective devices (Scales & Laupacis, 2007). Once the decision has been made, technology assessment should remain an ongoing effort because future innovations may make the chosen technology obsolete. Technology assessments should be as innovative as the technology itself, and the CNS assessment in the clinical setting, which is often less than an ideal environment, is as valuable as the assessment

EXHIBIT 23.6B SELECTED SOURCES OF EVIDENCE FOR TECHNOLOGY ASSESSMENT

Name	Web Site	About
The Association for the Advancement of Medical Instrumentation (AAMI)	http://www.aami.org	Purpose is to increase understanding and beneficial use of medical instrumentation; AAMI provides continuing education, conferences, certification, and publications of technical documents, periodicals, books, and software
U.S. Agency for Healthcare Research and Quality (AHRQ)	http://www.ahrq.gov	Technology Assessment Clinical Practice Guidelines
National Guidelines Clearinghouse™	http://www.guideline.gov	An initiative of AHRQ and U.S. Department of Health and Human Services. Resource for evidence-based clinical practice guidelines
National Quality Measures Clearinghouse™ (NQMC)	http://www.qualitymeasures. ahrq.gov/	Public repository for evidence-based quality measures and measure sets
Emergency Care Research Institute (ECRI)	https://www.ecri.org/Pages/ default.aspx	Nonprofit organization that provides independent evidence: standards, rules, and regulations for the use of technology that affects health; medical device hazard and recall information, management tools, guidelines, and customized consulting; information resources for patient safety, technology planning, and assessment, acquisition and management
U.S. Food and Drug Administration (FDA) Center for Devices and Radiological Health (CDRH)	http://www.fda.gov/cdrh/	Provides important information for device evaluation, human factors, safety news, recalls, medical device reporting, recent medical device approvals, and postmarketing surveillance
National Library of Medicine (NLM)	http://www.nlm.nih.gov/	PubMed—a service that includes over 17 million citations from MEDLINE and other journals from the 1950s. Includes full-text articles and related resources; Health Services/Technology Assessment Text (HSTAT)—a free Web-based resource of full-text documents that provides information for health care decision making for health care providers, researchers, policy makers, and consumers
National Information Center on Health Services Research and Health Care Technology (NICHSR)	http://www.nlm.nih.gov/ nichsr/	To improve the organization and dissemination of results of health services research; includes practice guidelines and technology assessments

completed in the controlled research environment (Eisenberg, 1999).

TECHNOLOGY IN THE CLINICAL SETTING

Technology has increased the complexity of nursing practice. Increasingly, medical devices require more and more nurse's attention and responsibility, which gives rise to an increasingly impersonal environment. Less time to interact with patients results in fewer patients in therapeutic relationships with their caregivers. Additionally, technology is no longer being applied just to the critically ill but to the chronically ill outside the intensive care unit (ICU). As a result, medical device monitoring becomes more important than monitoring

EXHIBIT 23.7 COMMON PROBLEMS UNCOVERED IN A TECHNOLOGY ASSESSMENT

EXHIBIT 23.7 COMMON PROBLEMS UNCOVERED IN A TECHNOLOGY ASSESSMENT

Problems
1. Technology underused
2. Device inappropriately used
3. Lack of compliance with guidelines or standards associated with use
4. Frequent repairs
5. Disorganized maintenance
6. Failure to monitor and replace outdated technology
7. In-services held at inappropriate times
8. Disorganized implementation plan
9. Slow engineering responses for problems
10. Failure to plan for upgrades

the patient (Bauld, Dyro, & Grimes, 2004; Laing, 1982; Sweeney, 1992).

What are the forces driving technology application outside the ICU? First, technology in many situations improves quality of life independent of the diagnosis or prognosis. However, experience suggests that fear of litigation may be the more common reason. Failure to use available technology appears to increase liability even when all the evidence suggests that application is not necessary, and overacting on information gained from a medical device may result in more harm than good. As a result, nurses practice in a clinical setting fraught with legal and ethical dilemmas (Bauld et al., 2004).

Evidence suggests that the future will be even more complex. New emerging technologies promise to radically change the environment of care. Some newer technologies include continuous ST segment monitoring, indirect continuous cardiac output, esophageal Doppler monitoring for hemodynamic assessment, continuous central venous oximetry, transcutaneous carbon dioxide monitoring, bispectral index monitoring for sedation, brain tissue oxygen monitoring, and computerized glycemic control (Albert, 2006; Arbour, 2006; Bader, 2006; Button & Keaton, 2006; Drew & Funk, 2006; Flanders, 2006; Goodrich, 2006; Headley, 2006; Hill & Klein, 2006; Prentice & Sona, 2006; Zwerneman, 2006).

With more medical devices in the clinical setting, there are more alarms in a changing geography that increasingly fails to support the visibility of patients. The challenge for the CNS is finding ways to assist nurses to safely respond to multiple alarms in environments saturated with interruptions and competing demands. Exhibit 23.8 describes the factors associated with failure

to respond to medical device alarms, which leads to alarms not heard or even ignored and increased risk of negative patient outcomes (Chambrin, 2001; Phillips, 2006).

The CNS can help nursing staff gain control over medical device alarms. To begin, list all equipment and alarms in the clinical setting. The list may include the following: emergency call light, nurse call light or signal, ventilator-cardiac-infusion pump alarms, and medical gas alarms. Second, discern all factors that inhibit responding appropriately to alarms. Factors may include staffing, workload, logistics, competency with use of the device, and lack of guidelines to minimize false and meaningless alarms (Phillips, 2006). Third, assess the culture within the clinical area. What are the roles, norms, and behaviors associated with clinical alarms? Does the staff work as a team in responding to alarms, or is each nurse responsible only for their assigned patient alarms? Based on this assessment, the CNS can develop meaningful guidelines and individual clinical skills to reduce the number of false and irrelevant alarms, which can reduce the likelihood of failing to respond to a true alarm (Phillips, 2006). Exhibit 23.9 describes a template that could be used to assess competency for medical device alarms and can assist the CNS to improve staff response to medical device alarms (Chambrin, 2001).

Another problem is the lack of standards for new technology. For example, only recently have standards of care been developed for ECG monitoring, which has existed in the clinical setting for nearly 40 years (Leeper, 2006). The CNS in collaboration with nursing staffs is in the best position to develop standards of care and protocols to minimize false alarms and provide support to staffs using the technology.

EXHIBIT 23.8 FACTORS ASSOCIATED WITH FAILURE TO RESPOND TO MEDICAL DEVICE ALARMS

Factors
1. Multiple competing alarms
2. Lack of standards for alarm response
3. Failure to customize alarm settings based on patient assessment
4. Lack of backup for primary responders
5. Staffing
6. Workload
7. Frequency of nuisance alarms
8. Frequency of clinically irrelevant alarms
9. Frequency of false alarms
10. Nursing unit culture
11. Disabling or silencing alarms

EXHIBIT 23.9 MEDICAL DEVICE ALARM COMPETENCY ASSESSMENT

Assessment

1. Customizes alarms based on nursing assessment
2. Checks alarm defaults
3. Knowledgeable of alarm limits
4. Sets the alarm limits when appropriate
5. Alarm audible within the ambient noise of the environment
6. Knowledgeable of the alarm significance
7. Knowledgeable of the implications of nonresponse
8. Demonstrates methods to decrease nuisance alarms
9. Shares responsibilities of responding to clinical alarms
10. Able to explain alarms to patients and families
11. Responds appropriately to clinical alarms

Concomitant with this transformation of patient care is the beginning of the disappearance of the paper medical record. Increased technology at the bedside has created a greater need for more information for an ever-increasing number of specialists providing care who work in ever-widening venues. The electronic medical record promises increased access to information, interconnection of clinicians, improved biosurveillance, and streamlined processes for collecting quality improvement data (Clancy, 2006a).

IT may be the most complex application health care has ever experienced. Until there is a standard template to structure health care information as well as access, data entry, and data transfer, information systems will remain more a problem rather than a solution for health care organizations. The dream of *integrating* primary, inpatient and outpatient care, lab results, tests, and procedures is still a dream. While the electronic record promises to reduce adverse events, evidence suggests that new, subtle, and systematic events will occur related to the linear design of computer programming that as of yet cannot capture the complex multitasking health care environment (Koppel, Metlay, & Cohen, 2005, Langley & Beasley, 2007; O'Malley, 2007). The generally poor customization ability of many IT systems makes adding and linking data fields very difficult. In an organization undergoing conversion to an electronic record, the CNS must be prepared to work intimately with programmers and staffs to enhance training, prevent workarounds, and correct errors in programming and design. The CNS can play an instrumental role in

supporting staffs and the organization implementing an electronic record.

TECHNOLOGY MAINTENANCE

The average academic medical center has over 10,000 medical devices, and hidden in every technology purchase is the cost of ongoing training and evaluation (Baretich, 2004; Bauld et al., 2004). Because few basic nursing programs offer technology theory and limited clinical experience with medical technology, the burden is further increased on the nurse educator and CNS to educate new and current employees on a limited budget (Krautscheid & Burton, 2003).

The goal of all medical device education is that the user must be able to operate or apply the medical device as intended and prevent adverse events associated with use (Bronzino, 2004; Murff, Gosbee, & Bates, 2007). Education is crucial to prevent improper and inappropriate use of medical devices. Annual staff surveys and critical evaluation of incident and anecdotal reports from *risk management* and *quality assurance* can provide the CNS a foundation for planning appropriate education. CNS collaboration with clinical engineers can further identify and eliminate gaps in knowledge or experience that could lead to injury (Bauld et al., 2004; Shepherd, 2004) .

Educational content may include medical device safety, proper set up, and indications and contraindications for use. Step-by-step demonstrations for small groups with return demonstrations *during* the class and *after* can increase staff confidence in use of the medical device. Use of simulators is another powerful method for training and can uncover latent design errors not uncovered during technology assessment (Murff et al., 2007). Computer-based training, newsletters, e-mail, video, and audiotapes, combined with super-user resources for clinical staff, can assist the CNS in preparing a competent and confident nursing staff (AACN, 1999; Bauld et al., 2004; Nelson & Blenkin, 2007; Sensmeier, 2007).

Despite education, quality control, preuse inspections, and trials of technology in the clinical setting, medical device failures still occur (Institute of Medicine, 1999). The vast majority of medical device errors are due to user error rather than medical device failure (Bauld et al., 2004). User errors are a function of the *interaction* of the *user* and the *device in the environment*. Powerful influences include noise, lighting, user fatigue and skills, competing demands, and patient acuity (Murff et al., 2007). Exhibit 23.10 summarizes factors associated with technology failure in the clinical setting (David et al., 2004; ECRI Institute, 2007).

EXHIBIT 23.10   REASONS FOR MEDICAL DEVICE FAILURES

Reasons

1. Failure to inspect and certify the device before use
2. Failure to have a medical device management program
3. Failure to verify that the vendor will deliver a complete system with necessary accessories and disposables
4. Failure to control risks associated with implementation
5. Lack of technical support
6. Failure to provide education to direct and indirect users
7. Failure to complete preventative maintenance
8. Failure to act on recalls
9. Failure of clinical engineering or biomedical technicians to listen to staff feedback
10. Failure to operate the equipment according to manufacturer's guidelines
11. Failure to complete postimplementation evaluations
12. Introducing medical devices without guidelines for users
13. Failure to ensure competency of users at introduction
14. Failure to ensure competency of users over time
15. Failure to modify guidelines with experience and from staff feedback

Every adverse event investigation requires that the CNS critically evaluate with an unbiased and nonjudgmental attitude (Bauld et al., 2004). Preservation of evidence and immediate documentation and recollection of the adverse event is necessary. Crucial observations include device settings, placement, accessories used, environmental conditions, condition of the device, and observations from any personnel in attendance. The investigation should be nonpunitive and supportive of the individuals involved, who are often severely traumatized by the event and even more traumatized by the subsequent investigation. The underlying principal of any investigation must be explicit to all involved, and that is: *Every* adverse event offers incredible opportunity for improvement of related policies and procedures associated with the medical device and, ultimately, improvement in nursing care.

THE FUTURE

The world market for medical products is approximately $150 billion, with pharmaceuticals accounting for $100 billion and $50 billion for medical devices. While technology is often blamed for the rising costs of health care, the market for medical devices continues to expand. Technology has improved health care in terms of access, quality, and efficiency. Technology has also extended the science and practice of nursing (David et al., 2004).

However, technology also threatens the profession of nursing. Intimate body care and sacred therapeutic relationships are increasingly being replaced with technical intimacy (Sandelowski, 2000; Schoenhofer, 2001). Overemphasis on technological competency has gradually eroded the nurse–patient dyad to the patient–technology–nurse triad. More often than not, the patient–nurse relationship occurs only if there is time left after required actions with technology are completed. Gradually, the nurse–patient relationship, which has the greatest lasting impact on the health care experience, is eroding (Sandelowski, 2000; Schoenhofer, 2001).

The increasing mechanistic view of human beings expressed as sole emphasis on outcomes and benchmarks implies that human beings are predictable and manageable (Mitchell, 2001). The increasing obsession with technology, task, and evidence-based practice is changing practice from holism to a biomedical paradigm. Nursing's commitment to honor, care, respect, and help persons under their care is gradually being lost (Mitchell, 2001).

The continuous technological transformation of health care provides promise and risk for nursing. There are four risks the CNS must continuously monitor and be prepared to address now and in the future to preserve the art and science of professional nursing practice.

First and foremost, beware of the promise that the technology permits the nurse to care for *more patients.* Evidence suggests that technology increases the need for *more nurses* related to maintenance, programming, troubleshooting, and differentiation of true and false alarms (Sandelowski, 2000; Schoenhofer, 2001). Furthermore, technology usually restricts patient mobility, thereby increasing the incidence of pressure ulcers, respiratory problems, falls, and stress for patients and families. More rather than less nursing care is usually needed to prevent these unfavorable outcomes (Sandelowski, 2000; Schoenhofer, 2001). Critical evaluation of technology impact on practice and patients can provide necessary evidence that supports appropriate nurse–patient ratios, which in turn supports nurse retention and safe patient care.

Even more dangerous is the assumption that technology can *substitute* for the judgment of a nurse. No technology, no matter how well designed or programmed, interfaced with a human being can discern all the sources of variance in the physiological and health care environments. Because all technology carries some degree of risk *and* error in application, nursing actions should be based on critical evaluation rather than unhesitating acceptance of technology-provided data (Rinard, 2001; Sandelowski, 2000). The CNS can provide critical advocacy for patients and nurses when technology is implemented through education, training, and development of practice guidelines that enhance decision making rather than replace it.

The increasing mechanization of health care is subtle and powerful. Technology has extended practice, but technology has also increased the risk of depersonalization for the patient *and* the nurse. Critical care environments where nurses are in continuous relationship with multiple technologies and one patient are particularly at risk. Depending on patient acuity, staffing, experience, and competency, the nurse–patient relationship is often sacrificed along with teaching, providing comfort, and presence to maintain the technology–patient interface safely (Sandelowski, 2000; Schoenhofer, 2001). The CNS can assist nursing to plan the best staffing, responsibilities, and training so that technology is not the exclusive recipient of nursing care (Brooten & Naylor, 1993; Darmondy, 2005).

The CNS must protect nursing at the bedside. Increasingly, nurses are doing the work of medicine, respiratory therapy, pharmacy, laboratory, and physical therapy, radiology, and nutrition services under the disguise of nursing care. Once the novelty of new technology wears off and risks are known, technology once exclusively under the prevue of a specific discipline is usually transferred to nursing *after* application to the patient because nursing is with the patient 24 hours a day (Sandelowski, 2000; Schoenhofer, 2001). Recent examples of technology transfer to nursing include extra corporeal membrane oxygenation, cardiac ventricular assist support, vascular sheath removal, renal replacement therapies, weaning from mechanical ventilation, and bedside laboratory analysis. As a result, nursing care increasingly is becoming more surveillance and less comfort, more troubleshooting and less touch, and technology-based outcomes rather than a healing therapeutic relationship.

The promises of technology—convenience, productivity, and access to information 24 hours a day, 7 days a week—have opened a Pandora's box of unimaginable consequences (Miller, 2007). It is increasingly difficult to separate human beings (patient or staff) from the technology in health care. Constant availability, multitasking, role expansion, and flattening of management hierarchies have nearly eliminated the *time* necessary for critical thinking (Miller, 2007).

Multitasking, which emerged from the computer sciences under the false conclusion that computers multitask, has become the norm for health care organizations. The reality is that while computers appear to be completing several tasks at once, the program only completes *one task at a time*. However, computer recovery *following* task completion is immediate, so the next task is completed without a break and seemingly simultaneous with the previous task.

Nurses multitask, caring for patients and responding to increasing numbers of interruptions including requests for information, families, and managing technology. However, recovery is not simultaneous, and evidence suggests that up to 23 minutes is required to get back to the primary task at hand after an interruption. The result is a neurologically stressful environment associated with tension, anxiety, and depression (Miller, 2007). In the future, the CNS will increasingly have to find ways to carve out time for nurses to use the nursing process.

Technological proficiency is an expression of nurse caring. Monitoring, interpretation of medical device data, and technological competency are critical elements of nursing care. However, without intentionality, compassion, confidence, commitment, and conscience, the nurse is only a robot, and the patient is only an object within a technology dense environment (Locsin, 2001b). The CNS must protect and make known nursing's contribution in technology-rich environments so that nurses do not become invisible, undervalued, and perceived only as an adjunct to medical and economic outcomes (Schoenhofer, 2001).

Technology is fleeting and ever-changing and is not owned by any one discipline. Some have suggested that in the future technology may free patients from their caregivers (Mitchell, 2001). This would result in an unimaginable transformation in health care. What then would be nursing's mission?

Technology has reshaped the aesthetics, politics, ethics, and roles in health care. Nurses, physicians, respiratory therapists, nurse's aids, patients, and families use stethoscopes, sphygmomanometers, infusion pumps, ventilators, and defibrillators at home, on the road, in the clinic, and the physician office. Cross training, personnel substitution, and role dilution are gradually rendering nursing invisible (Sandelowski, 2000). The CNS is the best advocate to make visible nursing's contribution to patient outcomes beyond the management technology. The CNS can help preserve the art and science of nursing practice in technology-rich environments through critical evaluation, advocacy, teaching, role modeling, consultation, and research.

Experience suggests that technology alone cannot heal, care, protect, or comfort. Without a committed, expert nurse able to balance caring and technology management *within* a nurse–patient relationship, patients become machines whose outcomes can be engineered. Patients are more than biology, disease, machinery, or treatment. Nurses are more than technology managers (Barnard, 2001). The CNS is in the best position to preserve nursing practice, protect vulnerable patients, and drive safe technology application that supports the most important relationship in health care: the nurse–patient relationship.

DISCUSSION QUESTIONS

1. How does technology impact your nursing practice?
2. What percentage of your practice is devoted to technology issues?
3. Technological proficiency has been described as evidence of a caring nurse. Do nurses believe this? Do you think patients also believe this?
4. In technologically rich environments, what can a nurse do to foster a personal and healing relationship with a patient?

ANALYSIS AND SYNTHESIS EXERCISES

1. Increasingly, complex medical informatics (electronic medical record, computerized physician order entry, electronic medication record) promise improved information accessibility and fewer errors. With these promises come the realities of monumental changes in health care culture, workflow, workload, and different errors. Locate a hospital in your area that has converted to the electronic medical record (EMR). Obtain an interview with a CNS who practiced through the conversion to the EMR. Discuss the following critical elements: staff training, relationships with IT staff, hardware and software decisions, access and integration of information, and changes in workflow. If the process could be done over, what would be different or the same?
2. Using the information provided in Exhibit 23.5, complete an assessment of one technology in a clinical setting. Based on your findings, where in the life cycle is the technology? Are upgrades or improved replacement technologies available? What are the implications of upgrading or replacement for nursing, patients, and the organization?

CLINICAL APPLICATION CONSIDERATIONS

1. Locsin (2001b) believes technological competency defines nursing practice. List the core competencies required for nurses where you practice. Which of these competencies require technology application? For each technology identified, describe the education, training, and competency assessment required for safe patient application. Next, determine

whether the technology increased or decreased nursing workload. Does nursing control the technology, or does the technology control nursing? If workload is increased, is this a function of complexity, patient acuity, or improper use? What could be done differently to reduce workload or improve nurse satisfaction?

2. Design and administer a survey of nurses regarding all technologies in a defined clinical setting. For each technology, assess the nurse's perceived competency with application, troubleshooting, alarms, and discontinuation. Based on staff feedback, develop interventions, which may include in-services, individual mentoring, developing super users as staff resources, writing procedures, or designing posters and/or information cards. Include an evaluation for each intervention.

ADDITIONAL HELPFUL RESOURCES

Abbey, J., & Shepherd, M. (1999). The Abbey-Shepherd Device Education Model. *Nursing and technology: Moving into the 21st century* (pp. 4189–4231). Annapolis, MD: HHS/FDA.

American College of Clinical Engineering. Retrieved January 9, 2009, from http://www.accenet.org/

Dyro, J. F. (1983). Depolarizing nursing and biomedical engineering. *Device Techniques, 4*(1), 9–10.

ECRI Institute. (1991). *Medical Device Problem Reporting.* Retrieved January 9, 2009, from https://www.ecri.org/PatientSafety/ReportAProblem/Pages/default.aspx

ECRI Institute. (1995). *Health Devices Inspection and Preventative Maintenance System.* Retrieved January 9, 2009, from https://www.ecri.org/Products/Pages/Health_Devices_System.aspx?sub=Device%20Safety

ECRI Institute. (2000). *Healthcare Standards Directory Online.* Retrieved January 9, 2009, from https://www.ecri.org/Products/Pages/healthcare_standards_directory.aspx?sub=Management%20Tools,%20Guidelines,%20and%20Standards

FDA Medical Device Classification System. Retrieved January 9, 2009, from http://www.fda.gov/cdrh/prodcode.html

Gardner, S., & Flack, M. (1999). *Designing a medical device surveillance network.* Washington, DC: U.S. Food and Drug Administration.

Howell, J. D. (1995). *Technology in the hospital—Transforming patient care in the early twentieth century.* Baltimore: The Johns Hopkins University Press.

Institute of Medicine. (1999). *To err is human: Building a safer health system.* Washington, DC: National Academies Press.

Institute of Medicine. (2001). *Crossing the quality chasm: A new health care system for the 21st century.* Washington, DC: National Academies Press.

Joint Commission on Accreditation of Health Care Organizations. (2001). *Revisions to Joint Commission standard in support of patient safety and medical/health care error reduction.* Chicago: Author.

Perrow, C. (1999). *Normal accidents: Living with high-risk technologies.* Princeton, NJ: Princeton University Press.

Wang, B., & Levenson, A. (2000). Equipment inclusion criteria: A new interpretation of JCAHO's medical equipment management standard. *Journal of Clinical Engineering, 25*(1), 26–35.

HELPFUL JOURNALS

Biomedical Instrumentation and Technology. http://www.aami.org/publications/BIT/.

Journal of Clinical Engineering. http://www.lww.com/product/?0363-8855.

PROFESSIONAL SOCIETIES

Association for the Advancement of Medical Instrumentation. http://www.aami.org/.

American Society for Healthcare Engineering. http://www.ashe.org/.

REFERENCES

Albert N. M. (2006). Bioimpedence cardiography measurement of cardiac output and other cardiovascular parameters. *Critical Care Nursing Clinics of North America, 18*(2), 195–202.

American Association of Colleges of Nursing (AACN). (1999). *Response to the Institute of Medicine report: To err is human: Building a safer health system.* Retrieved January 9, 2009, from http://www.aacn.nche.edu/publications/positions/whitepaper.htm

Arbour, R. (2006). Impact of bispectral index monitoring on sedation and outcomes in critically ill adults: A case series. *Critical Care Nursing Clinics of North America, 18*(2), 227–241.

Bader, M. K. (2006). Recognizing and treating ischemic insults to the brain: The role of brain tissue oxygen monitoring. *Critical Care Nursing Clinics of North America, 18*(2), 243–256.

Baldwin, D., Bingham, J., & Connors, H. (1996). *Teaching with technologies. Distance education strategies report.* Kansas City: University of Kansas Medical Center.

Baretich, M. (2004). Equipment control and asset management. In J. Dyro (Ed.), *Clinical engineering handbook* (pp. 122–123). Boston: Elsevier Academic Press.

Barnard, A. (2001). On the relationship between technique and dehumanization. In R. C. Locsin (Ed.), *Advancing technology, caring and nursing* (pp. 96–105). Westport, CT: Auburn House.

Barnard, A., & Cushing, A. (2001). Technology and historical inquiry. In R. C. Locsin (Ed.), *Advancing technology, caring and nursing* (pp. 12–21). Westport, CT: Auburn House.

Bauld, T., Dyro, J., & Grimes, S. (2004). Clinical engineering and nursing. In J. Dyro (Ed.), *Clinical engineering handbook* (pp. 321–327). Boston: Elsevier Academic Press.

Bronzino, J. (2004). Clinical engineering: Evolution of a discipline. In J. Dyro (Ed.), *Clinical engineering handbook* (pp. 3–7). Boston: Elsevier Academic Press.

Brooten, D., & Naylor, M. D. (1993). The role and functions of clinical nurse specialists. *Clinical Nurse Specialist, 25*(1), 73–78.

Button, E., & Keaton, P. (2006). Glycemic control after coronary artery bypass graft: Using intravenous insulin regulated by a computerized system. *Critical Care Nursing Clinics of North America, 18*(2), 257–265.

Canlas, J., Hall, J., & Shuck-Holmes, P. (2004). Medical device design and control in the hospital. In J. Dyro (Ed.), *Clinical engineering handbook* (pp. 346–349). Boston: Elsevier Academic Press.

Chambrin, M. C. (2001). Alarms in the intensive care unit: How can the number of false alarms be reduced? *The Critical Care Forum, 5*(4), 184–188.

Clancy, C. (2006a). *Accelerating the adoption of health information technology. Testimony before the Senate Committee on commerce, science, transportation subcommittee on technology, innovation, and competitiveness.* Agency for Healthcare Research and Quality, Rockville, MD. Retrieved January 9, 2009, from http://www.ahrq.gov/news/test062106.htm

Clancy, C. (2006b). The 1.6 trillion dollar question—If we're spending so much on healthcare, why so little improvement in quality? *Medscape General Medicine, 8*(2), 58.

Darmondy, J. V. (2005). Observing the work of the clinical nurse specialist. *Clinical Nurse Specialist, 19*(5), 260–268.

David, Y., Judd, T., & Zambuto, R. (2004). Introduction to medical technology management practices. In J. Dyro (Ed.), *Clinical engineering handbook* (pp. 101–107). Boston: Elsevier Academic Press.

Drew, B. J., & Funk, M. (2006). Practice standards for ECG monitoring in hospital settings: Executive summary and guide for implementation. *Critical Care Nursing Clinics of North America, 18*(2), 157–168.

ECRI Institute. (2007). *Critical care safety: Essentials for ICU patient care and technology.* Retrieved January 9, 2009, from http://www.ecri.org/criticalcare

Eisenberg, J. M. (1999). Ten lessons for evidence-based technology. *Journal of the American Medical Association, 282*(19), 1865–1869.

Flanders, S. A. (2006). Continuous ST-segment monitoring: Raising the bar. *Critical Care Nursing Clinics of North America, 18*(2), 169–177.

Gaev, J. (2004). Technology in health care. In J. Dyro (Ed.), *Clinical engineering handbook* (pp. 342–345). Boston: Elsevier Academic Press.

Goodrich, C. (2006). Continuous central venous oximetry monitoring. *Critical Care Nursing Clinics of North America, 18*(2), 203–209.

Harding, G., & Epstein, A. (2004). Technology procurement. In J. Dyro (Ed.), *Clinical engineering handbook* (pp. 118–122). Boston: Elsevier Academic Press.

Haselkorn, A., Rosenstein, A. H., Rao, A. K., VanZuiden, M., & Cove, M. (2007). New technology planning and approval: Critical factors for success. *American Journal of Medical Quality, 22*(3), 164–169.

Headley, J. M. (2006). Arterial pressure-based technologies: A new trend in cardiac output monitoring. *Critical Care Nursing Clinics of North America, 18*(2), 179–187.

Heidegger, M. (1977). *The question concerning technology and other essays.* New York: Harper and Row.

Hill, K. M., & Klein, D. G. (2006). Transcutaneous carbon dioxide monitoring. *Critical Care Nursing Clinics of North America, 18*(2), 211–215.

Institute of Medicine, Committee on Quality of Health Care in America. (1999). *To err is human: Building a safer health system.* Washington, DC: National Academies Press.

Keller, J. (2004). Comparative evaluations of medical devices. In J. Dyro (Ed.), *Clinical engineering handbook* (pp. 366–368). Boston: Elsevier Academic Press.

Koppel, R., Metlay, J. P., & Cohen, A. (2005). Role of computerized order entry system in facilitating medication errors.

Journal of the American Medical Association, 293(10), 1197–1203.

Krautscheid, L., & Burton, D. (2003). Oregon education-based technology needs assessment: Expanding nursing education capacity. *Technology in Nursing Education.* Retrieved January 9, 2009, from http://www.oregoncenterfornursing.org/docu ments/Tech_Assessment.pdf

Laing, G. (1982). The impact of technology on nursing. *Medical Instrumentation, 16*(5), 241–242.

Langley, J., & Beasley, C. (2007). Health information technology for improving quality of care in primary care settings. *Agency for Healthcare Research and Quality, Publication No. 07–0079-EF.* Retrieved January 9, 2009, from http://healthit.ahrq.gov/portal/server.pt/gateway/PTARGS_0_1248_661809_0_0_18/AHRQ_HIT_Primary_Care_July07.pdf

Lanzafame, R. J. (2006). Issues in the acquisition, development and use of technology in health care. *Journal of the Society of Laparoendoscopic Surgeons, 10*(4), 401–408.

Leeper, B. (2006). Monitoring and hemodynamics. *Critical Care Nursing Clinics of North America, 18*(2), xiii–xiv.

Locsin, R. (2001a). Introduction. In R. C. Locsin (Ed.), *Advancing technology, caring, and nursing* (pp. xxi–xxvi). Westport, CT: Auburn House.

Locsin, R. (2001b). Practicing nursing: Technological competency as an expression of caring. In R. C. Locsin (Ed.), *Advancing technology, caring, and nursing* (pp. 88–95). Westport, CT: Auburn House.

Matuszewski, K. A. (1997). A primer on the assessment of medical technologies. *Pharmacy Practice Management Quarterly, 16*(4), 53–65.

Mitchell, G. J. (2001). Pictures of paradox: Technology, nursing and human science. In R. C. Locsin (Ed.), *Advancing technology, caring, and nursing* (pp. 22–40). Westport, CT: Auburn House.

Miller, H. (2007). *The siren song of multi-tasking.* Retrieved January 9, 2009, from http://www.hermanmiller.com/hm/content/research_summaries/pdfs/wp_SirenSong.pdf

Murff, H. J., Gosbee, J. W., & Bates, D. W. (2007). *Chapter 41. Human factors and medical devices.* Agency for Healthcare Research and Quality. Retrieved January 9, 2009, from http://www.ahrq.gov/clinic/ptsafety/chap41a.htm

Nelson, D. L., & Blenkin, C. (2007). The power of online role-play simulations: Technology in nursing education. *International Journal of Nursing Education Scholarship, 4.* Retrieved January 9, 2009, from http://www.bepress.com/ijnes/vol4/iss1/art1/

O'Malley, P. (2007). Computerized provider order entry and prescribing and evidence for safe practice. *Clinical Nurse Specialist, 21*(3), 139–141.

Phillips, J. (2006). Clinical alarms: Complexity and common sense. *Critical Care Nursing Clinics of North America, 18*(2), 145–156.

Prentice, D., & Sona, C. (2006). Esophageal doppler monitoring for hemodynamic assessment. *Critical Care Nursing Clinics of North America, 18*(2), 189–193.

Richter, N. (2004). Evolution of medical device technology. In J. Dyro (Ed.), *Clinical engineering handbook* (pp. 339–341). Boston: Elsevier Academic Press.

Ridgway, M., Johnson, G., & McClain, J. (2004). History of engineering and technology in health care. In J. Dyro (Ed.), *Clinical engineering handbook* (pp. 7–8). Boston: Elsevier Academic Press.

Rinard, R. G. (2001). Technology, de-skilling and nurses. The impact of the technologically changing environment. In R. C. Locsin (Ed.), *Advancing technology, caring, and nursing* (pp. 68–75). Westport, CT: Auburn House.

Rosen, R., & Gabbay, J. (1999). Linking health technology assessment to practice. *British Medical Journal, 319*(7220), 1292.

Rosenstein, A. H., O'Daniel, M., & Geoghan, K. (2003). Assessing new technology: How are other hospitals facing the challenge? *Healthcare Financial Management, 57*(10), 70–74.

Sandelowski, M. (2000). *Devices and desires: Gender, technology, and American nursing (studies in social medicine).* Chapel Hill: The University of North Carolina Press.

Scales, D. C., & Laupacis, A. (2007). Health technology assessment in critical care. *Intensive Care Medicine, 33*(12), 2183–2191. Retrieved January 9, 2009, from http://springerlink.com/content/p3751tg86943311p/

Schoenhofer, S. B. (2001). Outcomes of caring in high-technology practice environments. In R. C. Locsin (Ed.), *Advancing technology, caring, and nursing* (pp. 79–87). Westport, CT: Auburn House.

Sensmeier, J. (2007). The future of IT: Aggressive educational reform. TIGER initiative preps nurses for healthcare's digital era. *Nursing Management, 38*(9, IT Solutions supplement), 2–8.

Shekelle, P. G., Morton, S. C., & Keeler, E. B. (2006, April). *Costs and benefits of health information technology.* Evidence Report/Technology Assessment No. 132. (Prepared by the Southern California Evidence-based Practice Center under Contract No. 290-02-0003.) AHRQ Publication No. 06-E006. Rockville, MD: Agency for Healthcare Research and Quality. Retrieved January 9, 2009, from http://www.ahrq.gov/downloads/pub/evidence/pdf/hitsyscosts/hitsys.pdf

Shepherd, M. (2004). Systems approach to medical device safety. In J. Dyro (Ed.), *Clinical engineering handbook* (pp. 246–249). Boston: Elsevier Academic Press.

Welter, L. O. (2004). The health care environment. In J. Dyro (Ed.), *Clinical engineering handbook* (pp. 11–14). Boston: Elsevier Academic Press.

White, G. (2007). The sky is falling . . . or maybe not: The moral necessity of technology assessment. *American Journal of Business Education, 7*(10), 20–21.

Wilson, D., Kumor, R., & Bar, A. H. (2007). Lasso runaway technology and supply chain costs. *Nursing Management, 38*(5), 25–30.

Zwerneman, K. (2006). End-tidal carbon dioxide monitoring: A VITAL sign worth watching. *Critical Care Nursing Clinics of North America, 18*(2), 217–225.

Interview or Interviewee: Essential Skills for the Clinical Nurse Specialist Employment Interview

Ann F. Minnick

THE INTERVIEW: AN IMPORTANT WAY TO INFORM A COSTLY DECISION

The chance to achieve a great match between the skills and interests of a clinical nurse specialist (CNS) and the demands of a position that requires CNS preparation can be won or lost in a single employment interview. This chapter considers both sides of the imaginary interview table because every CNS will apply for a position and almost every CNS will at least participate in, if not lead, CNS employment interviews.

The selection of the wrong person for a CNS post will cost an organization thousands of dollars in direct costs and, potentially, millions of dollars in indirect costs. Before one dismisses this assertion, consider the source of these costs. Direct costs include all expenses related to the search process. Examples are orientation time, recruitment costs, termination costs, and possible settlement costs if an employee leaves (or is asked to leave) soon after employment. Indirect costs could be in the millions if the CNS's poor practice leads to the adoption of ineffective policies and procedures, poor staff education, or incorrect modeling of patient care that results in poor outcomes and/or lawsuits. Making

the right decision can result in an institutional gain of impressive amounts. Hiring a CNS who can help staff revise a clinical practice with the result of a shortened length of stay for persons with high-volume diagnoses is but one example of how this can occur.

The CNS applicant has a considerable financial and professional stake in making the right employment decision. The position may require relocation and all of its attendant expenses, the full costs of which are almost never completely recovered by the employee. Leaving a position in a short time usually results in no accrual of retirement benefits. For example, leaving three positions in under a year during a 30-year CNS career means a loss of at least 10% of one's employer retirement benefits because many employers do not make or match contributions until the first full year of employment has passed. In real dollars, the loss is perhaps greater if these changes occur early in a career because the power of long-term investment is lost. Adding to the seriousness of the CNS's employment decision are indirect costs. One of these indirect costs may be future marketability. Employers are interested in a work history that demonstrates some stability. They also are interested in professional growth. Taking a position that one leaves quickly or that provides no growth opportunities could result in the CNS losing opportunities for career advancement.

USING THIS CHAPTER FOR BEST RESULTS

The interview is one of the best ways to match applicants and positions. It is, therefore, a situation in which both the employer and the potential employee use interview skills to determine if a match exists. Although recognizing this duality, this chapter uses the term *interviewer* for the employer and *interviewee* for the CNS applicant. To conduct an interview that results in the best assessment of the match between interviewee and the position, interviewers and interviewees should review both roles.

After considering the ways in which CNS interviews differ from those at the staff nurse level, this chapter describes process and content activities for interviewers and interviewees during the preinterview, interview, and postinterview periods. The sections review general principles of interviewing and those specific to the CNS interview. Checklists or interviewer and interviewee activities are provided at the end of the chapter.

SPECIAL CONSIDERATIONS IN THE CNS INTERVIEW PROCESS

There are many excellent references regarding general interview techniques and guidelines (Cardinal, 2003; Howell, 1999; Murphy, 2006; Puetz, 2005; Yate, 2006), but the nature of the CNS position requires special considerations. Although nurses will probably have had extensive experience in interviewing and being interviewed for staff nurse positions, three important aspects of any CNS position must be recognized in planning and executing the interview process. The first aspect is the interdisciplinary nature of a CNS position. Although staff nurses interact with other disciplines, the CNS is one of the key nursing representatives in interdisciplinary standard setting and achievement. The CNS position also requires skill in the communication of the scientific developments and emerging viewpoints of other care providers to an institution's nursing staff as well as sharing nursing developments with other disciplines. The interview process must, therefore, be structured to allow the person responsible for making the hiring decision to evaluate the candidate from the perspective of interdisciplinary colleagues. The applicant must have the opportunity to evaluate the structures and tone of interdisciplinary contact.

A second aspect of the CNS role that influences the interview is the position's emphasis on accomplishing quality improvement, educational, and/or research projects rather than the patient care assignments that are common for staff nurse positions. The extent to which the CNS applicant wants independence in project selection, design, and execution will play an important role in the applicant's assessment of the position. Employers may also have specific projects related to the accomplishment of strategic plan objectives that should be explained during the interview process. The extent to which the applicant's and employer's project interests and institutional targets mesh must be established early in the interview process.

The third aspect that makes the interview for a CNS somewhat different from other nursing positions comes from the 1990s when CNS positions were (or were perceived to be) the first nursing positions sacrificed during labor reductions. In institutions where CNS positions were sacrificed, the CNSs were not effectively documenting impact on patient outcomes, including cost savings, cost avoidance, and revenue generation. Although the situation has improved, it is imperative for the CNS applicant to ask about the availability/accessibility of patient outcome and cost data in order to document the CNS's contribution to cost savings, cost avoidance, and revenue generation. Applicants cannot expect nor employers guarantee life-long employment, but a clear understanding of how the position is supported and its holder evaluated is essential.

PREINTERVIEW PREPARATIONS: THE INTERVIEWER

Throughout the remainder of the chapter, the term *interviewer* is used to simplify the presentation although the interview process is assumed to involve multiple interviewers based on the intra- and interdisciplinary responsibilities of the CNS, as well as the multiple reporting structures that might be attendant to a position with multidepartment funding sources. The lead interviewer is defined as the person who has direct hiring authority and coordinates the interview process.

Interviewer Decisions

As soon as the recruitment process begins, the lead interviewer needs to make some basic decisions. First, determine who needs to interview the candidate. Then, for each interview, decide when it should be conducted, what the goal of the interview is, and the what role the interviewer plays in making a final selection. Although these plans may change as the interview process evolves, the lead interviewer's completion of these duties will ensure that the process makes the most of every moment spent with the candidate. To select the interviewers, consider the groups with whom the CNS will work. A common mistake is to underestimate the importance of staff nurse involvement in the selection process. Staff nurses will be important colleagues of the CNS. Excluding them from the interview process may be construed as an attempt to hide a staff problem.

If the list of potential interviewers has grown long, the lead interviewer must decide if a staggered interview process would be helpful. For example, the lead interviewer might conduct a preliminary interview, and then, based on its outcome, schedule an inclusive series of interviews. One can also consider scheduling more than one interview at a time. If this is done, pairing interviewers of similar interests is essential.

The order of an interview series can be crucial to a productive interview experience, especially if one hopes to maintain the independence of multiple interviewers' opinions. Proper sequencing can also help determine how well an applicant listens to and synthesizes organizational issues. For example, if an early interviewer describes a major issue influencing CNS practice at the institution, a subsequent interviewer could lead the interview in a direction that requires some synthesis of possible solutions. The capacity of a CNS applicant to learn throughout the interview process may be one indication that the applicant has the skills required by the position.

Timing is also a consideration if a decision has been made to conduct single interviewee–multiple interviewer sessions. An interviewer should not interview a candidate without a full interview schedule, positions goals, role and job description information, and the applicant's resume. If this information is not available to all interviewers, the interview should be rescheduled.

Review the Position Description and Create a Project Summary

There is probably no better way to lose a qualified CNS applicant than to send him/her on a round of interviews in which the interviewers either profess that they know nothing about the position or portray the position's main duties at polar extremes. Implementing the following suggested activities can help avoid these situations.

The lead interviewer must begin the position review process for two reasons: (1) It is a statement of what the position entails should legal questions be raised about how the hiring process eliminated or selected certain candidates, and (2) it serves as a basis for multiple interviewers to reflect on the minimal skills and abilities needed to succeed in the position. Most important, the position review clarifies what the person responsible for making a hiring decision wants. Examples of questions to ask during this review include: Are the educational criteria sufficient? Is familiarity with systems no longer in use at the hospital listed as a job requirement?

What does the description say about reporting responsibilities? How is the position evaluated? Is the position description open to negotiation with the applicant? If so, which elements can be negotiated? Is travel between hospitals within the system required? Approximately how often will such travel be necessary? For more, see Exhibit 24.1.

The typical institutional description of the CNS position does not have sufficient detail to serve as the basis for an interview for a specific CNS job. For example, during the first year, a neonatal CNS's position-related goals may involve initial project goals to help staff prepare for magnet status application, assisting nursing school faculty in arranging clinical teaching opportunities, and launching a new "baby life flight" program. Another main responsibility of the CNS during the same year may be launching an intraoperative safety program. Human resource departments counsel against making rigorously individualized position descriptions for legal and regulatory reasons. Very detailed descriptions also limit expectations about the flexibility required in the rapidly changing health care environment and, thus, changing demands within the health care institution. Position descriptions for CNSs should be consistent with the National Association of Clinical Nurse Specialists (NACNS) *Statement on Practice and Education* (2004).

EXHIBIT 24.1 CNS POSITION ATTRIBUTES

Desired Attributes
1. Consistency with personal and professional values
2. Opportunities for professional growth
3. Opportunities to utilize best skills
4. Resource availability
   a. Personnel, nursing
   b. Personnel, nonnursing
   c. Equipment
   d. Financial
   e. Staff support
5. Working conditions
   a. Temporal, including schedule
   b. Spatial
   c. Physical
   d. Safety measures
   e. Over all milieu
   f. Travel expectations
6. Compensation
   a. Benefits
   b. Salary
   c. Incentives/bonus plans
7. Organizational stability
8. Common understanding among interviewers of
   a. Strategic goals/reporting
   b. Relationship(s) and evaluation mechanisms

The position description should cover the three spheres of influence and be written in terms that allow for the dynamic flow and emphasis from sphere to sphere consistent with institutional need.

To assist in identifying specific expectations of the CNS, the lead interviewer can draft a description of current and planned projects related to the CNS position. Sharing this description with other interviewers provides an opportunity for all to clarify the CNS position-specific job expectations. In a shared governance or matrix institution, the lead interviewer would anticipate that these discussions may result in additional iterations of the description. In hierarchical organizations, the lead interviewer would benefit from the responses of the potential interview team.

Essential Versus Ideal Skill Sets: A Basis for the Interview Report Form

The position description review and the drafting of the description of current and future projects may result in the realization that the position seems to require skills that no one person can possess. To address this problem, the lead interviewer needs to identify the position's essential skills versus those that are ideal for the position. Other interviewers may assist the lead interviewer in this determination. These skills can then be listed on the interview report form. The lead interviewer may ask each interviewer to concentrate on a specific skill, thereby avoiding the possibility that essential skills are never probed during the interview process. The product of all these deliberations should be an interview report form that allows the interviewer to evaluate the applicant on the essential skills and to describe any ideal skills noted during the interview.

Update One's Knowledge of the Labor Market

Prior to conducting any interviews, the lead interviewer must contact the human resource department for information about supply and demand for CNSs locally and outside of the region. If the organization is small, that is, a practice, reviewing one's state's fair employment practice site will be helpful. Knowledge of the market includes understanding CNS employment patterns and the terms being offered by the market. During the interview itself, one will need to be prepared to evaluate applicants' employment condition requests against the broader hiring market.

The lead interviewer should not assume the role of a compensation and benefits officer but should be prepared to discuss: (1) the potential for an employment contract or other safety net provisions, (2) institutional commitments to health and safety with emphasis on

those issues most likely to arise in the CNS's specific clinical area (Hess, 2005), (3) general educational and professional benefits (e.g., opportunity to work with well-known experts or gain experience in certain procedures), and (4) unusual benefits. An example of an unusual benefit is the provision of full college tuition for an employee's children. Although compensation and benefits are often discussed at the time an offer of employment is made, in competitive markets this information may need to be presented early during the interview process to maintain an applicant's interest. If the CNS position is a split clinical–educational position, the lead interviewer needs to be familiar with the general process for determining faculty rank. Details must be handled by the school or college.

Spend Interview Time Wisely

To avoid using precious interview time in relaying facts, the lead interviewer should assemble a package of information about the job description, the facility, its operations, and relevant projects that may not be available on the institution's Internet site. The packet should also include the interview schedule. The lead interviewer must consider the multidisciplinary perspective when providing this information. The CNS applicant will want to know, for example, about resident and fellow roles and personnel availability. Each applicant scheduled for an interview should receive the same information in the interest of fairness. Care must be taken to avoid sending competitive or financially sensitive information. At a minimum, the titles and departments of interviewers should be clearly listed on the interview schedule. Including contact information on the schedule can assist with questions that an interviewee may have after the interview.

As with other nursing positions, the provision of general information that is available on Web sites to CNS applicants is not recommended. An applicant can demonstrate motivation and critical thinking skills by collecting and analyzing this material and using the information to ask pertinent questions during the interview process.

Review Legal and Ethical Responsibilities

Beyond knowledge of federal and state standards regarding the fair treatment of applicants regardless of race, religion, gender, age, and ethnicity, the entire interview team must have a basic understanding of questions related to disability that may be asked. The human resource office is a common source for information about these issues. They may subscribe to newsletters such as "The Fair Employment Practices Guidelines" that can help clarify any issues. The interview process must be as similar as possible for each candidate to avoid any hint of preferential treatment. The lead interviewer's circulation of the interview evaluation form will help make the interview process similar for each candidate.

The lead interviewer is responsible for honoring any agreements with applicants regarding the timing of reference checks and current employment verification. Although some interview experts suggest doing this prior to an initial interview, understandable concerns about premature disclosure of interest in a new position contradicts this advice for CNS professionals. The placement of nurse licensing information online in many states has, however, made it possible to verify discreetly registered nurse licensure, advanced practice, and citizenship status.

Prepare Questions Before Reviewing the Applicant's Resume

Human resource research has produced conflicting results regarding the extent to which resume review leads to self-fulfilling prophecy during an interview (Dougherty, Turban, & Callender, 1994). For example, does reading the resume and finding out the applicant trained with the same people as the interviewer lead to automatically assuming competency questions can be omitted in the interview? Preparing questions that probe for essential qualities and specific skills prior to reviewing the resume may help prevent this phenomenon. After reading the resume, plan probing questions for each major area.

Exhibit 24.2 presents examples of several approaches to question development. Prior to the interview, inexperienced interviewers should practice asking these questions with a frank, experienced colleague acting as the interviewee. For more potential general questions use a computerized search engine with the key words "interview questions."

Consider the Impressions You and Your Organization Project

Much has been written regarding applicant dress for job interviews, yet interviewees are also judging the professionalism, courtesy, and mannerisms of their potential employer and coworkers (Howell, 1999; Puetz, 2005). Attention to basic hospitality measures (e.g., taking the applicant's coat and offering a beverage), use of the applicant's preferred name, and focus on the applicant (as opposed to the most recent e-mail message on a desk screen) are minimum standards that must be observed. The day may be an exceptionally busy one, but the interviewer must try to observe the duck principle (all paddling must be confined to below the surface). Be sure the support staff know who the candidate is and the appointment time. If the applicant will need to

wait for you, be sure the staff know where to seat the applicant.

The choice of interview area and seating arrangements (across a desk, facing chairs, chairs around a table) convey information about the organization and the interviewer. The choice will also likely influence the openness of the exchange with across-desk interviews being most likely to elicit formal responses. Asking the interviewee some questions during a facility tour or a meal are excellent ways to elicit more spontaneous responses. In some situations, the initial interview must be conducted by telephone. Ensuring that the telephones provide clear and reliable connection is recommended. Speaker phones often have unpleasant and sound-distorting qualities. During an initial interview, eliminating such distractions is important for building rapport.

PREINTERVIEW PREPARATIONS: THE INTERVIEWEE

This section is written based on the assumption that the interviewee has identified the potential position through an organized search. Steinmiller (1999) suggests a CNS new graduate begin the process during the last year in school. Steps include determining career goals and rewards and developing networks of professional contacts at professional meetings.

Determine Attributes

Before you go to your interview, determine the attributes of the ideal CNS position, and then determine the essential attributes for your consideration of a position. Use the attributes suggested in Exhibit 24.1 and add your own. If you decide something is essential, write a description of why. Writing your rationale will help you judge if the attribute is really essential or preferred. Write possible questions next to each attribute so that you will be prepared to phrase your query in a professional and effective manner.

Consider Your Strengths and Weaknesses

Before you apply for a position and again after you receive detailed information about the job, but before the first interview, review how the experience and skills you bring match the CNS position. If you are especially strong in meeting one of the requirements, plan how you will highlight this without bragging. For example, one might say, "In my last position, I led two quality improvement efforts on my unit that reduced renal patient readmissions by 12%." Keep the statement objective,

EXHIBIT 24.2 INTERVIEWEE QUESTION DEVELOPMENT

Desired Skill	Sample Questions
Values/Organizational Orientation	Describe who the CNS's customers are. Describe your customer orientation. What kind of organizational milieu best facilitates your work style? What kinds of organizational values may be antithetical to your own? Tell me about some times you exceeded a position's regular expectations. Why? What values do you believe are most important for your employer to model? What values do you believe are most important for a CNS to model? What organizational characteristics give you the most pride in your employing organization?
Analytic Ability	[After describing a clinical problem], how would you recommend the CNS proceed and why? What clinical issues have you analyzed? What were the results? [After describing a problematic clinical situation], what are the issues to be addressed? Why? How would you define the central problem?
Listening/Personnel Assessment/Group Dynamic Ability	How do you gain insight about others? Tell me about challenges you have experienced in leading meetings. How did you address them?
Communication Skills	What is your strongest communication method? What have others said about your writing? Describe business plans/quality improvement plans and reports you have developed. Tell me about your speaking style.
Communication Skills (continued)	What techniques are you most or less likely to use in meetings? When you are the convener? When you are a participant?
Motivation/Determination	Describe the most difficult professional goal you ever achieved. Why was this important to you? Describe the most difficult professional goal you have not yet achieved. Why is it an important goal for you? What interests you most about this position? What would you like to achieve in your professional life during the next 3 to 5 years? When things are not progressing as planned? What is the first thing you are likely to do? What professional organizations do you plan to influence? How? In what roles?
Work Ethic	Describe a typical day's work for a CNS in this position. What would constitute too much work? Not enough?
Work Ethic (continued)	On occasion, sustained extraordinary effort is needed in the role of a CNS. Describe the longest period you have had to exert such effort and why. Describe the work ethic you expect of others.
Efficiency	Describe how you approach a new project. What project management framework(s) do you rely on? How would you describe your approach to personal productivity? Describe your orientation toward deadlines. What efficiency measures are applicable to a CNS position?
Teaching Skills	What teaching methods suit you best? What methods don't suit you? How do you assess professional learners' need for content? What about nonprofessionals?

EXHIBIT 24.2 INTERVIEWEE QUESTION DEVELOPMENT (*CONTINUED*)

Desired Skill	Sample Questions
	What learning evaluation methods are you most familiar with?
	What online and/or simulation programs have you used or developed?
	Describe your professional responsibilities for nursing students.
Economic Awareness	Describe your project budgeting skills.
	What productivity measures do you think should be applied to this job?
	What would be major line items in a unit training program for [describe a project]?
	Describe an experience you have had in developing a revenue stream.
Risk-Taking Tolerance	Describe a professional risk you have taken. Why did you take it?
	What happened as a result?
	What would others tend to say about your overall risk tolerance?
Clinical Skills/Awareness of Current Science	Tell me about the last health care article you found provocative for our area of practice. What was interesting to you about it?
	How do you stay current in our field?
Personnel Management	Describe your personnel management style.
	How have you dealt with underperforming project team members in the past?
Personnel Management (continued)	How would you improve the performance of project personnel who do not report to you?
	What reward structures do you think are effective? Why?
Research/Quality Improvement	Which research/quality improvement skills do you have experience with? In what kind of projects? What was your level of responsibility/independence?
	Describe your ability to participate in research. What roles are you competent to assume and why?
	Describe the uses and abuses of benchmarking in quality improvement.
	Describe guidelines, protocols, or other standardized clinical initiatives with which you have experience. Did you design any of these?

and provide measurable outcomes. If you have no experience in an area, indicate your willingness to learn and be ready to present ideas about how you will master the area. Some positions, for example case manager, require CNS preparation but emphasize only specific CNS skills (Tahan, 1997). Consider if these specific skills are your strong point or ones you wish to develop. In addition, some positions may result in a different weighting of the needed skills. A family practice position will emphasize small organization skills more than a large medical center (Cardinal, 2003).

Know Your Worth

Although salary and benefits are usually discussed late in the interview process, review the labor market and compensation situation with regard to your desired compensation level. You will only get one chance to negotiate a salary and benefit package and must be prepared. If this comes up early in the interview, you may also feel that there are certain benefits or salary ranges that are essential. It is better to communicate any non-negotiable demands early in the process. For example, if you must work 4 days per week, clarify this.

To assess the benefit package, it is often possible to compare and contrast benefits offered by institutions that employ CNSs by visiting the employment section of their Web sites. Most of these are open to nonemployees. Salary statistics are compiled by many professional, governmental, and private organizations. For example, Salary.Com provides salary data for national and metropolitan areas. According to this Web site, as of September 2006, the national median salary for a CNS was $76,672; the 25th quartile was $70,832 or less and the 75th quartile began at $82,512. One should also consider that some benefits are not likely to be listed on a general Web page. In some institutions, bonuses or performance incentives are used to reward a CNS's contributions toward strategic goals. If travel between sites is required, favorable reimbursement rates or provision of a car might be possible.

If the position will involve teaching students, review the associated school's faculty appointment and promotion guidelines. Most are now online. Depending on long-term career goals, attainment of faculty rank can be important.

Secure and Review Information

The serious interviewee will expect to have some input into the interview process, so secure and review information regarding the interview process, the institution, its operational and financial stability, and the position description ahead of time. If the interview schedule does not include opportunities to meet with key personnel, you should discuss your request with the institutional contact well before the interview date. Operational and financial stability can be preliminarily assessed by reading the annual report. These are often available online.

Review the Resume You Submitted and Bring Extra Copies

The interviewers' questions will, for the most part, come from what you included or omitted in this document. For example, your resume may state you worked for 6 months on an oncology unit. The interviewer is probably going to probe why you left after such a short period of time. Bringing extra resumes is suggested because there is always a possibility in a multi-interview situation that someone has misplaced or forgotten to bring their copy of your resume.

Plan Your Appearance and Refine Any Distracting Mannerisms

Interviewers' impressions are formed by overall appearance, including clothing and grooming. An interviewing rule of thumb for the professional is to choose clothes that are consistent with business attire, not business casual. Visit your public library or bookstore for manuals on projecting a powerful, professional image. For example, a midcalf floral print dress with wide portrait collar trimmed in lace may be formal enough to wear to a worship service, but it does not project power. Men may find themselves taken less seriously if they choose to come to the CNS interview in a polo shirt, sports jacket, and pressed chinos. Grooming issues center on cleanliness and neatness. Hair, beards, make-up, and nails are major areas for grooming attention. Friends can be an important resource in identifying potentially distracting mannerisms. Fidgeting, saying "you know," and tapping one's foot needs to be curtailed to present a mature image appropriate for the advance practice nurse.

Plan a preinterview regimen that provides the sleep and food needed to sustain energy during the interview process. If meals are a part of the process and you have food restrictions, plan how you will accommodate them.

Practice asking questions of interviewers and giving responses to interviewer's questions with trusted colleagues. See Exhibit 24.2 for practice items and techniques. Search the Internet for practice questions and answers. Enter the term "interview questions" to find sites supported by employment agencies that provide typical interview questions.

Ethical and Legal Considerations

During the interview process, the organization may share confidential information regarding performance, finances, or planned competitive initiatives well beyond what may be shared when applying for a staff nurse position. The interviewee must be careful not to share this information with persons outside the organization and to determine with whom within the organization the information can be shared. Not every level of an organization is given the same level of information.

In some cases, the CNS may be asked to sign a nondisclosure agreement before or during the interview process. This is most likely to happen when a patient care technology is under development by a medical center or through partnership with a proprietary company, and the CNS will be involved in implementation or evaluation. Read the entire statement before deciding if you will sign.

Another ethical consideration concerns the acceptance of an offer to interview. Interviewing a CNS candidate requires the investment of expensive professional time as well as staff resources. Interviewing "just for the practice" is stealing from the institution.

THE INTERVIEW

Interview Topics/Content: The Interviewer

A review of the human resource literature and consideration of the nature of CNS positions indicate that specialty clinical skills are only a small part of what makes a candidate a good match for the position (Cardinal, 2003; Howell, 1999; Strasser, 2005). The following areas are just as important and should be used as guides for interview content: problem-solving/analytic skills, communication and listening skills, motivation/determination especially in terms of long-term career plans, work ethic/dedication/reliability, efficiency, teaching skills, economic awareness, and risk-taking tolerance (see Exhibit 24.2).

In addition to the topics of interest to the interviewer are those of the interviewee. The interviewer is reminded to review the job aspects in the interviewee section and be prepared to discuss them.

The final interview content area is the negotiation of the next steps in the selection process. The interviewer needs to indicate who will contact the applicant regarding the next steps and when and how the contact will be made. The interviewer must not assume the decision is the institution's alone. At the end of the interview(s), the interviewer should probe the applicant's continued interest in the position and resolve any unanswered questions.

Interview Content: The Interviewee

The CNS interviewee needs to assess, at a minimum, the following aspects of the position: organizational goals and the relationship of these goals to those of the CNS position, reporting relationships, position span of control, inter- and intradisciplinary support mechanisms, opportunities for career growth, position rewards, and evaluation philosophy. Take a small form listing these topics to the interview to remind you about them. Write brief notes at the end of the interview for follow-up and clarification if time permits.

If the next steps in the selection process are not outlined by the interviewer, the interviewee should ask who will be responsible for conveying the information and approximately when this will occur. If the interviewee had another job offer or anticipates one before the date provided by the interviewer, this basic information needs to be shared.

INTERVIEW PROCESS TECHNIQUES

The following techniques can be used by any interviewer or interviewee. Facility in using the techniques and choosing the best one for a given situation requires practice, not memorization. Mock interview sessions in which the techniques are implemented are suggested.

80/20 Rule

This well-known rule is based on the belief that 20% of an interview should be spent in asking questions and 80% spent in listening to answers to achieve a real understanding of the candidate's fit with the position (Yate, 2006). Obviously, if both parties in an interview take this approach, it is counterproductive. The rule does, however, raise one's awareness that questions and answers are both important parts of an interview. Commenting on every answer wastes time and is not necessary. In most cases, the interviewer controls the pace and emphasis areas of the interview and can be expected to come closer to the 80% listening and 20% asking proportion. The listening/asking proportion for the interviewee should be approximately reversed. Given the interviewer and interviewee will be speaking often, awareness of the physical and psychic energy required for what may be a full day of interviews dictates careful planning for rest and nourishment before the interview process begins.

Sequence Themes

Consider the themes you wish to explore, but before you consider the forms the questions for each theme will take, determine if there is a preferable order for the themes. For example, an interviewer might wish to explore goal orientation before analytic ability. An interviewee may ideally sequence items about nursing staff project readiness before moving on to a sequence of questions about multidisciplinary commitment.

Behavior-Based Interviewing

This approach centers the interview questions on behaviors instead of beliefs. CNS position interviews require exploration of both behaviors and beliefs, but because past behavior is often the best predictor of future actions, emphasis on behavior-oriented questions is important.

Controversies in Structured and Unstructured Approaches to Interviews

There has been much controversy regarding which approach produces an optimal hiring decision (Carson, Carson, Fontenot, & Burdin, 2005; Hough & Oswald, 2000; Schmidt & Zimmerman, 2004; Strasser, 2005). The structured approach includes not only an established set of questions but also benchmark answers. The same question order is followed with each candidate. The chief advantage of this method is the ability to compare all applicants to an ideal. The unstructured approach, asking questions in different ways and in a different order, allows the interviewer to assess specific issues and pursue unanticipated avenues of interest. Given the lack of consistent scholarly evidence to support the superiority of either approach, some combination of techniques might be advised.

Closed-Ended, Open-Ended and Multilayered Questions

Closed-ended questions produce little information. Yate (2006) has suggested that this technique be used only to query about a commitment (asking if interviewee wishes to continue with the process after an initial day of interviewing) or clarification of a factual item. The open-ended approach forces the respondent to elaborate on their approach to or their experience in a given situation.

The multilayered approach is often misunderstood. Asking a person about three or four things within the same question ensures an incomplete answer to at least one aspect of the question and is not truly multilayered interviewing. An example of a poor attempt at multilayered questioning is: "Tell me about your philosophy of nursing, and how this has been influenced by your past clinical experiences, and how you resolved philosophical conflicts, and how it influenced your productivity." This is an example of a poorly framed question. Effective layering refers to the practice of asking a series of questions that produce in-depth revelations about some aspect of the person being interviewed, not imbedding multiple questions in one statement.

Conversational Issues

The nurse who participates in an interview can benefit from the redirection skills developed in basic psychiatric nursing when dealing with an interview participant who is overly talkative, always off topic, very flustered, or stressed. This training can, however, backfire if the nurse employs these skills as if the interview were a therapeutic encounter. The main goal in an interview is to assess applicant fit, not heal or comfort.

If an unexpected or controversial question is asked, the responder should remain composed and answer tactfully. One can calmly point out the inappropriateness of the question and thereby refuse to answer (Andrica, 2000). If someone (usually the interviewer) asks an unusual or shocking question, pause and reconsider what is being asked. You may need to ask that the question be rephrased. Many questions seem to be sensitive but are legitimate, for example, why there are work record gaps on the resume or why the position has been open for a long period of time. Honest yet concise answers are best in these circumstances.

The Importance of Observations

The interview process is not a strictly verbal exercise. The participants must exercise their observation skills to detect the extent to which what is said is consistent with what is seen. This detection process is especially important to the interviewee who will have few opportunities outside the interview process to verify information. Observation is also useful in gathering information that cannot be obtained through verbal exchange. For example, the interviewee can often make observations about institutional attention to patient comfort, equipment, availability of computer stations, and interactions between disciplines as she or he walks to another interview.

POSTINTERVIEW CONSIDERATIONS: THE INTERVIEWER

There are three major activities postinterview. The first is providing any follow-up information promised to the applicant. The second is writing an evaluation of the applicant based on the interview. If a form has not been provided by the lead interviewer, the interviewer can

format the evaluation based on the position description. Each point on the job description can serve as an opportunity to write an account of answers and behavior noted during the interview. This approach has the advantages of consistency in the evaluation of every candidate and clarity regarding information the interview did or did not uncover.

The interview report should conclude with a recommendation regarding next steps. This recommendation need not be a simple hire–do not hire dichotomy. One's level of enthusiasm and supporting rationale for the candidate's selection should be indicated in the case of a recommendation for hire. The rationale for a "do not hire" recommendation should also be given. In some cases, the recommendation may be that a conclusion cannot be reached and that further evaluation is needed. If so, be clear about the additional information needed to make a decision.

The third action, informing the applicant of the institution's decision, is usually the lead interviewer's responsibility given the professional nature of a CNS position. In some areas, the competitive environment has necessitated that a telephone call replaces a letter. E-mail is another option, but many experienced interviewers prefer the opportunity for further clarification that the telephone provides.

POSTINTERVIEW CONSIDERATIONS: THE INTERVIEWEE

If the interview experience has led to the decision that the position would be a poor match from the interviewee's perspective, communicating this to the lead interviewer within 2 to 3 days is courteous. The time period is suggested because it gives the applicant time to carefully review her/his reaction, but it is not so long as to result in additional institutional costs.

Regardless of the outcome of the interview, the interviewee indicates professional respect by sending a written note of thanks to the lead interviewer (Rollet, 2005). The content can include praise for an aspect of the interview process (e.g., the thoughtfulness of the scheduling, the degree to which all aspects of the CNS position were explored, the opportunity to meet the inter- as well as intradisciplinary team). The note should also refer to some issue or conversation that arose during the interview to indicate your continued interest in the position.

There has been some debate about sending a note to each interviewer if multiple interviews were conducted. For example, a CNS interview schedule may cover 2 days and interviews with 15–20 people. If one can write a note that reflects on the individual interview and/or help of the interviewer, one should do so regardless of the number of people involved. If the interviewee accepts

EXHIBIT 24.3 CNS INTERVIEW ACTIVITY SUMMARY

Stage of Process	Interviewer	Interviewee
	■ Determine interview schedule, goals, decision makers ■ Review position description ■ Create a project summary ■ Determine essential skill set ■ Review labor market including salaries and benefits ■ Create a standard package of information for each candidate ■ Ensure all interviewers have reviewed ethical and legal requirements of interviewing	■ Determine the ideal CNS position and the essential attributes for your consideration of the position ■ Consider your strengths and weaknesses ■ Acquaint yourself with the salary and job market for the position. What, if any, are your nonnegotiable demands? ■ Educate yourself about the interview process, the institution, and the position ■ Maximize your first impression by planning your appearance and approach to the interview
Preinterview	■ Prepare and distribute interview evaluation sheets ■ Alert staff to interview schedule and attend to hospitality issues	■ Consider possible ethical and legal issues that could arise in the interview
Interview	■ Address all relevant content areas listed in Exhibit 24.1 ■ Before concluding the interview, address next steps in the process	■ Assess relevant content areas including organizational goals, reporting relationships, span of control, support, career growth, rewards, and evaluation philosophy ■ Clarify next steps and responsibilities
Postinterview	■ Provide necessary follow-up information to the applicant ■ Write an evaluation of the applicant and interview and make a recommendation for hire/do not hire ■ Inform the applicant of the decision/next steps	■ Send note of thanks to lead interviewer and any other appropriate contacts ■ Communicate your continued interest (or lack of interest) in pursuing the position

the position, these people become coworkers who will already mark you as a courteous person. If the CNS does not accept or is not offered the position, there is a high likelihood of meeting again in some professional capacity. A few moments spent in being courteous can add one small but important block toward building a career network.

Boyle has written a humorous yet salient top 10 list of reasons to rethink a CNS position based on the interview experience (Boyle, 1998). These include: (1) lack of a job description; (2) staff nurse–type expectations of the CNS; (3) never meeting a staff nurse; (4) CNS position role confusion, especially on the part of physicians; (5) expectations that the CNS is a professional committee member and jack of all trades; (6) three or more bosses; (7) a culture that does not value formal education; (8) lack of an evaluation strategy; (9) everyone talked about themselves and found out nothing about you; and (10) the director/VP of nursing has no idea what the CNS position entails.

SUMMARY

Attention to detail can ensure that an interview provides valuable data regarding the extent to which there is a good fit between a CNS candidate and a position. Exhibit 24.3 summarizes activities by stage of interview and can serve as a helpful checklist. Each CNS position is uniquely configured and each candidate has different position priorities. Individualizing the ideas presented in this chapter and using the suggested techniques can make the interview process more productive for the CNS candidate and the institution.

DISCUSSION QUESTIONS

1. How can one determine the extent to which structured and unstructured interview techniques should be used when you conduct an applicant interview?

2. At what point, if any, does interviewing to elicit stress on the part of the interviewee become unethical? Specify the ethical principles that guide your position.

3. A CNS works at a faith-based institution that has specific criteria and structures regarding the kind of care specific patients can and cannot receive. When and how in the interview process should this be raised with the interviewee?

4. A person's resume has been checked prior to the interview, and it appears the nature of the person's experience may be overstated. It is only an hour before the scheduled interview. Discuss the principles that might assist an administrator in determining the true extent of the person's experience. Discuss if there would be any difference in the principles selected if this was to be a multiperson interview situation.

5. A CNS administrator notes that the interview results reported by two CNSs and the unit physician director reach different conclusions and recommendations regarding a candidate. How should the CNS respond to these differences and make a decision about the candidate? What is the rationale for your approach? If you would recommend another series of interviews as part of your answer, what principles would best assist in the decision-making process? Who should conduct these interviews?

EXERCISES

1. You are a CNS interviewee and have just been asked by the unit's physician director if you plan on getting pregnant soon. Role play how you would respond.

2. You have just completed a series of interviews with the other CNSs at the institution. There are large discrepancies in what they tell you about the role of the CNS at the institution, the fiscal stability of the position, and the description provided by the lead interviewer. Role play how you would establish what the situation really is.

3. With a partner, conduct a preinterview telephone call making arrangements for a CNS interview. If you are in the same room, turn your backs to one another so there is no nonverbal feedback. After completing the "call," each person should discuss the topics, information, and personal impressions he/she believes were conveyed in the mock planning call. If this is a class room exercise, observers should discuss which preinterview tasks were completed and which remain to be achieved.

Exercise 4 requires partners. If possible, the interviews should be audiotaped. The tapes should be reviewed using Exhibits 24.1, 24.2, and 24.3 as guides.

4. Pretend to be a CNS director. Conduct one interview with a CNS colleague who will pretend to apply for a position at your institution. You may use information from a typical CNS position at your institution or fabricate the job requirements and other factual information suggested in the preinterview phase. Reverse positions and become the interviewee. You should play your part at the experience level you currently have attained. The career goals and ideal and acceptable job situations should be those you aspire to at this time.

REFERENCES

Andrica, D. C. (2000). Answering tough questions on interview. *Nursing Economics, 18*(1), 45.

Boyle, D. A. (1998). Top ten reasons to rethink taking that clinical nurse specialist position. *Clinical Nurse Specialist, 12*(3), 93.

Cardinal, P. (2003). Questions you should ask when hiring. *Family Practice Management, 10*(6), 46–48.

Carson, K. D., Carson, P. P., Fontenot, G., & Burdin, J. J., Jr. (2005). Structured interview questions for selecting productive, emotionally mature, and helpful employees. *Health Care Manager, 24*(3), 209–215.

Dougherty, T. W., Turban, D. B., & Callender, J. C. (1994). Confirming first impressions in the employment interview: A field study of interviewer behavior. *Journal of Applied Psychology, 79*(5), 659–665.

Hess, A. K. (2005). Health & safety: Ensure a long and safe career: Inquiring about health and safety during your next job interview. *American Journal of Nursing, 105*(6), 96.

Hough, L. M., & Oswald, F. L. (2000). Personnel selection: Looking toward the future—remembering the past. *Annual Review of Psychology, 51*(1), 631.

Howell, S. B. (1999). It's a match! *Nursing Management, 30*(2), 25–29.

Murphy, M. (2006). Hiring IQ improve your record. *Leadership Excellence, 23*, 11.

National Association of Clinical Nurse Specialists. (2004). *Statement on clinical nurse specialist practice and education* (2nd ed.). Harrisburg, PA: Author.

Puetz, B. E. (2005). The winning job interview: Do your homework. *American Journal of Nursing, 105*(Suppl. 1), 30–32.

Rollet, J. (2005). After the interview. How to stay in touch while waiting for an offer. *Advanced Nursing Practice, 13*(8), 74.

Schmidt, F. L., & Zimmerman, R. D. (2004). A counterintuitive hypothesis about employment interview validity and some supporting evidence. *Journal of Applied Psychology, 89*(3), 553–561.

Steinmiller, E. A. (1999). Finding the job you want, or, how a girl from Nebraska ended up in Philadelphia. *Clinical Nurse Specialist, 13*(2), 49–50.

Strasser, P. B. (2005). Improving applicant interviewing—Using a behavioral-based questioning approach. *American Association of Occupational Health Nurses Journal, 53*(4), 149–151.

Tahan, H. A. (1997). Hiring case managers: The role of the candidate and the interviewer. *Nursing Case Management, 2*(2), 85–92.

Yate, M. J. (2006). Hiring the best. *Electric perspectives.* Retrieved January 9, 2009, from http://findarticles.com/p/articles/mi_qa3650/is_200603/ai_n17180853/print

Entrepreneurship and Intrapreneurship in Advanced Nursing Practice

Maria R. Shirey

The United States has approximately 25 million small businesses and 10.5 million self-employed individuals (National Association of the Self-Employed, 2004). Small businesses employ 45% of the total U.S. private payroll and consistently over the last decade annually generated 60% to 80% of all net new jobs (U.S. Chamber of Commerce, 2006). It is obvious that small business owners and entrepreneurs contribute greatly to the social and economic growth of the nation. Collectively, the small business owners' economic power base positions this group as a significant voice shaping national policy decisions. Unfortunately, nurse entrepreneur representation in this influential contingency is virtually nonexistent. Much of the reason for lack of nurse entrepreneur presence has to do with reluctance to new ways of thinking, either as a result of limited knowledge of nurse entrepreneurship, lack of empowerment, or lack of "what if" thinking that challenges the status quo. Nurses in advanced practice have a keen understanding regarding the care needs and gaps evident in today's health care systems. Understanding the clinical nurse specialist's (CNS's) potential to seize the opportunities and bridge those gaps is a first step in unleashing entrepreneurial talent. The purpose of this chapter is to explore nurse entrepreneurship as a viable option for the CNS. Seeing nurse entrepreneurship within the realm of possibility provides opportunity to consider new ways of thinking, a new way that positions the CNS to change the status quo, improve health care delivery for the populations they serve, and to do so in *their* unique way. Leading a resurgence of nurse entrepreneurship

for the profession offers control over nursing practice and ultimately a chance to achieve greater personal and professional satisfaction as well to contribute toward greater societal good.

DEFINITIONS

Entrepreneurship

Entrepreneurship refers to the practice of starting new organizations or businesses generally in response to identified market opportunities. One definition of *entrepreneurship* (there are many) is that it is "a way of thinking, reasoning, and acting that is opportunity obsessed, holistic in approach, and leadership balanced" (Timmons & Spinelli, 2007, p. 79). Central to the entrepreneurship concept is the creation and recognition of opportunities inclusive of the will and initiative to seize those opportunities (Timmons & Spinelli). Although entrepreneurship often refers to the actual creation of a new and small business, the term goes beyond this narrow conceptualization. Drucker, in his classic book *Innovation and Entrepreneurship* (1985), describes entrepreneurship as a distinct feature of an individual or of an institution. This expanded notion of entrepreneurship takes into account that in order for businesses to remain vital in the marketplace, people within business entities must always search for change, embrace it, and exploit it as an opportunity.

The term *entrepreneurship,* coined by French economist Jean-Baptiste Say (Drucker, 1985), originates from the French word *entreprendre* meaning "to undertake" something. Motivation for entrepreneurship involves the desire to create something new that can exploit opportunities. To be an entrepreneur requires using a distinct skill set that may be learned. The entrepreneurial mindset includes the ability to deal with uncertainty and the aptitude for taking complex goals and breaking these into manageable sequential steps that an individual can diligently address and systematically complete. Entrepreneurs are conscientious risk takers who are driven by a vision of something better. They make decisions based on intuition and data analysis, assuming full risk and benefit from all aspects of their ventures. Overall, entrepreneurship creates value for society and individuals. It serves as an engine for job creation and economic growth for the future. Success as an entrepreneur also facilitates philanthropy to benefit mankind.

The study of entrepreneurship in the business world dates back to the 18th century and to the early work of French economist Richard Cantillon (Falcone & Osborne, 2005). An understanding of entrepreneurship is credited to the 1950s work of Austrian economist Joseph Schumpeter and to the more contemporary work of multiple scholars, including Peter Drucker (1985) and Jeffry Timmons (Timmons & Spinelli, 2007). Although the scientific study of entrepreneurship is prevalent in the business world, its study is far less prominent in health care. In nursing, only a small body of empirical literature is available to examine entrepreneurship as a phenomenon in the profession (Shirey, 2007).

Intrapreneurship

Intrapreneurship refers to the practice of a person utilizing entrepreneurial skills and approaches within a company. Pinchot and Pellman (1985) define *intrapreneurship* as behaving like an entrepreneur to "turn ideas into realities inside an organization" (p. 16). Intrapreneurs are generally independent thinkers who are known as "the dreamers who do" (p. 16). Fundamental to intrapreneurship is the notion of corporate renewal that involves using innovation and creativity to convert dreams or ideas into ventures yielding tangible results. Large organizations need intrapreneurs in order to retain their innovation edge and, thus, their competitive advantage. As such, these organizations depend on employees to spawn businesses within the business. The motivation for intrapreneurship is to challenge the status quo. Intrapreneurs and entrepreneurs both share a similar "can do" mindset.

The term *intrapreneurship,* coined by Pinchot and Pellman (1985), is based on an article in *The Economist* written by Norman Macrae, the journal's editor. Macrae

(1982) was of the belief that dynamic corporations of the future needed to experiment with alternative and better ways of doing things to stay "on their toes" and remain in competition with themselves. Based on the success of their original research and crediting Macrae for his influence, Pinchot and his associates developed the concept of intrapreneurship and published the classic book *Intrapreneuring in Action* (1985).

Intrapreneurship can be a rewarding career in and of itself, or it can be the initial step toward entrepreneurship. In intrapreneurship, the intrapreneur works inside an organization and answers to an authority figure within that organization. The entrepreneur, on the other hand, is self-employed and generally is the person running the company. According to Pinchot and Pellman (1985), intrapreneurship provides the best of both worlds: a smart way to learn entrepreneurship, but doing so using someone else's money and existing supportive structures. Intrapreneurship can be fulfilling for individuals who work within an organizational culture of innovation. In the absence of an innovative organizational culture, the intrapreneur may be at risk for frustration that becomes counterproductive to personal and organizational outcomes.

Nurse Entrepreneur

A nurse entrepreneur is a nurse who is "proprietor of a business that offers nursing services of a direct care, educational, research, administrative or consultative nature" (International Council of Nurses [ICN], 2004, p. 4). Nurse entrepreneurs may also be individuals who invent or patent new products, services, or devices. Regardless of the entrepreneurial activity, nurse entrepreneurs are usually self-employed individuals who have nurse control over practice and are directly accountable to the clients they serve. Nurse entrepreneurship ventures may include independent nursing practices, nurse-owned businesses, or consulting firms. Ideas for nurse entrepreneur ventures emerge from the ability to forecast and respond to health care needs and gaps in services or products. The scope of nurse entrepreneurial practice largely depends on the economic infrastructures (reimbursement systems) and legal/regulatory requirements of the health care industry.

Nurse Intrapreneur

A nurse intrapreneur is a nurse who is a salaried (or hourly) employee within a health care setting "who develops, promotes, and delivers on innovative health/nursing programs or projects" within the employment setting (ICN, 2004). Nurse intrapreneurs have control over their practice to the extent that is allowed within their employment arrangement. Nurse intrapreneurship ventures may include establishing a nurse-led clinical service, developing a new product line for a hospital, or championing a Magnet-designation journey for a health care system. Ideas for nurse intrapreneurship ventures emerge in response to or in anticipation of a health care or organizational need. The scope of nurse intrapreneurial practice depends not only on economic infrastructures and legal/regulatory requirements of the health care industry, but also on the organizational culture of the employing agency. For example, an individual with an entrepreneurial mindset employed within a rigid and hierarchical organization may be assigned responsibility for creating a new service or product. Although the nurse intrapreneur should be able to decide what projects to undertake, the employment relationship may dictate which projects the nurse intrapreneur will pursue. In an organizational culture where innovation is not valued, the nurse intrapreneur with new and enterprising ideas may be seen as more of a liability than an asset. In many ways, a stifling organizational culture can potentially squash the entrepreneurial spirit and derail the related intrapreneurial activities.

Entrepreneurship Versus Intrapreneurship

In summary, entrepreneurship and intrapreneurship are similar yet different concepts. Entrepreneurs are self-employed individuals running their companies, whereas intrapreneurs are still company employees given some degree of freedom to run a particular aspect of a program or subsidiary. Entrepreneurs assume the risks and benefits of a new venture, while intrapreneurs assume some level of risk within the safety net of a larger company. Entrepreneurs generally build organizational structures and processes from scratch, whereas intrapreneurs benefit from the support of existing structures (technical support, finance department, human resources department, existing marketing and sales support).

Although the terms are different, the principles underlying effective entrepreneurship and intrapreneurship ventures in nursing (and business) are very similar (ICN, 2004). Specifically, the mindset and skill set to succeed as either an entrepreneur or intrapreneur are the same. For this reason, this chapter primarily focuses on entrepreneurship, understanding that the principles presented are also valid for intrapreneurship.

BACKGROUND

Historical Overview

Florence Nightingale is largely credited with founding the nursing profession in 1854 (Dossey, 2000). Her original vision for nursing was one much ahead of her time and one that integrated a sense of service, duty, and nonconformity with the practices of the day. Although Nightingale may not have identified herself as an entrepreneur (women of her social stature could not work for financial remuneration), she in fact met many of the elements of a nurse entrepreneur (minus the remuneration piece). Nightingale was certainly *the* change agent who brought forth a new way of thinking, reasoning, and acting that was opportunity obsessed, holistic in approach, and leadership balanced.

Nurse entrepreneurship, that which goes beyond the philanthropic efforts of Nightingale's day, dates back to the turn of the 20th century (ICN, 2004). In the 1870s, formal education for nurses in North America was available only within training schools in hospitals. These hospital programs admitted women for a 2-year program (later 3 years), qualifying them upon graduation to practice as nurses inside the private homes of the sick or, to a lesser extent, to work as superintendents or head nurses in hospitals (Schorr & Kennedy, 1999). Private duty nurses went from case to case, living in the homes of their clients for the duration of their patient care responsibility. In this framework, private duty nurses practiced as independent contractors providing one-to-one nursing care within the scope of practice at the time. Private duty nursing was the main form of work available to nurses for the first 50 years of the profession. In many ways, private duty nursing was the precursor to nurse entrepreneurship as we know it today.

The establishment of public health nursing and visiting nurse associations in the 1890s gave graduate nurses a new venue for paid work and self-sufficiency, one not available through private duty nursing. As the reputation of hospitals improved in the early 1900s, patients went there more readily during times of illness (Schorr & Kennedy, 1999). This increasing shift in care from the home to the hospital resulted in many private duty nurses agreeing to take on "special cases" in hospitals. The nation's economic situation in the 1920s resulted in scarce opportunities for private duty nursing work. By the 1930s, hospital staff nursing (general duty) replaced private duty nursing as the major form of nursing work in the United States (Schorr & Kennedy). Although private duty nursing continued (as did the evolution of public health and visiting nursing) beyond the 1930s, this form of independent practice was no longer the professional mainstay.

Until World War II, most nursing professionals had been independent private duty nurses. The social and economic changes following World War II led to a shortage of nurses and institutionalization of nursing practice. These dynamics resulted in role and educational setting changes for nurses (Schorr & Kennedy, 1999), as well as increases in governmental funding to produce more nurses to meet postwar demand. In the 1950s, early discussions about entry into practice surfaced, followed by significant advances in nursing and health care in the 1960s. By 1965, the American Nurses Association (ANA) had adopted the position paper on nursing education identifying the baccalaureate degree as the basic foundation for professional nursing practice (Schorr & Kennedy). Concurrently, there was a boom in hospital building, emergence of specialty nursing practice (intensive care units begun), and introduction of the advanced practice nurse (APN). Although many nurses were now employed within the hospital setting, a new breed of nurse entrepreneurs was emerging in the form of the APN.

The 1980s saw significant reimbursement changes for health care as well as a major nursing shortage. Nurses working long hours of overtime with acutely ill patients and now better educated, more empowered, and wanting autonomy and control over practice began leaving hospitals, some to become entrepreneurs. These nurse entrepreneurs set up their own successful staffing agencies, home health agencies, educational services firms, nursing centers, and private practices. Concurrently, the explosion of nursing research accelerated by the creation in 1985 of the National Center for Nursing Research (now the National Institute for Nursing Research, or NINR) contributed to greater visibility for nursing and to documenting the profession's many contributions to society and to health policy development.

The 1990s and beyond have seen many of the conditions of the 1980s revisited, yet, more accentuated. A more profound nursing shortage is currently evident in the United States. Health care restructuring efforts have further constrained nursing practice in hospitals (where most nurses still work), resulting in nurses caring for more acutely ill patients and working under conditions that threaten health care quality and patient safety. Combined with the aging U.S. population; greater demands on the existing health care delivery system; explosion in science, technology, and knowledge; plus the empowerment of women (95% of nurses are women), these changes provide fertile opportunities for nurse entrepreneurship ventures. The fact that APNs are better educated, more highly valued, and more universally respected uniquely positions them to leverage their talents to advance their passion for quality patient care. Seizing the opportunity to reap the benefits of current social, political, and economic dynamics is the sign of a true entrepreneur. APNs now more than ever are in a position to reclaim their priorities, advance the profession's caring covenant, and do so as nurse entrepreneurs.

Prevalence

Statistical data to quantify the number of nurse entrepreneurs is difficult to obtain because different definitions are used to identify what constitutes a nurse entrepreneur. In general, 0.5% to 1% of working nurses

are nurse entrepreneurs (ICN, 2004). Nurse entrepreneurs appear to be more plentiful in geographic areas in which a public demand for nurse entrepreneurs is evident. Nurse entrepreneur–friendly areas include those in which the legal right to practice is not challenged, direct third-party reimbursement exists, and access to support services and a referral base prevail. In geographic areas in which the role of the entrepreneur has been seen and experienced closely, it is more likely that new entrepreneurs will emerge (Veciana, 2007). An example of such an area for nonnurse entrepreneurs exists in California's Silicon Valley. No comparable geographic area, however, is noted for nurse entrepreneurs who appear to be scattered throughout the United States. It follows, then, that nurses who grow up or practice in environments that nurture entrepreneurship (such as in a family business or in a business incubator organization) may be more inclined toward entrepreneurship. This supports the notion that to grow more nurse entrepreneurs means that they must be cultivated within the profession and through interdisciplinary collaboration. A return to nurse entrepreneurship as a prevalent form of practice, however, demands a major paradigm shift for most nurses.

THEORETICAL SUPPORT

Theoretical Approaches to Entrepreneurship

Entrepreneurship as a field of study is very broad, and to date, the entrepreneurship domain lacks one unifying conceptual framework (Shane & Venkataraman, 2007). No one theory prevails, rather many theories are evident (see relevant literature review for expanded discussion of the evidence in support of theory). Theoretical approaches to the study of entrepreneurship (Veciana, 2007), however, may be classified into a matrix (Table 25.1) consisting of three levels of analysis (micro, meso, macro) and four major approaches (economic, psychological, sociocultural, managerial). An extensive discussion of all the theoretical approaches is beyond the scope of this chapter. For purposes of this chapter, primary focus is given to the individual unit of analysis (micro level) and the combination of both the psychological (who the entrepreneur is) and managerial approaches (what the entrepreneur does). The rationale for selecting the micro level and psychological/managerial approaches is two-fold. First, CNS practice and development of the role focuses first on the individual. Because entrepreneurial behavior can be learned, it is important to understand the characteristics that define an entrepreneur (psychological approach) and what the entrepreneur does (managerial approach). Second, providing a fundamental understanding of what entrepreneurs are like and what they do facilitates movement to the next stage in personal development that involves *how* to become an entrepreneur and implement the entrepreneurial process.

The Timmons Model of the Entrepreneurial Process

Overview of the Model

The Timmons Model of the entrepreneurial process (Figure 25.1) is one conceptual framework originating in the business academic world and field tested and refined over several decades of research (Timmons & Spinelli, 2007). This holistic framework incorporates thinking from the economic, psychological, sociocultural, and managerial theoretical approaches as well as from systems theory. The framework derives from the principle that change is dynamic, normal, and healthy. This principle is consistent with research that indicates the major task in society and especially in the economy is to affect sustainability by doing something different as compared to doing better than is already being done (Drucker, 1985).

The Timmons Model (Figure 25.1) consists of a foundation, a founder, key elements, influential forces, important inputs, and one guiding map. The model emphasizes a managerial approach to entrepreneurship that is consistent with the definition that entrepreneurship is opportunity obsessed (economic theory), holistic in approach (systems theory), and leadership balanced (leadership/management theory). The significance of the model is that it provides guidance in executing the entrepreneurial process in venture creation.

Sustainability is the foundation upon which the model is built. Sustainability involves the capacity to endure and to do so in a way that does not harm the environment, the community, or society. A common myth about entrepreneurship is that it only exists for monetary gain. Although wealth creation may be one consequence of entrepreneurship that enhances sustainability, pursuing a passion for achieving greater good is a more powerful motivator.

An entrepreneurial venture originates with the dreams or ideas of the company founder, the lead entrepreneur who starts the business. The founder operates much like a juggler balancing the dynamic interplay of

25.1 | Theoretical Approaches to the Study of Entrepreneurship

LEVEL OF ANALYSIS	APPROACHES			
	ECONOMIC	**PSYCHOLOGICAL**	**SOCIOCULTURAL**	**MANAGERIAL**
MICRO (Individual level)	■ Entrepreneurial function as fourth factor of production. ■ Theory of the entrepreneurial profit. ■ Theory of occupational choice under uncertainty.	■ Traits theory. ■ Psychodynamic theory.	■ Margination theory. ■ Role theory. ■ Network theory.	■ Leibenstein's x-efficiency theory. ■ Behavioral theory of the entrepreneur. ■ Modes of new enterprise creation. ■ Modes to become an entrepreneur.
MESO (Corporate level)	■ Transaction cost theory		■ Network theory. ■ Incubator's theory. ■ Evolutionary theory.	■ Modes of new enterprise success and failure. ■ Corporate entrepreneurship.
MACRO (Global-country level)	■ Schumpeter's theory of economic development. ■ Theory of the endogenous regional development.	■ Kirzner's entrepreneur theory.	■ Weber's theory of economic development. ■ Theory of social change. ■ Population ecology theory. ■ Institutional theory.	

From "Entrepreneurship as a Scientific Research Programme" (pp. 23–71), by J. M. Veciana, 2007, in A. Cuervo, D. Ribeiro, and S. Roig (Eds.), *Entrepreneurship: Concepts, theory and perspective.* Berlin: Springer.

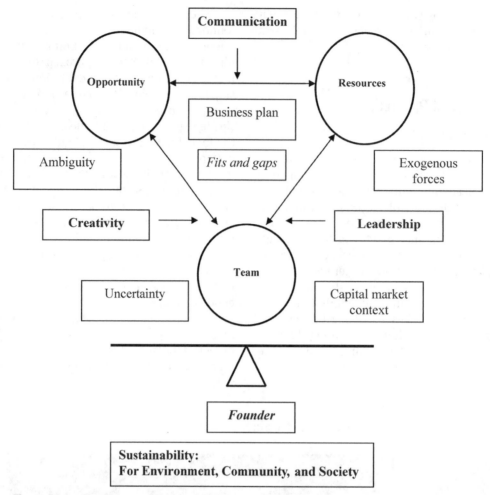

Figure 25.1 **The Timmons Model of the entrepreneurial process.**

From: *New Venture Creation: Entrepreneurship for the 21st Century* (7th ed.), by J. A. Timmons and S. Spinelli, 2007, New York: McGraw-Hill. Reproduced with permission.

three key elements in the changing environment: the entrepreneurial team, the opportunity, the resources. The entrepreneurial team consists of individuals who will assist the founder in seizing the business opportunity in order to achieve the organizational mission, vision, and goals. The opportunity consists not only of that good idea upon which the business was built, but also all other opportunities that will arise within the business environment. The resources refer to the inputs needed to assist the founder and the entrepreneurial team to maximize the business opportunity. These resources include not only money, but also such components as people, raw materials, and technology.

The founder's major job is to take charge of the success equation. That is, this individual is tuned into various influential sources and the changing dynamics created by both ambiguity and uncertainty in the external environment. The founder also tunes into the capital market context to size up competitive challenges, changes in the marketplace, financial risk, and other exogenous forces of a legal or regulatory nature.

In effect, the founder manages and redefines the risk-reward equation all with an eye toward sustainability. To do this, the founder uses important inputs of leadership, creativity, and communication skills to execute the conceived business plan (or guiding map) while also balancing the key elements and their related forces within the model.

Interaction of Component Parts

The major driving force of the Timmons Model is value creation (Timmons & Spinelli, 2007). The process is opportunity-driven and guided by the lead entrepreneur and the entrepreneurial team. The entrepreneurial process is resource parsimonious and creative and depends on the fit and balance of component parts that are integrated, holistic, and sustainable. Components of the Timmons Model are controllable in that they can be assessed, influenced, and modified at any stage of venture growth. Founders as well as investors in a venture carefully analyze components of the model to determine business risk and improve the venture's chances for success.

The entrepreneurial process begins with first an opportunity. Successful entrepreneurs and investors understand that a good idea is not necessarily a good opportunity (Timmons & Spinelli, 2007). Over time, entrepreneurs learn to identify which ventures to pursue and which to drop. According to Timmons and Spinelli, a good opportunity is one that has four major characteristics. First, the product or service creates or adds value to a customer or end-user. Second, the product or service either solves a significant problem or meets a want or need. The customer or end-user must also be willing to pay a premium for the product or service. Third, the product or service has robust market size (large enough with reachable customers), significant margins (40% or more), growth potential (20 + % growth), and strong and early free cash flow potential (recurring revenue, low assets, and low working capital). Lastly, there is a good fit with the founder, the entrepreneurial team, and the marketplace along with an attractive risk–reward equation.

One of the most common misconceptions among untested entrepreneurs is that all the resources including money must be in place to ensure venture success. In fact, the business literature suggests that thinking money first is a big mistake, primarily because money follows a high potential opportunity conceived and led by a strong management team (Timmons & Spinelli, 2007). Success stories abound of entrepreneurs who start significant businesses out of their garages using minimal resources to grow phenomenal products and services. Frugality in resource utilization at the early stages of a business may indeed provide a competitive advantage.

The entrepreneurial team is a key component of the entrepreneurial process. Success of a good idea rests squarely on the quality of the entrepreneurial team. Finding the right team members and achieving synergy between the business idea, the marketplace, the founder, and the entrepreneurial team are essential. To maximize success of the venture, a leader needs to be authentic (Shirey, 2006), a learner and teacher, resilient, and someone who builds an entrepreneurial culture and organization (this requires cultivating intrapreneurial activities). The entrepreneurial team needs to be competent, confident, motivated to excel, committed, creative, and courageous. Together all parties need to be passionate about the venture, comfortable with ambiguity and uncertainty, flexible under varying conditions, opportunity obsessed, and receptive to open lines of communication.

Besides the key elements of opportunity, resources, and the entrepreneurial team is the importance of fit and balance between and among forces in the model. It must be noted in the model (Figure 25.1) that opportunity, resources, and the entrepreneurial team are all represented in circles of identical size. The dynamics of the entrepreneurial process are effective when each of the three key elements remain in balance. For example, an opportunity that is too large, has very limited resources, and is directed by a weak entrepreneurial team may not result in a most effective entrepreneurial process. Likewise, the same could result if the opportunity is too small despite adequate resources and a capable entrepreneurial team. The founder ultimately must balance all the elements, being cognizant of not only fit and balance, but also of substance and timing. Success in this balancing act requires both analytical ability and intuition (sometimes acting on incomplete information) in order to create and sustain the ideal dynamics consistent with achieving the most effective entrepreneurial process.

Stages of Venture Growth

The entrepreneurial process and the creation of new ventures occurs within the backdrop of five stages in venture growth: research and development, start-up, high growth, maturity, and stability. Venture growth follows a theoretical view of gestation (growth, development, change) manifested by specific stages, distinct boundaries, and crucial transitions. Each stage also has implications for the type of financing commonly seen.

Stage 1, of venture growth is the research and development (R & D) stage, sometimes called the nascent stage. This stage begins with the discovery of the business opportunity and continues until the business is launched. The R & D stage can be as short as a few months or last years. Research suggests that if the business idea does not become a going concern within 18 months, likelihood that the start-up business will launch falls dramatically (Timmons & Spinelli, 2007). At this stage, the business venture usually includes a single aspiring entrepreneur and a small team exploring the business idea and doing due diligence. Financing at this stage usually comes from the aspiring entrepreneur's personal funds or from some type of seed money (investor, grants, loans).

Stage 2, the start-up stage, covers the launching of the business up to the first 3 years of operation. The failure rate for businesses at this stage exceeds 60% (Timmons & Spinelli, 2007). This explains why this stage is the most risky and thus requires the exhaustive drive, energy, and talents of the business founder and the entrepreneurial team. During the start-up stage, the business interacts with a critical mass of people (customers, vendors, investors, and competitors). It is during this time that customer confidence and competitive resilience are established. Crucial transitions seen in this stage include rapid growth in both sales and employees. The founder and members of the entrepreneurial team support the employee base by doing whatever is needed to grow the business. Financing at this stage is usually from the lead entrepreneur's personal funds (or loans), private investors (friends or family) or venture capitalists.

Stage 3, the high growth stage, usually covers from year 4 to year 10, although the length of this stage varies by company. Growth in sales and employees continues. Changes in the management mode are some of the most difficult transitions seen in this stage. As the business grows, the founder finds it increasingly difficult to both grow the company and manage the day-to-day operations. The founder begins to relinquish power and control, delegating more authority to others. Much of the founder's focus is in the short-term strategic planning needed to rapidly meet the overwhelming demands of the marketplace. Financing at this stage may come from the sale of new equity (initial public offering [IPO] or stocks) by the firm to public investors. An IPO allows the company to tap into a wide pool of stock market investors to provide significant capital that gets reinvested into the business. Investors have no further claim over the capital, but they do have a claim to future profits distributed by the company.

Stage 4, the maturity stage, lasts from 10 to 15 years and varies by company. The maturity stage is no longer about survival, but rather about steady and profitable growth. As the business continues to grow and stabilize (stage 5, beyond 15 years), major crucial transitions include shifts in management (now founder manages managers), potential erosion of founder creativity, and additional working capital needs for renovation, expansion, or reinvention. Without a significant renaissance and corporate energy at stage 5, the founder and entrepreneurial team's hard work may be at risk. Company growth at stage 5 requires corporate renewal or intrapreneurial efforts that should have been in place all along. Financing for company renewal efforts may come in the form of another public offering. In the absence of renewal efforts, the company could position itself for either a sale or be forced into liquidation. In the event of a sale, business owners should ideally have had an a priori harvest strategy in place to capture maximum value from the business.

In summary, the 5 stages of venture growth bring to bear different time periods, unique conditions, and crucial transitions. Given what is empirically known about the stages of venture growth, the pattern is predictable and informative. Learning from this science, the lead entrepreneur navigating the 5 stages of growth needs to know these stages are akin to periods of wonder (R & D stage), blunder (start-up stage), thunder (high growth stage), plunder (maturity), and asunder or renaissance of wonder (stability stage; Marram, 2003). During the wonder stage, companies experience great uncertainty about their survival. The blunder stage causes many companies to stumble and fall. The thunder stage allows for significant growth and the evolution of a strong management team. The plunder stage experiences robust cash flow. Lastly, asunder dictates that the company will either renew itself or risk decline.

RELEVANT LITERATURE

The business literature in entrepreneurship is well-grounded in an amalgamation of research and theory that draws from a variety of disciplines. This relevant review of the literature addresses empirical findings at the micro level of analysis (individual) and focuses on the psychological and managerial theoretical approaches (see Table 25.1).

General Entrepreneurship

Micro Level Psychological Approach

Traits theory, a psychological approach, focuses on who the entrepreneur is and what characteristics define them to identify a profile of the person who decides to create a new enterprise. A synthesis of the literature suggests that the main psychological traits and motivations of the entrepreneur are apparent in a mostly distinct profile (Veciana, 2007). Although there is not an absolute and neat set of behavioral attributes that separates entrepreneurs from nonentrepreneurs, the research shows that the entrepreneur is usually intrinsically motivated and has a higher internal locus of control. Entrepreneurs have a common way of thinking or mindset that exemplifies a strong need for independence and achievement. They have a propensity for moderated risk taking and the ability to trust their intuition. Entrepreneurs are unsatisfied with the status quo and, because of their high tolerance for ambiguity, can readily navigate in times of turbulence and great complexity.

In exploring motivators for self-employment, particularly in women and specifically addressing the "push and pull" debate, research suggests that women seek self-employment as a result of intrinsic motivation or "pull" factors (Hughes, 2003). Women entrepreneurs are primarily motivated by a desire for challenge, positive work environments, independence, and meaningful work. One-third of the 61 participants in the Hughes study were motivated to pursue self-employment as a result of critical economic constraints ("pushed" due to corporate restructuring and downsizing). Although the "pulled" entrepreneurs reported higher levels of satisfaction than did the "pushed" entrepreneurs, overall the levels of satisfaction for both groups were reported to be very high. Interestingly, the "pushed" to self-employment group in this study underwent what the researcher termed an "ideological pull," resulting in the "push" entrepreneurs expressing reluctance to return to paid employment (Hughes).

The study of the entrepreneur's profile has also led to creation of a taxonomy of entrepreneurs, which further differentiates between high and low innovation entrepreneurs (Manimala, 1996). High innovation entrepreneurs fall into one of seven subtypes: inventor/tinkerer, adventurer, searcher/problem solver, gap filler, social visionary, opportunity grabber, and specialist pioneer. The low innovation entrepreneurs, on the other hand, fall into one of six subtypes: chance entrant, agent turned producer, concession grabber, obsessed producer, ancillary/imitator, and nonpioneer niche holder. The commonality that all entrepreneurs have is that they collectively are innovative. The high versus low distinction within the taxonomy, however, suggests that the high innovation entrepreneurs are more proactive in executing the entrepreneurial process.

Scientific research in the entrepreneurial area of traits theory was very common in the 1970s, 1980s, and 1990s, but attention to this type of research has declined in recent years. That much is already known about the entrepreneurial psychological profile partially explains the decline in this type of research (Veciana, 2007). What is currently known about the entrepreneur's psychological traits and motivations contributes to the understanding of the skills and abilities that can be taught to foster entrepreneurial behaviors.

Micro Level Managerial Approach

Behavioral theories of the entrepreneur, a managerial approach, focus on what the entrepreneur *does* rather than what the entrepreneur *is* (psychological approach). Synthesis of the literature suggests that entrepreneurial behaviors demonstrate seven distinct abilities (Veciana, 2007). These entrepreneurial behaviors include the abilities to search and gather information, identify opportunities, deal with risk, establish relationships and networks, and make decisions under uncertainty and ambiguity. Additionally, entrepreneurs have leadership ability as well as the ability to learn from experience and to bounce back quickly from failure.

The entrepreneur's behavior is said to be a reflection of the individual's personal motivations that, in turn, are dependent on environmental characteristics (Stevenson & Jarillo, 2007). This psychosociological point of view was pioneered by David McClelland's 1961 best-selling book, *The Achieving Society*. McClelland's seminal work helped to explain why some societies exhibit high economic and social growth, attributing such growth to the need for achievement. McClelland's research provided the foundation to explain how the environment affects the practice of entrepreneurship.

Beyond the influence of personal motivation on behavior is the understanding that the nature and existence of the managerial team affects the likelihood of positive outcomes in entrepreneurship (Stevenson & Jarillo, 2007). The work by Timmons and Spinelli (2007), as captured in the Timmons Model of the entrepreneurial process (Figure 25.1), explains and supports the importance of the managerial behaviors of *both* the lead entrepreneur and the entrepreneurial team. Entrepreneurship within this framework is more than just starting up a new business; it is also a mode of management (beyond traditional management) designed to relentlessly pursue opportunities and achieve desirable results. Accordingly, Timmons and Spinelli identify five broad competencies of entrepreneurial management to include: (1) skill in building an entrepreneurial culture (intrapreneurship rises to the top here); (2) leadership, vision, and influence; (3) helping, coaching, and conflict management; (4) teamwork and people management; and (5) other management competencies, including but not limited to marketing, operations/production, finance, law and taxes, project management, negotiations, and information technology.

Nurse Entrepreneurship

Although anecdotal publications on nurse entrepreneurship abound, few research-based articles are available in the literature. A synthesis of the empirical literature on nurse entrepreneurship practice suggests that the first article was published in 1998, and most studies are small ($n = 4$ to 59) and exploratory in nature (Shirey, 2007). The studies available report on nurse entrepreneurship in the United States (Elango, 2007; Roggenkamp & White, 1998), Australia (Wilson, Averis, & Walsh, 2003, 2004), and the United Kingdom (Austin, Luker, & Ronald, 2006). What is empirically known from these studies falls into the categories of the micro level psychological and managerial approaches. Motivation and traits of the nurse entrepreneur as well as the skill set of the nurse entrepreneur have been studied using qualitative research designs.

Micro Level Psychological Approach

Motivation for the nurse entrepreneur includes key drivers, business factors, and personal factors (Shirey, 2007). Drivers that motivate nurse entrepreneurs are a love of nursing, self-efficacy as nursing professionals, a desire to make a difference, influence of family (Roggenkamp & White, 1998), and the ability to see opportunities (Elango, 2007). The love for nursing comes from professional experience in traditional practice settings such as hospitals. Most nurses have 3 to 15 years nursing experience before they become self-employed as entrepreneurs (ICN, 2004). The self-efficacy results from professional competence and confidence developed over years of practice. Given their love of nursing and their expertise in the field, nurse entrepreneurs feel they have the unique abilities and strong beliefs that can make a difference in the lives of their clients. Support from family has been shown to be a strong motivator to leave traditional nursing practice settings. A small qualitative study ($n = 4$) by Roggenkamp and White, 1998 reported that in 3 of 4 participants, the entrepreneurial shift came as a result of personal reinvention and a desire to have more time with family. Nurse entrepreneurs identified changing demographic trends and opportunities within health care facilities as factors that encouraged their decisions to become entrepreneurs.

The business factors primarily address the perceived enablers and disablers to nurse entrepreneurship. Nurse entrepreneurs report factors that facilitate entrepreneurship are enablers, and these include outside assistance during start-up, mentors, the need to make change (boredom and burnout), and some critical life event (Roggenkamp & White, 1998). A significant disabler or factor that hinders nurse entrepreneurship includes perceived lack of business skills, particularly in the areas of finance, billing and collections, law, regulation, and operational management of a business. Overwhelmingly, nurse entrepreneurs report that their traditional nursing education (at any level) does not prepare them for practice in nontraditional roles such as nurse entrepreneurship. Nurse entrepreneurs report a lack of connectivity between nurse entrepreneurs. Additionally, they report a lack of not only professional and collegial support for private practice, but also experiencing negative attitudes of other health care professionals toward nurses in private practice (Wilson et al., 2004).

The personal factors that motivate nurse entrepreneurs include their commitment to a quality mission and their desire to stay close to their clients. These personal factors are identical to the factors that motivated early nurse entrepreneurs to engage in case-by-case care and hold firmly to practice as private duty nurses. This ability to stay close to the client and focus on mission over profit is seen by nurse entrepreneurs as a higher order reward.

The profile of the nurse entrepreneur incorporates characteristics of the traditional business entrepreneur. That is, nurse entrepreneurs are opportunity driven, goal directed, risk taking, creative, assertive, and have strong leadership abilities. Research suggests other important characteristics of the nurse entrepreneur include accountability, commitment, perseverance, good self-esteem, and determination to succeed (Wilson et al., 2003).

The finding by Hughes (2003) in the business world that entrepreneurs follow the "pull" route to entrepreneurship is consistent with the nurse entrepreneurship empirical literature. Most nurses reportedly go into business not because they are unemployable (argument for "pushed" entrepreneurs), but rather because they seek to make a difference in their own way ("pulled" entrepreneurs; Wilson et al., 2003).

Micro Level Managerial Approach

Nurse entrepreneurs report clinical practice, consultancy, or education as their primary work domain, also identifying research as a less important aspect of the role (Wilson et al., 2004). Consultancy is the most reported nurse entrepreneur activity and is also the most lucrative. Although what nurse entrepreneurs actually do in the role is not mostly managerial, they identify operational and managerial competencies as important for success in the role.

Overall, nurse entrepreneurs report their operational and managerial competencies in venture creation to be weak (Elango, 2007; Wilson et al., 2004). Perceived lack of business skills, particularly in finance, legal issues, and running the day-to-day operations of a business are nurse entrepreneurship disablers. Nurse entrepreneurs may see that knowledge of business is not their forte, nevertheless, they still have the "can do" mindset to see threats as opportunities and to move forward to correct the perceived deficiencies. Nurse entrepreneurs also realize the difficulty of learning the requisite business skills while simultaneously running the day-to-day operations of a new business (Roggenkamp & White, 1998).

Experienced nurse entrepreneurs suggest the need to improve not only planning and management skills, but also networking abilities (Wilson et al., 2004) because these are used daily in the role. To facilitate nurse entrepreneurship, collegial working relationships with peers are essential. The loosely connected and underdeveloped field of nurse entrepreneurship, however, makes executing the role more difficult (Shirey, 2007).

ROLE OF THE NURSE ENTREPRENEUR

Scope of Practice

Nurse entrepreneurs practice in a variety of settings, and the scope of practice is broad. As self-employed nurses, entrepreneurs can legally offer any service that falls within the practice of nursing and does not infringe on the legislated responsibility or the exclusive practice of another health discipline (ICN, 2004). Nurse entrepreneur roles and work settings vary with public demand for services. Increasingly, nurse entrepreneurs use their expertise to develop ventures that not only meet the needs of clients, but also are professionally and personally fulfilling.

Roles for nurses as entrepreneurs are diverse and can include being a clinician/practitioner, teacher, consultant, therapist, researcher, case manager, writer, expert witness, business owner, partner, franchise operator, or niche provider. In all roles, nurses combine standard business practices with application of the nursing process to provide a unique product or service that improves the health status of the populations served.

Issues

Ethical Considerations

High ethical standards and integrity are crucial to the long-term success of the entrepreneurial venture. As nurse entrepreneurs, integrity and transparency must guide the multiple roles of business owner, employer, practitioner, and corporate citizen. This obligation requires congruence between the entrepreneur's values and the goals of the business and mandates both a macro and a micro approach. From the macro approach, the nurse entrepreneur establishes the business organization's guiding values and creates an organizational culture that supports ethically sound behavior. The nurse entrepreneur personally models high ethical standards and instills in all employees a sense of shared accountability to uphold those standards. From a micro approach, the nurse entrepreneur as health care provider sets fees for services expecting a profit, but also follows principles of fairness and just value. The nurse entrepreneur realistically presents expected benefits of the business services and follows strict guidelines for open disclosure of any conflicts of interest. Business decisions are patient-centered and focus on doing the right thing, while also providing quality services consistent with evidence-based practice and appropriate standards of care. The nurse entrepreneur as employer pays employees fair wages, provides employees with a healthy work environment for practice, and meets all legal, tax, and regulatory requirements of the business and the industry.

Economic Considerations

Nurse entrepreneurs starting a new venture face an uncertain future with potential fluctuations in income and lack of job security. For this reason, due diligence is an important concept for aspiring nurse entrepreneurs to comprehend. Prior to launching a new venture, the nurse entrepreneur should at a minimum make a determination as to whether the business opportunity meets the criteria for a "good" opportunity. The business concept needs to be explored with the advantages and disadvantages of the potential venture clearly understood. To minimize risk, enhance knowledge and critical thinking about the venture, and to ensure sources of external funding (small business grants or venture capital), the aspiring entrepreneur should develop a business plan. In addition to positioning the entrepreneur for external funding, development of a business plan forces the entrepreneur to consider multiple potential issues and challenges related to the venture.

Nurses considering an entrepreneurial venture must explore any personal turmoil regarding business (money issues) and traditional nursing forces (caring issues). Nurse entrepreneurs "are usually able to reconcile these competing forces by reinforcing their ability to be mission-driven and envision their unique potential for making a difference in the lives of clients" (Shirey, 2007, p. 234). Because traditional hospital-based nursing care does not usually isolate costs, charges, and revenue for nursing services, most nurses have difficulty quantifying the economic value of nursing services. Lack of experience with this cost/charge/revenue equation makes it difficult for nurses to develop an equitable fee for services structure. When calculating fees, the nurse entrepreneur must take into account multiple factors: complexity of the task, professional responsibility implied by the service, level of expertise required inclusive of costs for subcontractors, and time involved to produce the product or service, plus travel, expense for equipment, supplies, and supportive staff needed. When pricing a product or service, the entrepreneur must be cognizant of the fair profit desired and the going market rate for the service. Hard decisions need to be made in terms of which products and services the nurse entrepreneur can afford to provide and still stay in business.

Legal and Regulatory Considerations

Prior to launching a new venture, the nurse entrepreneur should obtain legal advice regarding many aspects of the business. Some legal and regulatory issues to consider include decisions regarding the company name, administrative offices for the business, ownership and protection of technology (trade secrets, patents, copyrights, trademarks), record keeping, security issues, insurance coverage (professional liability, general liability, director's and officer's liability, umbrella coverage, property and casualty, worker's compensation, business interruption, life and disability insurance for key company officers, health, retirement), and permits to operate the business, file claims (provider number), or get paid for services (tax identification number). A full discussion of all the legal and regulatory issues the entrepreneur must consider is beyond the scope of this chapter. For purposes of this section, only the decision regarding the business organizational structure is briefly presented. Selecting the organizational structure for the business (sole proprietorship, partnership, limited liability company or corporation) is an important decision that has economic, tax, and liability implications.

A sole proprietorship exists when an individual goes into business for him or herself (Weaver, 2005–2007). To form a sole proprietorship requires no state or federal filing requirements. The business owner still must comply with all state, local, and/or federal obligations for licensure, business permits, tax payments (property, payroll, sales taxes), and other requirements and regulations. A sole proprietorship is not a separate and distinct legal entity from the owner; in essence, business owners do business in their own name. The main advantage of this type of organizational structure is that it is the easiest way an individual can operate a business. There are no legal formalities to forming or dissolving a sole proprietorship. For tax purposes, income flows on a cash basis directly to the business owner who then reports the income (including business losses and profits) in an individual income tax return and is taxed at the self-employment rate. Setting up a sole proprietorship is inexpensive, proving beneficial for start-ups with limited capital. The major disadvantage of a sole proprietorship is that the business owner is personally liable for all debts and actions of the company. Another disadvantage is that a sole proprietorship will likely have a hard time raising capital for the business.

A general partnership is formed when two or more people operate a business together and share in the profits and losses (Weaver, 2005–2007). Most states require general partnerships to file a certificate of partnership (or its equivalent) with the appropriate state agency. Individuals in general partnerships are taxed as a sole proprietorship. The business owner obligations (in this case multiple partners) are the same as in a sole proprietorship except that with a general partnership, the management responsibilities may be divided. The advantages of a general partnership include having a shared financial commitment, pooling of expertise, and limited start-up costs. The disadvantages include finding a partner who shares a similar vision and goals for the business, partners have personal liability for business debts and liabilities, and there might be difficulties in attracting investors in the business.

A limited liability company (LLC) is a separate legal entity that limits the liability of its members (the multiple owners). In an LLC, company profits and losses are passed through the business and taxed on the member's individual tax return. The major advantages of the LLC are that members get the tax advantage of a partnership, while also having the limited liability benefits of the corporation. Members in the LLC can either manage the LLC or hire a management group to run the company. Members also can split the profits and losses any way they wish. Forming an LLC is more complex than a sole proprietorship in that it requires the development

of a charter document (Articles of Organization) for filing in the appropriate state. A disadvantage of the LLC is that some states impose income or franchise taxes on LLCs or require payment of state annual fees to operate in that state. The LLC requires the development of a written operating agreement, a document similar to a partnership agreement. Another potential disadvantage of the LLC is that because it is a relatively new type of business entity (Weaver, 2005–2007), there is not much legal precedent available to help owners make predictions on legal disputes.

The corporation is the oldest and most prestigious legal entity, one that is separate from its owners (Weaver, 2005–2007). Like LLCs, corporations limit the personal liability (debts, legal claims, other obligations) of the owners (called shareholders). The major advantage of a corporation is its tax advantages and protection of individual liability. The corporation's debt is not considered that of its owners. The major disadvantage of the corporation is that they are the most expensive to form, and they are subject to complex tax rules. Governance in corporations is more formal, complex, and expensive. Management within a corporation requires officers and directors with their roles specified in the corporation bylaws. Corporations may have shareholders that would require development and adherence to a shareholder agreement. The corporation must be established in accordance with the applicable laws of the jurisdiction in which the entity is formed and will require development of a charter document (Articles of Incorporation).

Personal Considerations

Before individuals decide to be nurse entrepreneurs, they must first ask themselves many personal questions: Is this what I *really* want to do? Do I have it in me to be a nurse entrepreneur? Am I willing to put in the long hours it takes to get this business off the ground and successful? Do I have the necessary support structures in place to help me pursue the nurse entrepreneurship journey?

Given that personal and professional isolation is a possible negative consequence of nurse entrepreneurship, individuals must explore this reality and develop proactive strategies to address this phenomenon. It may be that the nurse entrepreneur can combat the isolation by becoming involved in multiple professional venues that not only keep the nurse entrepreneur socially and professionally connected, but also allow for networking that provides exposure and a potential business referral base.

Maintaining a quality professional practice will also require the nurse entrepreneur to stay abreast of standards of practice and health policy matters related to the business and the specific industry. This requires the nurse entrepreneur to actively engage in ongoing professional and career development efforts plus also become involved in specific advocacy issues related to the nurse entrepreneur's business and industry.

APPLICATION TO CNS PRACTICE

At first glance, the role of nurse entrepreneur may appear overwhelming. CNSs, however, have an advantage primarily because their current role as advance practice nurses requires many of the elements of entrepreneurship. In looking at the definition of entrepreneurship, CNSs already have a level of proficiency in being opportunity obsessed, holistic in approach, and leadership balanced. CNSs continuously look at ways to improve the health status of the populations they serve. By virtue of their education and experience, CNSs are routinely astute regarding improvements in processes and systems that "raise the bar" for advanced nursing practice. From the holistic perspective, CNS practice addresses the whole of the human experience while also incorporating complexity, systems thinking, and learning from multiple disciplines. Working within all three spheres of influence (patient/client, nurses/nursing practice, and organization/systems), CNSs engage in interdisciplinary collaboration to achieve desired outcomes (National Association of Clinical Nurse Specialists [NACNS], 2004). CNSs also use their leadership skills on a daily basis to skillfully communicate, educate, and anticipate the future accurately (NACNS).

What CNSs lack and what nurse entrepreneurship research confirms is that aspiring nurse entrepreneurs need a better understanding of the requisite business management skills (finance/managerial accounting, business law, strategic planning, and operations management) to run the day-to-day operations of a business. This skill set certainly can either be taught or found in a capable business partner. Through proper guidance and mentorship, CNSs can gain the requisite business knowledge and savvy to complement their nursing knowledge, further broaden their sphere of influence, and maximize their value as nurse entrepreneurs. Early in the CNS role what aspiring nurse entrepreneurs need is a road map that directs them on *how* to become nurse entrepreneurs. Such a road map, albeit in an abbreviated form, may be found in Exercise 1 of this chapter.

EVALUATION

Measurement Outcomes

Although CNSs have a long history as health care providers, their unique contributions to patient care and the resultant nurse-sensitive outcomes they generate are not fully understood (Dayhoff & Lyon, 2001). CNS practice affects three spheres of influence, and it is through these spheres that CNS core competencies and actions are thought to affect CNS outcomes (NACNS, 2004).

The nurse entrepreneur outcomes documented include the establishment of nurse run businesses founded upon the entrepreneur's clinical expertise, business ventures making a difference, desired lifestyle for the entrepreneur, achievement of desired working relationships, emergence of expert status, and leaving a legacy for the profession. Because the nurse entrepreneur studies cited used nurse participants (non-CNSs) with competencies similar to those of the CNS, the study findings could be generalizable to the CNS population of entrepreneurs (Austin et al., 2006; Elango, 2007; Roggenkamp & White, 1998; Wilson et al., 2003, 2004). Further research is needed to study the practices of CNSs who are also entrepreneurs in order to establish the hypothesized relationships.

The more extensive business entrepreneurship (nonnursing) research literature documents additional nonfinancial and financial benefits of entrepreneurship at the various levels of analysis (micro, meso, macro; Luke, Verreynne, & Kearins, 2007). Nonfinancial benefits of entrepreneurship in the business literature include independence, autonomy, competitive advantage, increased market share, employment, and increased standard of living. The financial benefits of entrepreneurship in the business literature include enhanced remuneration from revenue, profits, cash flow, and return on investment. It would also be prudent to study the relationship between CNS core competencies and the entrepreneur outcomes documented in the business literature. It may be hypothesized that the relationships documented for nonnursing entrepreneurs will also hold for the CNS entrepreneur.

CONCLUSIONS

Pursuing nurse entrepreneurship is not an easy professional path, and it is not for everyone. When chosen, the entrepreneurship journey has the potential for having great impact on individuals and communities. That entrepreneurship significantly fuels economic growth is a powerful statement. That it makes a meaningful contribution to society is a profound and sobering reality. CNSs possess a unique skill set, knowledge base, and abilities that position them well for nurse entrepreneurship practice. Taking the step toward CNS entrepreneurship practice offers the opportunity to liberate the CNSs unique nursing knowledge and to deploy it for potential betterment of both distinct populations and society at large.

Exercise 1. How to become a nurse entrepreneur: A step-by-step approach.

I. Step 1

A. Conduct a self-assessment that compares the knowledge, skills, and abilities of the aspiring nurse entrepreneur with that of the established nurse entrepreneur identified in the literature. Use the following parameters for the assessment:
   1. Expertise in area of professional passion for making a difference.
   2. Sense of self-efficacy (competence, confidence, connectedness).
   3. Support systems available (mentors, coaches, family) to pursue goals.
   4. Business skills and knowledge about finance, law, regulation, general management, and the operation of a business.
   5. Ability to see and seize opportunities.
   6. Ability to be goal directed, committed, and determined to succeed.
   7. Risk-taking abilities, tolerance for uncertainty and ambiguity, and personal resilience.
   8. Sense of creativity and innovativeness.
   9. Leadership, communication, and networking abilities.
   10. Assertiveness, self-discipline, and personal directedness in achieving a desired future.
B. Begin self-awareness exercise to identify personal and professional passions that could potentially become a nursing business. Conceptualize the business ideas inclusive of the potential market, resources, and services.

II. Step 2

A. Develop a self-improvement plan based on findings from the self-assessment.
   * Note: Nurse entrepreneurs advocate learning the requisite business skills *prior* to and not concurrent with launching a new business. Learning these skills requires tapping into available resources within the community, books, and/or online.

III. Step 3

A. Identify mentors or a personal coach to help develop or support the aspiring nurse entrepreneur in implementing and critiquing progress with the self-improvement plan.

IV. Step 4

A. Utilize a current employment setting or external community volunteer role as a training site to practice and develop the identified nurse entrepreneur

knowledge, skills, and abilities needed. This may involve taking the challenge to be an intrapreneur in the current employment setting and volunteering for projects and assignments that develop the needed skill set.

V. Step 5

A. Revisit findings from the self-awareness exercise to reconnect with earlier thoughts of the potential nursing business venture.
B. Reassess viability and configuration of this option now that a self-improvement plan, personal coach, and practice with the nurse entrepreneur skill development have taken place.
C. End this step with reconfiguring and shaping the potential business idea inclusive of product or service to be provided and having an idea as to the business name, logo, and color scheme for the business and promotional materials.

VI. Step 6

A. Write the business plan for the proposed venture. If assistance is needed to develop this plan, tap into resources of the U.S. Small Business Administration (SBA), either online or at a local community office.
B. Develop an action plan that addresses each component of the business plan.
C. Identify members of the entrepreneurial team, including a strong management team.

VII. Step 7

A. Seek legal and/or accounting advice regarding what type of organizational structure to pursue (sole proprietorship, partnership, limited liability corporation, corporation) and assistance in ensuring that the appropriate local, state, and federal licenses, permits, and registrations have been accounted for and incorporated into the business plan.
B. Register the strategically conceived (name captures the unique services of the business) Internet domain for the future business Web site.

VIII. Step 8

A. Using information from steps 6 and 7, determine sources of funding (personal, loan, equity, grant, venture capitalist) for business venture.
B. Proceed to finalize the sources of venture funding.
C. Establish business relationship with a bank and a banker.
D. Open two business checking accounts at the selected bank: a payroll account and a business operations account. Seek assignment of a designated account executive and sign up for minimum account balance protection.

E. Concurrent with opening the checking accounts, an accounting system will need to be developed including a chart of accounts to keep track of business income and expenses. A separate payroll system to keep track of employee hiring documents, time cards, payroll checks for employees, payroll records, payroll taxes, and related reporting systems (weekly, monthly, quarterly, annual) are also needed. A competent individual will either need to be hired or subcontracted to maintain the appropriate record-keeping and accounting systems for both business and payroll functions.

IX. Step 9

A. File for appropriate legal structure for the business, taking into account that the more complex the organizational structure, the longer the lead time to finalize the requirements for the organizational structure.
B. Concurrently submit for the appropriate tax identification (federal, state, local) and provider numbers.

X. Step 10

A. Establish the business location for the administrative offices. Find the appropriate office space, furniture, equipment, technology (hardware, software programs, data protection and back-up protocols, filing systems), and communication (land phones, cell phones, standard phone service, long-distance service, high-speed Internet service, answering service, fax machines, photocopiers, scanners, postage meter) systems for the business start-up. Office, business, and medical supplies will also need to be purchased.

XI. Step 11

A. Commission development of the business logo along with business stationery, business cards, informal note cards, and related promotional materials. Using the business logo, order appropriate building signage and telephone directory advertisements for the business. Concurrently, have available a preliminarily developed Web site using the preobtained business domain. The nurse entrepreneur should not be too concerned if the initial Web site is not as elaborate as ultimately desired; there is time later to refine the virtual business presence.

XII. Step 12

A. Design office systems with internal controls to address the various aspects of the business: client services and core operations, business/finance/accounting services and operations, and human resource functions. This will require development of multiple policy and procedure manuals and related forms to address client care (patient flow, standards of practice, quality assurance, documentation of services), business office operations (billing and collection procedures, accounts payable, accounts receivables, financial management and reporting), and personnel policies (employment application procedures, hiring policies, training and education programs, record keeping).
B. Purchase all necessary insurance as specified in the business plan.

XIII. Step 13

A. Begin recruiting, interviewing, and screening potential new employees needed for the business start-up.

XIV. Step 14

A. Establish a short "soft opening" period for the business as a means to fine-tune operations prior to a "grand" opening.
B. Make necessary improvements following evaluation of soft opening.
C. Have developed and ready to launch the business marketing and advertising campaigns. Launch these campaigns to coincide with the end of the "soft" opening.
D. Aggressively pursue the marketing and advertising campaign to procure new clients and begin establishing a referral base for future clients.

XV. Step 15

A. Hold "grand" opening for the business.
B. Make necessary improvements following evaluation of grand opening.

XVI. Step 16

A. Design continuous quality improvement program to regularly monitor key aspects of the operation:
   1. Clients: Are patients satisfied? Are those who are sending clients satisfied? What can be done better and how? Are we meeting regulatory standards and/or expected standards of care?
   2. Business/accounting: How are we doing with our billing and collections? What are the trends we see? What can we do better and how?
   3. Human resources: How are our employees doing? Are they competent and adequately trained? Are they engaged and happy? What could we do better and how?

XVII. Step 17

A. Frequently tap into the business support team (attorney, accountant, banker, management team, employees, clients) for advice and suggestions for improvement.

B. Frequently review the business plan and assess progress.

C. Continue to work, work, work, evaluate, improve, and reevaluate.

XVIII. Step 18

A. Seek advice from potential sources outside of the business support team: advisory board, community representatives.

XIX. Step 19

A. Promote the business within the community and beyond through involvement in civic activities and the chamber of commerce.

B. Extend involvement to national venues through speaking and writing engagements.

XX. Step 20

A. Conduct a full-scale evaluation of the business annually and make timely modifications as needed.

B. Plan for the future, following yearly strategic planning sessions and taking into account the stages of venture growth.

DISCUSSION QUESTIONS

1. How should entrepreneurship concepts be introduced into the CNS curriculum? To address the learning needs of a CNS considering entrepreneurship as a part of the CNS role, what would you envision the curriculum to look like for the 21st century?

2. Conceptualize a business venture, and apply and explain the Timmons Model for the first 5 years of the new venture.

3. Think of a successful nurse entrepreneur you know, and identify that individual's knowledge, skills, and abilities (KSA). Compare these KSAs with the available nurse entrepreneur empirical evidence in the literature. What additional research questions related to nurse entrepreneur (individual) attributes and actions would you generate? Any other research questions related to the nurse entrepreneur's interactions with groups (meso level) and organizational systems (macro level)?

4. Using the unique CNS lens, identify 10 gaps in patient/client care that could be addressed through CNS intervention. Generate a list of as many possible CNS-related new ventures that could address the identified gaps in patient/client care.

5. Identify the entrepreneurial culture at your current organization. What strategies would you utilize to change or enhance the entrepreneurial culture at your current organization? Is it possible? Why or why not?

6. Why is the entrepreneurial team/lead entrepreneur relationship so important in the entrepreneurial process? Considering your past experiences leading a team, what strategies as a lead entrepreneur would you contribute to the effective dynamic of the entrepreneurial team? Why?

NURSE ENTREPRENEUR RESOURCES TO EXPLORE

Books

1. Allen, K. (2002). *Entrepreneurship for dummies.* New York: Wiley.
2. Avillion, A. E. (2005). *Nurse entrepreneurship: The art of running your own business.* Minneapolis: Creative Health Care Management.
3. Bemis, P. A. (2007). *Self-employed RN: Choices, business aspects, and marketing strategies.* Rockledge, FL: National Nurses in Business Association, Inc.

Journals

1. *Wall Street Journal* (http://online.wsj.com/public/us)
2. *Entrepreneur Magazine* (http://www.entrepreneur.com/)
3. *Harvard Business Review* (http://hbr.harvardbusiness.org/)
4. *Journal of Entrepreneurship* (http://joe.sagepub.com/)
5. *Entrepreneurship Theory and Practice Journal* (http://www.wiley.com/bw/journal.asp?ref = 1042–2587)

Web Sites

1. National Nurses in Business Association: http://www.nnba.net/index.htm
2. National Association of Independent Nurses: http://www.independentrn.com/
3. Nurse Entrepreneurship Network: http://www.nurse-entrepreneur-network.com/

REFERENCES

Austin, L., Luker, K., & Ronald, M. (2006). Clinical nurse specialists as entrepreneurs: Constrained or liberated. *Journal of Clinical Nursing, 15,* 1540–1549.

Dayhoff, N. E., & Lyon, B. L. (2001). Assessing outcomes in clinical nurse specialist practice. In R. M. Kleinpell (Ed.), *Outcome assessment in advanced practice nursing* (pp. 103–129). New York: Springer.

Dossey, B. M. (2000). *Florence Nightingale: Mystic, visionary, healer.* Springhouse, PA: Springhouse Corporation.

Drucker, P. F. (1985). *Innovation and entrepreneurship.* New York: Harper Business.

Elango, B. (2007). Barriers to nurse entrepreneurship: A study of the process model of entrepreneurship. *Journal of the American Academy of Nurse Practitioners, 19,* 198–204.

Falcone, T., & Osborne, S. (2005). *Entrepreneurship: A diverse concept in a diverse world.* Retrieved January 25, 2009, from http://www.sbaer.uca.edu/research/usasbe/2005/pdffiles/papers/21.pdf

Hughes, K. (2003). Pushed or pulled? Women's entry into self-employment and small business ownership. *Gender, Work and Organization, 10,* 433–454.

International Council of Nurses. (2004). *Guidelines on the nurse entre/intrapreneur providing nursing service.* Geneva: Author.

Luke, B., Verreynne, M. L., & Kearins, K. (2007). Measuring the benefits of entrepreneurship at different levels of analysis. *Journal of Management and Organization, 13*(4), 312–330.

Macrae, N. (1982). *Intrapreneurial now.* Retrieved January 29, 2009, from http://www.intrapreneur.com/MainPages/History/Economist.html

Manimala, M. J. (1996). Beyond innovators and imitators: A taxonomy of entrepreneurs. *Creativity and Innovation Management, 5,* 179–189.

Marram, E. P. (2003). *Managing the growing business: Six stages of growth.* Retrieved January 25, 2009, from http://homepage.cem.itesm.mx/maria.fonseca/master/documents/Growth.pdf

McClelland, D. C. (1961). *The achieving society.* Princeton: Van Nostrand and Company.

National Association of Clinical Nurse Specialists. (2004). *Statement on clinical nurse specialist practice and education* (2nd ed.). Harrisburg, PA: Author.

National Association of the Self-Employed. (2004). *2004 Future entrepreneur: America's young entrepreneurs trend data at-a-glance.* Retrieved October 12, 2007, from http://www.nase.org/fey/youngentrepreneurs_stats.htm

Pinchot, G., & Pellman, R. (1985). *Intrapreneuring in action: A handbook for business innovation.* San Francisco: Berrett-Koehler Publishers.

Roggenkamp, S. D., & White, K. R. (1998). Four nurse entrepreneurs: What motivated them to start their own businesses. *Health Care Manage Review, 23,* 67–75.

Schorr, T. M., & Kennedy, M. S. (1999). *100 years of American nursing: Celebrating a century of caring.* Philadelphia: Lippincott.

Shane, S., & Venkataraman, S. (2007). The promise of entrepreneurship as a field of research. In A. Cuervo, D. Ribeiro, & S. Roig (Eds.), *Entrepreneurship: Concepts, theory and perspective* (pp. 171–184). Berlin: Springer.

Shirey, M. R. (2006). Building authentic leadership and enhancing entrepreneurial performance. *Clinical Nurse Specialist, 20,* 280–282.

Shirey, M. R. (2007). An evidence-based understanding of entrepreneurship in nursing. *Clinical Nurse Specialist, 21,* 234–240.

Stevenson, H. H., & Jarillo, J. C. A paradigm of entrepreneurship: Entrepreneurial management. In A. Cuervo, D. Ribeiro, & S. Roig (Eds.), *Entrepreneurship: Concepts, theory and perspective* (pp. 155–170). Berlin: Springer.

Timmons, J. A., & Spinelli, S. (2007). *New venture creation: Entrepreneurship for the 21st century* (7th ed.). New York: McGraw Hill.

U.S. Chamber of Commerce. (2006). *Work, entrepreneurship, and opportunity in 21st century America.* Retrieved January 25, 2009, from http://www.uschamber.com/NR/rdonlyres/egd6apsvvwg333lvhlomles6lietyvlomlujv4o65b6z7jns4f7nsac6wry5hs6fldzwko5zwt6bwueo4e7gu6pyb2g/21st_final.pdf

Veciana, J. M. (2007). Entrepreneurship as a scientific research programme. In A. Cuervo, D. Ribeiro, & S. Roig (Eds.), *Entrepreneurship: Concepts, theory and perspective* (pp. 23–71). Berlin: Springer.

Weaver, J. W. (2005–2007, Dunlap, Grubb & Weaver, PLLC.). *A start-up businesses guide to choosing the right form of entity (S-Corp, LLC or Sole-Proprietor).* Retrieved January 25, 2009, from http://www.hg.org/article.asp?id=4790

Wilson, A., Averis, A., & Walsh, K. (2003). The influence on and experience of becoming nurse entrepreneurs: A Delphi study. *International Journal of Nursing Practice, 9,* 236–245.

Wilson, A., Averis, A., & Walsh, K. (2004). The scope of private practice nursing in an Australian sample. *Public Health Nursing, 21,* 488–494.

Billing and Reimbursement Issues

Susan Dresser

The U.S. health care system is undergoing tremendous reform driven by the demand for patient safety, reduced costs, improved effectiveness, greater quality, and streamlined efficiency. Clinical nurse specialists (CNSs) are clinical experts in the diagnosis and treatment of illness, the promotion of health, and the delivery of evidence-based nursing interventions (American Nurses Association [ANA], 2004). They function independently to provide theory and evidence-based care to patients in facilitating the achievement of health goals, and they work to advance nursing practice, improve outcomes, and provide clinical expertise to effect system-wide changes to improve programs of care (ANA, 2004; Lyon, 2002; Lyon & Minarik, 2001a, 2001b). By virtue of these characteristics and their understanding of systems processes and ability to reduce fragmentation of care, CNSs are ideally positioned to respond to these challenges by demonstrating the provision and coordination of high-quality, evidence-based, cost-effective care.

Pursuing reimbursement from third-party payers is a relatively new opportunity for CNSs and one that demands additional educational preparation beyond the basic CNS graduate program, as well as hands-on experience. As a provider of health care to Medicare and other third-party payer beneficiaries, CNSs will need to become knowledgeable about state and federal reimbursement laws, payment structure, rules, and regulations.

In order to monitor and influence health care debate and legislative efforts pertaining to advanced practice nursing and reimbursement, CNSs must have a solid understanding of the Medicare program as well as state and federal practice regulations for advanced practice nursing reimbursement (Minarik, 2000). Findings from a recent study of practicing CNSs' knowledge of Medicare structure and processes revealed that while

53% of the respondents ranked knowledge of Medicare as very important to extremely important to CNS practice, 66% of the respondents rated themselves as only "minimally expert" in knowledge of Medicare content (Zuzelo, Fallon, Lang, & Mount, 2004). This study further indicated that while CNSs were generally aware of Medicare structures and processes, many had basic knowledge deficits relating to reimbursement processes and lacked an understanding of federal regulations recognizing CNSs as advanced practice nurses (APNs) who could become Medicare providers. These findings support the need for CNS graduate programs to incorporate content pertaining to health care financing and reimbursement processes and for individual responsibility in seeking out this information.

Maneuvering the complex and dynamic system of rules and regulations characteristic of Medicare and health care financing and provider reimbursement can be overwhelming and frustrating, but it is necessary in order to receive appropriate reimbursement. This chapter provides a brief overview of the historical and legislative background leading to the current recognition of advance practice registered nurses (APRNs) as Medicare providers and focuses on specific information related to coding, billing, and reimbursement processes as they pertain to the CNS.

HISTORICAL BACKGROUND OF REIMBURSEMENT

The goal of third-party reimbursement for nursing coincides with the profession's long-standing struggle for recognition and autonomy dating back to some of the early efforts of support made by the ANA in 1948

(Griffith, 1984). Achieving provider recognition is believed by many to be critical for the recognition and survival of a health care profession. Public support for and confidence in nursing's ability has been demonstrated time and again as evidenced by the results of an ANA survey of the attitudes of the American public toward the nursing profession (Phillips, 1987). This national poll revealed that 68% of those surveyed believed nurses had the education to play a greater role in health care than they were currently permitted to do, and 85% to 96% of the respondents believed that with special education nurses could prescribe routine prescription drugs, conduct physical examinations, deliver babies, and provide home health care services and psychotherapy. Equally significant was that 80% believed that health care costs could be lower if more services were provided by nurses (Phillips, 1987).

Historically, special interest groups have prevailed upon policy makers of all branches of the government to influence and determine health policy relating to what can be done in health care, who is allowed to do it, who bears the cost for it, and who receives payment. In this political battleground, physicians have long been the dominant and most successful participants. Jacox (1997) provided a historical overview of the social, political, and economic influences that have defined the health care reimbursement system over the past 50 years. A previous analysis of the roles of advanced practice registered nurses by Barbara Safriet, as cited by Jacox, noted that physicians were the first health care providers to acquire legislative recognition of their practice. Safriet noted that the expansive definition of medical practice combined with the usual provision making it illegal for anyone not licensed as a physician to carry out any acts included in the definition, resulted in a preemptive strike by the medical profession to totally occupy the health care field, at least for any activity that could be deemed diagnosing, treating, prescribing, or curing.

Nurses and other providers of health care would be forced to "carve out tasks or functions from this all-encompassing medical scope of practice in seeking legislative recognition of their own professional roles, no matter how traditional or long-standing their activities" (Jacox, 1997). Physicians have used their political strength over the years to influence reimbursement policy and payment rules and regulations. One obvious outcome has been that only those who performed the service could be reimbursed. Over time, nursing has responded to a system that markedly favored physicians by launching deliberate and aggressive grass roots campaigns to gain provider recognition and reimbursement for APRNs.

The Omnibus Budget Reconciliation Act (1989) first opened the door to give APRNs the opportunity for reimbursement, although it was restricted to those nurses collaborating with physicians and practicing in rural areas. CNSs who provided care to Medicare patients in nonrural areas could only receive reimbursement by an indirect means known as "incident to" payments. These services had to be billed under a physician's Medicare number, and the CNS had to be an employee of the physician. The reimbursement went to the physician. Inadequate direct federal reimbursement continued to represent a significant barrier to the utilization of APRNs until 1998. The landmark Balanced Budget Act (BBA) of 1997 was signed into law by President Bill Clinton granting provider status to CNSs regardless of geographic location or practice site, thus, increasing billing and reimbursement opportunities. Effective January 1, 1998, this legislation removed the barriers to direct reimbursement and created numerous opportunities and challenges for CNSs and other APNs to be recognized as health care providers (BBA, 1997). For the first time, APRNs could be identified in the reimbursement process as the providers of care, even if not supervised by a physician, as long as services were performed in collaboration with a physician. By billing under their own names, APRNs were now able to make visible financial contributions in health care organizations. The definition of physicians' services was broadened with this legislation to include CNSs whose:

> services which would be physicians' services if furnished by a physician . . . and which are performed by a clinical nurse specialist or a nurse practitioner. . . . working in collaboration with a physician . . . which the nurse practitioner or clinical nurse specialist is legally authorized to perform by the State in which the services are performed , and such services and supplies furnished as an incident to such services as would be covered . . . if furnished incident to a physician's professional services, but only if no facility or other provider charges or is paid any amounts with respect to the furnishing of such services. (BBA, 1997)

As a result of this law, CNSs became eligible to submit claims to Medicare and receive direct reimbursement from Medicare at 85% of the current physician fee as stated in Medicare's physician fee schedule.

INTRODUCTION TO THIRD-PARTY PAYERS

There are four major categories of third-party payers that CNSs should be familiar with, including: government entities, such as Medicare and Medicaid; managed care organizations; businesses that contract for specific services; and commercial indemnity insurance companies. Each of these groups has their own set of rules and criteria defining reimbursement policies and fee schedules. Most payers base their payment amount in reference to the Medicare physician fee schedule. Third-party payers will reimburse for physician services that are provided by a CNS if the services provided are within the scope of practice of the CNS and the payers' rules are adhered to. Inconsistency in states' laws regarding APRNs combined with considerable differences in third-party payers' reimbursement policies for APRNs' services make the pursuit for reimbursement a challenge. The Centers for Medicare and Medicaid Services (CMS) of the U.S. Department of Health and Human Services (HHS) has developed detailed policies and rules governing the reimbursement of providers that are sometimes used as the standard by other reimbursement entities. CNSs must possess a sound knowledge and understanding of the structure, regulations, and reimbursement rules for each of the third-party entities with whom they are contracting.

MEDICARE

Medicare, the largest single health care payer, was created as part of the Social Security Act of 1965 and is the federal health insurance program for the elderly and disabled. It is administered nationally by CMS and locally by Medicare carrier agencies (Buppert, 2004). Previously known as the Health Care Financing Administration (HCFA), CMS operates as an agent of the federal government and interprets Medicare laws and awards contracts on a state or regional level to manage billing and reimbursement programs. Medicare carriers are private local companies under contract with CMS to pay Medicare Part B bills (Minarik, 2000). Medicare funds pay for medical services under two programs: Medicare Part A covers inpatient hospital services, hospice, skilled nursing facilities, and some home health care; Part B covers outpatient hospital services, laboratory charges, medical equipment and supplies, and the services of physicians and other selected providers such as CNSs and nurse practitioners. CNSs bill Medicare under Part B, and Part B payments are then administered by the local Medicare carriers.

The CMS Web site (http://www.cms.hhs.gov/) provides valuable educational resources, but unfortunately, it is a complex maze of information. To help navigate through the vast amount of material, CMS has created the Medicare Learning Network (MLN), which features the Advanced Practice Registered Nursing & Physician Assistants (APRN/PA) Web page. This dedicated Web page is for Medicare fee-for-service (FFS) APRNs and PAs who provide services to Medicare beneficiaries. From this Web page, you can access and review the Medicare FFS program topics in order to remain current in your knowledge of policy and operational updates specific to APRNs and PAs. One of the educational resources featured on this Web page is the APRN/PA

Web-Based Training Program—this interactive learning program provides definitions of and qualifications of the APRN/PA provider types, describes collaboration/supervision requirements for reimbursements, lists the Medicare billing requirements, and identifies links to Medicare manuals and other resources. This Web page is regularly updated and should be reviewed often for timely and reliable information from the MLN. The MLN also offers *The Guided Pathways to Medicare Resources Basic Tutorial*—a guided tour through the basic resources that help providers to understand and navigate the Medicare program. This tutorial utilizes an animated highly interactive *road trip* simulation to incorporate education resources into a structured format that provides information on coding, billing, forms, documentation, and numerous Medicare topics of interest for new and experienced providers.

MEDICAID

Medicaid is also a federal program administered by each state that provides coverage to low-income individuals and families, the elderly, and disabled. Each state establishes its own Medicaid rules under federal guidelines. APRNs can become Medicaid providers. Medicaid reimburses APRNs at 70% to 100% of rates set for physicians. For the rate that is applicable to a certain state, contact the state Medicaid provider agency. To apply for a Medicaid provider number, complete an application from the state Medicaid agency. Billing Medicaid patients requires the submission of the CMS 1500 form.

COMMERCIAL INDEMNITY INSURERS

An indemnity insurer is an insurance company that pays for the medical care for those it insures but does not deliver the health care. Provider charges are submitted directly to the insurance company (Barone & Paniagua-Ramirez, 2006). Commercial payers generally reimburse at a rate from 65% to 100% of their physician fee schedule rate. Unlike Medicare, commercial physician fee schedules vary and are negotiable. These insurers present a different challenge for coverage of medical services provided by APRNs but not because they fail to cover APRN provided services; most of them do. The problem is that there are a large number of commercial insurers in the market, and they may all have different policies for how services provided by an APRN are covered and how claim forms should be completed and submitted. The first step for a provider is to determine which commercial insurers are prevalent in your geographic and practice area. Next, you should make a list of all of the health care plans, including the addresses and telephone and fax numbers. Contact each entity by phone, requesting the name of the person responsible for credentialing, and inquire whether a provider number is required. When contacting to determine their policy on coverage be sure to phrase your questions with terminology that they will understand. An application to become a provider will have to be completed for each entity.

MANAGED CARE ORGANIZATIONS

Managed care organizations (MCO) are insurers that provide both the health care services and payment for the services provided. It is an umbrella term that includes organizations such as health maintenance organizations, physician hospital organizations, and provider-sponsored organizations. Some APRNs have been accepted on the provider panel of certain MCOs. This membership qualifies the APRN as the designated primary care provider, placing full responsibility for the patient's primary care upon the APRN (Buppert, 2004). Call the provider relations department for each MCO for which admission as a provider is needed, and request an application for admission to the panel of providers. If the application is rejected, note the reason and consult state insurance law if applicable.

THE PROCESS FOR OBTAINING REIMBURSEMENT

Physicians, APNs, and other health care providers must enroll in the Medicare program by completing form CMS-855I in order to be recognized as a provider of services. This form can be found on the CMS Web site and downloaded at http://www.cms.hhs.gov/cmsforms/downloads/cms855i.pdf. Prior to enrolling in Medicare, you must first obtain a national provider identifier (NPI). The federal NPI is the health care provider identification system adopted by HHS as part of the implementation of the Health Insurance Portability and Accountability Act (HIPAA), and it replaces the previously used health care provider identifiers. The CMS Web site has an NPI Web page providing information and an overview of the NPI program, regulations, application, and guidelines, which can be downloaded at: http://www.cms.hhs.gov/NationalProvidentStand/.

In the past, CNSs would have had to complete applications to get a unique provider identification number (UPIN), a Medicare number, and a Medicaid number, and then apply to each individual provider for a separate provider number. Now the NPI number will be used for all future billing transactions. A copy of the NPI notification letter must be included in the application to Medicare. The enrollment application is used to collect the required documentation to ensure you are qualified and eligible to enroll as a Medicare provider and includes authentication of professional licenses, the NPI notification letter, evidence of national certification, and documentation of a collaborative practice agreement with a physician regardless of whether or not it is required by your state.

Third-party payers vary in their requirements for credentialing for reimbursement so, it is necessary to be knowledgeable about the specifics of each payer. For services of a CNS to be covered by Medicare, the CNS must meet the following qualifications:

1. Hold an active license as a registered nurse authorized to perform the services of a CNS in the state where he or she practices;
2. Have a master's or doctoral degree in a defined clinical area of nursing from an accredited educational institution; and
3. Hold current certification as a CNS from an appropriate certifying body that has established standards for CNSs and that is approved by the secretary of HHS. (Medicare Benefit Policy Manual, 2008)

The following organizations are currently accepted by CMS as national certifying bodies for CNSs at the advanced practice level:

1. American Nurses Credentialing Center
2. Oncology Nurses Certification Corporation
3. American Association of Critical Care Nurses
4. National Board on Certification of Hospice and Palliative Nurses
5. Pediatric Nursing Certification Board
6. National Certification Corporation for Obstetric, Gynecologic and Neonatal Nursing Specialties (Medicare Benefit Policy Manual, 2008)

A qualification for continued participation as a provider in the Medicare program is to maintain current knowledge of the program rules. The health care provider who does not adhere to the rules may likely experience denied payments, reduced payments, demand for repayment of funds already paid, and investigation and charges of billing abuse or fraud. Medicare's rules are extensive and subject to frequent changes, and the rules relevant to CNSs are in multiple locations.

A number of regulations govern health care reimbursement for all providers with additional requirements for APNs. The first and most basic requirement for reimbursement is that payment is made *only* for those services that are defined as *physician services* by current procedural terminology (CPT) codes (BBA, 1997). These terms will be defined and discussed later in this chapter.

To determine whether the CNS is providing *physician services,* the following questions must be answered.

Is the Service to Be Performed One That Would Be a Physician's Service if Performed by a Physician?

Medicare defines physicians' services as the professional services performed by a physician or physicians for a patient including diagnosis, therapy, surgery, consultation, and care plan oversight. Consult the current CPT manual to determine the physician service components of the various procedures. CPT is a manual of procedure codes published by the American Medical Association (AMA, 2008). To gain an understanding of how physicians' services are described, it would be helpful to briefly scan the manual. Compare the service the CNS wishes to provide with the descriptions of service provided in the manual. For example, if the service to be provided is consultation, find the CPT codes for consultation, found in the "Evaluation and Management" section of the manual. The physician service components of consultation listed in the manual are: history taking, examination, and medical decision making. The manual defines medical decision making as diagnosing and selecting management options. Analyze whether the service the CNS provides or wishes to provide fits with the components of physician service described in the manual.

Is the Service to Be Provided by the CNS Covered by Medicare?

Certain physician services are not covered by Medicare. For example, regular physical examinations, health maintenance screening, and counseling for well patients are physician services, but Medicare does not cover these services. To obtain a list of noncovered services, refer to your local Medicare carrier.

Is the CNS Authorized to Perform the Service Under the State Law Governing CNS Scope of Practice?

CNSs' authority to practice varies greatly from state to state. To bill Medicare for a service, the CNS must be authorized to perform that service under state law. As an example, to perform a consultation, the CNS must have authority under state law to take a history, perform an examination, and diagnose and select management options. Examples of some of the services a CNS may provide (if authorized under the scope of their state license) that are considered physician services

include: assessing the patient's risk factors for indications of developing medical problems, diagnosing the medical problem(s), creating a plan of care, ordering applicable tests, providing selected treatments, counseling the patient, physical examinations, interpreting X-rays, and other independent evaluations and treatments of a patient's condition (Medicare Benefit Policy Manual, 2008).

The definition of collaboration defers somewhat to state law to define the exact collaborative arrangement. *Collaboration* is defined as a process in which the CNS works with one or more physicians to deliver health care services within the scope of the practitioner's expertise, with medical direction and supervision as provided for in jointly developed guidelines or other mechanisms as provided by the law of the state in which the services are performed (BBA, 1997). States vary in their requirements for collaboration between a physician and CNS. When a CNS practices in a state that requires physician collaboration, Medicare requires nothing beyond what the state requires. However, some states do require CNSs to have a collaborative agreement with a physician, and while Medicare generally defers to state law requirements, federal law requires that a CNS billing Medicare have a collaborative relationship with a physician. If you are a CNS in a state without specific collaborative requirements for CNSs, you will be required to document your scope of practice and indicate the relationship you have with physicians to deal with any issues outside your scope of practice (Federal Register, 1998). Reimbursable physician services must also be medically necessary, accurately documented in the medical record, actually provided, and provided by a CNS with a Medicare provider number (Buppert, 2002; Richmond, Thompson, & Sullivan-Marx, 2002).

The most lucrative reimbursement rate, 100% of the physician rate, is allowed by Medicare rules under the "incident to" billing—submitting bills under a physician's provider number for services provided by a supervised employee—under certain circumstances. To submit bills under the "incident to" provision, certain rules must be followed. If an APRN and a physician work together to provide physician services, the services can be billed under the physician's provider number in order to receive the full physician fee under the Medicare provision for "incident to" billing. However, certain rules must be followed when billing services under the "incident to" provision.

1. The services are an integral, although incidental, part of the physician's professional service.
2. The services are commonly rendered without charge or included in the physician's bill.
3. The services are of a type commonly furnished in physician's offices or clinics.

4. The services are furnished under the physician's direct personal supervision and are furnished by the physician or by an individual who is an employee or independent contractor of the physician.
5. Direct supervision does not require the physician's presence in the same room, but the physician must be present in the same office suite and immediately available.
6. The physician must perform "the initial service and subsequent services of a frequency that reflects his or her active participation in the management of the course of treatment" (Frakes & Evans, 2006, p. 557).

The physician or other provider under whose name and number the bill is submitted must be the individual present in the office suite when the service is provided. Care for patients in the hospital complicates billing because "incident to" billing is not allowed in the hospital setting. Additionally, a hospital-employed APRN cannot bill for any inpatient services provided if the hospital receives Medicare reimbursement for the APRN's salary (Buppert, 2005).

Providers who wish to bill Medicare Part B must submit the bill using a CMS-1500 form. CMS-1500 forms can be purchased from local business forms supply companies, or they may be ordered from the U.S. Government Printing Office, Superintendent of Documents, Washington, DC 20402. Orders may be charged to a credit card by calling 202-512-1800 (Baradell & Buppert, 2003). In addition to patient identification information, the bill must include a procedure code, a diagnosis code, and the provider's name and provider number. Medicare requires the use of *International Classification of Diseases*, 9th Revision (ICD-9) codes for coding medical diagnoses.

CODING

The goal of obtaining a thorough understanding of the complexities of coding and the required documentation is beyond the scope of any single publication. This chapter is designed to provide CNSs with a beginning knowledge of medical billing and reimbursement. To avoid legal pitfalls and allow for appropriate and timely reimbursement of services provided, CNSs are strongly encouraged to read authoritative work carefully; utilize audio conferences, CDs, and tapes; or attend a national specialty specific coding and billing conference provided by coding experts to become proficient.

Medicare and Medicaid are billed using the Healthcare Common Procedure Coding System (HCPCS). The HCPCS encompasses two independent and different sets of codes referred to as Level I Current Procedural Terminology (CPT) codes and Level II State codes. The CPT coding system is an information management system developed by the AMA in 1966 that is widely utilized by third-party payers (Baradell & Hanrahan, 2000). CPT codes are developed, maintained, and copyrighted by the AMA. As the practice of health care changes, new codes are created for new services, existing codes may be revised, and outdated unused codes are discarded. Literally thousands of codes are in use, and they are updated annually. Development, review, and maintenance of these codes is overseen by editorial boards at the AMA, and the publications of the software, books, and manuals needed by those who use them brings an estimated $70 million in income to the AMA each year (Torrey, 2008). A fee is associated with each CPT code. The fee for each CPT procedure under Medicare is based on established relative value units (RVUs) that take into consideration professional work involved, practice expenses, and liability insurance. CPT codes are organized into various categories and levels. To determine what services can be billed for under Medicare Part B, APRNs must understand the coding system. Individual providers are reimbursed under the CPT codes, which are a uniform five-digit numeric coding system for submitting medical claims. These codes describe levels of medical and diagnostic services and procedures and the level of complexity of care provided (Buppert, 2005). The purpose of the terminology in the CPT is to provide a uniform, consistent language that will accurately describe medical, surgical, and diagnostic services and, thus, provide an effective means for reliable nationwide communication among providers and payers.

Level II codes are nationally standardized state codes maintained by the CMS and applied by each state. Level II codes are also five digits and begin with a letter followed by a four-digit number, for example, H4008. Level II codes are often used by providers billing the state Medicaid agency for services provided to Medicaid beneficiaries. HCPCS refers to both Level I and II codes.

When billing for a patient's visit, codes are chosen that best represent the services provided during the visit. The HIPAA legislation of 1996 specified that all medical billing be accompanied by an applicable primary medical diagnosis code derived from ICD-9. ICD9-CM coding is an international disease classification system that groups related disease entities and conditions for the purpose of reporting statistical information. Coders rely on the documentation in the record to determine what codes to assign for services provided. The responsibility for capturing accurate diagnosis and procedures, in particular principal diagnosis, lies with the provider, not the coder. As a general rule, you want to code to the highest level of specificity so that you are providing the most complete diagnostic information about a patient and to capture severity of illness. CPT codes have to match up with their diagnosis codes—that is, all CPT procedure codes must point to a diagnosis. The combination of the ICD-9 code (why the service was necessary) with the CPT code (what service was provided) paints the complete picture of the patient encounter.

CPT coding is fairly easy in terms of supplies or procedures. However, coding becomes trickier when it comes down to the evaluation and management decisions. APRNs must base their choice of procedure code on the extent and complexity of the evaluation and management (E & M) services provided—generally the more complex the work performed, the higher the level of code the service is eligible for. The patient history, examination, and medical decision making are the key components that serve as the main driving force in determining E & M code selection. The documentation of the work done must support the level chosen because it would be inappropriate to bill a higher level of E & M when a lower level of service is provided or necessary.

Using the presenting illness or complaint as a guiding factor and clinical judgment, the provider can determine the level of complexity needed for each of the three key elements of service to be performed. Medicare's *Documentation Guidelines for Evaluation and Management Services,* which most private payers depend upon to a large degree, divides documentation of E & M services into three key elements of service: history, exam, and medical decision making. When billing for E & M, specific documentation guidelines must be adhered to, and the work performed must be clearly defined. E & M documentation and coding is one of the most important components in the billing process. The most recent E & M documentation guidelines are from 1995 and 1997, and either one may be used as a reference. Many people find the 1995 guidelines less cumbersome and easier to understand. In order to properly document and code for the work that you do, it is important to take the time to study the CPT manual and the documentation guidelines for evaluation and management. The documentation requirements necessary for the key element of *patient history* vary depending upon which level of history the provider determines is needed. Each of the levels require an increasing amount of detail to and are divided into problem focused, expanded problem focused, detailed, or comprehensive. The history is composed of three different sections: history of present illness (HPI), review of systems (ROS), and past, family, or social history.

As an example, in order to meet the documentation requirements for a *detailed history* on a new office patient (Level III 99203), the provider would have to perform an assessment and document the patient's chief complaint, an extended history of present illness (four or more elements), an extended review of systems (two or more systems), and a pertinent past, family, or social history (one or more history areas).

Within the second key element of an E & M service is the *examination.* The provider needs to document the extent of the examination performed. The levels of E & M services are again based on four types of examinations: problem focused, expanded problem focused, detailed, and comprehensive. The complexity and extent of the examination will depend upon the clinical judgment of the provider, the patient's history, and the nature of the presenting problem. The provider may not need to perform a detailed exam in a short visit or with a straight forward complaint. Essentially, there are two basic types of examinations that a provider can perform during a visit: general multisystem, which involves one or more organ systems or body areas; and a single-organ system examination, which involves a more extensive examination of a specific organ system.

Medical decision making, the third key element of an E & M service, involves the integration and consideration of three different components: number of diagnoses or treatment options that must be considered, amount and or complexity of data reviewed, and the risk of complications or morbidity and mortality (Buppert, 2004). Four different levels of medical decision making in the E & M descriptors are recognized as shown in Table 26.1: straightforward, low complexity, moderate complexity, and high complexity.

There are five major coding guidelines for billing for evaluation and management:

1. A billable visit requires face-to-face contact between a patient and a provider.
2. A billable visit requires association with an ICD-9 medical diagnosis.
3. The level of service is determined by the extent of history taking, physical examination, and medical decision making.
4. The documentation must reflect the level of care billed.

TIPS FOR ACCURATE AND TIMELY REIMBURSEMENT

CNSs will often be employed by a hospital or medical practice group that has an existing coding and billing staff. Coders attempt to keep current with the frequent CMS changes as they relate to billing and coding. Communication between coders and providers is essential to ensuring the accuracy of coding. Coders have an extensive knowledge of reimbursement, documentation requirements, and coding and can be one of the best resources for questions. Networking with other CNSs and APRNs who are already recognized Medicare providers can facilitate the process of learning, reduce frustration, and provide opportunities for sharing methods of productivity tracking and outcomes. Common provider

26.1 | CPT Code Examples

INITIAL NEW OFFICE PATIENT VISITS: CPT CODES AND REQUIRED DOCUMENTATION

E/M Code:	99201 Level I Problem focused	99202 Level II Expanded problem focused	99203 Level III Detailed	99204 Level IV Comprehensive	99205 Level V Comprehensive
History					
Chief complaint	Required	Required	Required	Required	Required
History of present illness	1–3 elements	1–3 elements	4 or more elements or 3 or more chronic diseases	4 or more elements or 3 or more chronic diseases	4 or more elements or 3 or more chronic diseases
Review of systems	NR	Problem pertinent 1 system	2–9 systems	10 or more systems	10 or more systems
Past history/ family history	NR	NR	1 element	3 or more elements	3 or more elements
Examination	1 system (1–5 elements)	2 brief systems (6–11 elements)	1 detailed system + 1 brief system (12 or more elements)	8 systems or 1 complete single system (comprehensive)	8 systems or 1 complete single system (comprehensive)
Medical Decision Making					
Risk of complication/ mortality	Minimal	Minimal	Low	Moderate	High
Diagnosis or treatment options	Minimal	Minimal	Low	Moderate	High
Data Reviewed	Minimal	Minimal	Low	Moderate	High
Time	10 minutes	20 minutes	30 minutes	45 minutes	60 minutes

Adapted from *1995 Documentation Guidelines for Evaluation and Management Services*, available at www.cms.hhs.gov/MLNProducts/Downloads/1995dg.pdf on the Centers for Medicare & Medicaid Services (CMS) Web site.

documentation errors include inconsistent documentation, incomplete documentation, undocumented care, failure to document chronic conditions, and illegibility. Incomplete or missing documentation could potentially compromise patient care and result in inaccurate data contributed toward research findings. CMS sends free e-mail alerts to its contracted members announcing updates, and it is imperative that CNSs are reviewing these updates and attending to detail to identify which ones will apply and affect their practice. As a provider of services, CNSs need to carefully monitor the financial impact of any Medicare reimbursement rules and rate changes that will potentially impact practice, opportunity, and revenue generation. Data on services

provided, charges, collections, and net income should be reviewed monthly to evaluate overall operations. One recommendation every provider should adhere to is a practice of performing routine chart audits. Conducting a chart audit is one of the best ways to uncover gaps between what you document and what you code. Inadequate documentation may be a cause for reimbursement denials or for inadequate reimbursement for the level of work provided. Poor documentation findings indicate that it is time to review the E & M documentation guidelines. Careful and accurate documentation and coding are vital skills for every provider to record the high-quality care provided for patients and to prevent undercoding or overcoding for the services provided. It is common for payers to reject claims from all types of providers for a variety of reasons, therefore, the APRN must get involved if this occurs by calling the third-party payer directly and resolving the issue. Direct participation will help develop a better understanding of the reimbursement process and covered benefits.

IMPLICATIONS FOR PRACTICE

CNS practice extends across three spheres of influence with a primary intent of achieving cost-effective improvement in patient outcomes. It is extremely important for CNSs to validate their contributions to the improvement of both clinical and economic outcomes. It is equally important, when looking at outcome measures in the context of billing for services under the traditional medical model, to carefully select outcomes to evaluate that will include those contributions that are clearly and purposefully reflective of the expertise of the CNS. CNSs that are being reimbursed must undoubtedly learn to track their productivity measures in terms of time and resource expenditure as compared to billable output. Relatively little research has been done on third-party reimbursement and CNSs, and no studies were found regarding outcomes of CNSs who were Medicare providers. Many CNSs perform the same procedures and services as physicians, and with direct billing, the opportunity exists to demonstrate the impact CNSs can have on generating revenue in addition to reducing costs and improving patient outcomes.

Historically, third-party payers provided significant financial support to hospitals by reimbursing hospitals for a percentage of their costs of providing care. Under the current prospective payment system, hospitals now receive a fixed reimbursement per patient discharge with no regard for actual hospital costs. As a result, hospitals have intensified efforts at minimizing costs by improving efficiencies of care delivery, decreasing patient length of stay, and other methods. This change in health care reimbursement practice, combined with the increasingly competitive environment for cost-effectiveness, growing public concerns for quality, projected physician shortages and expanded reimbursement opportunities for APRNs, has created a favorable climate for CNSs to demonstrate their expertise and cost-effectiveness of services. Our model of health care reimbursement has historically been based upon the medical model of illness management. This is in contrast to a more holistic nursing model of wellness, health maintenance, and preventive care that a CNS can provide. While both models have some similarities, such as the assessment of the patient's presenting complaint, the nursing model utilized by a CNS would integrate and synthesize data drawn from additional sources, including the patient's perspective of the illness, contributions of nondiseases etiologies, and influences of the patient's culture, family, and beliefs to arrive at a diagnosis. The plan of care developed from a CNS's advanced nursing perspective would incorporate the medical model interventions of medications, laboratory work, and procedures as well as nursing interventions to include the patient, family, community, and support.

SUMMARY

As advanced practice nursing gains a foothold in the reimbursement arena, the value of the CNS as a quality health care provider will continue to grow. CNSs can positively influence their economic viability within the health care system by providing high-quality reimbursable services and by properly defining, describing, and documenting the services they provide in accordance with the guidelines articulated in the CPT codes. While many of the services provided by a CNS may not be currently classified as physician services but rather fall under the category of "integrative or nursing services," their value will continue to grow as their cost-effectiveness is further realized. Some integrative CNS role functions may actually be billable as a physician service such as "coordination of care," but the CNS who bills for this must be prepared to defend how this is a physician service instead of a nursing service. Those CNSs considering becoming recognized providers of health care must be prepared to invest considerable time and energy into learning the rules, regulations, and requirements for practice, billing, and reimbursement. Now, more than ever before, reimbursement for health care services is heavily scrutinized and regulated by law. Although it is a somewhat difficult process, it is important that CNSs gain a good understanding of the regulations, terminology, and legalities surrounding reimbursement, even if you are not currently working in a position where you are being reimbursed. Take advantage of resources such as coding and billing seminars and conferences, continuing education programs, journal articles, and coding and billing experts.

DISCUSSION QUESTIONS

1. How would clinical judgment and critical thinking be utilized by a CNS in determining an appropriate E & M service level?
2. How could a CNS document the cost-effectiveness of his/her practice?
3. Does current entry-level education prepare CNSs to perform the skills necessary for reimbursement of professional services?

4. Describe ways that the CNS could integrate quality measures with the required documentation for reimbursement.
5. How could a CNS capitalize on current Medicare reimbursement opportunities in the areas of chronic illness and preventive services?
6. In what ways could a CNS work with a nurse executive to develop and propose reimbursement demonstration projects?
7. In what ways could a CNS work collaboratively and strategically with other stakeholders to expand reimbursement opportunities to include integrative and advanced nursing interventions?

ANALYSIS AND SYNTHESIS EXERCISE

1. Using the following case study and the previously supplied documentation guidelines, what level would be appropriate to bill for this patient visit?

A 58-year-old male presents to the office with a chief complaint of productive cough, mild dyspnea, fatigue, and fever to 101 degrees. His symptoms have been present for the past 3 days, and when over-the-counter cold medications were having no effect, he decided to seek medical attention. He denied any recent changes in weight but noted a loss of appetite. He denied any episodes of chest pain or discomfort. He has no significant past medical history, is a nonsmoker, takes no medications, and has no known drug allergies. On initial examination, he was pleasant; alert; oriented X 3; pupils were equal, round, and reactive to light and accommodation; conjunctiva were clear; throat mildly red; room air pulse oximetry was 96%; his blood pressure was 120/73; pulse was 98 and regular; and respirations were 20 and unlabored. Neck was supple, without lymphadenopathy, no jugular venous distention. He was febrile with a temperature of 101 degrees. Lung examination revealed the presence of right lower lung crackles with rare wheeze, with decreased breath sounds in this area as well. Heart sounds were crisp and regular without murmur, rub, or gallop. Extremities were warm, without clubbing, cyanosis, or edema. Pedal pulse were 2 + bilaterally, radially pulses were 2 + bilaterally. Abdomen was soft, flat, and nontender with active bowel sounds and no masses.

Laboratory studies revealed WBC of 15.6 with a left shift, sodium of 140, potassium of 4.5, BUN of 22, and creatinine of 1.0. Chest X-ray revealed a right lower lobe infiltrate.

2. Medical decision making:

Based upon the history, physical examination, lab work, and chest X-ray, this patient appears to have pneumonia, and it is most likely community-acquired pneumonia because he has no recent history of hospitalization.

There does not appear to be any newly discovered health problems other than the pneumonia. Based upon the presentation described, the patient does not appear to have a severe enough illness to necessitate admission to the hospital. In this case, based upon the information provided, the patient can be allowed to go home and start oral antibiotics, encourage fluids, and then reevaluated to see if he is improving. Lack of improvement at the follow-up visit would be an indication for hospitalization, as would deterioration while being treated.

REFERENCES

American Medical Association. (2008). *Current procedural terminology*. Chicago: Author.

American Nurses Association. (2004). *Nursing: Scope and standards of practice*. Washington, DC: Author.

Balanced Budget Act. (1997). U.S. Public Law 105–33: Title IV—Medicare, Medicaid, and Children's Health Provisions, Subtitle F; Chapter 1—Services of Health Professionals; Subchapter B—Other Healthcare Professionals, Section 4511.

Baradell, J., & Buppert, C. (2003). Billing for psychiatric clinical nurse specialists services within the Medicare program. *Topics in Advanced Practice Nursing eJournal, 3*(1).

Baradell, J., & Hanrahan, N. (2000). CPT coding and Medicare reimbursement issues. *Clinical Nurse Specialist, 14*(6), 299–303.

Barone, C., & Paniagua-Ramirez, C. (2006). Coding and reimbursement. *AACN Advanced Critical Care, 17*(2), 116–118.

Buppert, C. (2002). Billing for nurse practitioner services: Guidelines for NPs, physicians, employers, and insurers. *Medscape Nurses, 4*, 1–14.

Buppert, C. (2004). Reimbursement for nurse practitioner services. In *Nurse practitioner's business practice and legal guide* (2nd ed., pp. 269–285). Sudbury, MA: Jones & Bartlett.

Buppert, C. (2005). Third-party reimbursement for nurse practitioners' services on trauma teams: Working through a maze of issues. *The Journal of Trauma, Injury, Infection and Critical Care, 58*, 206–212.

Federal Register. (1998). *Final rule on nurse practitioner, clinical nurse specialist, physician assistant, certified nurse-midwives and Medicare billing* (section 410.76, pp. 58863–58912). Retrieved January 26, 2009, from http://www.gpoaccess.gov/fr/retrieve.html

Frakes, M. A., & Evans, T. (2006). An overview of Medicare reimbursement regulations for advanced practice nurses. *Nursing Economic$, 24*(2), 59–65.

Griffith, H. (1984). *A case study of the implementation of legislation providing direct third party reimbursement for services of nurse practitioners in Maryland*. Unpublished doctoral dissertation, University of Maryland, Baltimore.

Jacox, A. (1997). Determinants of who does what in health care. *Online Journal of Issues in Nursing, 2*(4). Retrieved January 26, 2009, from http://www.nursingworld.org/MainMenuCategories/ANAMarketplace/ANAPeriodicals/OJIN/TableofContents/Vol21997/No4Dec97/DeterminantsofWhoDoesWhatinHealthCare.aspx

Lyon, B. L. (2002). What to look for when analyzing clinical nurse specialist statutes and regulations. *Clinical Nurse Specialist, 16*(1), 33–34.

Lyon, B. L., & Minarik, P. A. (2001a). Statutory and regulatory issues for clinical nurse specialists (CNS) practice: Ensuring the public's access to CNS services. *Clinical Nurse Specialist, 15*(3), 108–114.

Lyon, B. L., & Minarik, P. A. (2001b). National Association of Clinical Nurse Specialists model statutory and regulatory language governing clinical nurse specialist practice. *Clinical Nurse Specialist, 15*(3), 115–120.

Medicare Benefit Policy Manual. (2008). *Covered medical and other health services* (section 210, chapter 15), Clinical Nurse Specialist Services. Retrieved January 26, 2009, from http://www.cms.hhs.gov/manuals/Downloads/bp102c15.pdf

Minarik, P. (2000). Pat Ford-Roegner—Solving Medicare reimbursement problems. *Clinical Nurse Specialist, 14*(4), 205–208.

Omnibus Budget Reconciliation Act of 1989, P.L. 101–239. Retrieved January 26, 2009, from http://www.ssa.gov/OP_Home/comp2/F101–239.html

Phillips, C. (1987). Reimbursement for nursing services revisited. *Nursing Economic$, 5*(5), 220–253.

Richmond, T., Thompson, H., & Sullivan-Marx, E. (2000). Reimbursement for acute care nurse practitioner services. *American Journal of Critical Care, 9*(1), 52–61.

Torrey, T. (2008). What are CPT and HCPCS codes? How do they affect your healthcare? *Patient empowerment.* Retrieved January 26, 2009, from http://patients.about.com/od/costsconsumerism/a/cptcodes.htm

Zuzelo, P. R., Fallon, R., Lang, C., & Mount, L. (2004). Clinical nurse specialists' knowledge specific to Medicare structures and processes. *Clinical Nurse Specialist, 18*(4), 207–217.

Regulatory and Professional Credentialing of Clinical Nurse Specialists

Brenda L. Lyon

The purpose of this chapter is to provide an overview of credentialing for advanced practice registered nurses (APRNs) and clinical nurse specialists (CNSs), in particular. Credentialing refers to the processes by which individuals and agencies are designated by a qualified agent as having met minimum standards and requirements at a specified time (American Nurses Association [ANA], 1979; Styles & Affara, 1998). Credentialing processes include both legal or regulatory mechanisms to authorize practice, such as licensure and registration, as well as professional mechanisms, including certification, privileging, and accreditation. The primary purpose of credentialing in health care is to help ensure public safety.

Credentialing is a dynamic and ever-changing area affecting CNSs and CNS practice. Understanding the requirements for various types of credentialing is essential for CNSs to legitimately establish themselves in practice. This chapter presents a discussion of the types of credentialing, including legal mechanisms that authorize an individual to practice, historical context, professional certification, accreditation of schools of nursing and privileging to practice within an institution. The chapter concludes with a section on current issues and future trends.

LEGAL AUTHORIZATION TO PRACTICE AS A REGISTERED NURSE AND CNS

The 10th amendment to the U.S. Constitution grants states the power to enact laws to protect the public.

Thus, states enact laws, also known as statutes. A statute is a formal written enactment of a legislative action that requires or prohibits something. The word *statute* is commonly used to differentiate between laws made by legislative action verses regulations issued by government agencies that have the power of law. A *regulation* is a form of secondary legislation promulgated by a government agency that is used to implement a primary piece of legislation appropriately. For example, rules and regulations are issued by state boards of nursing to implement the state's nurse practice act (statute) governing the practice of nursing. The legal authorization to practice can be granted via licensure or registration (National Council of State Boards of Nursing [NCSBN], 2005; Lyon & Minarik, 2001).

Licensure

Licensure is the legal authorization to practice a profession within a designated scope of practice. Typically, but not always, licensure not only prohibits the use of a designated title, such as Registered Nurse or RN, or Clinical Nurse Specialist or CNS, but it also prohibits someone who does not meet the requirements from practicing within the designated scope of practice. The purpose of licensure is to protect the health, safety, and welfare of the public by ensuring a minimal level of professional competence. Licensure requirements include the educational requirements that must be met and the means by which the individual must demonstrate minimal competency to begin practice as a licensed practitioner. Licensure occurs at and is regulated at the state level.

Licensure laws delegate the responsibility for enforcement to state administrative agencies. The agency responsible for regulating the practice of nursing is each state's respective state board of nursing. The statutory law in each state governing the practice of nursing is commonly known as the nurse practice act. Nurse practice acts and related rules and regulations can be accessed via each state board of nursing's Web site.

History of RN Licensure

Prior to discussing licensure as it pertains to CNSs as APRNs, it is important to discuss the history of RN licensure and the RN scope of practice. Knowing the history helps to put into context the evolution of current interest in and concerns about requiring CNSs to obtain a second license to practice as a CNS.

The first three laws governing the practice of nursing (Nurse Practice Acts) were passed and signed into law in the same year in the following states: North Carolina (March 2, 1903), New Jersey (April 7, 1903), and New York (April, 20, 1903). These statutes established the title RN because these initial laws established the *registration* of nurses. The first recognition of nurses did not specify a scope of practice but did set out the educational requirements (diploma) to distinguish between the educated nurse and the untrained nurse. The rest of the continental states followed suit over the next 20 years (Driscoll, 1976).

The following sequence of significant events chronicled by Veronica Driscoll, the executive director of the New York State Nurses Association (NYSNA), provides an informative progression in the evolution of New York's Nurse Practice Act, which led the way for other states. The years of persistent and compelling work by leaders in the NYSNA to advance the definition of registered nursing practice, despite incredible obstacles created by both the medical community and hospitals, was remarkable.

After 8 years of attempts, the 1903 the New York Nurse Practice Act was amended in 1920 to require licensure of nurses to protect the title *registered nurse* and to identify trained attendants as a second level of nursing. *Trained attendants* eventually evolved into licensed practical nurses (LPNs) or, in some states, licensed vocational nurses (LVNs). For the next 13 years, NYSNA leaders worked to amend the nurse practice act to define the registered nurse and require licensure for RNs who work for hire. Finally, on April 6, 1938, an amended Nurse Practice Act was signed into law by the New York governor. The definition of a registered nurse was:

A person practices nursing as a registered professional nurse within the meaning of this article who for compensation or personal profit performs any professional service requiring the application of principles of nursing based on biological, physical and social science, such as responsible supervision of a patient requiring skill in observation of symptoms and reactions and the accurate recording of the facts, and carrying out of treatments and medications as prescribed by a licensed physician or by a licensed dentist and the application of such nursing procedures as involves understanding of cause and effect in order to safeguard life and health of a patient and others. (Driscoll, 1976, p. 59)

The 1938 definition of a registered nurse clearly limited the practice of registered nursing to charting and the implementation of delegated medical regimens. All states followed this lead and adopted similar definitions of the RN, limiting the legal scope of practice to delegated activities. In 1969–1970, NYSNA leaders recognized the limitations of the definition of an RN in not delineating the independent nature of *nursing* functions in the context of the nursing process. Input was sought from both members of the association and from legal counsel. Legal counsel advised NYSNA that "independence of the nursing function is conditional upon the specification of the diagnostic privilege within the legal definition" (Driscoll, 1976, pg. 59). As a result, the Special Committee to Study the Nurse Practice Act proposed the following definition:

The practice of the profession of nursing as a registered professional nurse is defined as diagnosing and treating human responses to actual or potential health problems through such services as casefinding, health teaching, health counseling, and the provision of care supportive and restorative of life and well-being. (Driscoll, 1976, p. 59)

Importantly, the definition shifted from defining a registered nurse to defining the *practice* of a registered nurse. Thus, the definition identifies the autonomous scope of RN practice as "diagnosing and treating human responses to actual or potential health problems." It is interesting to note that this language from 1970 remains as the definition of RN practice in the ANA's *Social Policy Statement* (2004b), changing only the word "problems" to "conditions." After considerable interprofessional conflict and challenges to the definition authorizing RNs an autonomous or self-directed scope of practice in addition to the safe and therapeutic implementation of delegated medical regimens, the legislative bill was signed into law by Governor Rockefeller in March of 1972 (Driscoll, 1976, p. 64).

Just as before, the rest of the states followed the lead of NYSNA and enacted essentially the same scope of practice for RNs over the next 8 years. Thus, the RN scope of practice in each state typically authorizes RNs to practice in an autonomous domain and a delegated domain. *Autonomous* means self-initiated actions, that is, does not require initiation or authorization from another source. The autonomous domain encompasses health assessment, derivation of nursing diagnoses, and the implementation and evaluation of nursing therapeutics/interventions. The delegated domain encompasses the safe and therapeutic implementation of delegated medical regimens. RNs make very important judgments about the medical condition of a patient, but they are not authorized under the RN license to *self-initiate* medical interventions, such as use of pharmacological agents in response to those judgments. However, RNs can and do implement medical therapeutics in response to their judgments regarding the medical condition of patients via delegation from physicians in the form of medical orders, protocols, or standing orders. Although there have been some challenges to the use of protocols or standing orders, the use of these mechanisms remain.

History of APRN Licensure

One of the most significant issues for CNSs and the National Association of Clinical Nurse Specialists (NACNS) from the late 1990s through 2008 has been whether or not to advocate for requiring CNSs to obtain a second license to authorize practice as a CNS. In large measure, the issue was imbedded in confusion arising from two very different definitions of "advanced practice nursing" or "advanced nursing practice" (Lyon, 2004). The first definition emanates from the work of Peplau (1965) and Styles (1996) and is focused on advanced nursing practice within the domain of nursing's autonomous scope of practice and the "How, When, and Where" aspects of implementing medical therapeutics. The advanced nature of nursing practice is reflected in a highly developed and specialized foundation in evaluation and use of theory and research that informs: (1) the differential diagnoses of problems that require nursing interventions, and (2) the decisions regarding the "how, when, and where" to ensure that the most therapeutic response is achieved while implementing delegated medical regimens. This view of advanced nursing practice is referred to as the nursing-focused definition. The second definition of advanced practice nursing, consistent with the ANA's definition contained in the *Social Policy Statement* (ANA, 2004b), is focused on expanding the autonomous domain of nursing into the medical domain of practice. That is, defining *advanced* nursing practice as the diagnosis and treatment of disease. This definition is referred to as the medical-focused definition (Lyon, 2004).

Consistent with the nursing-focused definition of advanced practice, the CNS role from its inception in the 1940s (discussed in chapter 1) was to improve the quality of *nursing* care provided to patients. The evolution of the nurse practitioner (NP) role began in the mid-1970s. During the late 1970s and through most of the 1980s, the activities of NPs were authorized via "additional acts," clauses added to nurse practice acts. That is, nurse practice acts were amended to include additional activities using such language as "performing acts approved by the board or by the board in collaboration with the board of medical registration" (Lyon, 1983, p. 10). For many years, these clauses were thought to be sufficient in authorizing activities that extended into the medical domain.

In 1986, the NCSBN adopted a position paper on advanced clinical nursing practice recommending that the preferred method of regulating advanced nursing be designation/recognition, also known as registration (NCSBN, 1993). This is the lowest form of authorization/ regulation of practice in that it does not require that the state board inquire into the competence of the RN and simply provides the public with information about nurses with special credentials. In 1991, the NCSBN conducted a survey of states to study the regulation of advanced practice nursing (1993). The study revealed a great deal of variation in the titles for advanced practice nurses and how they were being authorized to practice, that is, varying from "additional acts" clauses to granting a second license with an additional scope of practice. At the same time, there was an increasing desire on the part of nurse practitioner organizations to enable NPs to diagnose and treat disease independent of physician supervision or collaboration. The 1993 NCSBN position paper recommended a definition of advanced nursing practice to encompass four roles: certified nurse anesthetists (CRNAs), nurse practitioners (NPs), certified nurse midwives (CNMs), and CNSs. Advanced practice was asserted to be based on the knowledge and skills acquired in a basic nursing education program, licensure as an RN, and a graduate degree with a major in nursing or a graduate degree with a concentration in an advanced nursing practice category such as anesthesia. The position paper also recommended that the title for advanced practice nurses be advanced practice registered nurse (APRN) and presented model legislative language that would require a second level of licensure for NPs and model administrative rules (NCSBN, 1993).

The variation in the forms of authorization and the qualifications to obtain authorization began to create significant state-to-state barriers for advanced practice nurses. During 1995, the NCSBN worked with NP organizations to begin to establish the criteria for professional certification exams to be legally defensible and psychometrically sound, thus, enabling certification exams to be used as a proxy for a second license exam for the advanced practice of nurse practitioners (NCSBN, 2008).

In 1998, the legislative/regulatory committee of NACNS conducted a critical analysis of state statutes and regulations governing CNS practice. The analysis found that 26 states had a CNS scope of practice and protected the title *clinical nurse specialists,* or CNS. That is, the only persons legally authorized to use the title or its abbreviation must have graduated, at a minimum, from a nationally accredited master's degree in nursing program that prepares CNS graduates. Of the 26 states, 10 required certification as a CNS in the CNS's designated specialty area. The remaining states either required certification in the specialty but not as a CNS, or provided a waiver of certification option when there was no certification exam available in the specialty or it did not require certification (Lyon & Minarik, 2001).

More recently, another survey of state statutes and regulations governing CNS practice found that 40 states recognize CNSs as advanced practice nurses. An additional 6 states recognize only psychiatric CNSs. Of the 40 states recognizing CNSs, 27 require certification at an advanced practice level, with 6 of those states offering other options for certification if not available to the CNS at an advanced practice level of the specialty. These options include certification in generic practice of the specialty, waiver, presentation of a portfolio, or an appeal process. In addition to the variability in regulatory requirements, there is also variability in titling, including such variations as CNS, APRN-CNS, APN-CNS, APN, APRN, and ANP (J. Rust, personal communication, December 1, 2008).

It is critically important that CNSs become intimately familiar with their respective state's nurse practice act and rules/regulations governing CNS practice as an advanced practice nurse. In states such as Michigan, where CNSs are not legally recognized, CNSs practice nursing in an advanced manner just as we did prior to the move to regulate CNSs. That is, CNSs practice under the authority granted via their RN license. Because the essence of CNS practice is in the advanced practice of *nursing,* there is no authority barrier to CNS practice as long as the CNS does not wish to diagnose disease and/or prescribe pharmaceutical agents. The primary difficulties with a state not legally recognizing CNSs are the inability to obtain third-party reimbursement for eligible CNS services and absence of title protection, meaning that persons not prepared as CNSs are not barred from using the title (Lyon & Minarik, 2001).

Registration

Registration is another form of legal or regulatory recognition of a practitioner whereby a government agency maintains an official roster of qualified individuals. This level of regulation does not require that the state board inquire into the *competency* of the practitioner, but it may require that the person seeking registration meet specified educational requirements and may also designate a scope of practice (Styles & Affara, 1998).

Legal Regulation and Professional Regulation

Legal regulation of the practice of nursing occurs via state boards of nursing and has the power of law. State boards of nursing are charged with the oversight responsibility for the persons it licenses or regulates and may bring sanctions against providers including, but not limited to, revocation or suspension of a license to practice.

Professional regulation occurs via the ANA's *Social Policy Statement* (2004b) and *Scope and Standards of Practice* (2004a) along with corresponding certification exams. The ANA scope and standards document spells out both the RN and the APRN scopes of practice, including CNS scope, as well as the standards of practice for both RNs and APRNs. In addition to the ANA standards of practice, many specialty organizations also have standards of practice that are congruent with the ANA standards but are specific to a specialty area of practice. Professional regulation does not have the power of law, however, scopes of practice and standards of practice are used in courts of law to help determine if a provider was practicing within his/her scope of practice and if the care provider met the standards of practice that would be expected from a reasonably prudent provider in a particular situation.

In addition to a CNS's respective state nurse practice act and the legal delineated scope of practice for the RN and CNS, it is imperative that the CNS be knowledgeable about the standards of practice. The standards for APRN practice provide the overarching framework for competency statements and, therefore, certification exams.

CERTIFICATION

Certification is a process whereby a nongovernmental agency or an association certifies that an individual has met predetermined standards or competencies specified by a profession for a specialty practice (Styles & Affara, 1998). The ANA initiated certification in nursing as an indication of excellence in practice. Certification for nurses to recognize excellence in practice was initiated in the mid-1970s through the ANA and the American Nurses Credentialing Center (ANCC) in the area of medical-surgical nursing. From the 1970s through the 1980s, many additional nursing organizations initiated certification exams to provide nurses an opportunity to demonstrate excellence in specialty areas of practice.

As noted earlier, in the mid-1990s, the NCSBN began to encourage the use of certification exams as proxies for licensure exams that would be required for APRNs to obtain a second license to practice in an APRN role.

When certification exams are used as proxies for licensure exams, a state board of nursing must be assured that the certification exam is both psychometrically sound and legally defensible to be used in regulation. To be psychometrically sound, there must be an adequate number of persons taking the exam to allow psychometric testing for reliability and validity. Many specialties do not have an adequate number of CNSs practicing in the area to be able to demonstrate psychometric soundness of an exam. To be legally defensible, the certification exam must test knowledge at a level corresponding to what is considered safe practice for an APRN who is entering practice after completion of an accredited graduate program. To ensure that exams are both psychometrically sound and legally defensible, certification exams offered by certifying bodies must be accredited by the American Board of Nursing Specialties (ABNS) or by the National Commission for Certifying Agencies (NCCA) for the certification exams to be used by state boards of nursing as a proxy for a licensure exam. The CNS certification exams for use in regulation can be found in Table 27.1. Currently, CNS certification is available through the ANCC in the following areas: adult health, pediatrics, psychiatric—adult, child/adolescent, and gerontology. Additionally, the American Association of Critical Care Nurses and the Oncology Nurses Association offer CNS certification exams. Due to the fact that many CNS specialty areas do not have a CNS certification exam, NACNS and ANCC have collaborated on the development of a CNS core certification exam to test competencies that are generic to the CNS role regardless of specialty. It is anticipated that this exam will be available to CNSs who do not have a certification exam available in their specialty in the fall of 2009 (ANCC, 2008; Goudreau & Smolenski, 2008).

Despite the fact that a certification program or exam might be accredited, it is the prerogative of each state board of nursing to determine which exams will be accepted for regulatory purposes. The NCSBN recommends the criteria to state boards of nursing to use when approving the use of a national certification exam to be used for regulatory purposes. One of the eligibility criteria to take a certification exam is that the applicant completed a minimum of 500 supervised clinical hours (NCSBN, 2002).

Once a CNS has obtained certification, the certification must be renewed at designated time frames, such as every 3 to 6 years with 5 years being the average (Goudreau & Smolenski, 2008). Most often the renewal involves presenting proof of continuing education units (CEUs) and additional academic or professional training along with a current curriculum vitae. If an APRN's certification lapses, it is generally necessary to retake the certification exam.

ACCREDITATION OF ACADEMIC PROGRAMS

Accreditation of master's level programs and soon doctoral level programs preparing APRNs is required to enable graduates to meet requirements for authorization to practice as an APRN. Accreditation is a voluntary, self-regulating, nongovernmental process that is designed to ensure a designated quality of education. The Commission on Collegiate Nursing Education (CCNE) and the National League for Nursing Accreditation Commission (NLNAC) are the two accrediting bodies

27.1 | Accredited Certification Programs for Clinical Nurse Specialists and Specialty Areas

American Nurses Credentialing Center http://www.nursingcertification.org/exam	Psychiatric-Adult CNS* Child/Adolescent CNS* Adult Health CNS* Gerontology CNS* Pediatric CNS*
Oncology Nursing Certification Corporation http://www.ons.org	AOCNS*
American Association of Critical Care Nurses Certification Board http://www.aacn.org	CCNS**

*ABNS Accredited
**NCCA Accredited

that accredit nursing educational programs. Both organizations use criteria for a evaluating educational programs. The CCNE uses *The Essentials for Masters Education for Advanced Practice Nursing* (AACN, 1996) approved by the American Association of Colleges of Nursing. This document stipulates that programs are required to use pertinent standards of practice for the particular role(s) of education in the program, for example the NACNS *Statement on CNS Practice and Education* (2004). The NLNAC has endorsed the NACNS statement for their use in the accreditation of programs preparing CNSs.

CREDENTIALING AND PRIVILEGING IN A HOSPITAL OR OUTPATIENT SETTING

Credentialing and privileging processes initially developed for physicians are now applied to APRNs, including CNSs, when a CNS desires the use of prescriptive authority within a health care organization. *Credentialing* is the process by which professionals provide evidence that they are qualified to perform clinical activities within a designated scope of practice. Although credentialing and privileging may occur within the same time frame, they are related but different operations. The primary intent of credentialing is to determine if the applicant will be authorized to practice within an organization, whereas the purpose of *privileging* is to outline the scope of practice activities that can be provided (Kamajian, Mitchell, & Fruth, 1999).

The responsibility for credentialing rests with the governing body of the institution, such as the board of directors or senior executive committee. Decisions are based on review and verification of information gathered in the credentialing process and recommendations of the medical staff regarding appointment and privileging.

CNSs, like other APRNs, are bound by internal and external mechanisms. Internal mechanisms influencing credentialing include an organization's mission, values, practice standards, multidisciplinary operations, and position descriptions. External mechanisms include nurse practice acts (scope of practice for APRN role), state board of nursing rules and regulations governing practice, the ANA and specialty organization standards of practice, and the ANA Code of Ethics (2001). The Joint Commission requires it's over 15,000 accredited health care organizations to assess and affirm the competency of all providers. Additionally, the Accreditation Association for Ambulatory Health Care (AAAHC) and the National Committee for Quality Assurance (NCQA) for managed care require affirmation of competency. The Joint Commission requires that the processes,

policies, and procedures of credentialing and privileging be well-defined, including specific time frames for response to applications.

Typical requirements for credentialing and privileging are: (1) licensure as RN and/or as APRN/CNS or CNS is in good standing, (2) proof of national certification as a CNS in specialty, (3) proof of education (graduate program transcript), (4) Drug Enforcement Agency [DEA] number, (5) summary of employment history, (6) membership in professional associations, (7) written collaborative agreement with physician if required in board of nursing rules and regulations, (8) photograph, and (9) references. Privileges to perform well-delineated diagnostic and/or therapeutic services are granted based upon each state's practice act scope of CNS practice, license, education, demonstrated competence, judgment, and the organization's clinical regulations.

It is the responsibility of the CNS to acquire and maintain all records that may be required as proof of meeting any credentialing requirements. A good practice is to keep a file folder in a safe place that contains all original documents. In addition to documents from outside sources, such as academic institutions, continuing education, and certification agencies, it is good practice to keep your curriculum vitae or resume updated yearly.

CURRENT ISSUES AND FUTURE TRENDS

After 4 years of collaborative effort by representatives from multiple nursing organizations on the APRN Consensus Work Group and the NCSBN, the Consensus Model for APRN Regulation: Licensure, Accreditation, Certification & Education was published (2008). The work was stimulated by the fact that there is no uniform model of regulation of APRNs across states. States vary in terms of legal scopes of practice, the APRN roles recognized, and criteria for entry into practice, including how competency is demonstrated. The Consensus Model defines APRN practice, including CNS practice, describes a uniform APRN regulatory model, identifies titles to be used (includes CNS), defines specialty, describes emergence of new roles and population foci, and presents strategies for implementation.

There are several important issues inherent in the model that will be grappled with by various APRN groups including NACNS and state boards of nursing over the coming years. One central issue is the requirement that all APRNs including CNSs obtain a second license to enter into practice as an APRN. Is a second license warranted and justifiable when a CNS's scope of practice does not include the independent diagnosis and treatment of disease? Additionally, the Consensus Model proposes that

APRN certification exams accepted as regulatory exams for initial licensure for each APRN role will only focus on one of six populations, including family/individual across the lifespan, adult—gerontology, neonatal, pediatrics, women's health/gender-related, or psychiatric—mental health. Therefore, CNS specialty areas other than adult and pediatrics or women's health would not be accepted for licensure purposes. Is testing a critical care CNS or an oncology CNS in adult—gerontological competencies sufficient for legal defensibility?

Regarding educational preparation of APRNs, the model has prescriptive curricular components, such as requiring: (1) that educational preparation be limited to one of the six population foci; (2) that three separate graduate level courses are taken in physiology/pathophysiology, advanced health assessment, and advanced pharmacology; and (3) that graduates be prepared with competencies to prescribe pharmacological agents even if such activities will not be part of the APRN's actual scope of practice or position responsibilities. Will these prescriptive educational requirements be accepted by the academic and regulatory communities? How will such prescriptive educational requirements be managed by graduate programs in nursing while maintaining the integrity and adequacy of curriculums in the preparation of CNSs?

Certification exams in specialty areas such as oncology and critical care may continue to exist, but they would not be acceptable for regulatory purposes, and educational preparation in such "sub" specialty areas could only occur built on the preparation for one of the population foci. There are important legal defensibility questions regarding the responsibility of state boards of nursing to assure the public of the competency of a critical care CNS or oncology CNS and testing only for adult—gerontology population-based competencies.

It is critical to recognize that the NCSBN and the APRN Consensus Group are not regulatory agencies. The NCSBN is a member association with each state board of nursing holding membership. The APRN Consensus Group is an informal group of representatives from various organizations. Neither the NCSBN nor the APRN Consensus Group can mandate changes in the regulatory arena. In order for the regulatory recommendations contained in the Consensus Model for APRN Regulation to take effect, each state would have to enact those recommendations in statute and in corresponding rules and regulations. Furthermore, each of the other areas, certification, accreditation, and education, would also have to comply. This is and would be a massive undertaking.

The Consensus Model document contains recommendations for a LACE (licensure, accreditation, certification, and education) structure to facilitate the collaboration of each area to assist in making the recommendations a reality. Representatives from each of the four prongs of LACE will comprise the structure to facilitate communication. It is hoped that the LACE mechanism will help in coordinating efforts to implement the Consensus Model recommendations by 2015. It remains to be seen if it is possible to actualize the recommendations as they now stand in all 50 states.

In addition to current trends and issues regarding credentialing of CNSs and including demonstration of competence, there is also the issue of continued competence. Credentialing for continued competence has been a long-standing regulatory issue. In 1995, the Per Health Professions Commission called for the implementation of mechanisms to assure the public of health care providers' continued competency. To date, a practitioner is determined to be competent on initial licensure or entry into practice, be that as an RN or as an CNS, NP, nurse midwife, or certified nurse anesthetist. However, 26 states require a designated number of CEUs for relicensure as an RN, and 27 states require certification to be recognized as a CNS, thereby requiring that the licensee meet the CEU requirements of the certifying body to renew certification.

Demonstration of continued competence is a thorny issue. Important aspects of the issue yet to be resolved include: (1) What is a legally defensible way for the practitioner to demonstrate continued competence? Some proposed mechanisms wrought with potential problems in legal defensibility include reexamination, peer review, client/case reviews, supervised practice, computer simulation testing, and employer skills testing; (2) Should basic competence or specialty competence be measured, and how do expected competencies differ based on years of experience?; (3) How will competency measurement be used in the workplace? and (4) What role does the employer have in ensuring continued competence?

SUMMARY

Credentialing is a dynamic and ever-changing policy arena affecting CNSs and CNS practice in particular. Legal and regulatory credentialing includes licensure and rules and regulations that have been promulgated by state boards of nursing as state agencies to implement statutes. Professional credentialing includes certification, accreditation, and institutional credentialing for practice privileges. Understanding the history of RN licensure and the legal authorization of nursing's autonomous scope of practice helps to illuminate some of the issues around whether or not CNSs who do not have or need prescriptive authority should be required to obtain a second license to practice. Currently, there is tremendous variation in the manner in which states legally recognize CNSs, variations in titles, and variations in requirements to obtain authorization to practice, including whether or not a certification exam is required.

The foundation for professional certification lies in the profession's standards of practice and the standards of practice for each of the CNS specialty areas. Historically, states requiring CNSs to be certified in their respective specialties as a requirement for authorization to practice has presented problems for CNSs in specialty areas where there are not a sufficient number of CNSs to make the creation of a certification exam economically feasible. Recognizing the need for a core CNS exam that would test for competencies generic to the CNS role regardless of specialty, NACNS has worked collaboratively with ANCC in the development of a core CNS certification exam.

Current developments and recommendations embodied in the Consensus Model for APRN Regulation are, in part, directed at trying to create more uniformity in the regulation of APRNs, including CNSs. It is yet to be determined if this effort will be successful.

It is the responsibility of the CNS to be familiar with his/her respective state nurse practice act, all applicable rules and regulations, and national standards for RNs and APRNs, specifically CNSs. It is also the responsibility of each individual CNS to maintain all documents related to credentialing, including proof of meeting requirements for certification and recertification, such as copies of CEU certificates (Joel, 2004).

It is hoped that every CNS will be actively engaged in staying abreast of both state and national level developments regarding CNS credentialing. The area of credentialing offers multiple opportunities for CNSs to become actively engaged in shaping the direction of the discipline and in the regulation of CNS practice in particular.

DISCUSSION QUESTIONS

1. Are CNSs legally recognized in your state? If so, what is the statutory language in the nurse practice act recognizing CNSs? Is the CNS scope of practice delineated in statute and/or in rules and regulations, and what is the scope of practice? What are the requirements to be recognized as a CNS in your state, and is the CNS title protected, that is, limited to only those who meet the requirements?

2. What is the difference between legal/regulatory and professional credentialing?

3. How can you access other states' nurse practice acts as well as rules and regulations?

4. What certification exam will you be taking, and what are the requirements to be eligible for the exam?

5. What are current issues in your state regarding credentialing of APRNs and CNSs in particular? Identify what local, state, and national level organizations you can join to remain informed about and influence developments in regulatory and professional credentialing of CNSs.

REFERENCES

American Association of Colleges of Nursing. (1996). *The essentials of master's education for advanced practice nursing.* Washington, DC: Author.

American Nurses Association. (1979). *The study of credentialing nursing: A new approach.* St. Louis, MO: Author.

American Nurses Association. (2001). *Code of ethics for nursing with interpretive statements.* Washington, DC: American Nurses Publishing.

American Nurses Association. (2004a). *Nursing: Scope and standards of practice.* Washington, DC: American Nurses Publishing.

American Nurses Association. (2004b). *Social Policy Statement.* Washington, DC: American Nurses Publishing.

American Nurses Credentialing Center. (2008). Retrieved January 11, 2009, from http://www.nursecredentialing.org/NurseSpecialties/CNSCoreExam.aspx

Consensus model for APRN regulation: Licensure, accreditation, certification & education. (2008, July 7). Retrieved December 1, 2008, from www.nacns.org.membersonly

Driscoll, V. M. (1976). *Legitimizing the profession of nursing: The distinct mission of the New York State Nurses Association.* New York: New York State Nurses Association Foundation.

Goudreau, K. A., & Smolenski, M. (2008). Credentialing and certification: Issues for clinical nurse specialists, *Clinical Nurse Specialist, 22*(5), 240–244.

Joel, L. A. (2004). Credentialing and clinical privileging. In L. A. Joel (Ed.), *Advanced practice: Essentials for role development* (pp. 136–154). Philadelphia: F. A. Davis Company.

Kamajian, M. F., Mitchell, S. A., & Fruth, R. A. (1999). Credentialing and privileging of advanced practice nurses. *AACN Clinical Issues, 10*(3), 316–336.

Lyon, B. L. (1983). *Nursing practice: An exemplification of the statutory definition—Indiana* [Monograph]. Birmingham, AL: Pathway Press.

Lyon, B. L. (2004). The CNS regulatory quagmire: We need clarity about advanced nursing practice. *Clinical Nurse Specialist, 18*(1), 9–13.

Lyon, B. L., & Minarik, P. (2001). Statutory and regulatory issues for clinical nurse specialist (CNS) practice. *Clinical Nurse Specialist, 15*(3), 108–114.

National Association of Clinical Nurse Specialists. (2004). *Statement on clinical nurse specialist practice and education* (2nd ed.). Harrisburg, PA: Author.

National Council of State Boards of Nursing. (1993). *NCSBN subcommittee to study the regulation of advanced practice: Position paper on the regulation of advanced practice nursing with model legislative language and administrative rules.* Chicago: Author.

National Council of State Boards of Nursing. (2002). *Criteria for APRN certification programs.* Chicago: Author.

National Council of State Boards of Nursing. (2005). *Nursing regulation and the interpretation of nursing scopes of practice.* Retrieved October 23, 2008, from https://www.ncsbn.org/364.htm

National Council of State Boards of Nursing. (2008). *History of APRN.* Retrieved January 11, 2009, from https://www.ncsbn.org/428.htm

Peplau, H. (1965). Specialization in professional nursing. *Nursing Science, 3*, 268–287.

Styles, M. M. (1996). Conceptualizing of advanced nursing practice. In A. C. Hamric, J. A. Spross, & C. M. Hanson (Eds.), *Advanced nursing practice: An integrative approach.* Philadelphia: Saunders.

Styles, M. M., & Affara, F. (1998). *ICN on regulation: Towards 21st century models.* Geneva: International Council of Nurses.

Student Clinical Experiences: Responsibilities of Student, Preceptor, and Faculty

Florence Myrick
Diane Billay

In the current health care environment, the role of the clinical nurse specialist (CNS) may be described as undergoing a significant renaissance in its evolution (Heitkemper & Bond, 2004). Indeed, there is considerable renewed interest regarding this particular role within the context of the nursing profession and the scope of practice that it entails. The CNS assumes a key position in various facets of health care delivery (Elliott, Gauthier, Mitchell, Oates, & Purdy, 2004). The nurse who is a CNS is required to possess not only a breadth but also a depth of knowledge and skill in a specialized area of clinical practice that can include gerontology, pediatrics, and oncology, to name a few. Key to that knowledge and skill is the preparatory process involved in educating individuals for this advanced role, and integral to that process is the preceptorship experience.

In this chapter, the authors provide an overview of the preceptorship approach to clinical teaching. In particular, they discuss the roles and responsibilities of the *student*, the *CNS preceptors*, and the *faculty*, or the triad of players integral to the context of the preceptorship experience, and they address specifically how the preceptorship experience contributes to the practical preparation of the CNS role.

PRECEPTORSHIP: A CONTEXTUAL PERSPECTIVE

Although preceptorship is often considered to be a recent educational phenomenon within the context of clinical teaching in the nursing profession, historically this is not an accurate reflection of its development and emergence as a viable teaching model (Backenstose, 1983; Myrick & Yonge, 2003). Indeed, one could describe preceptorship as having its roots in Florence Nightingale's day when "it was expected that the first-year practical training of nurses would occur in the hospital setting under the direct guidance of those nurses who had been trained to train" (Myrick & Yonge, p. 92). Nursing students were taught in hospital schools of nursing in which the apprenticeship approach to the clinical preparation of nursing students was provided. While this particular approach to the clinical preparation of nursing students was considered to be an effective one, a concern began to emerge recognizing that the educational needs of the students were often treated as secondary to patient care needs. Thus, a move commenced to transfer the education of nurses from the hospital setting to the postsecondary environment so that student learning needs could take priority in the educational process and in the preparation for professional nursing practice. In the 1950s and the 1960s, the transfer of nursing education to postsecondary institutions thus became a reality with students now beginning to be taught in universities, colleges, and technical institutions (Myrick & Yonge). And, with this transfer from the hospital setting to the postsecondary institutions, there began to emerge a different set of challenges to the nursing educational process.

Because nursing students were now being prepared away from the clinical practice setting, challenges began to develop in the guise of inadequate clinical preparation. Employers began to voice their concerns and educators their frustrations. In her seminal work on this issue, Kramer (1974) coined the phrase "reality shock" to describe the comparative inability of nurses to assume full patient care responsibility immediately upon graduation. A major thrust thus commenced to resolve this particular dilemma. Out of these developments emerged the preceptorship model, a model designed to facilitate and enhance student learning in the clinical practice setting and socialize students successfully into the professional role of the registered nurse (Myrick & Yonge, 2005). The preceptorship experience evolved into one that would assume a key contribution to the clinical preparation of registered nurses not only in undergraduate nursing education but also in advanced practice roles such as the CNS and the nurse practitioner (NP).

PRECEPTORSHIP: THE TRIAD

Educationally, preceptorship is an approach to teaching and learning that affords individual students the opportunity to work directly with expert practitioners or nurses in the clinical or community practice setting. It provides a one-to-one relationship with an expert in the field who can act as a resource, role model, facilitator, and guide throughout their entire clinical or practicum experience. "Such pairing intends to foster professional socialization, enhance learning, promote critical thinking, cultivate practical wisdom, and facilitate competence" (Myrick & Yonge, 2005, p. 3). The National Association of Clinical Nurse Specialists (NACNS; 2004) concurs that, through peer review and the establishment of a network of CNS colleagues who can serve as resources for continuing development and professional collaboration, preceptorship socializes the CNS student to professional practice. Key to the success of the preceptorship approach to clinical preparation is the triad or the individuals who are directly involved in the experience. This triad includes the student, the preceptor, and the faculty.

The Student

The student in the preceptorship relationship is often referred to in the literature as the *preceptee*. For the sake of clarity of discussion, however, the authors will use the term *student* throughout the chapter. The role of the CNS student is central to the preceptorship experience. In this approach to their educational preparation, graduate students are socialized directly into the advanced role of the CNS. In their role, students are required to assume particular responsibilities germane to the context of the preceptorship relationship.

CNS students who enter into a preceptorship experience at the graduate level present with a different demographic than do their counterparts in the undergraduate program (Myrick & Yonge, 2004). For example, graduate students "tend to arrive at the [preceptorship] experience with a certain level of expertise and a measure of respect in their own right" (p. 378). In their prior roles, these students have proven themselves to be valuable members of the health care team, and thus, they function most effectively in situations that afford them the respect and recognition for the experience with which they arrive to their student role. In a study carried out to examine the process used to enhance the critical thinking ability of graduate students in the preceptorship experience, such respect and value by the preceptor in particular figured prominently in the success of the experience. Conversely, the lack of such respect and valuing on the part of the preceptor was found to be responsible for an unsuccessful experience. This observation was reflected in the comments of a student in the study who stated, "I do think the relationship is seminal to the whole process . . . without that, forget it. There's no learning. I think it's the relationship first and foremost" (Myrick & Yonge, p. 374).

Over time it has often been an assumption that a teacher, in this case a preceptor, teaches or tells while the CNS student listens or assumes the role of a passive recipient of the knowledge and expertise that is being relayed. Such an assumption is, however, an erroneous one. In order for a learning experience to be an authentic one, both the teacher/preceptor and the student must assume active roles in the teaching and learning process. "Learning is about being actively involved in what could be described as a discovery process. [Learning] is about being introduced to new ideas and different ways of doing things or about acquiring a new way of looking at an old idea" (Myrick & Yonge, 2005, p. 105). Being an active participant requires considerable commitment on the part of both the student and the preceptor.

Students in the CNS preceptorship experience are being prepared at the advanced practice level and are thus required to be well-prepared prior to arriving to the nursing unit to provide advanced patient care. It is important that they be clear about the learning goals that need to be achieved throughout the practicum and at the completion of the preceptorship experience. Each CNS student needs to discuss these goals with the preceptor immediately upon commencement of the experience so that both student and preceptor are clear on each other's expectations. While this may appear to be a common sense statement, it is surprising how often confusion can arise as a consequence of discrepancies between student expectations and those of the preceptor. In administering their advanced nursing care under the tutelage of the preceptor, CNS students are required to use various sources of knowledge. They need to be clear about the specific objectives of their care, prioritize appropriately, and carry out patient care in a safe and competent manner reflective of an advanced practitioner. They also need to demonstrate effective communication and engage in reflective practice. Students need to demonstrate a strong sense of commitment to their role in the preceptorship experience. They are expected to adhere to ethical and nursing standards of practice; be respectful in their interactions with colleagues, patients, and families; be knowledgeable about their scope of advanced practice regarding their student role; and demonstrate prudent judgment in their clinical decision making.

The CNS as Preceptor

In the study previously alluded to (Myrick & Yonge, 2004), it was found that the preceptor student relationship is pivotal to a successful preceptorship experience. In the same study, it was also found that preceptors who are flexible, trustworthy, who create an environment that fosters student questioning, and who themselves are open to different ways of approaching a particular situation were found to be facilitative in their role. In light of such findings, it is thus incumbent upon the preceptor to draw on such behaviors to promote a successful and effective experience.

In the preceptorship experience, the preceptor assumes a multifaceted role that entails role modeling, facilitating, guiding, and prioritizing (Myrick, 2002; Myrick & Yonge, 2005), while at the same time demonstrating the following characteristics: clinical expertise; leadership; collaboration and consultation skills; professional attributes such as honesty and personal integrity, confidence, willingness to take risks and be wrong, self-review, and the ability to value and support diversity; and providing professional citizenship for the specialty (NACNS, 2004). The impact of preceptor behavior on student learning cannot be overestimated. Even at the graduate level, the preceptor is regarded as the role model to whom students look for guidance to inform their thinking and practice. For example, in the study alluded to on graduate student preceptorship, one of

the students was heard to state the following: "When I have the opportunity to watch her work, I'm constantly thinking about what is she doing, how did she think about this, what are the beliefs informing this. How would I do it differently, do I agree, do I disagree, all of those kinds of things" (Myrick & Yonge, 2004, p. 376). Another student in the same study intimated, "She's [preceptor] a master clinician and my learning and my development come from watching her" (p. 376).

In facilitating student learning in the preceptorship experience, the preceptor essentially paves the way for the various experiences throughout the clinical practicum. What this means is that together with the student, the preceptor draws on both of their previous experiences to provide meaningful learning in teaching and in validating psychomotor competencies, promoting enhancement of clinical judgment and decision making, and in providing immediate feedback that is constructive and affirming (Myrick & Yonge, 2005). Facilitating the student experience entails preceptor collaboration with the student by discussing and delineating specific goals that need to be accomplished. It is not about direction, it is about collaboration, which is accomplished when the CNS preceptor role models the three CNS practice spheres of influence, specifically the patient/client sphere, in which the goal of care is to decrease or prevent symptoms/suffering and improve functioning; nurses and nursing practice sphere, in which the role of the CNS is to advance nursing practice and improve patient outcomes by updating and improving norms of care and by using standards of care that direct clinical actions; and the organization system sphere, in which the CNS articulates the value of nursing care at the organizational, decision-making level and advocates for professional nursing (NACNS, 2004).

In guiding the preceptorship experience, the CNS preceptor essentially shows the student the way to achieve success in their role through modeling the five domains explicit to this advanced practice role: practitioner, consultant, educator, researcher, and leader (Canadian Nurses Association [CNA], 2003). As the expert practitioner to whom the student seeks guidance, the preceptor acts as a safety net. In a preceptorship study, one student was heard to say, "I guess you'd call her [preceptor] a safety net because if you need help or you need a question answered you have someone right there" (Myrick, 2002, p. 160). The preceptor through guidance helps to tailor or shape student assignments to respond to their individual learning goals and expectations. The preceptor is integral to the student's success.

The ability to organize one's patient workload is critical to the success of nursing care. At the graduate level it is no different. Priority setting is a critical feature of competent advanced nursing practice. While the students in the CNS preceptorship may have had previous nursing experience, they are now new to their current role and, thus, need to be provided with the support to be able to learn to prioritize in their new role. Again, it is important that such support be provided with respect and in an affirming manner so that the student can be not only competent but also confident in their new role.

The preceptor acts as evaluator of student performance. The role of evaluator is often sited by many preceptors as being the most challenging aspect of their role. For example, it is not often comfortable to provide feedback that may be less than flattering, thus, it is important how such feedback is provided. All feedback needs to be affirming rather than dismissive. Students must come to understand the areas of their performance that require improvement but at the same come away from such feedback with their dignity intact. It is in this role that the preceptor can draw on the experience and expertise of the faculty to assist them in the evaluation process, particularly with regard to giving and receiving feedback.

The Faculty

Frequently when one thinks of preceptorship, one thinks of the student and the preceptor. The role of the faculty, however, is also pivotal to the preceptorship experience. While the faculty is not and should not be in the forefront of the preceptorship experience, the faculty person acts as an important resource to the student and preceptor alike regarding the teaching and learning process. The faculty brings knowledge of the educational process. It is the faculty who must act as liaison between the clinical and the academic settings. It is important that the faculty meet with the preceptor and the student at the commencement of the preceptorship experience and throughout its trajectory. Availability and accessibility are important characteristics of the faculty role. Although, as previously stated, the faculty is not actively involved in the clinical aspect of the preceptorship experience, she/he is still responsible for ensuring that the experience is progressing in an appropriate manner, that the learning expectations of the student are being met, and that the educational goals and objectives of the learning institution are being achieved. It is within the purview of the faculty to clarify questions related to the educational perspective, to maintain open lines of communication among all three members of the preceptorship triad, and, if required, discuss any potential teaching strategies that might assist in contributing to the success of the preceptorship experience. The faculty also seeks ongoing feedback from the preceptor regarding student performance, provides feedback to the preceptor regarding his/her performance throughout the experience, responds immediately to any student or preceptor concerns, and provides input to students with regard to how best they can fulfill their role in the

preceptorship experience. Lastly, the faculty assumes the ultimate responsibility for the final evaluation and grading of the student's clinical performance. Such evaluation and grading is derived directly from the ongoing and final evaluation of the preceptor.

The Staff

As with the faculty, the role of the staff is often not regarded as being part of the preceptorship experience. The role of staff, however, as with the preceptorship triad, is significant to the success of the preceptorship experience. For example, if the staffs are not receptive to or accepting of the student to the unit, the preceptorship experience can prove to be a difficult one for all involved. On the other hand, when the staff accept the student as part of the team and provide them with the appropriate support, the learning experience becomes invaluable. The staff can act as resource to both the preceptor and the CNS student. In their role, staff can facilitate the preceptor in his/her selection of patient assignments and learning experiences for the student. They can provide assistance when required, and they can contribute to the overall success of the preceptorship experience (Myrick & Yonge, 2005).

PRECEPTORSHIP: THE PROCESS

The process that transpires in graduate education can be considered and anticipated to be different from that which occurs in undergraduate education (Myrick & Yonge, 2004). The graduate learner is one who: (a) generally presents with professional as well as personal experience; (b) is committed to the pursuit of a career, thus the pursuit of graduate education; (c) is seeking advanced theoretical knowledge and skill; and (d) is pursuing an advanced level of clinical practice. In light of these differences, one must assume that the process that evolves in the preceptorship experience in graduate education is also different than that which occurs in an undergraduate preceptorship experience.

In a recent study conducted to explore how the critical thinking ability of graduate nursing students is enhanced in the preceptorship experience, the researchers found that a complex interpersonal dynamic occurs between the graduate student and the preceptor that is key to the enhancement of critical thinking and ultimately to the success or failure of the preceptorship experience (Myrick & Yonge, 2004). The researchers termed the process *the relational process*. The findings from this study are used by the authors to provide a theoretical framework for discussing the teaching and learning experience of the CNS student while in the preceptorship relationship.

As with any relationship, the preceptorship experience can be a challenging one fraught with a variety of tensions, not the least of which can be interpersonal. Consider, for example, the fact that the preceptorship relationship essentially brings two complete strangers together to work closely on a day-to-day basis in what can be described at best as one of the most anxiety provoking situations there exists vis à vis life and death circumstances (Myrick & Barrett, 1994). Thus, it stands to reason that the one-to-one relationship that transpires between the student and preceptor would figure prominently. In the study alluded to (Myrick & Yonge, 2004), several students in the study indicated that the one-to-one relationship between student and preceptor is critical. How that particular relationship evolves determines not only how well the student develops but also how it contributes to their sense of professional competence. Both the student and the preceptor alike bring with them their own individual stories, both personal and professional.

In that same study, students expressed a sense of vulnerability in their role. For example, one student observed, "I think just being vulnerable and taking a risk, and then the fear of getting squashed" (Myrick & Yonge, 2004, p. 374). From such a comment, we can ascertain how important it is for preceptors to create a learning environment in which students are affirmed in their role and become empowered as opposed to invalidated. The approach of one preceptor in that same study reflected that supportive role, "I am very much aware of the students' experience, their previous experience. I usually start by exploring some of their experience so that they feel like I am acknowledging and accepting that" (p. 376).

If students are to progress in their preceptorship experience, they must feel that they are being treated with respect and that they feel a sense of safety and trust in their preceptor. In preceporting students, preceptors who are successful in their role project a respectful attitude toward their students, a respect that is reflected in their authenticity or their genuine appreciation for the experience and knowledge that the students themselves bring to the experience. Throughout the preceptorship experience, students also need to feel that it is safe for them to be able to express their ideas, to ask questions, and to challenge the different ways of doing things; for such a process to occur, the students need to feel that they can trust their preceptors (Myrick & Yonge, 2004). It is through the approach and demeanor of the preceptor that the student gauges exactly how safe it is to be able to enter into the process in a legitimate way. If such an approach is lacking, it is possible that the student will essentially shut down or present in a manner that is not indicative of their actual potential. For example, a graduate student was heard to say the following, "you have to feel safe and then you can feel challenged, and

then you can be challenged, because it's not about the person, it's about the ideas" (p. 377).

In order to facilitate the process of teaching and learning within the context of the preceptorship experience, there are several strategies of which the preceptor can avail (Myrick & Yonge, 2005). Some of these include such approaches as the use of one-to-one preclinical discussions with the student. Such discussions allow both the preceptor and the student to review the nursing care that will be required for the shift, delineate expectations for the day, address any questions or concerns of both parties, and clarify any areas of confusion regarding nursing care. Postclinical discussions are also an important aspect of the preceptorship experience. Such discussions provide an opportunity to evaluate the achievements of the day, extrapolate the positive aspects of the student's performance, examine areas that need improvement, and again, deal directly with any questions or concerns that may arise.

PRECEPTORSHIP: THE OUTCOMES

The goal of the preceptorship experience is to prepare the CNS student for competent advanced nursing practice. To that end, in this section specific outcomes of the CNS preceptorship experience are discussed, in particular: (1) socialization into the CNS role, (2) clinical proficiency, and (3) leadership, collaboration, and consultation.

Socialization Into the CNS Role

As preceptor, the CNS is integral to socializing the student into the role of an advanced practice nurse. The preceptor achieves this socialization process by: (1) demonstrating the art of advanced nursing practice, (2) fostering student critical thinking, (3) role-modeling effective communication, (4) exhibiting effective time management while working concomitantly with his/her case load and the student, (5) acting as an example for appropriate conflict resolution skills, and (6) nurturing and encouraging the CNS student to achieve success.

Demonstrating the Art of Nursing

Key to the CNS preceptorship experience is the preceptor's ability to demonstrate and articulate the art of nursing within the context of advanced nursing practice. Such practice reflects the values, attitudes, and beliefs of the discipline and profession of nursing as evidenced throughout the provision of nursing care. Such practice also accommodates the personal and emotional aspects of care and the unspoken, intuitive, and immeasurable facets intrinsic to humane nursing care. The art of nursing encompasses not only the everydayness of advanced practice, such as the completion of a detailed history and physical examination of a patient, or the determination of a series of treatments for a patient, but the art of nursing also encompasses the unspoken aspects of care, such as the intricate nature of performing a bed bath, wiping a fevered brow with a face cloth, or comforting a delirious elder just by the placing on of hands. In other words, the CNS preceptor daily mirrors the intricacies germane to the art of nursing indicative of CNS best practice.

Fostering Student Critical Thinking

A second important student-centered outcome associated with professional role socialization entails the fostering of student critical thinking. Learning is an active process that involves student engagement in all aspects of the learning environment. This active engagement involves preceptor questioning for the purpose of ascertaining the student's ability to be able to analyze/deconstruct, synthesize, and evaluate various patient situations. Indeed, it is incumbent upon the preceptor to ask the student "why" questions in order to develop insights into the thought processes used by a student in different clinical situations. Interwoven throughout this questioning process is an expectation that the student retain a healthy skepticism about knowledge acquisition. Stated differently, while it is important to ask probing questions, it is also important to remain skeptical about the answers. For example, just because a preceptor/physician/professor states something as fact, it is prudent for the student to be able to be confident enough to also question, a confidence that contributes to safe, competent, and humane nursing care.

Role-Modeling Effective Communication

Communication may be described as "a reciprocal sharing of ideas, opinions, information, and emotions. However, unless knowledge or information is presented and received, communication cannot and will not occur" (Myrick & Yonge, 2005, p. 123). The preceptor, thus, to be an effective communicator must have the ability to articulate clearly and directly. For, it is through effective communication that the preceptor and the student can develop an understanding and appreciation of one another. Indeed, effective communication is important to a successful preceptor–student relationship.

The preceptor must be able to demonstrate and role model effective communication skills if he/she is to encourage the same in the student. How the preceptor communicates is an important component of the role, particularly in influencing the student's preceptorship experience. Primarily, there are three types of communication: verbal, nonverbal, and paraverbal. In the preceptor–student relationship, it is important

that the preceptor be always aware of the manner in which she/he verbally communicates with the student who, despite the fact that they are experienced nurses, can still feel vulnerable in the student role. Because of this vulnerability, students can be predisposed to greater sensitivity with regard to verbal communication. Interestingly however, nonverbal communication comprises 55% to 65% of all communication (Cantor, 1992). Body language, gestures, and facial expressions are critical to effective communication. Paraverbal refers to "the way you make words sound—angry, happy, determined, sad, etc." (Cantor, 1992, p. 18). These three forms of communication are integral to the professional socialization of the student in the practice setting.

Efficient Time Management Skills

While working with a patient and student, the preceptor faces many professional challenges. One of these challenges involves efficient time management, in particular, when balancing the role between preceptor and caregiver. Each of these roles is discretely time consuming and complex. It is the ability of the preceptor in the situation that leads to a successful balancing of these complex roles through efficient time management. The ideal would be a reduction of the preceptor caseload so that the preceptor can effectively nurture the student in an appropriate manner and thus socialize the student effectively. The reality of the hospital/learning environment, however, is such that the preceptor workload tends not to be lessened but rather is often increased as a result of working with a student. Staff support thus becomes even more important to the success of the preceptorship experience in this instance. How well the preceptor balances his/her own workload is also reflected in how well the student develops and enhances his/her own ability to manage time effectively. Because the preceptor is an experienced practitioner, he/she can facilitate the student in contending with the ongoing patient assignments. As already discussed, effective communication is central to the relationship and, indeed, is critical in facilitating and guiding the student in developing their time management abilities.

Promoting Conflict Resolution

"The word conflict refers to discord or friction, and is something that often cannot be avoided" (Myrick & Yonge, 2005, p. 114). Owing to the nature of preceptorship vis à vis two strangers working closely together in a one-to-one relationship in what could be described as dire circumstances, it is not surprising that conflict can occur. Such conflict can derive from but is not limited to differences in working, personality, and learning styles. When confronted with a conflictual situation, it is important for the preceptor and the student to: (a) address the problem directly, (b) discuss their individual understanding and interpretation of the situation, (c) ensure that the preceptor and the student both have an opportunity to be heard, (d) seek clarity based on preceptor and student feedback, (e) jointly develop a plan specifically outlining each other's expectations, (f) delineate timelines for change to occur, and (g) resolve the conflict constructively (Myrick & Yonge, 2005). Do not ignore the conflict.

Supporting the CNS Student

The unwavering support of the preceptor in the practice environment is integral to student socialization. As previously alluded to, the relationship between the student and the preceptor is critical to the success of the preceptorship experience. To that end, the preceptor assumes a supportive role and, in that role, acts as facilitator and guide. As a facilitator, the preceptor draws on his/her experience and expertise to assist students in achieving their objectives. The preceptor needs to adopt a collaborative approach when instructing, ensure that the students are well-prepared for patient assignments, adopt a positive attitude toward the student, and encourage open communication. In guiding the student, the preceptor provides patient assignments appropriate for the student's capabilities, advises on the best way the student can improve his/her competencies, helps the student in developing their problem-solving and clinical decision-making skills, and paves the way for new experiences (Myrick & Yonge, 2005).

Clinical Proficiency

The attributes that distinguish a CNS from a registered nurse are many and varied. One such attribute is clinical proficiency within the context of advanced nursing practice (NACNS, 2004), which is a key focus in the preceptorship experience. According to NACNS, the CNS possesses clinical expertise in the specialty, conducts his/herself in a professional manner, adheres to the code of ethics delineated for nursing practice, and demonstrates professional citizenship. The CNA (2003) also identifies similar attributes, including expertise, leadership, consultancy, educator, and researcher.

According to the CNA (2003), the CNS demonstrates proficiency through their ability to readily assess clients and intervene in complex health care situations within the selected clinical specialty. While engaged in the preceptorship experience, the CNS student observes and learns from the preceptor by participating in and conducting assessments and by using an evidence-based approach to the provision of care (NACNS, 2004). In the preceptorship experience,

the CNS student is facilitated and guided in making differential diagnoses and in providing treatment in the most effective and clinical proficient manner. The preceptorship experience provides the CNS student with the opportunity to learn best practice regarding the promotion of quality client care and the advancement of nursing practice (CNA, 2003). The preceptorship experience promotes disciplined inquiry through the use of critical thinking, advanced decision making, and the synthesis of knowledge in the practice setting. Opportunities are also provided that allow for exposure to the research process and innovative patient care practices.

Leadership, Collaboration, and Consultation

According to NACNS (2004), the CNS provides clinical leadership by acting as a resource, facilitator, coordinator, role model, and advocate, as well as being a skilled communicator and educator. Fundamental to the preceptorship experience is a focus on these CNS capabilities as well as the provision of opportunities for students to enhance their ability to work collaboratively with others. The preceptor role models, facilitates, and guides students in developing their leadership skills and in working collaboratively with nursing colleagues and members of other disciplines for the betterment of the client (Myrick & Yonge, 2004). The preceptor also fosters collaboration through active teamwork with others and, in that context, promotes the students' ability to develop consultation skills to give and receive professional assistance (NACNS, 2004). The preceptor promotes the use of advanced knowledge, skills, and judgment to enhance client care and deal with complex and challenging clinical and social situations (CNA, 2003). Consultation is directed toward a multifaceted range of needs, including patient-related issues, staff education, program development, development of best practice guidelines and professional practice models, system change strategies, and professional development (NACNS, 2004).

The preceptorship experience is apropos for CNS students in developing professional integrity, promoting self-confidence, and increasing an awareness of their own strengths and areas that require further development with regard to clinical competence. It also affords students opportunities to cultivate the ability to embrace and support diversity (NACNS, 2004). Fundamental to the nursing care provided throughout the preceptorship experience are the following principles: respect for individual uniqueness, an appreciation for patient autonomy, a belief in the patient's right to a dignified life and death, and the delivery of safe and equitable patient care (NACNS, 2004).

CASE STUDY

The scope of CNS practice is reflected in three spheres of influence and includes: (1) the patient/client, (2) the nurses and nursing practice, and (3) the organization/system (NACNS, 2004). According to NACNS, the goal of CNS practice is to achieve effective and efficient patient/client-centered care, while at the same time also influence the practice of other nurses and health care organizations to support nursing practice.

The three spheres of CNS influence provide an organizing framework with which to describe core CNS competencies. To explicate these fundamental core competencies and to provide practical knowledge, or "how to" guidance, related to each sphere, three interwoven case studies are presented within the context of the preceptorship experience, and they appear in *italics* throughout this next section. These exemplars highlight the specific outcomes for each sphere. Each case study involves: *Steven*, a 30-year-old CNS student engaged in his final practicum experience prior to graduating with a Master's of Nursing (MN); *Yvette*, a preceptor with 15 years experience as a master's prepared CNS and who has preceptored 10 CNS students during her CNS career; and *Mike*, the patient.

Patient/Client Sphere of Influence

In this sphere of influence, the goal is to decrease or prevent symptoms and improve a patient's functioning. The preceptor role models for the student appropriate advanced level knowledge and skills necessary to assess, diagnose, and treat the ill patient and, as appropriate, the family and/or community. Depending on the student's learning style, learning can occur through a variety of modes. It can happen via direct, hands-on experience, which can be achieved by performing a targeted history and physical examination and then relaying the findings to the preceptor. Students also can learn through observation, which is achieved when the student directly observes, for example, the preceptor gathering swabs necessary to rule out a sexually transmitted infection. At the completion of the physical examination, the student and preceptor then discuss the case as a postconference. The student could learn by listening and discussing. Thus, an appropriate approach of the preceptor in this instance would be to discuss with the student a specific case to determine whether or not the student is adept at diagnosing and treating a complex patient. Perhaps the student is a kinesthetic learner, which implies that he/she learns best through movement. Whether the movement is related to tracing objects or making

notes and then rewriting them, the preceptor should acknowledge this learning style and accommodate the student accordingly.

Scenario 1

Steven is acquiring considerable knowledge and practical experience throughout this preceptorship placement. He finds Yvette, his preceptor, to be knowledgeable, enthusiastic, an excellent patient educator, and an exceptional facilitator of his learning. Today, he and Yvette are facing a particularly busy day. Yvette has informed Steven that Mike, a single 50-year-old male, is a newly admitted patient to the surgical unit and is to be treated with intravenous antibiotic therapy for multiple abscesses to both of his forearms and his left calf, and he requires a multifaceted approach to his nursing care needs. For the past 3 years, since his wife died, Mike has injected morphine, and the nursing staff on the surgical unit feel that their collective knowledge regarding the effective care of a patient such as Mike is limited. They have, therefore, requested that Yvette and Steven provide them relevant evidence-based information about injection drug users.

Patient/Client Outcomes of CNS Practice

According to NACNS (2004, p. 28), there are 16 outcomes of CNS practice listed under the patient/client sphere of influence. These include the following:

1. Phenomena of concern requiring nursing interventions are identified
2. Diagnoses are accurately aligned with assessment data and etiologies
3. Plans of care are appropriate for meeting patient needs
4. Nursing interventions target specified etiologies
5. Programs of care are designed for specific populations (e.g., vulnerable groups such as injection drug users, geriatrics, oncology)
6. Prevention, alleviation, and/or reduction of symptoms, functional problems, or risk behaviors are achieved
7. Nursing interventions, in combination with interventions by members of other disciplines, result in synergistic patient outcomes
8. Unintended consequences and errors are prevented
9. Predicted and measurable nurse-sensitive patient outcomes are attained through evidence-based practice
10. Interventions have measurable outcomes that are incorporated into guidelines for practice
11. Collaboration with patients, nursing staff, as well other health care professionals, occurs as appropriate
12. Desired measurable patient outcomes are achieved

13. Innovative educational programs for patients, families, and groups are developed, implemented, and evaluated

14. Transitions of patients are fully integrated across the continuum of care to decrease fragmentation

15. Reports of new clinical phenomena and/or interventions are disseminated through presentations and publications

16. Interventions that are effective in achieving nurse sensitive outcomes are incorporated into guidelines and policies

Mike's well-being and recovery is contingent upon nurses understanding the intricacies involved in caring for a patient who uses drugs as a means of coping. Steven knows that caring for Mike will be a challenge because he has never cared for an injection drug user before, so his learning curve will be great. As Steven develops a nurse–patient relationship with Mike, he understands he will have to identify: (a) care need requisites specific to Mike; (b) care plans and interventions appropriate to Mike's needs; (c) relevant consultation with other health care professionals/specialists to reduce/address Mike's needs; (d) achievement of measurable, patient-centered outcomes; (e) specific appropriate educational initiatives needed to ensure humane, ethical, and nurturing manner; (f) care needs of each family member; and (g) available policies and/or position statements that address patients in Mike's situation.

Application of CNS Outcomes to Scenario

The outcomes addressed in this scenario include: diagnosis, planning, and identification of outcomes; interventions; and evaluation.

Steven and Yvette enter Mike's room and immediately Steven begins his assessment of Mike. Because Steven knows the competencies of CNS practice as outlined by NACNS, he understands his assessment will include the following (2004, pp. 29–30): (1) conducting comprehensive, holistic wellness, and illness assessments using known evidence-based techniques, tools, and methods; (2) obtaining data about context, such as disease, culture, and age-related factors, along with data related to etiologies necessary to formulate differential diagnoses; (3) identifying the need for new or modified assessment methods or instruments within a specialty area; and (4) before designing new programs, identifying, collecting, and analyzing appropriate data on the target population (in this case, injection drug use) that serve as the basis for demonstrating CNS impact on program outcomes.

Mike is sitting in bed with several pillows propping his back, his face is clean-shaven, and his hair is neatly combed. Steven looks at Mike's bright blue eyes and observes that Mike is staring intently at both he and

Yvette. Mike is frowning. Both Yvette and Steven have smiles on their faces, and their postures are relaxed. Yvette introduces herself as the CNS for the surgical units and introduces Steven as the CNS student working with her. Mike allows both Yvette and Steven to shake his hand. Steven notes that Mike's skin feels smooth and warm to touch. Yvette begins speaking with Mike and explains both their roles in his care and that they are there to obtain a health history and to conduct a physical exam. During the brief time Yvette speaks with Mike, Steven notes that both of Mike's hands are clenched on the bed sheets and he wonders if Mike is in pain from the abscesses located on his limbs. Steven remembers that a history can be unreliable when obtained from someone who chronically uses morphine. With that in mind, Steven sits down on a chair next to Mike's bed and begins his assessment.

The questions Steven asks Mike about the abscesses include the following: when the abscesses first formed; location; presenting symptoms; quality; radiation; setting; timing, including onset, duration, and frequency; severity, noting if the abscesses are getting better, worse, or staying the same; aggravating factors; relieving factors; associated symptoms; and meaning for the patient. Additional components of the health history that Steven assesses include: past health, including childhood illnesses, accidents or injuries, hospitalizations or operations, allergies, and current medications; family history; a review of systems; a functional assessment, including asking questions related to self-esteem/self-concept, activity/exercise, sleep/rest, nutrition/elimination, interpersonal relationships/resources, coping and stress management, personal habits, environment/hazards; and Mike's perception of his health status. The answers elicited by asking questions related to interpersonal relationships/resources, coping and stress management, personal habits, and perception of health provide for Steven and Yvette a good snapshot into the past and current life of Mike. Specifically, this information provides Steven with insights into Mike's level of education, coping skills, social roles, support systems, past and current stresses in Mike's life, the last time Mike injected morphine, how much he injected and where, how frequently Mike typically injects in a day, how the morphine makes Mike feel, and whether Mike has tried any other drugs, such as marijuana, amphetamines, cocaine, and so forth.

As a CNS student, Steven is knowledgeable about the six CNS competencies as outlined by NACNS (2004, p. 30). Specifically, Steven knows he must complete the following processes: (1) synthesize and assess data, and develop differential diagnoses of illness problems; (2) draw conclusions about individual or aggregate patient problems with etiologies amenable to nursing interventions; (3) describe problems in context, including variations in normal and abnormal symptoms, functional problems, or risk behaviors inherent in disease, illness, or developmental processes; (4) plan for systematic investigation of patient problems needing clinical inquiry; (5) predict outcomes of interventions relative to prevention, remediation, modification, and/or resolution of problems; and (6) anticipate ethical conflicts that may arise in the health care environment and plan for resolution.

Results of the health history include the following pertinent information about Mike. History of present illness: There are a total of five abscesses located on his four limbs. Specifically, there is one abscess located on each of the following: his right forearm, left forearm, and right calf; and there are two abscesses located on his left calf. This is the first incidence of abscess formation for Mike, and he is worried about the condition of his skin and the pain he is experiencing as a result of the wounds. Mike acknowledges that just recently he used one of his own dirty needles and then a few days later his abscesses began to form and have since become worse over these past several weeks. Mike denies any history of childhood illnesses, accidents or injuries, allergies, or current use of prescribed medications. As well, Mike's family history is unremarkable. A review of systems reveals an unremarkable history except for the following: head—experiencing frequent severe headaches; skin—he has problems concealing his track marks from his coworkers and parents; neurological—Mike states he is sad but denies any thoughts of killing himself.

The results of Mike's functional assessment were unremarkable except for the following: sleep/rest—Mike indicated to Steven that he has been suffering from insomnia for the past 6 months; nutrition/elimination—Mike acknowledges a poor nutritional intake; interpersonal relationships/resources—Mike reports a strained relationship with his two parents and informs Steven that his wife of 30 years died 3 years ago, and since then his life has been "hell on earth." Since his wife's death, Steven states that he has just wanted to be "left alone"; coping and stress management—Mike reluctantly acknowledges his inability to feel happy and appears to be in constant emotional pain. Mike has not sought counseling; personal habits—Mike admits to his cocaine use, which involves injections three to four times a day, injecting each time between 30 mg to 60 mg to whatever vein is available, yet surprisingly, his using has not yet significantly affected his work life. Mike always uses sterile needles and supplies except for the one time. He tells Steven that on the anniversary of his wife's death he goes on a "bender" and will inject multiple times, usually until his parents come to his house to "smarten him up"; perception of health—Mike states he is ready to accept help to deal with his cocaine use and wants to attend a residential rehabilitation program.

Upon a comprehensive examination of all systems, no abnormalities are detected except with the following

areas: mental status, specifically his mood and effect, and skin. Regarding Mike's mental status, his appearance, behavior, cognition, and thought processes are examined. Specifically, Mike is alert, oriented, cooperative, and shows signs of acute distress because he is clenching at his bed sheets with both hands and is frowning. He appears clean, and when asked " how do you feel today?" Mike's facial expression changes to a frown, tears gather in his eyes, and he states, "I am sad and also in pain from these sores on my body." Mike denies any thoughts of suicide. His speech is appropriate, and his recent and remote memory is intact.

The examination of his skin reveals the following: color is light brown, warm to touch; turgor is good. Lesions are noted to the following: Right and left arms reveal one lesion to each region; to the left calf there are two lesions evident. A detailed description of each lesion will not be provided.

Steven is pleased that his assessment and physical examination of Mike only took 1 hour. Upon completion of the session, Mike was looking tired. Now that the assessment and physical examination are complete, Steven must determine the differential diagnosis and the interventions required for Mike's care. In terms of differential diagnosis, the following are discussed with Yvette: anxiety, ineffective individual coping, impaired adjustment, as well as damaged skin integrity, pain, and increased risk for infection. Based on the results of Steven's assessment and physical examination of Mike, Yvette agrees with Steven's differential diagnoses.

In accordance with approaching a patient intervention, Steven reviews NACNS's five competencies of CNS practice, which include: (1) selection of evidence-based nursing interventions for patients/clients with a focus on the etiologies of illness or behaviors; (2) development of interventions that enhance the attainment of predicted outcomes while minimizing unintended consequences; (3) implementation of interventions that integrate the unique needs of individuals, families, groups, and communities; (4) collaboration with multidisciplinary professionals to integrate nursing interventions into a comprehensive plan of care for the enhancement of patient outcomes; and (5) incorporation of evidence-based research into nursing interventions within the specialty population (2004, pp. 30–31).

Based upon these competencies, Steven, together with Mike's input, determines that appropriate interventions regarding Mike's treatment will include the following:

1. Wound care *including a course of intravenous antibiotic therapy followed by oral antibiotics, as well as appropriate dressing choices for abscesses.*
2. Pain control *appropriate to his level of pain. Mike will require higher than usual doses of analgesic.*

3. *A consult to* psychiatry *to ascertain the appropriate medications necessary to treat Mike's anxiety; referral to a residential drug treatment program to help Mike address and appropriately cope with the death of his wife.*

4. A dietician *to help Mike remain nutritionally fit.*

5. Patient education *regarding safe injection of drugs—choosing a vein, how to keep veins healthy, how to stay healthy while injecting, etc.*

6. Staff education *involving knowledge about the injection drug user, information pertinent to sexually transmitted infections, specifically HIV and Hepatitis C, and pain control for the person involved with illicit drug usage.*

7. Social support *or resources provided to the family, in particular the names of agencies that can be accessed by the family to help them cope with Mike's illnesses, which may include respite, support groups such as Narcotics Anonymous, and so forth.*

The final competency of CNS practice is evaluation (NACNS, 2004, p. 31). Just as it is vital to assess, plan, and implement care for a patient, it is also vitally important to evaluate the outcomes of the care provided. NACNS details six competencies of CNS related to evaluation of care. These include: (1) selection, development, and/or application of appropriate methods to evaluate outcomes or nursing interventions; (2) evaluation of the effects of nursing interventions for individuals and populations of patients/clients with regard to clinical effectiveness, patient responses, efficiency, cost-effectiveness, patient satisfaction, and ethical consideration; (3) collaboration with patients and other health care professionals, as appropriate, to monitor progress toward outcomes as needed; (4) evaluation of the impact of nursing interventions on fiscal and human resources; (5) documentation of outcomes in a reportable manner; and (6) dissemination of the results of innovative care, as appropriate.

Steven understands that once Mike is discharged from the surgical floor for admittance to the residential drug treatment program, he will not be able to follow-up with Mike's medical or emotional progress. Mike, however, has not yet been released from the surgical unit, so Steven will continue to monitor Mike's health status based upon the evaluation competencies as stated previously.

Nurses and Nursing Practice Sphere of Influence Outcomes of CNS Practice

Nursing is a practice profession. To that end, the CNS advances nursing practice by improving patient outcomes and by updating and improving norms and standards of patient care. Vital areas in which the CNS exerts influence include: development of policies,

procedures, and protocols that ensure nursing practice is evidence-based; role-modeling best practice to colleagues and nursing personnel; consultation; and education, all of which directly influence patient care outcomes (NACNS, 2004).

Scenario 2

Steven is amazed at how quickly the practicum is progressing, to the point at which he cannot believe he has only 2 weeks left with which to learn from Yvette. Mike's healing is progressing well. During the course of the past 2 weeks Mike has made great progress with his wound care *and, beginning 2 days ago, he even now carries out his own dressing changes. Mike's wounds have almost healed, so he is now taking oral antibiotics. Other aspects of his care have progressed as well: two members from the acute* pain *service—the physician and the nurse practitioner—have visited Mike and have written orders indicating what narcotic Mike should receive, the appropriate dosage, frequency, and so forth. Observing the physician and nurse practitioner working together was a great learning experience for Steven because he was able to witness how members of this service positively interact with Mike, the nursing staff, Yvette, and the physicians on the surgical unit. In addition, this experience provided a great opportunity for Steven and the pain service NP to begin* staff education *regarding appropriate pain control measures for injection drug users such as Mike; Steven visits with the* dietician *twice a week, and together they have devised a realistic plan to continue improving Mike's nutritional status, even while attending the residential drug rehabilitation center; every Monday, Wednesday, and Friday morning Mike speaks with the* psychiatrist *about all aspects of illicit drug use, positive coping strategies, and Mike's grief about his wife's death, to name a few; the unit-assigned social worker has been consulted to refer Mike's mother and father to a Narcotics Anonymous support group. The social worker has proved invaluable to his parents and their road to recovery.*

Outcomes of CNS Practice

According to NACNS (2004, p. 31), there are 13 outcomes of CNS practice related to this particular sphere:

1. Knowledge and skill development needs of nurses are delineated
2. Evidence-based practices are used by nurses
3. The research and scientific base for innovation is articulated, understandable, and accessible
4. Nurses are able to articulate their unique contributions to patient care and nurse-sensitive outcomes
5. Nurses are empowered to solve patient care problems at the point of service

6. Desired patient outcomes are achieved through the synergistic effects of collaborative practice
7. Nurses career enhancement programs are ongoing, accessible, innovative, and effective
8. Nurses experience job satisfaction
9. Nurses engage in learning experiences to advance or maintain competence
10. Nurses use resources judiciously to reduce overall costs of care and enhance the quality of patient care
11. Competent nursing personnel are retained due to increased job satisfaction and career enhancement
12. Educational programs that advance the practice of nursing are developed, implemented, evaluated, and linked to evidence-based practice
13. Nurses have an effective voice in decision making about patient care

Application of CNS Outcomes to Scenario

During his interactions with Mike, the nurse practitioner, and the physician, Steven determines that his knowledge is lacking in the area of injection drug use and sexually transmitted infections. After discussing with Yvette his intention to access seminal peer-reviewed journals addressing addictions and epidemiology, Steven visited the university library. There was nothing Steven enjoyed more than to perform hand searches of the library stacks because he usually found exciting articles relevant to the topic he was searching. In this case, Steven found four seminal articles addressing the psychology of addictions, and he found three excellent articles addressing current research findings on sexually transmitted infections. The discovery of the articles greatly informed his current knowledge in these areas and helped him to better understand Mike's circumstance.

To fulfill one practicum objective, Steven proposed to Yvette that he would provide for the unit's health care team a 40-minute in-service on best practices related to the following topics: the culture of drug use and current knowledge on sexually transmitted infections, specifically HIV and Hepatitis C. Yvette was in total agreement, as was the unit manager. As a result, Steven prepared, with input from Yvette, one newly hired staff nurse, and Mike's psychiatrist, a PowerPoint presentation addressing these topics.

The in-service went well. In attendance were 25 staff, including the unit pharmacist, the pastor, 3 newly hired nurses with various levels of clinical experience, the unit dietician, 2 physiotherapists, 4 interns, 2 medical residents, and 11 staff nurses, including nurses from the emergency department and the medical units. After the in-service, the 3 newly hired staff nurses approached Steven and congratulated him on a job well done. They told Steven that if this in-service reflects the caliber of future in-services, they were going to enjoy working on the surgical unit. Yvette was proud of the scholarly

presentation Steven presented to the attendees because she knew that the information shared and discussed with the group would ultimately benefit patients who experience care-related situations similar to Mike.

This outcome includes assessment; diagnosis, outcome identification, and planning; intervention; and, evaluation of the effects. Under *Assessment: Identifying and Defining Problems and Opportunities*, NACNS (2004, pp. 32–33) delivers six competencies:

1. Uses/designs methods and instruments to assess patterns of outcomes related to nursing practice within and across units of care
2. Uses/designs appropriate methods and instruments to assess knowledge, skills, and practice competencies of nurses and nursing personnel to advance the practice of nursing
3. Identifies, in collaboration with nursing personnel and other health care providers, needed changes in equipment or other products based on evidence, clinical outcomes, and cost-effectiveness
4. Gathers and analyzes data to substantiate desirable and undesirable patient outcomes linked to nursing practice
5. Identifies interpersonal, technological, environmental, or system facilitators and barriers to implementing nursing practices that influence nurse-sensitive outcomes
6. Collaborates with nurses to assess the processes within/across units that contribute to barriers in changing nursing practices

The unit manager (UM) on Yvette's surgical floor was very encouraging of Steven. Indeed, the UM understood that many nurses on the surgical unit lacked knowledge related to caring for injection drug users and people who engage in a high-risk lifestyle, so she wanted these nurses updated on current best-practices related to these areas of care. To that end, the UM knew Steven would present an excellent, evidence-based discussion regarding these topics because he had direct access to resources such as the library and clinical experts in the area of drug use, and he could access practice leaders at the state board office to ascertain the legal/ethical knowledge required to care for patients in Mike's situation. He would also visit one local inpatient rehabilitation facility and speak with an addictions counselor about typical plans of care withdrawal, the psychosocial aspects of addictions, and so forth. Because the UM wanted this topic addressed with the nursing and allied health staff, she asked two of the newly hired nurses to accompany Steven when he visited the addictions counselor.

It was advantageous that the UM had the full support of the hospital administration and the staff nurses because if she did not have that support the in-service would likely not occur due to barriers such as: staff

*bias related to injection drug use and a mistaken be-
lief that injection users should not be given narcotics
because doing so would contribute to drug use, to name
a few. Yvette knew that there were some nurses who
were judgmental toward this vulnerable population, but
she hoped that with time and education these nurses
would see things her way, which, in essence, was to be
patient-centered.*

Under Diagnosis, Outcome Identification, and
Planning (NACNS, 2004, p. 33), seven competencies are
identified:

1. Drawing of conclusions about the evidence-base and
   outcomes of nursing practice that require change,
   enhancement, or maintenance
2. Identification of desired outcomes of continuing or
   changing nursing practices
3. Anticipation of both intended and unintended consequences of change
4. Incorporation of clinical and fiscal considerations in
   the planning process for product and device evaluation
5. Plans for achieving intended and avoiding unintended outcomes
6. Plans for using facilitators and overcoming barriers
   for changing nursing practice and incorporating new
   products and devices
7. Consideration of resource management needs when
   weighing the benefits of changing practices

*The day after the in-service, Steven met with Yvette and
the UM to discuss the completed evaluation forms he
had recently received. There were several key themes
identified that would be addressed by the unit nurse
educator at a later date. The five themes pertained to:
(a) a pervasive lack of knowledge on the part of the
nurses related to "what is an addict," specifically, how
one defines an addict and what might an addict medically resemble; (b) treatments a person who uses drugs
should receive while in hospital, what does withdrawal
look like; (c) the amount of analgesic that a drug user
can receive for pain control; (d) services that are available in the community for drug users; and (e) what the
names of commonly abused substances and the concomitant signs/symptoms of (over)use.*

Under Intervention: Developing and Testing
Solutions, NACNS (2004, pp. 33–34) identifies eight
competencies:

1. Anchors nursing practice to evidence-based information to achieve nurse-sensitive outcomes
2. Mentors nurses to critique and apply research evidence
   to nursing practices
3. Works collaboratively with nursing personnel to
   implement innovative interventions that improve
   outcomes

4. Implements interventions that are effective and
   appropriate to the complexity of patient care problems
   and the resources of the system
5. Develops and implements educational programs that
   target the needs of staff to improve nursing practice
   and patient outcomes
6. Assists staff in the development of innovative, cost-
   effective patient programs of care
7. Mentors nurses to acquire new skills and develop
   their careers
8. Creates an environment that stimulates self-learning
   and reflective practice

*Yvette was proud of Steven. The in-service was well-
received by all who attended because he: set up the room
so that the tables/chairs were arranged in a circle, engaged the participants by encouraging everyone to ask
questions, encouraged participants to discuss individual
experiences of caring for patients who inject drugs and
who live a high-risk lifestyle, and provided opportunities for participants who were less likely to speak up to
engage in the in-service by asking them to write responses
on the white board. At the completion of the in-service,
Steven challenged all attendees to reflect on the goal of
the in-service and the content discussed. Steven requested
that each participant determine at least one strategy he/
she would use to humanely and effectively care for a
person who uses drugs, but he realized that realistically
some attendees would not follow his suggestions. Some
would, however, and those individuals would be the
catalysts for change.*

Under Evaluation of the Effects, NACNS (2004,
p. 34) identifies four competencies:

1. Evaluates the ability of nurses and nursing personnel to implement changes in nursing practice, with
   individual patients and populations
2. Evaluates the effect of change on clinical outcomes,
   nurse satisfaction, and collaboration with other
   health care disciplines
3. Documents outcomes in a reportable manner
4. Disseminates results of changes to stakeholders

*This is Steven's last week of his preceptorship experi-
ence. He and Yvette just completed a meeting with the
faculty/tutor, and everything went well. There were no
surprise revelations from Yvette or the faculty member,
as should never be the case. This week Steven will work
with the nurse educator and Yvette to determine if the
in-service actually resulted in a positive outcome, specifically, was the desired effect achieved, that is, a better
understanding of injection drug use by the health care
team members?*

*Yvette has a long and collegial history with the
nurses and other health care staff on the unit, so she
knows which natural leaders to approach to ascertain*

if the in-service was beneficial. If it was, she wanted to know why and how so, but if it was not, she would want to know why and why not, and how could the in-service be improved. For all intents and purposes, the in-service was highly regarded, but there were two key areas to improve. First, the nurses would have liked a handout detailing the kinds of drugs typically abused, their side effects, withdrawal symptoms, and a discussion regarding the differences between the culture of acute care facilities and the culture of the street or people involved with high-risk lifestyles because they note that while Mike does live a risky life style, he is not a typical "user." Normally, the patients who the nurses treat are more immersed in the "street" lifestyle (drug-seeking behavior) to the point at which the acute care culture clashes with the culture of the street.

Organization/System Sphere of Influence

This sphere "is critically important in the complex health care systems of today" (NACNS, 2004, p. 19). The role of the CNS is to communicate the value of nursing care at the organizational level where decisions are being made that affect patient care. In addition, he/she promotes and advocates for the profession of nursing (NACNS, 2004).

According to NACNS (2004), "the CNS influences the trajectory of care from admission through to discharge in order to assist the patient in achieving the desired outcomes after discharge and to minimize recidivism and readmission" (p. 20). Indeed, once a patient is admitted to a health care facility it is the focus of the CNS to ensure that all patient care needs are competently managed and to plan for all immediate and potential care needs for when the patient is discharged back to the community. However, in order to provide the necessary services and care that patients require, administration must provide the CNS with mechanisms by which the CNS can collect and analyze data to document the impact of nursing practice on outcomes (NACNS, 2004). Another focus of the CNS is to develop and then establish health care policies so that effective and efficient patient-centered care occurs.

Scenario 3

On the day of his admission, Mike's discharge planning began. As previously illustrated, Yvette and Steven, along with Mike and other members of the health care team, were busy planning for Mike's eventual discharge from the surgical unit to a residential rehabilitation facility. However, along the way many care concerns had to be addressed, such as the rehabilitation facility to which Mike would be discharged and the earliest intake date.

Resulting from Mike's time spent on the unit, several policies were developed by Yvette and Steven. Each of the new policies addressed the care needs of the injection drug user/street-involved person and specifically addressed pain control, stigmatization, and preconceived ideas of health care workers regarding this vulnerable population, wound care, withdrawal from narcotics, grief/grieving, social networking, and psychiatric consult.

Outcomes of CNS Practice

According to NACNS (2004, p. 34–35), there are 13 outcomes of CNS practice:

1. Articulation of clinical problems within the context of the organization, mission, culture, policies, and resources
2. Continuous patient care processes that benefit the system
3. Integration of change throughout the system
4. Policies that enhance the practice of nurses individually as members of multidisciplinary teams
5. Innovative models of practice that are developed, piloted, evaluated, and incorporated across the continuum of care
6. Development and implementation of evidence-based, best practice models
7. Articulation of nursing care and outcomes at organizational decision-making levels
8. A common vision of practice outlines shared by stakeholders, such as nurses, other health care professionals, and management
9. Decision makers within the institution who are informed about practice problems, factors contributing to the problems, and the significance of those problems with respect to outcomes
10. Patient care initiatives that reflect knowledge of cost management strategies
11. Patient care programs that are aligned with the organization's strategic imperatives, mission, vision, philosophy, and values
12. Staff adherence to regulatory requirements and standards
13. Policy-making bodies that are influenced to develop regulations/procedures to improve patient care and health services

Application of Outcomes to Scenario

As mentioned previously, Steven in consultation with Yvette identified the following clinical issues associated with Mike, their 50-year-old patient who has been an injection user for less than 5 years: multiple abscesses located on all of his limbs that required antibiotic treatment; a consult with a psychiatrist who will assist Mike in dealing with his immediate addiction and the grief experienced because of his wife's death; the unit nutritionist, who will assist Mike in maintaining his nutritional status; and the pain service team, who together with Mike will help to ensure appropriate pain control measures are used in Mike's care. In addition, Steven developed, implemented, and evaluated an in-service targeted toward all health care disciplines, but in particular, targeting front-line nurses who would care for injection drug users.

As a result of Steven's in-service, the hospital administration developed several policies and procedures reflecting evidence-based, best practice models when caring for injection drug users in inpatient units as well as in the emergency department. Indeed, given the inner-city location of this hospital, and with the implementation of the policies and procedures, the administration has seen a decline in patient admissions to the hospital as well as a decreased patient stay by this vulnerable population. The reasons for these outcomes are: emergency department health care staff appropriately administer narcotic analgesics, instead of underadministering same; front-line nurses choosing appropriate, cost-effective wound care products to treat abscesses; front-line health care workers markedly improve understanding of the complexities of care involved in caring for this population, the immediate need to consult psychiatry to treat dual diagnosis (treat mental health issues as well as drug use–related issues), and to consult the dietician upon admission to a hospital unit; and, the understanding that this population group must be treated humanely and with respect.

This outcome includes assessment; diagnosis, outcome identification, and planning; intervention; and evaluation of the effects. Under Assessment: Identifying and Defining Problems and Opportunities, NACNS (2004, pp. 35–36) delivers six competencies:

1. Uses system-level assessment methods and instruments to identify organization structures and functions that impact nursing practice and nurse-sensitive patient care outcomes
2. Assesses the professional climate and multidisciplinary collaboration within and across units for their impact on nursing practice and outcomes
3. Assesses targeted system-level variables, such as culture, finances, regulatory requirements, and external demands, that influence nursing practice and outcomes
4. Identifies relationships within and external to the organization that are facilitators or barriers to nursing practice and any proposed change
5. Identifies effects of organizational culture on departments, teams, and/or groups within an organization
6. Monitors legislative and regulatory health policy that may impact nursing practice and/or CNS practice for the specialty area/populations

During the planning phase for the in-service, Steven benchmarked with several national and international organizations whose mandates for the treatment of drug use are imbedded in the philosophy of harm reduction. Specifically, Steven wanted to produce an in-service that focused on the humane treatment of people who use illicit drugs. To that end, Steven contacted two Canadian harm reduction programs, one European-based program, as well as two U.S.-based programs and asked each program manager to e-mail/mail him copies of their program's philosophy of care, mission statement, program expectations/outcomes, and any educational reference materials, such as pamphlets, videos, and so forth, that were free of charge, to assist him in planning for the in-service. Because the in-service would be videotaped, Steven knew that all staff who could not attend could view the video at a later date. As well, the administration along with the nurse educator guaranteed that every newly orientating staff member would view the video during organization orientation.

Under Diagnosis, Outcome Identification, and Planning, NACNS (2004, p. 36) identifies five competencies:

1. Diagnoses facilitators and barriers to achieving desired outcomes of integrated programs of care across the continuum and at points of service
2. Diagnoses variations in organizational culture (e.g., values, beliefs, or attitudes) that can positively or negatively affect outcomes
3. Draws conclusions about the effects of variance across the organization that influence outcomes of nursing practice
4. Plans for achieving intended system-wide outcomes, while avoiding or minimizing unintended consequences
5. Draws conclusions about the impact of legislative and regulatory policies as they apply to nursing practice and outcomes for specialty populations

Yvette is proud of Steven and the video/in-service he produced as part of his preceptorship experience. Not only did he identify the organization-wide need for best practice–related policies and procedures for injection drug users, but he also, then, benchmarked with noted national and international harm reduction programs to learn best practices related to drug use. As a long-term employee of an inner city hospital, Yvette is very familiar with the players within the system who consistently erect barriers when a patient-centered initiative is implemented that might be perceived by those individuals as risky and "outside the box." Yvette was not worried that Steven's educational initiative would fail because she was a recognized practice leader in the hospital and would "spread the word" that the video must be reviewed by all nurses, and hopefully all other disciplines, because the content was patient-centered, *educated the front-line staff on an important topic, and, from an ethical and moral standpoint, it was the right thing to do.*

Under Intervention: Developing and Testing Solutions, NACNS (2004, p. 36–37) identifies 11 competencies:

1. Develops innovative solutions that can be generalized across differing units, populations, or specialties
2. Leads nursing and multidisciplinary groups in implementing innovative patient care programs that address issues across the full continuum of care for different population groups and/or different specialties
3. Contributes to the development of multidisciplinary standards of practice and evidence-based guidelines for care, such as pathways, care maps, benchmarks
4. Solidifies relationships and multidisciplinary linkages that foster the adoption of innovations
5. Develops or influences system-level policies that will affect innovation and programs of care
6. Targets and reduces system-level barriers to proposed changes in nursing practices and programs of care
7. Facilitates factors to effect program-level change
8. Designs strategies to sustain and spread chance and innovation
9. Implements methods and processes to sustain evidence-based changes in nursing programs of care, and clinical innovation
10. Provides leadership for legislative and regulatory initiatives to advance the health of the public with a focus on the specialty practice area/populations
11. Mobilizes professional and public resources to support legislative and regulatory issues that advance the health of the public

The wonderful aspect of this video, in Yvette's opinion, is that it can be used across differing units, ethnic populations, and specialties. Indeed, the video is a wonderful teaching tool for not only the inpatient units but also for outpatient services and community settings as well. Just the other day, a CNS from a hospital in another part of the city called wanting access to the video: This CNS wanted it so she could teach front-line nurses involved in community outreach about drug use by patients. As well, an emergency nurse practitioner at the hospital, after viewing the video, began to develop pathways and care maps specifically addressing this vulnerable population. Yvette has also contacted the faculty member contact and insisted that together with Steven they submit abstracts to present at conferences related to harm reduction, clinical evidence-based best practice, education-focused best-practice, and leadership focused best-practice.

Under Evaluation of the Effects, NACNS (2004, p. 37–38) identifies seven competencies:

1. Selects evaluation methods and instruments to identify system-level outcomes of programs of care
2. Evaluates system-level clinical and fiscal outcomes of products, devices, and patient care processes using performance methods
3. Uses organizational structures and processes to provide feedback about the effectiveness of nursing practices and multidisciplinary relationships in meeting identified outcomes of programs of care
4. Evaluates organizational policies for their ability to support and sustain outcomes of programs of care
5. Evaluates and documents the impact of CNS practice on the organization
6. Documents all outcomes in a reportable manner
7. Disseminates outcomes of system-wide changes, impact of nursing practice, and CNS work to stakeholders

Yvette, Steven, and the faculty member have just finished discussing the content of Steven's final evaluation. Needless to say, Steven passed his final preceptorship experience with honors. At this meeting, Steven disclosed to Yvette that prior to being a BScN-prepared registered nurse he was a teacher at an inner-city high school, which, in hindsight, did not surprise Yvette. Yvette believes that not only is Steven an excellent CNS clinician, but he is a superb educator, as well: two qualities that will enhance the care he provides to and for his future patients/families.

It was evident by the quality of the in-service Steven provided to the health care staff that he had read and synthesized the contents of the NACNS (2004) document. Steven clearly demonstrated the need for: the hospital administration to "buy in" to the education initiative; benchmarking with seminal organizations clearly advocating for the principles of harm reduction; Yvette to positively influence all front-line staff and advanced practice nurses to attend the session and view the video; effective evaluation methods to be used to identify strengths and areas for improvement of the in-service and video; and the evaluation of current policies and procedures related to the care of vulnerable populations, such as injection drug users.

SUMMARY AND CONCLUSION

This chapter has provided an overview of the preceptorship experience within the context of CNS student education. Preceptorship is an important approach to teaching and learning in the clinical/community practice settings. It provides a connection between the theoretical and practical aspects of advanced practice nursing, and in so doing, it continues to further strengthen the profession and discipline of nursing.

REFERENCES

Backenstose, A. G. (1983). The use of clinical preceptors. In S. Stuart-Siddall & J. M. Haberlin (Eds.), *Preceptorship in nursing education* (pp. 9–20). Rockville: Aspen Systems.

Canadian Nurses Association. (2003). *Position statement: Clinical nurse specialist*. Ottawa, ON: Author.

Cantor, J. A. (1992). *Delivering instruction to adult learners*. Toronto: Wall & Emerson.

Elliott, H., Gauthier, P., Mitchell, M., Oates, S., & Purdy, N. (2004). The clinical nurse specialist. *Registered Nurses Association of Ontario (RNAO) Practice Page, 4*(3). Retrieved January 9, 2009, from http://www.rnao.org/Storage/13/726_Practice_Page_CNS.pdf

Kramer, M. (1974). *Reality shock. Why nurses leave nursing*. St. Louis: Mosby.

Heitkemper, M. M., & Bond, E. F. (2004). Clinical nurse specialists. State of the profession and challenges ahead. *Clinical Nurse Specialist, 18*(3), 135–140.

Myrick, F. (2002). Preceptorship and critical thinking in nursing education. *Journal of Nursing Education, 41,* 154–164.

Myrick, F., & Barrett, C. (1994). Selecting clinical preceptors for basic baccalaureate nursing students: A critical issue in clinical teaching. *Journal of Advanced Nursing, 19,* 194–198.

Myrick, F., & Yonge, O. (2003). Preceptorship: A quintessential component of nursing education. In M. H. Oermann & K. T. Heinrich (Eds.), *Annual review of nursing education* (vol. 1, pp. 91–107). New York: Springer.

Myrick, F., & Yonge, O. (2004). Enhancing critical thinking in the preceptorship experience in nursing education. *Journal of Advanced Nursing, 45*(4), 371–380.

Myrick, F., & Yonge, O. (2005). *Nursing preceptorship. Connecting practice and education*. Philadelphia: Lippincott Williams & Wilkins.

National Association of Clinical Nurse Specialists. (2004). *Statement on clinical nurse specialist practice and education* (2nd ed.). Harrisburg, PA: Author.

Exemplars of the Clinical Nurse Specialist Role in a Variety of Settings

Hospital-Based Clinical Nurse Specialist Practice

Katie Brush
Theresa Murray

Editors' Note: This chapter reflects the clinical practice of two critical care nurses. Katie Brush's practice was in an academic teaching hospital; Theresa Murray's practice is in a community hospital. Ms. Brush became gravely ill and passed away unexpectedly before the publication of this book. The editors extend condolences to her family and many friends.

CARE OF A COMPLEX TRAUMA PATIENT IN AN ACADEMIC TEACHING HOSPITAL

Katie Brush

The surgical intensive care unit (SICU) in an academic medical center can be a challenging environment. As a clinical nurse specialist (CNS), I need to balance the multiple challenges of the environment with the constant shuffling of priorities created by complex patient physiological demands and psychosocial needs. And, while I can do many things, as a CNS it is important to remember to work through unit staff nurses. Working through staff nurses helps facilitate adherence to a change in the plan of care, provides opportunities to teach the nurses and other providers about caring for acutely ill patients, and moves practice forward by using principles of evidence-based practice. What follows is a case example of CNS practice involving an acutely ill patient in an academic teaching hospital.

CASE EXEMPLAR

A female patient was admitted to the SICU following major trauma. She suffered pelvic fractures, a right acetabulum fracture, a right wrist fracture, sternal fracture, and a head injury. This patient case is a good example of the many ways a CNS supports the care of a patient with complex needs related to multiple trauma.

The patient experienced intermittent periods of intracranial instability as demonstrated by her intracranial pressure (ICP) waveforms. Staff nurses in the SICU learn ICP waveform analysis during unit orientation; however, the ability to actually analyze and interpret waveforms as they are occurring takes practice. To further develop staff skill in waveform interpretation, I use actual patient situations to validate comprehension. Using real patient experiences to build skill with staff is one way a CNS contributes to quality nursing care and improved patient outcomes. Over the course of ICP monitoring, I lead many discussions about waveform interpretation with nurses, neurologists, and resident physicians.

The patient initially had a subarachnoid bolt placed. Later, the bolt was removed, and she had a ventriculostomy placed to allow for drainage and maintenance of a stable pressure in the ventricular space. Upon arrival early one morning, I found a physician resident attempting to resecure the drain to the patient's scalp, explaining that overnight the patient began draining blood-tinged cerebral spinal fluid (CSF), and he was unable to irrigate the catheter. The clinical situation indicated emergent need for a computed tomography (CT) scan. I worked with the staff nurse to contact the attending physician, explain the problem, obtain orders for the test, and prepare the patient for transport. Transport was complicated by pelvic traction. The staff nurse had never removed pelvic traction before. I directed the actions of the staff nurse and a patient care assistant, and the traction was removed while taking care not to move (not to abduct or adduct) the patient's leg while transferring to the stretcher. The patient had a severely fractured acetabulum in combination with her open book pelvic fracture. We discussed the possible worsening of her acetabular injury and the potential for misalignment of her pelvic fracture if the leg were not kept straight. The patient was transferred successfully. As a result of the scan, interventions were put in place to clear the ventriculostomy so that ICP would not exceed the normal range.

The day after the CT scan, the patient had an external fixation device placed in her anterior pelvis to stabilize the fractures. Although a difficult process, the external fixation device would give the patient much more stability as healing proceeded. Upon making rounds in the unit, the same staff nurse I helped with the pelvic traction asked me to assess wounds around the patient's external fixation device. The external fixation pins had caused tearing of the skin around the pin sites. We discussed a plan of care. Noting that the current type of dressing kept moisture continuously against the patient's skin, we discussed other dressing options, materials, and techniques. I role modeled how to problem solve by talking out loud while using a decision tree–type algorithm, including various dressing choices available. We reviewed each dressing choice until we came to a single dressing that was absorbent and would turn into a gel as it soaked up serous fluid, thereby decreasing the amount of fluid on the patient's skin. This problem-solving model led to a best practice decision for the patient. It is important to note that the staff nurse sought my help on the second day based on a positive interaction with me on the first day. Staff want and need clinical support and will seek out a CNS who they perceive to be helpful. I believe the two critical elements to being perceived as helpful from the staff's perspective are clinical expertise and a nonjudgmental bearing.

Feeling confident about the dressing decision, the staff nurse asked me to examine the patient's labia and noted a significant amount of serous discharge coming from her vagina. Together we identified tears in the labia, most likely the result of positional edema. We made a wound care plan to treat the tears. We then reviewed the chart to determine if the patient had a pelvic exam upon admission. I explained to her that the vagina is often the "forgotten organ" in pelvic fractures, whereas the urethra and rectum are always examined. Severe vaginal tears can occur in open-book pelvic fractures and can go untreated unless the trauma is identified in an examination in the emergent part of the admission.

Determining that a pelvic exam was not completed, the staff nurse took responsibility for calling the trauma team. Not only had I helped ensure appropriate care for this trauma patient, but I educated and empowered the staff nurse. Empowering the staff nurse with knowledge and skill is one of those all too often invisible contributions CNSs make to quality patient outcomes.

At one point in the patient's stay in the SICU she required an urgent magnetic resonance imaging (MRI) to evaluate a changing neurological status. The radiology technicians were concerned about placing the patient into the MRI machine with a Steinman pin in the pelvis. I showed the technicians how to use a magnet to test metal for iron, which would put the patient at risk in the MRI. It would be very unusual for any device today to contain iron because most are made of other metals, such as titanium. However, the technicians' concerns were valid: placing a patient with an implanted device that contained iron could result in significant injury to the patient and to the staff because the MRI could literally pull the device out of the patient's body. I took advantage of the teaching opportunity, gave the technicians a pacemaker magnet, and had them hold it to the Steinman pin to determine if the magnet was attracted to the pin. As anticipated, there was no attraction, but this was a wonderful demonstration and one that took advantage of a teachable moment.

This exemplar described just a few days in the care of a severely traumatized patient. Within the example, I have been able to demonstrate competencies in CNS practice across three spheres of influence: the patient, the nurses, and the system. In this example, the care occurred in an academic teaching hospital. What makes teaching hospitals unique is the presence of students and new practitioners, all needing support and guidance as they complete formal education and begin clinical practice. A CNS in this setting not only helps ensure safe, quality care for patients but is in the position to influence the practice of beginners by establishing practice patterns that can last a lifetime.

CARE OF A COMPLEX SEPTIC PATIENT IN A COMMUNITY-BASED HOSPITAL

Theresa Murray

Community hospitals are admitting and treating very ill patients, which places demands on nurses to keep up with emerging clinical needs and new care techniques. Sepsis has been around forever; however, increasing emphasis on morbidity and mortality in light of patient safety has made sepsis a focus of renewed interest. This exemplar describes how a hospital-based

CNS developed a program to reduce sepsis across a community hospital network of five hospitals.

Sepsis is the 10th leading cause of death in the United States. Sepsis begins as a seemingly harmless infection and spreads to the entire system, causing life-threatening changes in physiology that can result in death if not recognized and addressed immediately. Patients can present from the community with infections such as pneumonia or a urinary tract infection (UTI). If a hospitalized patient develops a systemic response to this previously localized infection, the result could be sepsis, severe sepsis, or septic shock. Organ failure and/or hypotension may develop, and the patient is suddenly in the intensive care unit (ICU) facing a complex and costly treatment plan.

In October 2006, I lead the initiative at the community-based hospital where I worked to develop a program for early recognition of sepsis. The clinical goal of the program was to increase the number of previously unrecognized local infections cases among newly admitted patients, provide early intervention, and prevent systemic sepsis with concomitant poor patient outcomes. The sepsis prevention program had several components, including a medical intervention protocol, nursing education, and medical record support.

Medical interventions for the sepsis protocol were developed in collaboration with the hospital's intensivist physicians. Scientific evidence for early intervention of sepsis was reviewed, and the work of Rivers and colleagues (2001) served as the guidelines for protocol development. The guidelines included a medical order set for the entire hospital network and was presented to the critical care committee at all network facilities for approval. The critical care committee includes intensivist physicians, emergency care and family practice physicians, ICU and emergency care unit management, the critical care CNS, and a pharmacist. After the guidelines and order set were approved, implementation with the staff began.

An educational program for nurses and nursing care personnel was developed and delivered in collaboration with unit educators. While the education program was eventually delivered to all nursing personnel, nurses working in medical, progressive, intensive, and emergency care departments were targeted to begin assessment for local infection and early recognition of indicators of systemic sepsis. For the target units, the CNS presented information at a regularly scheduled intensive care/progressive care unit team day. The presentation stressed the need to screen patients twice a day and reviewed the approved order set for the treatment of sepsis. A media presentation was developed and placed on a laptop computer secured to a rolling cart. The media presentation toured all the units as a portable and flexible education program. It stressed screening patients once a day and, if positive, contacting the patient's physician and requesting a code blue nurse consult.

Simultaneous to the educational sessions, I worked with the information technology (IT) department to create and install a hospital-wide sepsis documentation tab in the electronic medical record. This tab facilitated just-in-time charting for easy identification of patients testing positive for infection upon admission. Also, this addition to the medical record supported electronic tracking of sepsis screening, reporting, and monitoring.

Clinical implementation began by having each patient admitted to the emergency department (ED) screened for infection. Next, the program moved to having all inpatient admissions screened. Patients screening positive were referred to the code blue team covering that particular hospital. The practice in the system is for each hospital to assign an ICU nurse to the code blue team for a shift to respond to patient emergencies in the hospital. Building in a code blue nurse consult call ensured that patients screening positive for sepsis were brought to the attention of the emergency team. The code blue team took responsibility for follow-up. Follow-up included initiating medical referrals and/or diagnostic testing and medical intervention. By identifying local infections in a proactive manner, patients have much better outcomes from their care.

Here's an example of how the screening process was implemented. A 62-year-old female with abdominal pain entered the ED from home at 6:30 p.m. and was admitted to a medical inpatient unit. Findings from her laboratory test arrived at the unit at approximately 9:00 p.m. The staff nurse evaluated the laboratory findings along with findings from the ED clinical assessment and determined the patient had a positive screen for sepsis. According to the information learned in the education sessions, the staff nurse knew she should call the code blue nurse. The code blue team nurse confirmed the positive sepsis screen and, using a protocol, began volume resuscitation, called the attending physician, and obtained a consult from the intensivist physician. The patient's condition continued to deteriorate; she was intubated and admitted to the ICU and placed under sepsis care within 45 minutes of a positive screen for sepsis. The next morning she went into surgery to correct a pancreatic abscess. With the source of infection controlled and adequate volume resuscitation, the patient improved significantly over several days and was discharged from the critical care unit to a medical unit within 7 days. This patient suffered no additional complications as a result of her treatment. Her sepsis treatment was more expeditious than prior to the implementation of the sepsis program. Without the programmatic approach to early sepsis identification, this patient may not have been identified until it was too late and would have likely suffered severe consequences from less than timely treatment.

Evaluating a system-wide initiative requires both outcome and process measures. In this instance, feedback about the educational sessions, data reflecting documentation of the screening, and reporting to the code blue team were all process measures. Findings of diagnostic laboratory studies and initiation of medical therapies are also examples of process measures. The clinical outcomes included mortality, days of care in the critical care unit, and overall cost per patient day.

Data for the past 3 years shows that, in 2006, sepsis was a widely and inappropriately utilized diagnosis. After initiating the sepsis screening program and associated educational efforts, the recorded number of cases dropped across the hospital network from over 700 to roughly 500 in 2008. This finding is attributed to more precise diagnosis of sepsis. At the same time, mortality rates dropped also, indicating that for the true cases, early intervention was indeed saving lives.

In this community hospital network, the CNSs were able to implement a screening and rapid intervention program using medical protocols, nurse education sessions, and an electronic medical record support. Clinical support was provided by an existing emergency team, which was able to initiate a rapid response intervention. By working at the system level to empower nurses, the hospital now provides screening and rapid response for local infections or early-stage sepsis, leading to greatly improved diagnostic precision and better patient outcomes.

REFERENCES

Rivers, E., Nguyen, B., Havstad, S., Ressler, J., Muzzin, A., Knoblich, B., et al. (2001). Early goal-directed therapy in the treatment of severe sepsis and septic shock. *New England Journal of Medicine, 345*(19), 1368–1377.

30

Clinical Nurse Specialist in Collaborative Private Practice

Jeffrey S. Jones

The purpose of this chapter is to briefly describe one type of clinical nurse specialist (CNS) private practice model. It is not meant to be an all-inclusive guide on how to set up your own business. Rather, it is a highlight of key points that were and still are essential to the ongoing success of this particular practice model. The intent is to motivate and inspire CNSs who desire a private practice by illustrating that such a private practice model is achievable.

DESCRIPTION OF POPULATIONS AND PRACTICE

Pinnacle Mental Health Associates, Inc., is a psychiatric CNS private practice offering primary outpatient mental health services for adults in Mansfield, Ohio. The practice offers mental health services (assessment, diagnosis, therapy, medication management, consultation, and supervision) designed to meet the needs of the adult working professional.

EMPLOYMENT STATUS

The practice is CNS-owned and operates as a professional S corporation (S corp.). A professional S corp. structure was decided upon after study of various business options (LLC, C corp., etc.) and consultation with a local business attorney. An S corp. allows the owners to share the profits and offers some tax advantages to the

owners in that they are able to report gains and losses on personal income tax. An S corp. structure also protects the owner's personal assets in the event of liability. The two CNS partners divide the duties of president, vice president, secretary, and treasurer. As owners they are also shareholders in the company. The business has a third employee who functions in a clerical capacity as an office manager and provides administrative support.

WORK ENVIRONMENT

The business suite is located in a professional office building in the heart of the city's business community. The professional environment was designed by the two owners. In collaboration with the building owner, the suite was redesigned to capture a very open, casual, warm, and homey feel. The intent was to distinctly not have a medical office appearance. Tan, earthy colors were chosen for the walls and carpet. A living room feel was accomplished by placing a modular couch and swivel chair in one corner and a table and chairs at the other. Fresh coffee and iced tea is always available for customers as they wait to be seen. A small kitchen nook also offers a choice of iced beverages to patrons. Numerous plants and other foliage augment the homey feel. The waiting area is open, with the receptionist in an island in the center where she freely interacts with patrons. The clinician's offices are at opposite ends of the suite and are professionally decorated in continuation of the relaxed homey feel. Plush couches, chairs, and a small but functional desk complete the scheme. Each office has a laptop because all the records are electronic. As the result of purposeful milieu management, the small workforce and comfortable surroundings create a relaxing and intimate environment.

PROFESSIONAL RESPONSIBILITIES

Typical daily duties include overseeing the day-to-day operations of the business. This includes but is not limited to managing cash flow, making decisions regarding the business, marketing, and negotiation of contracts with outside entities such as the Department of Corrections and local mental health centers. The actual clinical work in the office may consists of assessment and diagnosis of mental health disorders; engagement in individual, family, or group therapy; prescription and management of medications; and liaison contact with other community linkage support services or referral entities.

PROFESSIONAL SUPPORT STRUCTURE

The structure of the business consists of two CNS partners, an office manager/clerical support person, and a collaborating physician. The physician is not physically located onsite but collaborates from a distance. The requirements of the collaborative agreement are met via monthly meetings with the physician for the purpose of case review.

FUTURE OPPORTUNITIES AND CHALLENGES FOR CNSs

Because advanced practice registered nurses (APRNs) are increasingly recognized as potential primary care providers, CNSs now have the opportunity to secure their place among their APRN peers. Even though CNSs are historically recognized as experts in a given area, there continues to be some resistance from the medical community and even some APRN colleagues in viewing the CNS as an APRN. This resistance is thought to be due to the prevailing, traditional medical model of primary health care delivery.

TAKING THE PLUNGE

As a CNS, you may have arrived at a point in your career where you have worked within an organization and have navigated downsizing, rightsizing, and many corporate changes. You may now be ready to make the

decision to create your own universe by practicing outside of the established medical community. Welcome to the ranks of CNS entrepreneurs who have established their own private practice.

Those who chose to take this route have several decisions to make. The first choice is whether or not to join an existing practice in a traditional office structure. This type of practice is most likely based on a medical model design. The second option is to open your own office. This option offers control to choose a nursing framework as a practice model. My partner and I chose the latter. Deciding on the second option grew out of past experiences trying to function as a CNS within a medical doctor (MD) or nurse practitioner (NP) dominated practice and medical model. CNSs think and practice differently than MDs and NPs because of the difference in CNS education. We both had reached a point in our career where we needed to be in an environment that reflected and supported the CNS practice model.

The next choice is deciding whether you want to establish a solo practice or work within a partnership. There are positives and negatives to either choice. Establishing a solo practice offers more control and autonomy, which some entrepreneurs need or find attractive. Going it alone, however, means that you shoulder the whole responsibility. This can be burdensome and very lonely. I chose to have a partner because I value the collegiality and peer support of another CNS. I also prefer a business model of shared responsibility.

Whether you chose a solo business model or a partnership model, you may also need to consider a collaborative arrangement with a physician if this is required in your state. The specifics of this will vary from state to state in terms of the language that is used to describe the relationship. The most common terms are collaboration or supervision. Our practice is in Ohio, where the relationship language is *collaboration*. Choosing a collaborating physician is as equally important as choosing a business partner. This decision should be guided by a sense of like-mindedness. Both the physician and the business partner need to have a clear understanding and appreciation for the scope of practice of CNSs and how it differs from NP-focused practice. It may be helpful at some point to gather information and evaluate personality traits through the use of such tools as the Meyers-Briggs Personality Inventory®. Additionally, and more specific to you and your business partner, it is important to invest time in evaluation of each other's entrepreneurial traits. A clear understanding of each other's perspective allows each person to know themselves, to know how they react under various circumstances, and to become familiar with their own particular strengths and comfort levels. Once these very basic but key steps are taken, you are ready to develop a business plan.

PUTTING IT ON PAPER

The development of a sound, well-structured business plan can open many doors for you as you proceed. When seeking advice and assistance from the local business community or lenders that will help with your financial needs, all will want to review your business plan. There are numerous books as well as free online resources concerning the construction of a business plan. Some have been written specifically for nurses. *Managing Your Practice—A Guide for Advanced Practice Nurses,* by Fitzpatrick, Glasgow, and Young (2003), is an excellent guide. Whatever source you use, the most common elements of a good business plan are:

1. Executive summary (including your mission statement)
2. Table of contents
3. Description of the practice
4. Products and services
5. Operations
6. Marketing plan
7. Assessment of competition
8. Risks
9. Finances (start-up costs, projected spreadsheets, etc.)
10. Milestones
11. Summary

Our business is a private mental health practice. As most owners do, we had many choices to make in order to set up the business. Meeting with an attorney who understands business law and the services you plan to deliver is essential in clarifying the advantages and distinctions among these options. After completing this step, our business decided to structure itself as a professional S corp. As previously described, an S corp. allows the owners to share the profits and also offers some tax advantages because each is able to report gains and losses on personal income tax. The other main advantage of an S corp. structure is that it separates and protects the owner's personal assets in the event of liability.

WHAT ARE NURSING SERVICES WORTH?

Now that you have a business plan and an attorney, the next step is beginning to explore your financial needs. This should begin in a meeting with an accountant that has had experience with servicing health care organizations. The accountant will help you refine elements of the business plan that may be unrealistic. This feedback will lead to the development of a more accurate financial spreadsheet. When this step is completed, you are ready to approach a lender.

This phase of the business experience for the CNS can be the most awkward. Nurses aren't inherently educated or acculturated to think of nursing services as independent and marketable commodities. More likely, nurses have adapted the identity of who they are and the service they provide from an organization or an MD provider. It is absolutely imperative that these false (and weak) notions about nurses and dependent nursing services be dealt with and refined before the beginning phase. Lenders want to know what experience you have, what has brought you to this point in your career, and what enables you to offer services independent of another entity. They need to see that you have confidence in your abilities, and they need to get a crystal clear idea of how you plan to succeed. This is precisely the time to drag out the power suit, brush up on your presentation skills, and do everything you can to sell yourself.

You may have to speak with several lenders before you find one willing to take the risk of investing in a start-up business. Securing the actual start-up funds should involve two products from the lender. The first should be a term loan to use for start-up essentials. The second should be a line of credit to cover operational costs until your cash flow is steady. Remember that over 50% of new businesses fail in the first year. The main reason this happens is that the business is undercapitalized at start-up.

Finding the right location for your business and beginning to market your services will take more time than you may think. Choosing just the right spot that fits your budget and also is convenient to the population you intend to serve is tricky. Marketing is also complicated. You can spend a lot of money on commercial advertising that may be wasted. Many marketing people will want to help you spend your money on advertising. It is wise to adapt a diverse approach. Here are some helpful tips.

- Know that the most powerful marketing tool is word of mouth so start networking early.
- Schedule yourself for speaking engagements that target the population you serve.
- Get the local newspaper interested; an in-depth interview about a nurse-run business is usually a newsworthy item.
- Develop a Web site for the business. This can be relatively inexpensive and a lot of consumers can get their information about you from the Internet. The Web site developed for our business can be used as an example: http://www.pinnaclemha.com/.
- Get interviewed on the local radio and TV station.
- Save the costly things such as print ads, flyers, and direct mailings to deploy closer to your opening. A successful marketing strategy is ongoing and never ends. It takes a long time for a community to remember that a new business is in town.

■ Set aside some of your budget each month to do some advertising. You may or may not get support from the medical and APRN community. Some communities are more receptive to others regarding CNSs in private practice. The name recognition of APRN is so closely linked with the NP/MD practice model that it may be difficult for other health care providers, including your own colleagues, to understand a practice model that is truly focused on advanced practice nursing.

Another consideration is the decision regarding how you will be reimbursed for your services. Will you apply for and become impaneled on all the major insurance plans? Will you accept Medicare and Medicaid? (If so, this process needs to start approximately 60 days prior to opening.) Will you accept credit cards? What current procedural terminology (CTP)-codes will you use to bill for services and how much will you charge? After carefully looking at various options, we decided to be a solely fee-for-service/out of network practice. We are not Medicare or Medicaid providers, although we do see a number of consumers with this type of coverage. They simply pay out of pocket. Consumers are charged the same rate for service as the marketable rate in comparable mental health care offices. As a courtesy to our customers, we do bill electronically for the service, but it is clearly explained that we are out of network and the copay may be higher. This practice model works for the market niche we target. Your practice may need to operate differently depending on the population you intend to serve.

COVERING YOUR ASSETS

A crucial but often overlooked aspect of owning a private practice is ensuring that you and the business are adequately covered regarding liability. It will be necessary to find an insurance carrier who will provide coverage not only to you and your partner as CNSs, but also who will cover the building or office suite for claims not related to malpractice. An essential aspect of this is finding a carrier that recognizes the CNS category in the APRN role. Some of the more prominent nursing malpractice carriers only recognize NPs, nurse midwives, and nurse anesthetists, placing CNSs under the NP category. If pressed, some of these carriers will write what is called a rider, acknowledging that you are a CNS and not an NP. While this may suffice in a court of law, from a legal perspective you would be better advised to procure a company that clearly recognizes the scope of practice of a CNS as unique and distinct from other types of APRN.

Finally, the day-to-day operations of the business will ebb and flow as the weeks go by. You will make daily decisions and the next week change your mind after learning from your mistakes. There are only a few absolutes in managing your own practice. As your business grows, it will become part of the community. Your business will develop a rhythm, and your attentiveness to that rhythm will provide you cues as to when to make changes to meet changing community needs. This may include augmenting services or implementing different marketing strategies.

TRUE AUTONOMY

The opportunity to function independently in a private practice setting can be an incredibly powerful and liberating one for CNSs. Free from the hospital structure that sometimes is unsupportive of the role of the CNS, you may find yourself wondering what took you so long to make the decision to become an entrepreneur. To be sure, this chosen path is not without its risks. Managing a business is time consuming and is a 24/7 job. Unless you have a large sum of money invested and available, you will potentially have to use your home and car for collateral. Relationships can be strained both personally and professionally. You may find days when you wonder if you have done the right thing. Then, you will see your next client. You will get to spend as much time with them as you want. You will get to focus on the health care that emphasizes preventative advanced practice nursing strategies. You will have a truly unhindered sense of the concept of the nurse–patient relationship. And at the end of the day, your last client will thank you for all you've done for them and will leave your office in a healthier state than when you first saw them a few months ago. It is then that you will become reinvigorated about the path you have chosen. You are practicing health care from a true nursing model, and you will remember why you became a nurse and a CNS in the first place.

REFERENCES

Barry, P. (2005). Questions and answers for the nurse psychotherapist in private practice. *Perspectives in Psychiatric Care, 41*(1), 42–44.

Cobb, M. A. (1998). CNS role in women's health promotion and maintenance in a collaborative practice. *Clinical Nurse Specialist, 12*(3), 112–116.

Davis, E. A. (1994). Factors influencing the implementation of the CNS role in a private practice working with a physician. *Clinical Nurse Specialist, 8*(1), 42–47.

Dayhoff, N. E., & Moore, P. S. (2004). Entrepreneurial dimensions of CNS practice. CNS entrepreneurship: Marketing 101. *Clinical Nurse Specialist, 18*(3), 123–125.

Dayhoff, N. E., & Moore, P. S. (2005). CNS entrepreneurs: innovators in patient care. *Sourcebook for Advanced Practice Nurses, 30*(1), 6–8.

Fine, S. (1997). *Developing a private practice in psychiatric mental health nursing.* New York: Springer.

Fitzpatrick, J. J., Glasgow, A., & Young, J. N. (2003). *Managing your practice: A guide for advanced practice nurses.* New York: Springer.

Hilderly, L. J. (1991). Nurse–physician collaborative private practice: The clinical nurse specialist in a radiation oncology private practice [Electronic version]. *Oncology Nursing Forum, 18*(3), 585–591.

Lesseig, D. Z. (1995). Private practice in Missouri: A CNS perspective. *Missouri Nurse, 64*(3), 6–7.

Lyon, B. L. (2003). Entrepreneurial dimensions of CNS practice. A clinical nurse specialist private practice in nursing. *Clinical Nurse Specialist, 17*(3), 131–132.

Nevada RNformation. (2004). *Collaborative and independent practice: Ongoing issues for nursing* [Electronic version; Brochure]. Nevada: Author.

Schulmeister, L. (1999). Starting a nursing consultation practice. *Clinical Nurse Specialist, 13*(2), 4–11.

Soehren, P. M., & Schumann, L. L. (1994). Enhanced role opportunities available to the CNS / Nurse Practitioner. *Clinical Nurse Specialist, 8*(3), 123–127.

Wilson, A., & Averis, A. (2002). Facets of private practice nursing: A conceptual model. *Collegian, 9*(2), 16–21.

Woodreuff, D. (2003). The metamorphosis of a CNS entrepreneurial business. *Clinical Nurse Specialist, 17*(6), 290–291.

31

Clinical Nurse Specialist Entrepreneurship: A Journey From Idea to Invention

Kathleen M. Vollman

In your nursing career, have you come across a product or service that you thought could be improved upon or changed? Perhaps you have even thought of something totally new that would help meet a health care need. What barriers exist that prevented you from exploring it further? As clinical nurse specialists (CNSs) we are presented with many unique opportunities to pursue entrepreneurial adventures and possess the necessary skill set to make it happen. What questions need to be asked and answered in order to motivate you to pursue your idea? I would like to share my journey of creating and marketing a frame to help turn and support a critically ill patient with acute respiratory distress syndrome (ARDS) into the prone position to help improve their oxygenation. The journey was a fascinating, challenging, sometimes exhausting, and absolutely rewarding life event when you take a product from the idea stage to market.

CRITICALLY ILL PATIENTS WITH ACUTE RESPIRATORY DISTRESS SYNDROME: MAKING PRONE MOBILIZATION SAFE

Discovering the impact of positioning on oxygenation in critically ill patients occurred early in my career. As a result of a review of the literature and my clinical experience, I discovered that a strategy of a 30-minute interval positioning from side to side for a patient with ARDS improved the patient's gas exchange (Ray et al., 1974). Therefore, when introduced to the concept of the prone position, several of the nursing staff were excited to try it. In the early 1980s, we were reaching for any treatment strategies that may impact a population with a 70% mortality rate. The challenge of positioning a critically ill patient prone with extensive tubes and lines without risking major complications posed a large obstacle to use of the prone position. I saw this challenge as an opportunity to make a patient care process better. My passion for the idea joined with the foundational information served as a strong basis for me to believe I could pursue this idea and actually make it work (Vollman, 2004). Ideas for successful inventions usually arise from solution development surrounding problems that exist in our everyday work and personal life. The concepts or ideas created need to come from our current knowledge, skills, or abilities. If an invention is launched in order to learn new skills the chance of success diminishes significantly (Zagury, 1993).

What is usually missing in most CNSs' toolkits, as was in my case, is the general knowledge and skills of business planning and financial management. However, there are many resources that can help CNSs, such as small business associations, local community colleges, professional associations, and Internet sites (Biel, 1994; Levy, 1995; Vollman, 2001, 2004). I took advantage of each of these to move from passion about an idea to product development. With considerable advice from family, friends, and colleagues, I developed a plan to further examine the concept of prone positioning. I designed and developed a support frame and procedure for prone positioning as part of my master's thesis, and then tested it with critically ill patients as described in this chapter.

PRACTICE INNOVATION

Producing the Prototype

A prototype is a workable model that can be tested and further developed. If you don't have the time, money, skills, or commitment to build or get your idea turned into a prototype the odds of licensing or bringing that idea to market are small (Levy, 1995). There are a number of ways to get prototypes built, including university engineering schools, prototype development businesses, and talented extended family members. A local inventors group may be an additional resource to help you find prototype makers within your community (Levy, 1995). I was fortunate enough to have a relative who was a mechanical engineer and believed he could build the frame I had in mind. The engineering schools may also be an economical way to develop your idea. Each semester engineering classes have projects they must design and develop. Why not have one of those project ideas be yours? In addition, many universities outside of the engineering department have formal programs designed to assist inventors with their ideas or patents. Whatever strategy you choose, remember you will move farther in the process with a tangible product that can be tested versus just an idea on paper (Biel, 1994).

The prone positioner's first prototype was built out of wood. Blueprints were developed from that model and changes were made to accommodate the technology of critical care during the turning procedure. The second prototype was manufactured together with a plastics company that works with prototypes. This prototype was used in a product evaluation study conducted at California State University in Long Beach with nursing students in a simulated critical care environment as the first phase of my master's thesis. The third prototype was made after changes in the design occurred based on the results of the product evaluation study and was used in the second phase of my thesis with critically ill patients.

Intellectual Property Protection

Once the idea is formulated, it must be analyzed to determine the level of protection that is required. There are three levels of protection for intellectual property (ideas). A copyright protects the tangible expression

of an idea. A trademark provides the owner with the right to exclude others from using confusingly similar product identification in commerce. A patent provides the owner with the right to exclude others from making, using, or selling the invention throughout the United States. A patent is the granting of intellectual property rights (Biel, 1994; Vollman, 2004). Think seriously before giving away an idea. Remember, an idea is intellectual property, or your brain trust, and any consideration of sharing that idea needs to be classified as a consultation that requires a fee.

I started protection of my intellectual property regarding the prone positioner idea very early in the process with documentation of the initial idea development and crude drawings. I had read somewhere about keeping an inventors log including a detailed description of the idea and drawings, and having the document witnessed by two people. Later, my patent attorney shared with me that this document was actually my first form of protection. Since June 8, 1995, the U.S. Patent and Trademark Office (USPTO) has offered inventors the option of filing a provisional application for patent, which was designed to provide a lower-cost first-patent filing in the United States. Applicants are entitled to claim the benefit of a provisional application in a corresponding nonprovisional application filed no later than 12 months after the provisional application filing date. The USPTO reminds inventors that any public use or sale in the United States or publication of the invention anywhere in the world more than 1 year prior to the filing of a patent application on that invention will prohibit the granting of a U.S. patent on it (USPTO, n.d.). The clearer your description and drawings, the stronger your protection will be. In addition, my attorney and I had the prototype manufacturer, the student nurse subjects, and my research assistants all sign 5-year confidential disclosure agreements before participating in the testing of the prototype in the product evaluation part of the study. A confidential disclosure agreement provided us with a way to protect the idea while working on the patent submission.

There are different types of patents, including a design, plant, and a utility patent (Levy, 1995). The prone positioner is a utility patent. A utility patent is granted for a new, useful, and nonobvious process, machine, manufactured article, composition, or an improvement on any of these. When beginning the patent process there are four steps to move through: a patent search, preparation and a file application, processing the application, and issuing the patent (Levy, 1995).

When I began the search for a patent attorney, I knew the process was expensive. My resources and family financial support were already being stretched by graduate school and prototype development. I was fortunate to be introduced to an attorney who was willing to take a student and work creatively to meet my legal needs in a cost-conscious manner (Vollman, 1999). In the patent search there were several patents that may be considered similar, making it necessary to document how the prone positioner was different. That step was successfully completed, and the utility patent was filed for in 1987. At that point, the positioner had patent-pending protection and could then be used in the second phase of my master's thesis examining the effect on oxygenation in critically ill patients using the prone positioner (Vollman & Bander, 1996).

The Cross Roads: A Crucial Decision-Making Point

As you are designing a plan to bring your idea to market, you will reach a crossroads. Do I produce the product myself, license it to a company, or seek out a company that helps inventors move their product to the market? Be cautious of taking your idea to an invention marketing company. Reputable invention marketing companies usually will not require any up-front fees and do not advertise on TV or radio, or in newspapers, direct mailers, or magazine ads (Levy, 1995). If you choose the do-it-yourself road, you will need to raise money and dedicate yourself to one single enterprise. If you decide on the licensing option, there are a number of strategies that can help make the pitch to a company stronger. Some of those strategies include a working prototype, patent protection, data on market size, selling impact, and potential cost to produce. The more homework done prior to the licensing pitch, the stronger your negotiating platform (Biel, 1994).

The preparation homework was done for the prone positioner. Abstracts, publications, and regional and national lectures to share the information about the science of positioning and the prone positioner were prepared. The road to licensing was hilly and full of curves, taking almost 7 years from completion of the study to signing a contract. I chose the licensing road because I knew I still wanted to be a practicing CNS and not a manufacturer. I began discussions with Hill-Rom, an international company that manufactures and distributes beds, support surfaces, and furniture in early 1996. I licensed my invention to Hill-Rom, and the Vollman Prone Positioner went on the market in January of 1997. I have maintained involvement through a consulting agreement in the marketing and education of the device and the science of prone positioning. Currently, the device is being used worldwide to help facilitate the turning and positioning of critically ill patients prone. The knowledge gained from this experience was invaluable in my role as CNS for the medical critical care service in a large urban hospital setting. I was heavily involved in evidence-based new product acquisition and standardization for materials that helped make it more efficient for the bedside nurse

to deliver nursing care. Part of the strategy to help get the product to market was submission of scientific abstracts for presentations at local, regional, national, and international conferences as well as numerous publications covering a wide variety of topics. As my comfort in those CNS competencies increased, I was able to help the staff submit papers and develop and present data on the care practice improvements we created, while helping them to develop professionally. The competencies developed during this process helped prepare me for a consultation business, but more importantly, they allowed me to excel as a unit-based CNS in changing processes and practices to improve patient outcomes (Dayhoff & Moore, 2002; Sao Lan, 2005).

Outcomes: Defining Success

I frequently get asked the questions, "How successful is the positioner?" and "Do you make a lot of money from it?" Every person defines success in a different way, and I would like to share with you how I define success with an e-mail I received from a patient that experienced use of the Vollman Prone Positioner.

> My name is JM and I had been admitted to the hospital with a severe case of streptoccocus pneumonia this past January, which resulted in some serious complications, including ARDS. Among the interventions that saved my life was the use of the prone positioner you invented, which had been procured but never had the chance to be used. It was the hospital's first use of the technique. I responded very well to it and survived the ordeal. I just wanted to drop you a note to thank you for your innovation. I am expected to make a full recovery and am well on the way to doing that now. I thought it might do you good to hear from a beneficiary of your device. Thanks again, and I wish you every success as you continue to make a difference in people's lives.

In addition to the personal rewards, the professional rewards were beyond anything I ever dreamed. As part of the inventing and licensing process, I created a consulting agreement for further refinement of the prone positioner and utilization of my expertise regarding the science of positioning critically ill patients. Through this process I have learned many skills, including contract negotiation, outcome measurement, cost/benefit analysis, and long-term project management. The experience served as a strong foundation for my CNS role in a large urban hospital setting as well as the consultation and speaking business that I began while working at the hospital (Vollman, 1999, Vollman & Bander, 1996). Through the journey, I developed a world-wide reputation for speaking and consulting on various pulmonary/critical care and professional nursing topics. In 2003, I launched the company Advancing Nursing, LLC, which is focused on creating empowered work environments for nurses through the acquisition of greater skills and knowledge to advance the profession of nursing. It has allowed me to meet many wonderful clinicians and influence evidence-based practice around the world.

I feel I am one of the most fortunate people in the world because I am living my dream and sharing my passion of questioning the status quo with other nurses and health care practitioners to make an impact in our patient's lives. The key is to be yourself and be faithful to your own muse while resisting the herd instinct. Take the chance of being an entrepreneur; you will never regret the journey.

REFERENCES

Biel, M. H. (1994). Nurse inventors: Turning ideas into products. *Dimensions of Critical Care Nursing, 13*(4), 202–206.

Dayhoff, N. E., & Moore, P. S. (2002). Entrepreneurial clinical nurse specialists: Innovators of patient care. *Clinical Nurse Specialist, 16,* 274–276.

Levy, R. C. (1995). *The inventor's desktop companion.* Detroit: Visible Ink Press.

Ray, J. F., Ost, L., Moallem, S., Sanoudos, G. M., Villamona, P., Parades, R. M., et al. (1974). Immobility, hypoxemia and pulmonary arteriovenous shunting. *Archives of Surgery, 109,* 537–541.

Sao Lan, J. I. (2005). Clinical nurse specialist entrepreneurship. *The Internet Journal of Advanced Nursing Practice, 7*(1).

U.S. Patent and Trademark Office. (n.d.). *Provisional application for patent.* Retrieved October 1, 2007, from http://www.uspto.gov/web/offices/pac/provapp.htm

Vollman, K. M. (1999). My search to help patients breathe. *Reflections, 25*(2), 16–18.

Vollman, K. M. (2001). Be an entrepreneur: Create opportunities for a new life adventure. *AACN News, 18*(4), 5.

Vollman, K. M. (2004). Nurse entrepreneurship through inventing: Taking an idea from birth to the market place. *Clinical Nurse Specialist, 8*(2), 68–71.

Vollman, K. M., & Bander, J. J. (1996). Improved oxygenation utilizing a prone positioner in patients with acute respiratory distress syndrome. *Intensive Care Medicine, 22,* 1105–1111.

Zagury, C. S. (1993). *Nurse entrepreneur: Building the bridge of opportunity.* Long Branch, New Jersey: Vista Publishing.

32

The Clinical Nurse Specialist in Industry/Business

Jane L. Bromund
Mary A. Short
Kathleen C. Solotkin

The clinical nurse specialist (CNS) in the pharmaceutical or medical device industry has far-reaching spheres of influence that encompass the client, nurse, and organization (Goudreau et al., 2007; National Association of Clinical Nurse Specialists [NACNS], 2004). Industry needs utilize the CNS skill set in a multitude of roles and settings that are often virtual. The CNS must have deep therapeutic knowledge of the patient population being served as well as how the pharmaceutical or medical device affects the patient. The patient population, under stringent privacy protection, is served from afar. Opportunities abound and most often focus on the patient with disease amenable to intervention in such areas as neuroscience, oncology, cardiovascular, critical care, women's health, endocrine disease including diabetes, and infectious disease.

Functioning in a global market, the emphasis is to understand the effects of the therapy across major ethnicities while targeting a vast population. The CNS is called upon to implement strategies in a wide variety of countries, cultures, and health care systems under different regulatory authorities around the world. Because the patient and provider are not located at the primary work site, the CNS must adapt to virtual methods of assessment and communication. Telecommunication is common and the industry CNS utilizes email, Web conferences, and teleconferences as primary modes of interaction. Face-to-face interactions often require travel with significant time zone changes and adaptation to different cultural

environments, languages, and traditions. At all points of development, safety and quality are at the forefront in the work of the industry CNS. The goal remains to achieve the best possible outcome for the patient by ensuring the right drug for the right patient at the right time, reinforcing the adage that what is good for the patient is good for the business.

The pharmaceutical and medical device industries have two primary functional divisions relevant to the roles a CNS might pursue: sales/marketing and medical. In addition, various other functional areas support the medical and marketing divisions including regulatory, data management, and governmental affairs. Work in any of these divisions can be within the scope of the industry CNS practice.

In the sales/marketing environment, one area of focus for the CNS is ensuring medical accuracy in promotion of approved drugs or devices. The CNS affects the patient through consulting with marketing personnel on the development of materials such as educational brochures, Web sites, and advertisements directed to the patient or health care professional. The CNS is uniquely qualified to help the sales and marketing staff in understanding the disease state and the impact therapy has on efficacy, safety, and quality of life. Sales/marketing associates for an industry CNS may be analogous to the nursing staff for a CNS in a hospital-based practice setting. An industry CNS may be called upon to advance the knowledge level of these associates from basic to advanced in a limited time frame, despite geographical constraints and often without the benefit of health care education or experience. The CNS illuminates important strategic considerations regarding patient and practitioner issues to enhance marketing's ability to positively impact health care.

In the medical division, the CNS has a key responsibility to protect patients' rights and safety in the development of clinically relevant research to address unmet medical needs. Deep therapeutic expertise, a core competency of the CNS role, is necessary to support product development and a clinically relevant research strategy (American Nurses Association [ANA], 2004; NACNS, 2004).

Data dissemination is another key responsibility of the CNS in the medical division. The CNS uses the ability to assimilate and communicate large volumes of complex information accurately to produce external scientific publications and regulatory documents. Examples of scientific data dissemination include abstracts, posters, manuscripts, and other medical response documents. Examples of regulatory documents include protocols, informed consent documents, clinical study reports, annual reports, and clinical trial registry summaries.

Developing relationships with key medical experts is another critical role of the CNS in industry. The CNS must establish and maintain contact with investigators and other leaders in the medical community. To do this, it is critical that the CNS maintain scientific expertise in order to provide deep and advanced disease state and product information. The CNS uses the feedback and insights gathered from medical experts to better inform research and overall strategic direction.

Within the organizational sphere, both the medical and marketing divisions use the leadership skills of the CNS to contribute to process improvement initiatives with the goal of decreasing the time and cost of bringing drugs and devices to the market. Leadership, knowledge, and communication skills are needed to influence across large multidisciplinary development teams and ultimately to communicate with the health care practitioners. The ability of the CNS to skillfully interpret the health care environment for the organization is highly valued. In industry, the CNS spheres of influence are very similar to those in a hospital-based practice (Zuzelo, 2003). Figure 32.1 illustrates the adaptation of the CNS spheres of influence to the industry environment and provides examples of key modes of influence.

Industry CNS Spheres of Influence

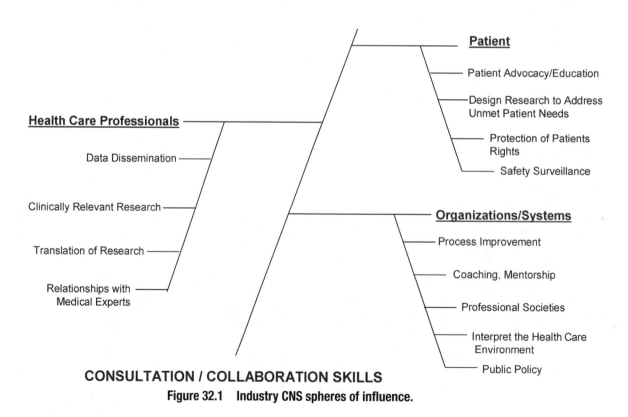

CONSULTATION / COLLABORATION SKILLS

Figure 32.1 Industry CNS spheres of influence.

EXPLORING CNS OPPORTUNITIES IN INDUSTRY

Industry is looking for individuals with advanced medically-related degrees to provide technical or therapeutic expertise, support research, assist in data dissemination, develop important relationships with health care professionals, and provide leadership across functional areas. Potential candidates include individuals with an advanced degree in a scientific discipline such as pharmacy, nursing, or other fields. In addition, several years of hands-on experience in a scientific field, clinical setting, or research setting, or pharmaceutical/device industry is often required. It is important to recognize that individuals with these qualifications are your competitors for industry positions and eventually your colleagues within industry. Highlighting your skill set as a CNS in your curriculum vitae, during the interview process, and eventually when collaborating with your industry colleagues is essential to success.

The CNS is uniquely prepared to function in a variety of roles in industry. The actual title of the roles may vary between companies and most have a career ladder similar to the clinical ladder in nursing. In general, these roles all require sound clinical judgment, demonstrated problem solving experience, and an appreciation of drug/device development and clinical research. Strong interpersonal skills, including negotiation, communication, and presentation skills, and an ability to operate in a multicultural environment are highly valued. Some examples of industry roles that may be of particular interest to advanced practice nurses are included in Table 32.1.

Therapeutic expertise is a core component of the CNS role, and that expertise is valued by industry. Pharmaceutical, medical device, and start-up biotechnology companies may have a narrow therapeutic focus. The key to success in gaining employment as well as

32.1 | Examples of Roles and Responsibilities

ROLE	RESPONSIBILITIES
Medical information associate	Reviews pertinent literature and communicates information with team Develops response documents to answer questions from health care professionals Trains business partners such as call center agents and sales representatives
Medical liaison	Field-based liaison between the company and key opinion leaders Reviews pertinent literature and communicates latest research
Clinical research scientist	Participates in the design and support of clinical trials in the target disease state Provides strategic input into data dissemination and medical/marketing needs Interacts with consultants and investigators Facilitates/develops publications Conducts medical review and approval of marketing and regulatory documents
Scientific communications/ medical writing	Coordinates/develops abstracts, posters, and manuscripts Authors regulatory documents such as protocols and clinical study reports
Regulatory affairs consultant	Liaison between the company and key regulators such as the Food and Drug Administration Participates in development of the product label and other documents Reviews marketing materials for compliance with regulations
Drug/product safety consultant	Monitors reports of adverse events and product complaints Participates in surveillance and risk management programs
Health outcomes liaison/ research scientist	Liaison between the company and key payer organizations and health technology assessment agencies Participates in development of formulary dossiers Conducts research on drug utilization and economic modeling/evaluation
Medical education consultant	Develops and coordinates education for industry business partners and health care professionals Evaluates applications for grant support of Continuing Medical Education

| Interviewing for an Industry Role

ACTIVITY	REASON
It is important to do thorough research before applying for a position in industry.	This will help you determine if a particular position interests you and if you have the qualifications necessary. Do not arrive for the interview unprepared.
Gain an in-depth understanding of the company's areas of interest, approved products, investigational products, and their product pipeline prior to interviewing for a position.	The company's Web site is a good place to start to gather this information. The investor section on the company Web site often contains a brief description of the product pipeline. Data on investigational products can often be obtained from clinical trial registries in the public domain, such as clinicaltrials.gov or from company registries.
Update your CV	Include all aspects of research and data dissemination in which you have participated. Ensure that your leadership strengths are clearly outlined in your resume.
Update your CV *(continued)*	Describe your previous roles in terms of project management, organizational, analytical, negotiation, and decision-making skills. Highlight situations where you created and maintained relationships with clinical or scientific thought leaders. Include any involvement in professional organizations or patient advocacy groups.
Provide a portfolio of your written work.	Include abstracts, posters, manuscripts, and patient education materials.
During the interview:	Be prepared to critique a research article or to demonstrate your presentation skills. As you discuss your experience, be as specific as possible about *your* key contributions to and results of the projects highlighted.

professional satisfaction in an industry role is aligning CNS therapeutic expertise to industry need. Table 32.2 provides suggestions for the industry application and interview process.

CHALLENGES TO THE CNS ROLE WITHIN INDUSTRY

Industry is a highly regulated environment. While the hospital-based CNS is regularly involved in preparation for inspections by The Joint Commission (formerly the Joint Commission on Accreditation of Healthcare Organizations) and other agencies, audit preparedness is an even more constant focus in industry. The CNS in industry must develop the regulatory mindset critical to protection of patient safety and patient rights, as well as the concept of fair balance in reporting research results and developing promotional materials. Presentations and publications are critiqued by medical, legal, and regulatory at a level of detail that is not often found in a clinical environment.

The CNS in industry rarely has direct patient contact. The patient remains the most important customer within industry; however, because the patient is further removed it can be easy to lose that patient focus. You may find that many of your industry colleagues do not have a clinical background and may not fully appreciate patient needs. Keeping the team focused on the patient is an area where the CNS can make a significant impact; however, the need to do so can also be a source of frustration.

Maintaining clinical expertise is an area of challenge for the advanced practice nurse in industry. Generally, outside employment must be reviewed for potential conflict of interest. Similarly, even scholarly work (manuscripts, presentations, etc.) completed outside of employment must be reviewed to ensure protection of the company's intellectual property.

Like many areas of innovation, bringing a pharmaceutical or a medical device to market takes many years and significant expenditure. Most pharmaceuticals in development do not end up as approved therapeutic agents. A CNS supporting early phase development may never see success because most compounds do not move forward into phase 3 trials. If a compound moves into phase 3, clinical trials may take years to complete and additional time is required for regulatory review prior to making an impact for the patient. In contrast, successes in the clinical role may come at a more rapid pace and be more tangible.

The likelihood that a CNS can remain in a specific therapeutic area is less in an industry setting compared to a clinical setting. When compounds do not meet expectations, entire therapeutic areas may be realigned or disbanded. Flexibility is required, and the learning agility of the CNS serves one well as a new area of therapeutic expertise must be developed to retain employment.

SUPPORT STRUCTURE IN INDUSTRY

Like the clinical environment, the industry environment will have a medical director, physicians, and colleagues of diverse allied health backgrounds. In many respects, navigating those interactions will feel familiar. However, the nonmedical, business colleague interactions may be more challenging. It is helpful to establish an informal network of individuals within the company that have a nursing background. Mentoring and coaching are expected behaviors of the CNS in industry, so networking is part of employment expectations. Continuing your involvement in nursing professional organizations is also important to maintain your therapeutic expertise and professional relationships.

CONCLUSION

Similar to the clinical setting, the role of the CNS has broad application in industry. The need for a professional that can integrate the systems of care and ensure patient safety exists in industry as well as in the clinical setting. The CNS is uniquely prepared to be successful in that role, and many opportunities exist in the industry environment for the CNS to optimize patient outcomes.

REFERENCES

American Nurses Association. (2004). *Nursing: Scope and standards of practice*. Washington, DC: Author.

Goudreau, K., Baldwin, K., Clark, A., Fulton, J., Lyon, B., Murray, T., et al. (2007). *A vision of the future for Clinical Nurse Specialists*. Retrieved January 26, 2009, from http://www.nacns.org/LinkClick.aspx?fileticket=7AX5Ga5RbTg%3d&tabid=117

National Association of Clinical Nurse Specialists. (2004). *Statement on clinical nurse specialist practice and education* (2nd ed.). Harrisburg, PA: Author.

Zuzelo, P. R. (2003). CNS practice: Spheres of influence. *Association of Perioperative Registered Nurses Journal, 77*, 361–372.

Exemplars of Clinical Nurse Specialist Practice in a Variety of Specialty Areas

Providing Pediatric Palliative Care in a Regional Children's Medical Center

Patricia O'Malley

PRACTICE OVERVIEW

Cindy Asher has provided expert clinical nurse specialist (CNS) practice at the Children's Medical Center in Dayton, Ohio, for 23 years. Cindy received a Bachelor of Science degree in nursing from Wright State University (Dayton, Ohio) and a Master of Science degree in nursing from the University of Cincinnati (Cincinnati, Ohio). Recognized as a local and regional expert for pediatric palliative care, Cindy's influence stretches from the bedside to the boardroom. This CNS drives best practices at end of life where time is short and the patient-family are extremely vulnerable. Within this acute care environment the needs of the child, family, and staff for comfort, meaning, and safety are overwhelming. Cindy demonstrates how CNS practice meets these critical needs through evaluation, consultation, mentoring, education, and advocacy.

CNS PRACTICE OVER TWO DECADES

Cindy has cared for children and families through the myriad changes that have occurred in CNS practice in the past 25 years. As a novice CNS, primary responsibilities were education and development of nursing staff. Over time, the boundaries dissolved between the classroom and the bedside, between nurses and physicians, between caregivers and management, and between staff and families. Years of dedicated practice and careful cultivation of professional relationships across the spectrum of care have allowed Cindy to cross freely across all levels of the organization to meet common goals of providing the best care to acutely ill children.

Pediatric practice like adult care has dramatically changed over the past 20 years. Medical and surgical units provide care for children that were once cared for only in the pediatric intensive care unit (PICU). Children in the PICU require complex technology-based care. With changes in reimbursement and expanding outpatient services, children once hospitalized are cared for at home.

Societal changes have dramatically impacted practice. Increasing numbers of blended and nontraditional families with deep economic or social needs drive the character of pediatric admissions. Children with insurance are more likely to be managed as outpatients. Children without insurance or poor social environments are more likely to be admitted. Cindy has observed a rise in depression and emotional problems in children, insured or not. Providing care for the body, mind, and spirit at a variety of developmental levels has become more intense and difficult.

Like adult settings, safety has become the core focus at all levels of care. Coupled with safety is a concentration on increasing regulations from accrediting agencies. Cindy's focus is integration of safety interventions in the fabric of care within the reality of the human condition or error.

CURRENT CNS PRACTICE

Cindy's office is in the middle of the fray. She was initially offered an office outside the inpatient units, but Cindy decided to maintain her position close to staff and patients. In this way, she is accessible to patients, families, and staff. Daily patient rounding provides infinite opportunities for mentoring staff, patient advocacy, and bringing best practices to the bedside. Staff advocacy is very important because Cindy believes CNS roles support and facilitate the expert practice of clinical nurses. Staffs seek her consultation, information, reassurance, and assistance in solving problems. Particularly satisfying is the mentoring of graduate students to the pediatric CNS role.

Holding on to gains made during continuous change and balancing availability to staff and patients with writing, teaching, research, and education best describes Cindy's current practice. Meetings and paperwork consume precious time yet are necessary part of the CNS role. Multitasking is required in order to balance organization and personal goals with day-to-day demands.

PEDIATRIC PALLIATIVE CARE

Palliative care began at Children's Medical Center within an endowed bereavement team. Over time, focus has changed from attention to outpatient palliative care with the goal of dying at home to increasing services for children who require inpatient care due to severity of symptoms and/or lack of human or material resources at home. Cindy provides pain and symptom consults within the interdisciplinary team to preserve the relationships of child and family with the primary nurse and to keep the child on their own unit. Monthly education and development of end-of-life order sets for children with any life-threatening or life-ending process supports clinical nurses and physicians on any unit to provide the evidence-based end-of-life care. Certainly this is strong evidence as to how the CNS role supports and extends the practice of the clinical nurse and facilitates desired outcomes.

Specialized education by the CNS is extended across the spectrum, from medical students to residents. Partnership with local medical centers and statewide groups such as the Ohio Pediatric Palliative End of Life Network (of which Cindy is the treasurer) helps drive best practices, federal and state funding, and grant writing. As a member of the board of directors for the Society of Pediatric Nursing, Sigma Theta Tau, and the American Society of Pediatric Nursing, Cindy is changing the landscape of end-of-life care for children—one bedside at a time.

Cindy further supports nursing practice by individual and group debriefings for staff and families during difficult cases or critical incident reviews. Staff can call a hotline 24 hours a day for any incident or difficulty. The CNS role is pivotal in helping staff respond to grief in themselves or others and to manage the stress of end-of-life care. As necessary, Cindy consults Employee Care for issues beyond end-of-life nursing care.

Based on experience and evidence, Cindy has developed procedural pain guidelines to guide practice in any setting to minimize pain and distress for children. Gradually, this CNS is moving staff through planned change to support family presence during resuscitation. The future holds more change with pending conversion to the electronic medical record.

THE FUTURE

Cindy's goals for the future are full of promise and obstacles. However, this CNS is undaunted. Pediatric palliative care must become more comprehensive and care more formalized to obtain reimbursement and funding to meet community needs. More CNSs are needed to meet staff and family needs.

After careful review of the content of doctor of nursing practice (DNP) programs, Cindy is not convinced that a DNP is required for the CNS role. Furthermore, Cindy believes that current DNP program content adds little beyond current clinical and academic preparation of the CNS. Cindy fears a requirement for a DNP may reduce the number of future CNSs so desperately needed for practice just as the nurse practitioner (NP) programs did in the past decade. She believes increasing interest in the CNS role for advance practice is based on the current health care system's needs as well as the reality of narrow boundaries of the NP role. While the NP role is very important, patients, families, and clinical nurses need the CNS role, which crosses freely across the endless networks in health care to drive expert nursing practice and positive patient outcomes. Though the DNP controversy continues, Cindy believes that nursing should focus instead on the resolution of entry into practice and the nursing shortage.

Cindy is an example of expert CNS practice. Her practice is based on the maxim that excellent nursing care is imbedded in relationships and nurses find satisfaction and purpose through these sacred relationships. Her dedication to the dying child and their family during the terminal phase of illness creates meaning, strength, and a sense of security for all involved in the child's journey. Cindy empowers rather than takes over for clinical nurses at end of life to protect the nurse–child relationship where safety and security rest. Her understanding of suffering, her ability to address unvoiced needs, and her competence and experience provide a rich foundation for end-of-life services at the Children's Medical Center now and in the future. This CNS personifies caring, compassion, and presence in a dark journey made light through the best nursing care.

34

Implementing a Comprehensive Bariatric Care Protocol

Kathleen D. Wright

PRACTICE OVERVIEW

While my primary responsibilities as a wound os-tomy continence (WOC) clinical nurse specialist (CNS) include providing direct services to patients, I also serve as clinical leader for a team of three board-certified WOC nurses with administrative accountability for our service line. Direct patient care is provided by the WOC team across a continuum of care from preventative to restorative in a community hospital with 150 acute care beds and an active out patient setting. Additional ser-vices are provided on a contractual basis for two long-term care settings, two home health agencies and a hospice. Indirect patient care activities include manage-ment of the service area's human and fiscal resources, and participating in organizational team meetings and committees such as product standardization and evalu-ation, health education, service excellence, and leader-ship coordination committees.

While direct patient care remains a central focus of this specialty practice, all three CNS spheres of influence are crucial to successful outcomes. The WOC nurses facilitate implementation and evaluation of pre-ventive skin care and wound management programs. The WOC nurses also provide individual bedside edu-cation as well as formal staff development programs to ensure appropriate implementation of patient-specific treatment recommendations. As research advances the science of the specialty and generates innovative interventions and products, system-wide policies and procedures are reviewed and revised to ensure state-of-the-art specialty care.

The setting's WOC nurses are all members of the Wound Ostomy Continence Nurses Society. The society provides the membership with an annual conference, professional best practice documents and online mem-bership forums to facilitate clinical problem solving and "group think" on timely topics. There is a regional and local affiliate of the national specialty organization, which provides opportunities for networking on a regular basis. Membership in the National Association of Clinical Nurse Specialists, the American Nurses Association, and Sigma Theta Tau provide a well-rounded perspective of the nursing profession with valued insights from other specialties and practice settings. The aging population and the increasing number of complications associated with diabetes and obesity provide both a challenge and opportunity to effectively address the demands for CNSs with an expertise in wound and skin care.

PROBLEM IDENTIFICATION

Obesity is epidemic in our country, with two-thirds of adult Americans overweight or obese. It is estimated that 5 to 10 million people in the United States suffer from severe or morbid obesity (National Center for Health Statistics). Obesity is reported as the second leading cause of preventable death, killing approxi-mately 400,000 Americans annually, and it is associated with more than 30 medical problems, including various dermatological conditions. This chapter discusses the WOC CNS's involvement in developing a bariatric care program in the community hospital setting.

The community hospital initiated the first bariatric surgery program in the state following extensive planning by a multidisciplinary team, which included the bariatric surgeons, CNSs, registered dietitians, certified social workers, and exercise specialists. Hospital-wide staff education and competency development focused on morbid obesity as a chronic illness with associated comorbidities, surgical risks and complications, postoperative care, cultural sensitivity, and access to size-appropriate equipment.

As the volume of bariatric patients increased, the WOC CNS identified a need to further standardize care for this population. Staff frequently requested consultations for specific information regarding equipment, such as weight limits on equipment and nursing interventions for the morbidly obese patient. One emergent weekend call came to the WOC CNS concerning a 750-pound patient scheduled to arrive in the emergency department whose ambulance stretcher was already bending beneath his weight. Another morbidly obese patient under the care of WOC CNS services for management of erythematous lower extremities due to chronic lymphedema became tearful as he told of being "wedged into a bedside chair" and of delays in toileting because staff could not access a bariatric commode. Safety issues were also identified. The extra-wide bariatric bed that had to be constructed in a patient's room would not fit through the doorway or onto the elevator, thus a transport stretcher or wheelchair had to be constantly available to prevent delays in testing, treatment, or potential emergency evacuation.

GOALS FOR PRACTICE INNOVATION

The CNS's goal was to develop and implement a comprehensive bariatric care protocol. The bariatric care protocol was holistic and addressed the multiple common clinical needs of this patient problem. In addition, the protocol promoted safety concerns for patients and staff by outlining the use of specially modified equipment. The protocol also promoted patient dignity as issues of stigma, shame, and embarrassment are common for this patient group.

INNOVATION SPECIFICS

The WOC CNS collaborated with the bariatric program director to develop a comprehensive bariatric care protocol (see Table 34.1).

The bariatric protocol outlines important assessment parameters to be considered upon the patient's entry into the facility's care. On admission, patients are assessed for weight and height. Body mass index (BMI) charts are available with the protocol for staff reference; patients with a BMI greater than normal are expected to be assessed for abdominal/hip girth related to ability for safe lateral repositioning or chair sitting. Caregiver risk for injury is closely linked to the patient's level of activity, with greater risk associated with lower patient activity, thus, this parameter is critical for planning both patient care and staffing assignments.

As with all patients admitted to the hospital, a comprehensive head-to-toe skin assessment is completed on the bariatric patient. Staff are expected to be particularly alert for common obesity-related skin complications, including candidiasis in the perineum area or skin folds, incontinence-related dermatitis secondary to inability to perform personal hygiene, pressure ulcers (including sites other than bony prominences), venous insufficiency/ulceration, and/or lymphedema in the lower extremities. After assessment, staff make note of urgent equipment needs, such as CPAP for preventing respiratory comorbidities, a bariatric walker to facilitate mobility, or a bariatric bedside commode for toileting.

After completing a comprehensive patient assessment, specific treatment plans and management guidelines are developed to address individualized patient needs. For patients > 204.6 kg (450 lbs) and/or those with significantly widened hip girth interventions might include obtaining size-sensitive equipment, including a bariatric bed. The protocol provides a guideline that the standard hospital frame is 39 inches in width and accommodates up to 204.6 kg (450 lbs). A bariatric bed, stored in the post-anesthesia care unit, can be accessed at all times for nonsurgical bariatric patients' admissions as needed. The protocol delineates the location of a wheelchair-accessible bariatric scale that can accommodate up to 454.4 kg (1,000 lbs), which is available in the day surgery unit.

To help ensure safe clinical care and patient dignity, staff in all patient care areas have access to bariatric blood pressure cuffs, bariatric patient gowns, and bariatric sequential compression boots. For patients requiring total or partial assistance with mobility, appropriate size-sensitive lift, transfer, ambulation, and transportation equipment is available. The protocol notes that the standard hospital stretcher accommodates up to 227.2 kg (500 lbs); both bariatric transport stretchers and bariatric wheelchairs are available. Patient lateral transfer devices can accommodate up to 363.3 kg (800 lbs) and are available on all acute care areas. The bariatric protocol also notes that an overhead lift device is available from the post-anesthesia care unit.

EVALUATION AND OUTCOMES

The bariatric protocol is available in the hospital policy and procedure manuals, accessible in each patient care area. Regardless of whether a facility has a surgical

34.1 | Bariatric Care Protocol Policy

TITLE: Bariatric Care	Policy #
	Database # 1965
CATEGORY: Protocol	Page: 1 of 3
OWNER: Kathy Wright	Effective: 10/03
MANUAL: Care of the Patient, DO-WOCN	Reviewed/Revised:
Committee Review: CCLC	
Signature: Vicki L. Allen, 08/11/04	Required Review: Every 3 years

PURPOSE:
To meet the physical needs of the bariatric patient promoting clinical safety and dignity.
NOTE: The word *bariatric* pertains to weight and is used in the field of health care to describe the treatment and management of weight. Weight is measured in kilograms. When referenced with a person's height it can be described in terms of body mass index (BMI) and categorized accordingly: normal (BMI 20–25), overweight (BMI 26–29), obese (BMI 30–39), morbid obese (BMI >40).

PERSONNEL:
All NMH patient care providers.

DESIRED PATIENT OUTCOME:
To ensure patient and caregiver safety, patient dignity, and emergency preparedness.

AREAS OF RESPONSIBILITY	CARE DIRECTIVES
Assessment	On admission, patient should be assessed for:
	1. Weight/height.
	2. Estimated abdominal/hip girth related to ability for safe lateral repositioning or chair sitting.
	3. Level of dependency
	A. Total assist
	1. Cannot support own weight and/or is uncooperative.
	2. Little to no upper body strength.
	B. Partial assist
	1. Able to bear weight but needs assistance more than supervision/instruction.
	2. Upper body strength.
	C. Independent
	1. Requires only supervision/instruction.
	2. Performs tasks safely with or without assistive devices.
	4. Skin complications
	A. Candidiasis within perineum or skin folds.
	B. Incontinence-related dermatitis secondary to inability to perform personal hygiene.
	C. Pressure ulcers.
	D. Venous stasis/lymphedema.
	E. Presence of or needs for specialized equipment, e.g., glucometer, C-PAP, walker, bedside commode.
Treatment/Management	1. For patients >204.6 kilograms (450 lbs) and/or significantly widened hip girth, consider the use of appropriate size-sensitive equipment:
	A. Bariatric bed (see Procedure # 922: Specialty Bed Rentals). Standard hospital frame is 39" in width and accommodates up to 204.6 kilograms (450 lbs).
	B. Bariatric bedside commode.
	C. Bariatric scale (wheelchair accessible and accommodates up to 454.4 kilograms [1,000 lbs], available from Day Surgery).
	D. Bariatric blood pressure cuff.
	E. Bariatric patient gowns.
	F. Bariatric sequential compression boots, e.g., Flowtrons, if ordered.
	G. Gradient sequential compression boots. Consult WOCN for appropriate placement.

(Continued)

34.1 | Bariatric Care Protocol Policy (*Continued*)

	2. For patients requiring total or partial assistance with mobility, appropriate size-sensitive lift, transfer, ambulation and transportation equipment should be used: A. Stretcher chair—Camtec Converta Litter available in ICU . B. Bariatric transport stretcher—Standard hospital stretcher up to 227.2 kilograms (500 lbs). C. Bariatric wheelchair. D. Bariatric walker. E. Hover Matt—accommodates up to 363.3 kilograms (800 lbs). Available on all acute care areas. F. Vertical lift device— Sit-to-Stand device available on PCU and MSU. G. Bariatric Hoyer/overhead lift device, available from PACU upon completion of Specialty Equipment Requisition form (see Patient Care Specialty Equipment policy and procedure).
Consultation/Referral	1. Wound ostomy continence nurse 2. PT/OT 3. Social worker/case management 4. Registered dietician 5. Bariatric program coordinator
Documentation	1. Clinical notes 2. Patient education form 3. Specialty equipment requisition form
Patient Education	1. Educate family/caregiver on safe and effective use of equipment.

bariatric program or not, ongoing attention to staff education and the organization's physical environment is central in identifying potential areas of risk and opportunities for improvements in meeting the needs of this special patient population. Providing care for morbidly obese patients will continue to present unique challenges to staff and patients not only for surgical bariatric patients but for all patients across the continuum of care (Wright, 2005). Access to equipment sensitive to a person's weight and habitus for purposes of mobility, lift/transfer, and testing is an important consideration for patient care staff. Development of an organization-wide protocol specifically designed to meet the needs of the bariatric patient was found to facilitate safe and dignified care for both patient and caregiver (Siewinski, 2003).

Many CNS competencies were operationalized in the design and development of this practice innovation. *Theoretical foundations* enabled the CNS to incorporate the obese patients' perspectives of care delivery into a protocol that would facilitate safe and effective self-care with dignity. Recognition of significant *phenomena of concern*, including potential skin breakdown, mobility limitations, and ineffective coping related to self-image prompted the use of validated measurement tools, for example, the Braden Skin Risk Assessment Tool and other evaluation methods to guide cost-effective patient care. Effective *teaching and coaching strategies* were utilized to facilitate synthesis of the bariatric protocol into staff practice patterns. Clinical inquiry and knowledge of technology, products, and devices combined with interdisciplinary consultation and systems thinking toward positive outcomes for the hospitalized bariatric patient (National Association of Clinical Nurse Specialists, 2004).

REFERENCES

Baptiste, A., & Nelson, A. (2004). Bariatric safety. *Advance for Nurses, 5,* 39.

Barr, J., & Cunneen, J. (2001). Understanding the bariatric client and providing a safe hospital environment. *Clinical Nurse Specialist, 15*(5), 219–223.

Gallagher, S. (2004). Obesity: Considering mobility, patient safety and caregiver injury. In W. Charney & M. Hudson (Eds.), *Back injury among healthcare workers: Causes, solutions and impact.* New York: Lewis Press.

Gallagher, S. M. (1998). Caring for obese patients. *Nursing, 28*(3), 98.

Gallagher, S., Arzouman, J., Lacovara, J., Blackett, A., McDonald, P., Traver, G., et al. (2004). Criteria-based protocols and the obese pateint: Pre-planning care for a high risk population. *Ostomy/Wound Management, 5,* 32–34.

Gallagher, S., & Gates J. (2003). Obesity, panniculitis, panniculectomy, and wound care: Understanding the challenges. *Journal of Wound Ostomy Continence Nursing, 30*(6), 334.

Gallagher, S., Langlois, C., Spacht, D., & Henns, T. (2004). Preplanning with protocols for skin and wound care in obese patients. *Advances in Wound and Skin Care, 17,* 436–443.

Garcia-Hidalog, L. (2002). Dermatologic complications of obesity. *American Journal of Clinical Dermatology, 3*(6), 497–506.

Hahler, B. (2006). An overview of dermatological conditions commonly associated with the patient with obesity. *Ostomy/Wound Management, 52*(6), 34–47.

Hill-Rom Bariatric Program. (2003, July). *Care of the severely obese patient.* Baltimore, MD: Author.

Lemiska, L. (2003). Meeting the needs of obese patients. In C. Milne, L. Corbett, & D. Dubuc (Eds.), *Wound, ostomy, and continence nursing secrets.* Philadelphia: Hanley & Belfus.

Mathison, C. (2003). Skin and wound care challenges in the hospitalized morbidly obese patient. *Journal of Wound Ostomy Continence Nursing, 30*(6), 78.

National Association of Clinical Nurse Specialists. (2004). *Statement on clinical nurse specialist practice and education* (2nd ed.). Harrisburg, PA: Author.

National Center for Health Statistics. *Prevalence of overweight and obesity among adults: United States.* Retrieved January 11, 2009, from http://www.cdc.gov/nchs/

Ryan, M. A. (2005). My story: A personal perspective on bariatric surgery. *Critical Care Nurse Quarterly, 28,* 288–292.

Siewinski, T. (2003). Evacuation of bariatric patients. *Advance for Nurses, 3,* 31.

Strumia, R. (2005). Dermatologic signs in patients with eating disorders. *American Journal of Clinical Dermatology, 6*(3), 165–173.

Wilson, J., & Clark J. (2004). Obesity: Impediment to wound healing. *Advances in Skin and Wound Care, 17,* 426–431.

Wright, K., & Bauer, C. (2005). Meeting bariatric patient care needs. *Journal of Wound Ostomy Continence Nursing, 32*(6), 402–406.

35

Improving Patient Pain Management Across a Health Care System

Mary Pat Johnston

PRACTICE OVERVIEW

As an oncology clinical nurse specialist (CNS) for a community-based, multisite regional cancer center in southeastern Wisconsin, I provide CNS services to four medical oncology clinics, three radiation oncology clinics, one dedicated inpatient unit, and a medical-surgical unit within three settings: a suburban 300-bed hospital, a rural 100-bed hospital with connected outpatient clinics, and two freestanding outpatient facilities. My primary responsibilities include: managing complex physical, psychological, social, and spiritual symptoms that people with cancer and their families experience through consultation and collaboration with other oncology nurses, physicians, and other interdisciplinary team members; mentoring new oncology nurses in caring for people with cancer and their families, as well as the administration of chemotherapy and biotherapy agents; designing and implementing oncology-specific education programs for ongoing continuing education and oncology-related competencies, such as preparation of staff for new and novel therapies in the cancer center, which includes the development of policies, protocols, preprinted order sets, and patient- and family-centered education materials; and leading performance improvement initiatives in the regional cancer center with an emphasis on the integration of an evidence-based practice and measurement of outcomes to promote patient safety and quality cancer care. Additionally, I provide CNS knowledge, skills, and expertise to organizational initiatives, such as implementation of shared practice through facilitation and

membership on several councils, professional development through a clinical advancement process, and evidence-based practice through integration of a model and promotion of nursing research. I hold an advanced certification in oncology nursing. As a volunteer, I have served the Oncology Nursing Society (ONS) in a variety of roles, such as president of the local chapter, member of a planning committee for the Advanced Practice Nurse (APN) Conference 2004, advisory panel member for Evidence-Based Practice Outcomes, project team member for the development of Putting Evidence Into Practice (PEP) Resources, member of the CNS Special Interest Group, and selected as member of the steering council, subsequently serving a 1-year term as chair.

PROBLEM IDENTIFICATION

Although The Joint Commission mandated health care organizations to create the infrastructure to develop, implement, and evaluate improvements in pain assessment and management, adopting these recommendations in clinical settings has been complicated (Berry & Dahl, 2000). The obstacles have been described as lack of education about appropriate pain assessment and management strategies, deeply held attitudes about pain, lack of awareness of the negative consequences of pain, and fears of patients and families, especially regarding pain medications (McCaffery & Pasero, 1999; Paice, Barnard, Creamer, & Omerod, 2006). With knowledge and expertise in cancer pain management as an oncology CNS and demonstrated leadership in a pain improvement initiative within the cancer center, the senior nurse executive asked me to co-lead the organization's implementation of the pain standards with the integrated care coordinator. To build the case for change, we identified data that already existed and determined other tools to obtain missing data, collaborating with staff nurses and other resources to obtain it from house-wide patient satisfaction surveys, chart audits, and patient surveys about their pain experiences. The engagement of other nursing staff and disciplines in data collection facilitated the transition of ownership from my project to everyone's project. The baseline data from one of the clinics within the cancer center indicated that only 66% of patients were assessed for pain. It was a startling finding for physicians and nurses, who believed that pain management was not an issue in our clinic. All of the results were presented to key stakeholders along with a plan for improvement. Other findings were that no consistent pain scale was utilized across the organization, myths and misconceptions about pain were pervasive as staff described the addictive behaviors of patients and difficulty accepting the patient's report of pain, and limited understanding of pain medications and equianalgesia. The cornerstone of the improvement plan was to develop and implement a pain resource nurse (PRN) program to create clinical resources, patient advocates, role models, and champions of change at the bedside.

GOALS FOR PRACTICE INNOVATION

While the overall goal was to improve pain management across our organization, the goals of this practice innovation were to provide specialized training in pain management to registered nurses (RNs) to advance the knowledge and skills of the nurse, who provides direct patient care, and to expedite implementation of the pain standards in the care of patients across the organization. The model of the PRN training course was first developed at the City of Hope National Medical Center in Duarte, California, as a 5-day course (Ferrell, Grant, Ritchey, Ropchan, & Rivera, 1993). Over the years, other organizations across the country have embraced this program as a means to improve pain management (Holley, McMillan, Hagan, Palacios, & Rosenberg, 2005; McCleary, Ellis, & Rowley, 2004; Paice et al., 2006). As the CNS leader, I developed a formal proposal and budget, identified potential funding sources, completed grant applications, cultivated enthusiasm among nurse staff for the program, and collaborated with two nurse educators, three staff nurses, and an integrated care coordinator. Based on previous work, experiences, and staff needs, I adapted the format to a 3-day training PRN

course and coordinated a follow-up plan for role implementation, support, and evaluation.

INNOVATION SPECIFICS

With the first course, participants were asked to complete an application for the program, meet eligibility criteria, and were selected by a committee to identify highly motivated nurses who not only would make changes in their own practice, but serve as change agents in their clinical areas for the implementation of pain standards. In addition, they completed pre- and postcourse knowledge and attitudes surveys. For our course, I identified topics, key objectives and content, internal and external faculty, and program agenda. I completed and submitted the application for nursing contact hours to enhance the professionalism of the program. Other members of the committee organized program logistics, posters, brochures, mailings, and announcements. One of the nurse educators and I created a logo for the course. The participants received materials including a course binder with handouts from the faculty lectures, key pain policies, current patient education materials, equianalgesic dosing chart, and other supplemental resources for reinforcement of training and tools for postcourse activities. The senior nurse executive for the organization was invited to provide closing remarks for the 3-day training program and celebrate with a reception that followed distribution of their training completion certificates. Other forms of recognition included PRN buttons, 8 x 17-inch posters individualized for their units or clinics identifying them as the PRN, and press releases in the organization's newsletters. Additionally, performance improvement initiatives were highlighted in newsletters or poster displays. After the course, participants developed an action plan for next steps in their clinical area, attended quarterly networking meetings and continuing education sessions for implementation of their new role within the first year, and evaluated participant and program outcomes. Based on PRN identified needs, an 8-hour advanced pain concepts course was added to update pharmacology, review equianalgesia, discuss case studies in complex pain, provide performance improvement data, and describe current initiatives in their clinical areas.

EVALUATION AND OUTCOMES

Our PRN program increased awareness about pain and pain management; dispelled myths; redefined expectations about pain assessment and management; and identified gaps in pharmacology knowledge, especially in regards to opioids and equianalgesia. With 40 participants in the inaugural course, the average precourse survey score was 80.4%, with a postcourse score of 89.9%. In 2006, 35 self-selected participants had an average precourse score of 58.9% and a postcourse score of 81.1%. PRN contributions have included revisions to policies, documentation tools, and discharge instructions; development of unit- or clinic-based newsletters, poster displays, learning boards, additional educational programs, and inservices; unit- or clinic-based performance improvement activities; and greater participation by PRNs in organizational pain initiatives, such as selection of new IV patient-controlled analgesia device. While these findings demonstrate an increase in knowledge, especially for later course participants, education alone does not change practice, underscoring the importance of mentoring experiences as the PRN implements this new knowledge and role. Clinical education programs such as the PRN program offer nurses the opportunity to discover what they do not know. As a CNS, I articulate the vision and identify the next steps for advancing nurse practice in the management of pain. At a time of rapid changes in technology, crises in the current health care environment, nursing shortages, and competition for resources, it is critical to provide mentoring experiences to support the integration of new knowledge and changes in practice. With more than 100 registered nurses trained as PRNs, my next steps will be to: (1) provide mentor training to current PRNs to foster their growth and development, (2) transition the initial PRN course to a 2-day program with an additional 1-day course approximately 6 months later, and (3) formalize quarterly networking and education sessions. The PRN program has been a catalyst for practice changes within our organization, identifying gaps in the care of patients experiencing pain, and has led to unit- or clinic-based and organizational performance improvement initiatives.

This chapter describes core CNS competencies in action, building on the foundation of expertise in oncology pain management, evolving into leadership for an organization's initiative, and demonstrating use of power among several spheres of influence (National Association of Clinical Nurse Specialists, 2004). Although the patient/client sphere grounded me, clearly, the nursing and nursing practice sphere and the systems/organization sphere were critical to implementation of a PRN program and integration of pain standards across the organization.

REFERENCES

Berry, P., & Dahl, J. (2000). The new JCAHO pain standards: Implications for pain management nurses. *Pain Management Nursing, 1*(1), 3–12.

Ferrell, B. R., Grant, M., Ritchey, K. J., Ropchan, R., & Rivera, L. M. (1993). The pain resource nurse training program: A unique approach to pain management. *Journal of Pain and Symptom Management, 8*(8), 549–556.

Holley, S., McMillan, S. C., Hagan, S. J., Palacios, P., & Rosenberg, D. (2005). Pain resource nurses: Believing the patients, and believing in themselves. *Oncology Nursing Forum, 32*(4), 843–848.

McCaffery, M., & Pasero, C. (1999). *Pain: A clinical manual* (2nd ed.). St. Louis: Mosby.

McCleary, L., Ellis, J. A., & Rowley, B. (2004). Evaluation of the pain resource nurse role: A resource for improving pediatric management. *Pain Management Nursing, 5*(1), 29–36.

National Association of Clinical Nurse Specialists. (2004). *Statement on clinical nurse specialist practice and education* (2nd ed.). Harrisburg, PA: Author.

Paice, J. A., Barnard, C., Creamer, J., & Omerod, K. (2006). Creating organizational change through the Pain Resource Nurse program. *Joint Commission Journal of Quality and Patient Safety, 32*(1), 24–31.

36

Leading Revisions of Neutropenia Practice Guidelines

Barbara Holmes Gobel

PRACTICE OVERVIEW

As an oncology clinical nurse specialist (CNS), I work in a large metropolitan medical center in the midwestern part of the United States. My scope of practice as a CNS includes two acute inpatient oncology units, including the specialties of hematology, general oncology, stem cell transplantation, and palliative care and hospice. The primary focus of my role is to advance nursing practice at the hospital. This is done through activities such as educational development of the nursing staff, updating oncology related policies and procedures, consultation on symptom management of patients with cancer, and supporting evidence-based practice via research activities and evidence-based journal clubs.

PROBLEM IDENTIFICATION

In my setting of care, one of the clinical concerns voiced by the nursing staff was about the benefit and necessity of our institution-specific practices and policies regarding the care of the patient with chemotherapy-induced neutropenia. Many of the nurses expressed concern about the restrictive nature of the neutropenic precautions (neutropenia is defined at this institution as an absolute granulocyte count of < 500 cells/mm^3) undertaken in the management of these patients, such as instituting a low-microbial diet when the patient becomes neutropenic; restriction of plants, flowers, silk flowers, and balloons on each of the acute oncology units; and the need for the use of masks when patients are outside of their patient care rooms. Patients also complained

about the restrictions related to their neutropenic conditions, particularly patients who underwent stem cell transplantation and were required to be in the hospital for lengthy periods of time, for example, not being allowed to have silk flowers or balloons in their room to brighten the environment. One of the outcomes of CNS practice in the nurses and nursing practice sphere of influence is that evidence-based practices are used by nurses (National Association of Clinical Nurse Specialists [NACNS], 2004). Based on this, I helped to establish the Neutropenia Journal Club, which was developed to review the evidence in the literature regarding the nursing management of neutropenic patients.

GOALS FOR PRACTICE INNOVATION

The goal of the Neutropenia Journal Club was to review the existing research regarding the nursing management of the patient with neutropenia and to develop proposed practice changes based on the existing evidence. The journal club developed the following question to guide their review of the evidence: "Are the current neutropenic precautions practices and policy and procedure evidence-based?" The journal club was made up of the CNS, staff nurses from each of the oncology units, staff educators from each of the oncology units, the infection control coordinator (a registered nurse [RN]), and the stem cell transplant dietician. The cochairs of the journal club were members of the institution's nursing research committee (the CNS and a staff educator).

A literature search was undertaken by the CNS with assistance from the staff educators and the hospital medical librarian. The topics that were searched included the areas of concern voiced by the nursing staff (e.g., general diet versus a low-microbial diet; restriction of plants, flowers, silk flowers, and balloons; and the need for masks worn by patients with associated neutropenia while outside of their patient room). The journal club met once a month for 10 months to review the literature and to develop practice recommendations.

Another outcome of CNS practice in the nurses and nursing practice sphere of influence is that knowledge and skill development needs of nurses are delineated (NACNS, 2004). CNSs are educated to review and critique the evidence (research) and help to translate the evidence into practice. "CNS practice is the translation of clinical expertise into nursing care provided either directly or by influencing nurses and nursing personnel through evidence-based nursing care standards and programs of care" (NACNS, pp. 5–6).

This was one of the goals of the CNS in this activity: to increase the research utilization skills of the staff nurse. The objectives of this goal were to identify and review a model of change for evidence-based practice and to help the staff to begin to differentiate the different levels of evidence that are presented via research findings. Articles to help meet these objectives were reviewed in the journal club meetings. The model of evidence-based practice that was chosen for review is one that is adopted by our institution for nursing research, the Rosswurm and Larrabee model (Rosswurm & Larrabee, 1999). This model takes the individuals involved in evidence-based practice changes from assessing the need for change in practice through integrating and maintaining that change in practice. See Exhibit 36.1 for a synthesis of the Rosswurm and Larrabee model of evidence-based practice.

The model for the levels of evidence that we reviewed and adopted is the Oncology Nursing Society (ONS) *Levels of Evidence* (See Table 36.1) (Ropka &

Spencer-Cisek, 2001). This model for levels of evidence was adapted from the Haydorn model of rating the quality of evidence for clinical practice guidelines (Haydorn, Baker, Hodges, & Hicks, 1996). Review of all articles was done at the journal club meetings. The journal club maintained a table for documentation of reviewed research studies, including such aspects as characteristics of the intervention, sample characteristics (e.g., age, gender, disease, and treatment characteristics), dependent and independent variables, prevention of infection in neutropenic patients, any special training that is required to deliver the intervention, results/conclusions, and the ONS evidence rating.

Another competency of CNS practice, Intervention: Developing and Testing Solutions, was also met by helping to develop the knowledge and skills of nurses, that is, to mentor nurses to critique and apply research findings to nursing practice.

LITERATURE REVIEW

Several articles were chosen to review as part of the Neutropenia Journal Club. One article of particular interest to the group was a systematic review of nursing interventions (Larson & Nirenberg, 2004) that summarized the evidence related to issues such as low-microbial diets, as well as protective clothing and environments of care of the neutropenic patient. The authors provided an overview of a Cochrane database of systematic reviews (high-level systematic reviews and meta-analyses) that were reviewed for clean food and water, protective environments and clothing, and skin care/oral hygiene. They reported that no recent studies were found that linked dietary restrictions with a lower risk for infection. They also reported that significant gaps exist between empirical evidence and those nursing interventions that may prevent infection in neutropenic patients.

INNOVATION SPECIFICS

An important outcome of CNS practice in the nurses and nursing practice sphere of influence is that nurses are able to articulate their unique contributions to patient care and nurse-sensitive outcomes (NACNS, 2004). After reviewing and compiling the data regarding the research findings about the care of the neutropenic patient, the members of the Neutropenia Journal Club then compiled a list of proposed practice changes (accepted practice changes are also included) based on the available evidence. See Table 36.2 for a list of neutropenia journal club proposed and accepted practice changes.

These proposed practice changes were then taken to a number of committees for approval by the cochairs

---

EXHIBIT 36.1 THE ROSSWURM AND LARRABEE MODEL FOR EVIDENCE-BASED PRACTICE

1. Assess need for change
2. Link problem, interventions, and outcomes
3. Synthesize best evidence
4. Design the practice change
5. Implement and evaluate pilot
6. Integrate and maintain practice change

Adapted from "A Model for Change to Evidence-Based Practice," by M. A. Rosswurm and J. H. Larrabee, 1999, *Image: Journal of Nursing Scholarship, 31,* 317–322.

36.1 | Oncology Nursing Society (ONS) Levels of Evidence

ONS LEVEL	LEVEL OF EVIDENCE SUBCATEGORY	EVIDENCE SOURCE	STRENGTH OF EVIDENCE
I – Research-based evidence	1	Meta-analysis or systematic reviews of multiple well-designed, randomized, controlled clinical trials	High
	2	Well-controlled, randomized clinical trials with adequate sample size	High
	3	Well-designed trial without randomization (single group pre/postcohort), time series studies	High
II – Research-based evidence	4	Well-conducted, systematic reviews of nonexperimental design studies	Moderate
	5	Well-conducted case–control study	Moderate
	6	Poorly controlled (flawed randomized studies) or uncontrolled studies (correlational descriptive studies)	Moderate
	7	Conflicting evidence or meta-analysis showing a trend that did not reach significance National Institutes of Health Consensus Report Published practice guidelines, for example by professional organizations, health care organizations, or federal agencies	Moderate
III – Non–research-based evidence	8	Qualitative designs Case studies, opinions of expert authorities, agencies, or committees	Low

From "Rating the Quality of Evidence for Clinical Practice Guidelines," by D. C. Hadorn, D. Baker, J. S. Hodges, & N. Hicks, 1996, *Journal of Clinical Epidemiology, 49,* 749–753. Adapted with permission of the author.

of the journal club. The nursing committees that the practice changes were taken to included the nursing research committee and the nursing practice committee. Because the policy that the group was seeking to change was a patient care policy, it was required to be taken to the patient care committee, the medical executive committee, and the infection control committee.

One of the CNS practice competencies is that of Assessment: Identifying and Defining Problems. The CNS is to identify interpersonal, technological, environmental, or system facilitators and barriers to implementing nursing practices (NACNS, 2004). Prior to taking the proposed practice changes to the various hospital committees, there was an attempt to identify system barriers, such as potential stakeholder issues. The journal club identified the primary stakeholders of these potential practice changes as the patients, the nurses, dietary, and the physicians. At the outset of the formation of the journal club, the CNS met with the cancer quality committee, which had oncologists as members of the committees, and informed them of the intent of the work of the journal club. This committee was an ideal communication conduit because there are many private practice and university-based oncology

physicians at this institution. Unfortunately, this committee disbanded for the period of time that the journal club met and no further formal communication vehicle was identified by the CNS, thus, one of the significant stakeholder groups was not kept informed of the progress of the journal club.

As the proposed practice changes were taken through the hospital committee structure it became apparent that clear and frequent communication with the physician group would have likely improved the flow through the committee structure. As there were no physician champions (e.g., committed stakeholder) of this project, it became evident that each of the physician-based committees required the information to be shared in a unique manner, from lengthy and narrative descriptions of the review of the literature to graphs and tables of the evidence. The journal club was asked to make calls to similar institutions to query about institutional practices regarding the care of the neutropenic patient. It was clarified to the committees that the journal club had undertaken an exhaustive review of the research, which included institutional surveys regarding care of the neutropenic patient, but this step was ultimately undertaken to gain the support of this important stakeholder group.

36.2 | Neutropenia Journal Club Proposed and Accepted Practice Changes (for the following patients: matched unrelated donor, allogeneic, autologous transplant recipients, and all other oncology/hematology neutropenic patients)

NEUTROPENIC MANAGEMENT PRECAUTIONS

Dietary Issues
1. General diet with safe food handling and safe food practices—including well-washed raw vegetables (except for tomatoes) and well-washed thick, smooth-skinned fruits, including salads.
2. Foods to avoid: Raw or uncooked meat or fish, deli meats, cheeses from deli, aged cheeses, fast foods, unpasteurized or raw dairy products, unpasturized beverages, raw honey, raw grain products, brewers yeast, unrefrigerated cream-filled products/desserts, all miso products, salad bars, cold smoked fish, pickled fish.
3. No leftovers older than 48 hours

Fresh Flowers/Plants
1. Acute oncology: Patients that are NOT neutropenic, defined as an absolute neutrophil count <500, are allowed fresh flowers and/or plants in their rooms. However, when the patient becomes neutropenic it is the responsibility of the staff to remove the plant(s) or fresh flowers from the patient's room and have a family member or friend take them home.
2. Stem cell transplant: All fresh flowers and plants are restricted

Silk Flowers/Balloons
1. All patients (including neutropenic patients) are allowed to maintain mylar balloons and silk flowers in their rooms at all times.

Masks
1. All patients (including neutropenic patients) are able to ambulate on their respective units without the use of high-efficiency masks.
2. All neutropenic patients are to wear a high-efficiency (N99) mask while off the unit at ANY time.

Oral Care/Personal Hygiene
1. Chlorhexidine mouth rinses should be eliminated from the floor stock, as well as chemotherapy order templates.
2. Bar soaps to be replaced with soap dispensers in all patient showers.

The approval process for the proposed practice changes took longer to get through the committee structure than it did for the 10 months of data collection and compilation of the evidence.

EVALUATION AND OUTCOMES

Two of the critical competencies of the nurse and nursing practice sphere of influence of the CNS are to disseminate results of changes to stakeholders and develop and implement educational programs that target the needs of staff to improve nursing practice and patient outcomes. Once the proposed practice changes were steered through the hospital committee structure and were approved, the CNS and the members of the journal club had the responsibility to disseminate these changes to the stakeholders.

Dissemination of this information required housewide education as the policy was changed from "Care of the Chemotherapy-Induced Neutropenic Patient" to "Care of the Neutropenic Patient." This required education of the practice changes to all of the patient care areas that attend to neutropenic patients, both inpatient and outpatient. Members of the journal club assisted

in educational programs regarding the changes in the care of the neutropenic patient. There is still a plan to change the educational materials that patients receive regarding management of neutropenia, including patient teaching sheets and the "Stem Cell Transplant Handbook," which patients undergoing this procedure receive prior to their stem cell transplant. Final policy changes were disseminated to all nurses, physicians, advanced practice nurses, and support services (e.g., dietary and social service) that care for the patient who experiences neutropenia.

DISCUSSION OF THE CNS CORE COMPETENCIES

Meeting the core competencies for CNS practice is vital to one's performance as a CNS. Listening to the needs articulated by the nursing staff and the patients for whom you care often guides the activities that you are involved in within this role. The information shared regarding the Neutropenia Journal Club demonstrates how the nurse and nursing sphere of influence competencies were met by one CNS in a medical center.

CNS core competencies provide the foundation for all CNS practice, regardless of specialty. The CNS should be able to actualize these competencies upon entry into the CNS role, based on one's educational preparation. Additional specialty practice competencies may be required.

REFERENCES

Haydorn, D. C., Baker, D., Hodges, J. S., & Hicks, N. (1996). Rating the quality of evidence for clinical practice guidelines. *Journal of Clinical Epidemiology, 49,* 749–753.

Larson, E., & Nirenberg, A. (2004). Evidence-based nursing practice to prevent infection in hospitalized neutropenic patients with cancer. *Oncology Nursing Forum, 31,* 717–723.

National Association of Clinical Nurse Specialists. (2004). *Statement on clinical nurse specialist practice and education* (2nd ed.). Harrisburg, PA: Author.

Rosswurm, M. A., & Larrabee, J. H. (1999). A model for change to evidence-based practice. *Image: Journal of Nursing Scholarship, 31,* 317–322.

Ropka, M. E., & Spencer-Cisek, P. (2001). PRISM: Priority Symptom Management Project Phase 1: Assessment. *Oncology Nursing Forum, 28,* 1585–1594.

Facilitating a Programmatic Approach to Children With Special Health Care Needs

Jo Ellen Rust

PRACTICE OVERVIEW

I am a pediatric clinical nurse specialist (CNS) with a clinical focus in pediatric neuroscience. I facilitate a program, *Children with Complex Care Needs,* at a midwestern quaternary/tertiary children's hospital/referral center in a large metropolitan city. Children with special/complex health care needs often have multibody system involvement leading to complex care scenarios. These children require health services more or less continuously across their lifespan from both generalist and specialist providers and are frequently hospitalized. As a group, they represent one of the most frequent recipients/consumers of pediatric health care services. We envisioned the concept of a multidisciplinary program to meet the particular needs of this population. Our program was developed to implement a system of care for the child with complex health care needs that is seamless, supportive, and safe—a program that brings the child's identified care providers and resources, including child/family, into "a circle of care." Program goals include:

1. Normalize the life of the child in a family and community,
2. Minimize the disruptive impact of the child's condition,
3. Foster the child's maximum growth and development,
4. Foster family-centered care,
5. Foster *medical home* concept,
6. Enhance cross-discipline and cross-service communication and collaboration,
7. Improve both patient/family and provider satisfaction, and
8. Maximize patient safety.

A criterion for referral is that a child be followed by two or more medical services/providers and hospitalized three or more times per year. Referrals are sometimes made on the basis of family need and can come from any provider, including nurses, social workers, physicians, speech therapists, or others. For each patient, the CNS assists the patient and family with a variety of needs, including but not limited to:

1. Direct patient care, synchronization between admitting and consulting services and with nursing staff, and confirmation that patients are admitted to a consistent unit as much as possible;
2. Access to physicians from the multiple services seeing the patient;
3. Coordination and management of medical information pertaining to the patient;
4. Education of family members regarding the diagnosis, treatment, and management of the patient's health condition;

5. Identification of and access to hospital and community-based resources according to the families' needs (social, educational, financial, and medical);
6. Resolution of patient and family complaints;
7. Facilitation of communication between multiple services, staff, and the family; and
8. Management of multiple sources of input for the development of care plans.

Problem Identification

The Epilepsy Foundation (n.d.) reports 300,000 people have a first convulsion each year: 120,000 occurring in persons under the age of 18, with between 75,000 and 100,000 involving children under the age of 5 who have experienced a febrile (fever-caused) seizure. About 200,000 new cases of epilepsy are diagnosed each year, with 45,000 cases in children under the age 15. Prevalence of active epilepsy (history of the disorder plus a seizure or use of antiepileptic medicine within the past 5 years) is estimated to be approximately 2.7 million in the United States, with 326,000 school children through age 14 having epilepsy. By 20 years of age, 1% of the population can be expected to have developed epilepsy. The basic, underlying risk of developing epilepsy is about 1%. Individuals in certain populations are at higher risk. For example, it is estimated that epilepsy can be expected to develop in:

- 10% of children with mental retardation,
- 10% of children with cerebral palsy,
- 50% of children with both disabilities,
- 8.7% of children of mothers with epilepsy,
- 2.4% of children of fathers with epilepsy, and
- 33% of people who have had a single, unprovoked seizure.

Among patients in the *Children with Complex Care Needs* program, the second most frequently affected body system is the nervous system. The third most commonly occurring patient problem across all body systems is a seizure disorder. During the early months of program development, while meeting with patients and families, I identified that education regarding seizures and the management of seizures in children was rudimentary and inconsistent across providers. Resources available through our outpatient pediatric neurology program were not well-known by the inpatient staff and therefore not utilized for patient and family education.

GOALS FOR PRACTICE INNOVATION

In addressing educational needs of patients and families related to epilepsy and seizure management, goals were created based on past comments on patient satisfaction questionnaires. The current goals are written from the patient/family perspective:

1. I will have all my questions answered to my understanding.
2. I will receive all necessary training to care for my child.
3. I will know who to contact for concerns.
4. I will know what my child will need at home, have the supplies I need, and know how to provide care.
5. I will know all others who will be helping me if needed at home.
6. I will understand effects of medications.
7. I will understand how to troubleshoot my child's care.

INNOVATION SPECIFICS

I contacted the pediatric neurology nurse clinician about jointly developing a class on the management of seizures in children for our patients and families. The clinical pharmacist, family resource center librarian, and our patient education coordinators were contacted to assist. With input from the pediatric neurologists, a 1-hour class designed to meet the parental/family expectations noted previously was developed.

The class content was designed to meet patients' and families' concerns through the following objectives:

- Understand the basic anatomy of the nervous system
- Describe what a seizure is
- List common causes of seizures
- Describe how we diagnose a seizure disorder
- Describe different types of seizures
- List risk factors that might trigger seizures
- Understand how seizures are treated with medicine
- Identify other treatment options for seizures
- Know how to care for your child during a seizure
- Work with your doctor to manage your child's seizures
- Know how to discover reliable resources
- Have access to contact information for providers

Our hospital is fortunate to have a family resource center, which includes the family education center. The center's goal is to foster and facilitate the independence of our patients and families. Our patient education coordinators facilitate a schedule of classes designed to meet this goal. They assisted in the implementation of the new class within the existing calendar; the course is offered twice a week, every Tuesday afternoon from 3:00 to 4:00 P.M. and Thursday morning from 10:00 to 11:00 A.M. (except holidays). Our content was tested for learner readability. The educational content was calculated at a Flesch-Kincaid Grade Level of 7.5. The content is presented by me (a CNS) and the neurology clinician together, or we rotate responsibility as our schedules require modification. We have also arranged for backup presenters from the pediatric neurology outpatient staff. The Spanish language patient educator has attended the course and can now provide the content to our Hispanic/Latino population as needed, or we arrange for an interpreter and extra class time if a family with limited English proficiency wishes to attend one of our regular sessions. The class is provided informally in a small, quiet, well-appointed room around a table and chairs. This format provides a relaxed atmosphere for learning away from the bedside. It can be presented at the bedside upon request via a laptop based on presenter availability. In addition to a copy of the PowerPoint slides used in the classroom, patients/families in attendance receive a Parents' Guide to Seizures and Seizure Medicines, a seizure diary, a glossary of terms, a list of available books on epilepsy, and a list of reputable Web sites on epilepsy/seizure disorders. Additional materials available include drug information sheets as desired, information on video EEG, and managing seizures at school.

A teaching record was designed to document the education within the classroom. This record is placed in the inpatient medical record where education can be reinforced by the inpatient staff prior to discharge. If the attendees are outpatient, the record is sent to the health information management department for placement in the patient's medical record.

EVALUATION AND OUTCOMES

The class is offered to the families and patients with a new diagnosis of seizure disorder as well as our long-standing families who were previously diagnosed. The class has been well-received by both groups. Families are encouraged to send grandparents or other family members, as well as others who interact with their child such as babysitters or teachers. The class often stimulates discussion or questions between families and their health care team as reported to us by medical providers.

All participants are asked to anonymously evaluate the class upon completion. Early feedback indicated the content was not presented in an interesting manner. To address this concern we added video streaming of various seizure types to the educational presentation. Subsequent feedback demonstrated that this addition corrected the problem, and evaluations are now stellar.

Class attendance can vary. The class is marketed by the family resource center through their flat screen communication boards, parent bulletin boards on patient care units, and the daily hospital e-newsletter. Additional marketing strategies include a pocket-size invitation to the class with class schedule, contact information, and location. This card is distributed to the inpatient families via the pediatric neurology faculty, residents, and the CNS. An additional card advertising available family resource center classes and time schedule is made available for use with all children with complex care needs and their families. Upon identifying its availability through the online marketing efforts or through one of our system employees, adult patients and families have also availed themselves of the class.

DISCUSSION OF THE CNS CORE COMPETENCIES

CNSs have as their principal focus nursing's unique scientific and practical contributions in the management of symptoms and functional problems to meet distinctively different societal needs at the individual, group, community, and health care institution levels. Within the patient/client sphere of influence, CNSs develop, implement, and evaluate innovative educational programs for patients, families, and groups. Access to health information and knowledge acquisition through patient/family education enhances the attainment of predicted outcomes while minimizing unintended consequences for patients and families. Within the nursing sphere of influence, the teaching record provides a collaborative guide for the synergistic effect of the classroom method with the educational reinforcement by the bedside nurse at the point of care. This work continues to solidify relationships between patients, families, and their providers by helping families better understand their child's condition and treatment plan, encouraging participative decision making, and increasing open, honest dialogue between all. Within the organizational sphere, variation in patient family knowledge acquisition was identified. Facilitators in the organizational structure like the family education center, and existing patient education materials were utilized. Content development and implementation required multidisciplinary linkages across medicine, nursing, pharmacy, patient education, and families. This class also provides a generalizable patient education program applicable across differing units, diagnoses, populations, or medical specialties along the full continuum of care (National Association of Clinical Nurse Specialists, 2004).

REFERENCES

Epilepsy Foundation. (n.d.). *About epilepsy: Epilepsy and seizure statistics*. Available from http://www.epilepsyfoundation.org/about/statistics.cfm; accessed January 11, 2009.

National Association of Clinical Nurse Specialists. (2004). *Statement on clinical nurse specialist practice and education* (2nd ed.). Harrisburg, PA: Author.

Psychiatric Consultation Liaison Clinical Nurse Specialist in the Acute Care Setting

Pamela A. Minarik

Psychiatric consultation liaison nursing (PCLN) practice integrates the psychiatric, psychosocial, and physical aspects of care in a systems approach. PCLN specialists practice in nonpsychiatric settings such as hospitals, long-term care facilities, rehabilitation centers, home care agencies, ambulatory clinics, private practices, and public health departments and may care for populations of any age. Usually, the PCLN specialist is in a staff or consultative position rather than an administrative position. The client of the PCLN specialist may be the person with actual or potential physical illness, family members, nurses or other clinicians, or the health care system itself. PCLN began in the United States but has grown internationally (Minarik & Neese, 2002).

The practice of most PCLN specialists involves direct and indirect care, the nurses and nursing practice sphere, the client sphere of influence, and the systems/organizations sphere of influence. Direct care psychiatric mental health nursing services emphasize coping responses to acute, catastrophic, chronic, and potential physical dysfunction; identification of undiagnosed psychiatric disorder; and preventive care to decrease the impact of distress and mental disorder. In addition, the practice includes the identification of behavioral, emotional, and cognitive manifestations of pathological physical conditions and collaboration with other health care disciplines in diagnosis, intervention, and evaluation. PCLN specialists use short-term, crisis-oriented mental health interventions and education to bridge the gap between psychiatric and physical nursing care (Minarik & Neese, 2002; Yakimo, Kurlowicz, & Murray, 2004).

Staff in nonpsychiatric settings often feel ill-equipped to deal with the demoralization and distress that are common with physical illness, patient behavior problems that complicate caregiving, conflicts with other staff members, and the multiple and rapid changes in contemporary health care (Yakimo et al., 2004). Lazarus's (1998) work on trivialization of distress is an important resource for understanding demoralization and distress common with physical illness. PCLN specialists have a multifaceted consultative practice that includes indirect interventions to help staff with these difficulties as well as consultation with managers regarding organizational issues, communication, and teamwork problems.

Sparacino and Cartwright (2000) described the relationship of CNS competencies and spheres of influence as follows: what a CNS does (the subroles of expert clinician, consultant, educator, and researcher, and possibly administrator) and how a CNS performs the role (CNS competencies) affects the practice setting through effective use of influence (spheres of influence). This chapter includes two vignettes to illustrate the range of PCLN CNS practice in relation to roles, competencies, and influence. The first vignette is of direct care and indirect care that involved the client sphere of influence and nurses and nursing practice sphere of influence. The second vignette is of indirect care involving the nurses and nursing practice sphere of influence and the systems/organizations sphere of influence.

MRS. LIU

The setting was a West Coast academic medical center where the PCLN CNS had practiced for over 10 years and was well-known. The referral to the CNS came from experienced adult intensive care unit (ICU) nurses who were caring for an elderly Chinese woman with cancer, Mrs. Liu, who was on a ventilator and communicating little. The nurses expressed the moral distress felt by the medical and nursing team who believed that further treatment was futile, but the family wanted everything done, particularly more chemotherapy. The team members experienced helplessness and distress when they encountered difficulty in helping the family to recognize and acknowledge the transition from possible recovery to acceptance of probable death (Robichaux & Clark, 2006).

Two granddaughters, who were acting as family spokespersons, conveyed the family's anger and distress, believing that the physicians and nurses were giving up too quickly in asking the family to agree to stop treatment and withdraw life-supporting interventions. They believed there was potential for recovery, and the staff believed the family did not understand the implications of the biomedical choices. Robichaux and Clark (2006), who conducted research on prognostic conflict at the end of life, found that family members are unprepared for the end-of-life decision-making role of families and, further, that acceptance of probable death was an evolving process that did not occur quickly. The staff and family, coming from different cultural perspectives, were not communicating well. The staff came from the culture of contemporary American biomedicine (Kleinman & Benson, 2006) and the family from the perspective of a multigenerational immigrant Chinese Buddhist family.

Goals and Description of Intervention

After initial assessment based on discussions with the nurses, the nurse manager of the ICU, and members of the ICU and oncology medical teams, the PCLN CNS determined initial goals for care of the Liu family were to first understand the family's viewpoint, preferences, values, and needs and then design interventions that would help the family reach a realistic understanding of Mrs. Liu's condition and help the staff provide care in a culturally and ethically appropriate manner (Institute of Medicine, 2000; Kleinman & Benson, 2006; Lipson & Dibble, 2005; Lipson, Dibble, & Minarik, 1996). The

immediate goal was to enhance communication among the people involved and for the health care providers to meet the family *where they were* instead of trying to push them to the biomedical perspective.

The CNS used the explanatory models approach that Kleinman and Benson (2006) called performing "mini-ethnography" (p. 1674). This approach involves asking about ethnic identity and determining whether it matters for the family and patient and then evaluating what is at stake in the illness episode. Following that, the focus is on the meaning of illness based on the explanatory models the patient and family members use to understand the illness episode. Explanatory models may or may not include the biomedical perspective. The next step is to consider the psychosocial stressors and supports in the patient's and family members' lives. Finally, an important step is to examine the influence of culture on clinical relationships, which includes the culture of biomedicine and questioning the view that technical expertise is the best answer.

The CNS facilitated meetings with the granddaughters, and the primary nurse focused on discovering the culture of the family, their explanation of Mrs. Liu's illness, family roles, and their expectations and hopes. Mrs. Liu had been responsible for care of the granddaughters through their childhood. They loved, respected, and honored her and demonstrated this in the ICU by visiting regularly and speaking up. After coming to the United States, Mrs. Liu had never learned English, did not speak Mandarin or Cantonese, and spoke only a dialect from her small village in China. In addition, Mrs. Liu was Buddhist, although the granddaughters were not, and other family members were nonpracticing. The granddaughters stressed the central importance for their grandmother and the family of making medical decisions in consideration of ancestors and future family generations, thus, they could not give up or make a decision to stop medical treatment and withdraw support. In addition, the granddaughters wanted to create an environment in the ICU room that would feel safe and comfortable for their grandmother.

The meetings facilitated by the CNS were followed by regular short meetings between the primary nurses and the granddaughters. The purpose of these meetings was to review nursing care with the granddaughters, help them gain a realistic picture of their grandmother's day-to-day care and condition, and begin to recognize probable death.

To improve communication between the ICU nurses and Mrs. Liu, the second intervention was a large chart created with common words and phrases about patient needs and nursing actions in the ICU and the equivalent term in the phonetically written Chinese dialect. This chart was a collaborative effort and gave the granddaughters a recognized role in patient care. It was posted in Mrs. Liu's room, visible to all health care providers and used to aid verbal communication.

To increase Mrs. Liu's comfort in the environment, her granddaughters brought in a familiar red blanket, which was kept on the bed by the nurses. The granddaughters also brought in familiar Chinese music, and the nurses took responsibility for playing it softly. The nurses felt they were able to do something, seemingly small, to meet important family needs.

Regular family meetings were held to enhance communication between the family (including the granddaughters, their father, and other family members), Mrs. Liu, and the medical and nursing staff. Because the nursing staff assumed responsibility for communication, the PCLN CNS participated in the family meetings irregularly. In these meetings, Mrs. Liu's condition and treatment plan were reviewed, and medical decisions were discussed. Family members conveyed the content of the discussions to Mrs. Liu and communicated to the staff their wish for continued chemotherapy. Although the medical and nursing teams believed treatment was futile, everyone agreed to one more trial of chemotherapy and, later, if that was not effective, to ending chemotherapy. Family meetings continued, and the family's urgency about more treatment lessened. The family began to feel listened to and understood, and they felt that everything that could be done was done. Eventually, Mrs. Liu was extubated without requiring the family to make a decision. The ICU team respected what was at stake for the family for ancestors and future generations. With her family present, Mrs. Liu died peacefully with the sounds of familiar music playing. Acknowledging cultural practices that were important to Mrs. Liu, her son accompanied her body to the morgue and then to the Chinese mortuary.

Evaluation and Outcome Information

Evaluation of Mrs. Liu's care did not focus on one provider but on the impact of the interdisciplinary team. Her dying process was not unnecessarily prolonged, but the family members were given time to understand and accept probable death. Her family members were satisfied with the quality of patient care and their inclusion in the process of decision making about the care. Finally, they felt that the process would be acceptable for ancestors and future generations of their family. The moral distress of the team was reduced, and nurses felt satisfied with the care provided.

CNS Core Competencies

CNS core competencies were essential to the successful outcomes. The PCLN CNS was known in the institution

as an expert clinician, effective consultant, collaborator, and clinical psychiatric nursing expert with a breadth of knowledge, an interest in culturally appropriate care, and an understanding of when to engage with staff and when to disengage and be a resource. Psychiatric nursing expertise was applied in direct care of Mrs. Liu's family. The PCLN CNS demonstrated expert teaching, role modeling, and coaching, especially about cultural factors, working with families, and ethical decision making at end of life. The CNS was a role model for the expert nurses, demonstrating the integration of theory and practice in culturally appropriate family-focused care.

"MEAT AND POTATOES": CREATING A PROFESSIONAL NURSING PRACTICE ENVIRONMENT FOR INPATIENT PEDIATRICS

Identification of Practice Problem

At a large East Coast academic medical center where the PCLN CNS had worked for 4 years and developed strong relationships with nurses, the CNS's overall goals were to improve the quality of care through improving the practice environment, as well as coaching staff through times of crisis and transition in the climate of financial challenges and constraints. The vignette described here involved the nurses and nursing practice sphere of influence and the systems/organizations sphere of influence. The request for consultation about systems change came from the administrative director for the pediatric nursing division.

Goals and Objectives for Practice Innovation

Formally titled "Creating a Professional Practice Environment" but usually known as "Meat & Potatoes" (M & P), the innovation was a performance improvement initiative in pediatric nursing using the Institute for Healthcare Improvement (IHI) Model for Improvement (IHI, 2008). The vision of the pediatric administrative director was the development of a Professional Practice Model that would enable the delivery of excellent nursing care and achieve outcomes of high patient, family, staff, and physician satisfaction; exceptional patient care; and decreased registered nurse (RN) turnover. The purpose was to transform the environment of low patient satisfaction, high nurse turnover, and fragmentation of care delivery that characterized the general pediatric inpatient units at that time and to develop unit-based leadership.

Under the leadership of the pediatric administrative director, the means of achieving the vision was the M & P committee, an intradisciplinary team of key pediatric stakeholders working together to create systems, tools, and supports using the IHI model with a guiding principle emphasizing fundamentals or "back to basics" (thus the name "Meat & Potatoes"). M & P was endorsed by the patient services leadership of the hospital. Leader sponsorship is critical to successful innovation in an organization (Pearson, 2002).

Description and Implementation of Innovation

Key aspects of the innovation were leader communication, the team, group work, a unit-based leadership model, the use of appropriate models for practice improvement and for group process, and the role of the PCLN CNS as consultant to the director and facilitator. Implementation began with clear communication from the pediatric administrative director to all pediatric nursing staff about the urgent need for change. The administrative director stated her guiding principles as follows: (1) staff wants to deliver exceptional care (positive expectations), (2) current systems get in the way, (3) no blaming (failure tolerant), (4) we possess everything we need to change, and (5) the people doing the work know what needs to change (emphasis on local innovation). She emphasized the patient as the center of care and support of clinical nurses, "real-time, real-life, on-unit support," as a goal. The administrative director manifested failure-tolerant leadership (Farson & Keyes, 2002), helping the staff overcome fear of failure and creating a culture of intelligent risk-taking. Her passionate articulation of her vision enabled the staff to clearly perceive the goal.

According to the IHI Model for Improvement, including the right people on a team is critical for success (IHI, 2008). Led by the administrative director, the M & P committee was composed of patient services managers, assistant managers, and clinical nurses from each unit; pediatric CNSs and clinical nurse educators (CNEs); a performance improvement coordinator; and a care coordinator. The PCLN CNS participated as facilitator. The inclusion of clinical nurses from all general pediatric units was essential for making sustainable change.

For 9 months, weekly M & P committee meetings focused on planning, implementation of pilot projects, evaluation, and revision, following the IHI Plan-Do-Study-Act cycle (IHI, 2008). Meetings were used for reporting and decision making. The meeting ground rules were: (1) no meetings without clinical nurses, (2) full participation, (3) come prepared and on time, (4) report, discuss, decide. The PCLN CNS, as meeting facilitator, maintained a safe environment and ensured that clinical nurses spoke and administrative leaders listened. Verbal contributions were balanced between clinical and administrative nurses.

Additional group work time was provided by a series of retreats for M & P committee members and unit-based nursing staff, based on retreat techniques and tools used previously by the PCLN CNS (Minarik & Catrambone, 1993). The purpose of the retreats was to develop plans and strategies for transformation of core practice elements that were thought most likely to result in improvement.

A sensitive area of implementation was the deployment of master's prepared CNSs and CNE resources throughout the pediatric service with balanced assignments to units as part of a unit-based leadership model, a new infrastructure for continuing support, and practice improvements. The M & P committee recognized the difficulty of changes involving trust, power, and personality and saw this topic as requiring an expert facilitator (PCLN CNS) to maintain neutrality and prevent personal attack. The PCLN CNS was sought as a mentor and trusted consultant by pediatric CNSs, CNEs, and managers during the pilot phase of the unit-based leadership model.

The IHI model and the Gibb model were utilized in M & P. The IHI Plan-Do-Study-Act cycle was used as the model to guide practice change. The PCLN CNS modeled group process facilitation and taught the Gibb model for trust building in organizational groups, group process skills, and specific skills for leading committees to key subgroup leaders, who were then independent in leading their work groups. A summary of the Gibb model, originally published in 1964, is available at http://www.cofe.anglican.org/info/educa tion/lifelong/sharedresources/resources/understand inggroups/theory1.pdf. A similar model is the Drexler/Sibbet Team Performance Model, which is available at http://www.grove.come/site/method_pm_tpm.html. Use of an explicit model for group trust building shared this knowledge with all members. In regular meetings with the administrative director, the PCLN CNS provided process consultation, explored feelings that arose, and coached the director in learning and trying new behaviors, as well as providing resources and ideas about change and transition (Bridges, 1991).

Evaluation and Outcome Information

Overall, the visionary leadership of the administrative director was crucial. Because M & P was collaborative among administrative and clinical nurses and the PCLN CNS, separating PCLN CNS impact from the impact of others was challenging. Essential to the outcome was the reestablishment of trust with front-line clinical staff, which began with developing trust at the committee level. The PCLN CNS as facilitator of the meetings and process consultant to the administrative director was essential for engaging clinical nurses.

At 6 months, the unit-based leadership model, including CNSs, CNEs, and nurse managers, was found to be effective in leading unit-based efforts to improve RN morale and satisfaction with nursing practice. Developing trust, working relationships, and the sense of being a leadership team took more time than expected. Trust and a safe environment were found to be necessary to raise issues of conflict.

The PCLN CNS initiated a discussion among M & P members about "group dose" based on the concept of "nurse dose" (Brooten & Naylor, 1995; Brooten & Youngblut, 2006). The discussion failed to determine hours needed, but important components of group dose were delineated. Components that constituted the necessary group dose for M & P can be summarized in three categories: composition of the group, face-to-face time, and outcomes. The inclusive group was composed of the stakeholders in pediatric nursing. Credibility for the process was enhanced by the numbers of clinical nurses involved. Face-to-face time was important in terms of establishing or reestablishing trust with front-line clinical staff and everyone hearing the same communication at the same time. Time pressure was avoided in recognition of the time needed for complex cognitive processing. Outcomes were identified with clear goals and expectations, were reported weekly with visuals, and were celebrated. The work was focused, with group rules and structure, clearly identifying problems and solutions. The members felt they were "on a mission." Nurses were excited about working together to improve professional practice and described the group development as going from not trusting to trusting and having fun.

Evaluations, including weekly reports, quarterly patient satisfaction survey results, and nurse turnover reports, were reviewed at the M & P meetings. Weekly progress reports enabled refinement of the implemented strategies. A nurse satisfaction survey was developed by nurses for post-implementation evaluations.

Professional nurses identified pride in professional practice as an outcome. At 4 months, RN vacancies dropped from 17% to 1.8%. Returning clinical instructors for prelicensure students remarked about the positive change in the culture of care. At 9 months, patients' ability to identify their primary nurse improved from 34% to 46%. Patient satisfaction scores showed an improving trend. Survey results showed that RN morale and satisfaction improved by 30%. The length of stay was stable below the organizational target. Finally, a direct correlation between patient satisfaction and RN satisfaction was demonstrated. The importance of the leader's commitment and involvement

at the unit level and the division level to effect changes in staff could not be overestimated. In summary, M & P was about developing leaders at all levels of the pediatric division.

CNS Outcomes and Competencies

PCLN outcome categories identified by Yakimo et al. (2004) are patient, family, staff satisfaction; changes in perceived work environment; measuring change within clients; and defining outcomes according to interest group. During M & P, data were collected measuring changes over time in satisfaction and RN vacancies, possibly a proxy for perceived work environment. These outcomes were presented differently according to audience—to the pediatric nursing staff with colorful graphs regularly over time and condensed in a PowerPoint summary presentation for the patient services leadership.

The major roles of the PCLN CNS were consultant, group process facilitator, coach, mentor, and teacher. The PCLN CNS served as a coach and mentor in leadership development, particularly for understanding stages of group process and the model of trust development in groups. The PCLN CNS encouraged celebration of accomplishments at the conclusion of each phase of the work, demonstrating effective management of change and transition.

CNS competencies demonstrated in M & P were psychiatric nursing practice expertise, a variety of consultative competencies as an internal consultant, expert teaching and coaching of administrators and staff, leadership competencies, and competencies in collaboration (Sparacino & Cartwright, 2000). Also contributory to successful outcomes were professional attributes of the PCLN CNS, such as honesty, personal mastery in managing emotions, and knowledge of personal strengths and weaknesses, which are enhanced and expanded as the CNS practices in the role (National Association of Clinical Nurse Specialists [NACNS], 2004). The PCLN CNS was seen as trustworthy, able to keep a confidence, able to maintain a neutral perspective in sensitive situations, able to produce results, and helpful in dealing directly with difficult issues.

SUMMARY

This chapter presented an overview of PCLN and illustrated the range of PCLN practice with two vignettes. The first vignette involved cultural factors, family concerns, moral distress, and end-of-life decision making in an ICU. The PCLN CNS demonstrated the integration of theory and practice in culturally appropriate family-focused care. The second vignette described a complex performance improvement practice innovation in a pediatric nursing division in a large academic medical center. Each vignette identified CNS roles and competencies essential to PCLN practice.

ACKNOWLEDGMENTS

The author thanks all of the patients, family members, nurses, health care providers, and others who have contributed so much to her development as a CNS. In particular, the author would like to acknowledge with gratitude the collaboration with the ICU staff and with Mary Beth Esposito-Herr, Diane Vorio, and the pediatric nursing staff. The author thanks Diane Vorio for her work on presentations of this material. This chapter is dedicated to the memory of Mary Beth Esposito-Herr.

REFERENCES

Bridges, W. (1991). *Managing transitions: Making the most of change.* Reading, MA: Addison-Wesley Publishing Company.

Brooten, D., & Naylor, M. D. (1995). Nurses' effect on changing patient outcomes. *Image—the Journal of Nursing Scholarship, 27*(2), 95–99.

Brooten, D., & Youngblut, J. M. (2006). Nurse dose as a concept. *Journal of Nursing Scholarship, 38*(1), 94–99.

Farson, R., & Keyes, R. (2002). The failure-tolerant leader. *Harvard Business Review, 80*(8), 64–71, 148.

Institute for Health Care Improvement. (2008). *How to improve.* Retrieved January 26, 2009, from http://www.ihi.org/IHI/Topics/Improvement/ImprovementMethods/HowToImprove

Institute of Medicine. (2000). *Working together: We can help people get good care when they are dying.* The National Academies Press. Retrieved January 26, 2009, from http://books.nap.edu/catalog.php?record_id = 9798

Kleinman, A., & Benson, P. (2006). Anthropology in the clinic: The problem of cultural competency and how to fix it. *PLoS Medicine, 3*(10), 1673–1676.

Lazarus, R. S. (1998). *Fifty years of research and theory by R.S. Lazarus: An analysis of historical and perennial issues.* Mahwah, NJ: Lawrence Erlbaum Associates.

Lipson, J. G., & Dibble, S. L. (Eds.). (2005). *Culture & clinical care.* San Francisco, CA: UCSF Nursing Press.

Lipson, J. G., Dibble, S. L., & Minarik, P. A. (Eds.). (1996). *Culture & nursing care: A pocket guide.* San Francisco: UCSF Nursing Press.

Minarik, P. A., & Catrambone, C. (1993). Collective participation in workplace decision making. In D. J. Mason, S. W. Talbott, & J. K. Leavitt (Eds.), *Policy and politics for nurses: Action and change in the workplace, government, organizations and community* (2nd ed., pp. 306–328). Philadelphia: W.B. Saunders Company.

Minarik, P. A., & Neese, J. B. (2002). Essential educational content for advanced practice in psychiatric consultation liaison nursing. *Archives of Psychiatric Nursing, 16*(1), 3–15.

National Association of Clinical Nurse Specialists. (2004). *Statement on clinical nurse specialist practice and education* (2nd ed.). Harrisburg, PA: Author.

Pearson, A. E. (2002). Tough-minded ways to get innovative (Best of HBR 1988). *Harvard Business Review, 80*(8), 117–124.

Robichaux, C. M., & Clark, A. P. (2006). Practice of expert critical care nurses in situations of prognostic conflict at the end of life. *American Journal of Critical Care, 15*(5), 480–491.

Sparacino, P. S. A., & Cartwright, C. C. (2000). The clinical nurse specialist. In A. B. Hamric, J. A. Spross, & C. M. Hanson (Eds.), *Advanced nursing practice: An integrative approach* (2nd ed., pp. 349–379). Philadelphia: W.B. Saunders Company.

Yakimo, R., Kurlowicz, L. H., & Murray, R. B. (2004). Evaluation of outcomes in psychiatric consultation-liaison nursing practice. *Archives of Psychiatric Nursing, 18*(6), 215–222.

Growing a Clinical Nurse Specialist Practice in a Rehabilitation Setting

Kathleen L. Dunn

Rehabilitation nurses assist individuals with disabilities or chronic disease toward maximal health through health restoration, maintenance, and promotion (Association of Rehabilitation Nurses, 2000; Mauk, 2000). The Association of Rehabilitation Nurses notes that "rehabilitation nursing is a philosophy of care, not a work setting or a phase of treatment" (p. 7). An advanced practice rehabilitation nurse "conducts comprehensive assessment and demonstrates a high level of autonomy and expert skill in diagnosis and treatment in the management of complex responses of individuals, families, groups and communities to health problems stemming from altered functional ability and altered lifestyle" (Association of Rehabilitation Nurses, 1996). The advanced practice nurse may also "direct care or manage systems of care for complex patient/family/community populations" (p. 6). This chapter discusses the clinical nurse specialist (CNS) role and practice as demonstrated through opening a new acute and rehabilitation spinal cord injury (SCI) unit.

PROBLEM

As an experienced SCI rehabilitation CNS, I was recruited for the CNS position at a new spinal cord injury and disease (SCI/D) unit in a Veterans' Affairs (VA) medical center. My first responsibilities were to develop essential clinical programs and support opening the unit,

a situation with both challenges and opportunities. A major challenge was my lack of experience working within the VA health care system. I also would be working with a nursing staff that had little or no experience in rehabilitation or SCI/D nursing, including registered nurses (RNs) and licensed vocational nurses (LVNs). The hospital did not employ nurses aides. Opportunities included the ability to help design a program and unit from the beginning, to expand my CNS practice, and to develop new staff in this specialty area. I would be establishing practice standards and norms, training new staff, and helping create a unit culture—all in addition to ordering specialty equipment and supplies to meet the needs of this patient population.

GOALS

The overall goal was to have the inpatient unit and home care program open within 3 months. To meet this goal, the following initiatives had to be completed:

1. Develop the new CNS position, including procedures for clinical consultation with nurses on other units caring for SCI patients.
2. Develop interdisciplinary policies and procedures, including admission criteria, scope of service, and procedures for admission, care coordination, and discharge.

3. Develop nursing policies and procedures specific to the program and unit, including standard procedures for everything from bowel, bladder, and skin management to management of complex medical emergencies such as autonomic dysreflexia.
4. Orient, educate, and train the entire interdisciplinary team.
5. Select and order equipment and supplies.
6. Develop a seamless system of care between the SCI/D clinic, inpatient unit, home care program, and our external and internal stakeholders.

IMPLEMENTATION/ MOVING FORWARD

I had just 3 months from starting the CNS position in a new, largely empty building to admitting the first patient. There was a long to do list. As a CNS new to the VA, I had to focus on developing working relationships that would be essential to the opening of the new unit. In addition to developing relationships with the new nurse manager and unit physician, this position would require frequent collaboration with other medical center CNSs and nurse managers, with staff in other areas of the hospital, and with the SCI/D center therapy, counseling, and administrative staff. I would also need to learn how to work with a physician's assistant (PA) on the inpatient unit (a new experience for me) and to develop relationships with discharge planners and case managers at local trauma centers as well as Department of Defense medical facilities in our region.

The acting nurse manager had been a professional colleague and friend for many years. Having her as my supervisor initially necessitated a change in our relationship; however, she was also experienced in the VA system and was invaluable to me in helping me learn both the formal and informal methods of getting the job done and the patients' needs met. She was a nurse practitioner (NP) with an extensive background of working with CNSs, and she was very comfortable with the CNS role. At the time there were four CNSs at this medical center, all unit-based. They were my major source of support and also a resource for learning how the informal chain of command worked—how things "really get done around here." I began participating on nursing service committees and task forces and collaborated on hospital-based special projects. I also spent a lot of time getting to know the SCI physician and PA. The acting nurse manager and I often discussed role boundaries and expectations for the nursing staff and the medical staff (including the PA). Initially, the PA wanted sign-off approval of nursing policies and procedures. We disagreed. Redefining and setting boundaries and clarifying roles continued through the first year.

Working with a nursing staff that had little or no experience in rehabilitation or SCI nursing was a challenge. Most staff had previous experience in medical-surgical or long-term care nursing only. Rehabilitation nursing requires a paradigm shift in perspective of the nurse–patient relationship and the roles of a nurse in teaching, coaching, and guiding versus direct care provider. Staff education had to emphasize cognitive/affective competencies as well as psychomotor competencies. Disability awareness training had to be integrated with learning skills such as body mechanics for transfers and bowel care. I was not able to participate in all the new nursing staff interviews. This meant that I did not meet most of the nursing staff until they began orientation, which made needs assessment much more difficult.

Emphasis was placed on key issues required for patient and staff safety, but quality of care also had to be addressed. Many of the orientation classes would be provided in an interdisciplinary group, so they needed to meet the needs of a varied staff. I worked extensively with the nurse manager, who had obtained information about similar orientation programs at other VA SCI centers and who also helped me identify guest faculty from both our facility and other VA SCI centers. Some of these presentations were scheduled prior to my hire; however, I became responsible for coordinating the presentations and bridging the gaps in content.

I had developed educational materials over the years, and while it was helpful to have a large collection of audiovisual materials, additional educational programs and materials had to be created. The medical center's media center helped with this and videotaped staff orientation presentations. I also ordered additional teaching materials, including videotapes, models, books, and journals, as well as equipment such as projectors and videotape players.

During orientation, key people from other hospital departments were invited, including other CNSs, staff from Prosthetics and Central Supply, and leadership from departments such as social work and psychology. The combined team orientation lasted a week, with an additional week for nursing staff only. Class formats included didactic presentations, skills labs, and disability "experiences," with ample opportunities for discussion and questions. The nursing classes consisted of specific nursing skills, such as intermittent catheterization, application of external condom catheters, and transfers skills, as well as classes on rehabilitation nursing theory, primary nursing, care planning, and working in an interdisciplinary team.

The unit was custom designed for SCI care, with large bathrooms that were fully wheelchair accessible; however, some important and necessary features were not included. A medication room was missing, hand-washing facilities were not available at the nurses station, and the space allocated for bowel care and showers was an outdated hold-over from old VA SCI unit designs. In addition, there were no plans for office space on the unit and no plans for a staff lounge and/or classroom. Working together, the acting nurse manager and I were able to have space reallocated and minor modifications made for all these needs. The shower/bowel care area was redesignated (though not remodeled) for equipment storage because the accessible bathrooms in each patient room were adequate. Our success was, in part, related to the manager's extensive experience in the VA system and her ability to work within her established networks/relationships. This experience underscored the need to put relationship building on the top of my priority list.

Rehabilitation care involves a lot of different specialized equipment and supplies; opening a new unit required evaluating and selecting these items. Some equipment was already in place, including beds, bedside stands, med carts, chart racks, and commode chairs. Upon further investigation, however, some of this was not appropriate for rehabilitation patients. The over-toilet shower/commode chairs, for example, did not fit the unit toilets. I found suitable replacements and was able to negotiate a trade-in of 15 previously purchased chairs for chairs that would fit over the toilets.

Other specialized patient equipment needs included hands-free nurse call bells, positioning and transfer equipment, and bathing assistance equipment. Specialized supplies had to be evaluated and ordered, such as external condom catheters, straight and indwelling catheters, urinary drainage bags, and wound care supplies. Vendors were contacted for samples, and I worked closely with the nurse manager of Central Supply to ensure sufficient supplies would be on hand prior to the opening of the unit.

I was responsible for developing many of the clinical policies and procedures. Some of this work could be based on previous experience, others were developed from the literature, and others were based on policies at other VA and private sector SCI centers. Collaboration with the SCI physician and other hospital departments was critical, and many meetings were needed to work out details. For example, a standard procedure and an accompanying nurse competency for managing episodes of autonomic dysreflexia (an emergency in SCI patients) was necessary to be able to respond appropriately and quickly to this emergency situation. Arriving at consensus on the protocol involved consideration of nursing scope of practice, level of practice competency, internal VA regulations, and state nurse practice guidelines, along with evidence-based best practices as described in the literature.

As CNS, I was designated to determine criteria for nurse competence. I developed both learning modules and competency assessment methods, including written tests, return demonstrations, and clinical case study simulations and methods for documenting and maintaining competency records.

Clinical policies and procedures were also needed for treatments and procedures such as intermittent catheterization programs, bowel care programs, and a self-medication program. These were developed collaboratively with appropriate disciplines and in compliance with both Veterans Health Administration (VHA) and hospital existing policies.

I would also be responsible for preadmission screening for those patients referred to the center for both acute care and rehabilitation following a new SCI. I designed screening forms, developed materials to give to referral sources about our program for both their information and patients and families, and arranged to make site visits to the referring facilities (if within the county) to assess the patient, provide information, and coordinate a smooth transfer. I worked closely with the SCI Chief so that we were in agreement on criteria for admission, assessment parameters, and appropriate medical stability for these patients. This involved making many phone calls to facilities referring patients out of the area and screening by phone when needed. I visited the local Navy hospital to establish a contact there with the appropriate case managers and social workers and to become familiar with their units and facility.

IMPLEMENTATION

The unit had to be ready for our first admission on Friday of the week the educational programs were completed. Organizing supplies and setting up rooms was a priority. As is typical for CNSs who focus on "making it happen," I found myself helping an LVN install patient televisions on Thursday afternoon. A good CNS has many diverse skills. Being mechanically inclined and having the ability to work with hand tools is a definite asset!

The first few patients admitted to the new SCI unit were medically stable and needed hospitalization only for tests and procedures. As the unit CNS, I worked side by side with the nursing staff, helping them develop competence and confidence. When the first emergency admission occurred at the end of the first week, I stayed on the unit for 14 hours to assist with management of the patient's pyelonephritis and autonomic dysreflexia. Over the next few weeks I averaged 10–12 hour days so that staff were adequately supported both in routine care delivery and with problem solving. I also consulted and made some home visits with our new SCI homecare nurse, and I consulted with the new SCI NP in the outpatient clinic to help them problem solve and develop increased expertise in SCI nursing. These were long and tiring days, but it was necessary in order for the unit to be successful.

EVALUATION AND OUTCOMES

We initially opened with 8 inpatient beds, and by the end of 3 months increased this to 15. By the end of 9 months, we had 18 inpatient beds open and had hired and oriented two more groups of staff including nurses, therapists, a physician, and another PA. Some staff found that SCI and rehabilitation nursing was not for them and left quickly. A few were found unsatisfactory and terminated. Several found that SCI and rehabilitation nursing was their calling and remained for many years.

Overall, staff believed they were well prepared to provide patient care, and they also noted how important it was to them to have ready access to CNS support when confronted with actual patient care situations that were unfamiliar or unanticipated.

The new nurse manager and I worked closely with other SCI center leadership staff to develop a unit culture and spirit of camaraderie. This spirit extended to unit-based social events such as potluck lunches and beach parties. We even obtained donated polo shirts with the unit logo for all the staff.

The first year was tough, with turnover of both medical and therapy leadership staff and some nursing staff. Feedback from patients was helpful to identify areas where we were meeting or exceeding the expectations of our clients and to identify areas for improvement. Care delivery was modified based on our assessment of what was and was not working, with frequent staff and patient input. We found that we needed frequent contacts with the medical staff and other leadership, so a SCI leadership committee was established to review progress toward unit goals and to work together on process improvement projects.

Materials developed for the initial orientation proved invaluable for use in subsequent orientations. I continued to use some of the videotaped lectures for a number of years until the content became dated, meanwhile developing more easily updated materials consistent with evidence-based practice.

I started screening new injury referrals as soon as we opened. I coordinated services with the discharge coordinator or social worker at the referring facility, with eligibility and the transfer coordinator at our hospital, and with external case managers for different insurances or the Department of Defense. The SCI physician accepted or declined these admissions based on my data collection and recommendations. While having a CNS perform screenings and assessments is not unique in the world of rehabilitation nursing, it is fairly unique within VA SCI centers. The ability of the CNS to both assess the patient and coordinate complex systems to achieve a smooth transition to our unit has been invaluable to the success of our program.

MY CNS PRACTICE TODAY

In the years that have passed since first opening the unit, my CNS role has evolved. Currently, I am also the case manager for new injury rehabilitation SCI patients (averaging 1–4 patients at a time on our 26-bed unit). I continue to coordinate revision of and development of evidence-based nursing policies and procedures and the SCI personal care attendant training program. I also implement SCI new nurse orientation and inservices, chair the SCI interdisciplinary patient/staff education committee, and serve on the hospital-wide patient education council. I coordinate the hospital-wide safe patient handling and movement program, review and approve all requests for specialty mattresses and beds for all system outpatients, and serve on the wound care task force. I provide direct care to patients, with a special interest in sexuality education and counseling. I coordinate and lead the SCI unit interdisciplinary weekly wound care rounds, and I also coordinate activities to meet Commission for Accreditation of Rehabilitation Facilities standards.

Since opening the unit 18 years ago, I have worked with six different SCI nurse managers, four different supervisors, and four different SCI chief physicians. Only three of the original staff nurses are currently working on the unit. I have had to learn to be flexible in working with other leadership staff with vastly different leadership styles and approaches to patient care. Being able to adjust to changes in leadership and personnel, with differences in philosophy and approach, while maintaining focus and commitment to rehabilitation nursing principles has remained a keystone to my practice.

My participation in national nursing and interdisciplinary organizations has resulted in invitations to present and publish nationally and internationally. I coordinate a panel of other SCI advanced practice nurses who answer health-related questions on a Web site for people with SCI (http://sci.rutgers.edu). I have represented both the Association of Rehabilitation Nurses and the American Association of SCI Nurses on the Steering Committee for the Consortium for Spinal Cord Medicine (which develops and publishes clinical practice guidelines). I serve on a national task force for implementation of safe patient handling and movement programs within the VA health care system and serve as a National Association of Clinical Nurse Specialists (NACNS) representative to the American Nurses Credentialing Center (ANCC) Core CNS Certification exam Content Expert Panel. In 2008 I was the first nurse inducted into the Spinal Cord Hall of Fame. With a new

SCI unit in the early planning stages, I am able to bring my years of experience and expertise to the table for a radically different and improved facility sometime in the future.

Opening a new unit and watching it grow and mature was one of the major accomplishments of my career. The CNS, as the clinical expert in specialty-focused advanced nursing practice, is ideally prepared to coordinate physical facility design, develop care delivery systems and processes, evaluate outcomes, and make continued corrections to adjust and adapt to new technology, science, and clinical evidence. My first and last passion is being a CNS in SCI rehabilitation nursing. Finding your passion, working in a stimulating environment with a network of peers, and making a difference for patient outcomes is the ultimate success in a nursing career.

REFERENCES

Association of Rehabilitation Nurses. (1996). *Scope and standards of advanced clinical practice in rehabilitation nursing.* Glenview, IL: Author.

Association of Rehabilitation Nurses. (2000). *Standards and scope of rehabilitation nursing.* Glenview, IL: Author.

Mauk, K. L. (Ed.). (2000). *Standards and scope of rehabilitation nursing.* Glenview, IL: Association of Rehabilitation Nurses.

Exploring Clinical Nurse Specialist Practice in the Emergency Department

Garrett Chan

OVERVIEW OF EMERGENCY NURSING AND EMERGENCY DEPARTMENT PATIENT POPULATIONS

Clinical nurse specialists (CNSs) in the emergency department (ED) are master generalists. CNSs in emergency care must be educated in many aspects of human physiology in addition to growth and development knowledge across the life span with expertise in several physiological, pathophysiological, psychological, social, and public health systems. Inherent in emergency clinical practice is a sense of uncertainty and unpredictability as patients arrive to the ED unannounced and with chief complaints rather than with diagnoses common in other practices in health care. Clinicians need to be prepared to care for anyone with any disease or injury process who present to the ED (Zink, 2006). Emergency nurses are trained to assess whether the patient has a life-threatening condition, to assist in making a diagnosis, and to initiate diagnostic and resuscitative interventions in an effort to stabilize the patient's condition (Newberry, 2003). Differential diagnosis is a cornerstone of emergency nursing practice. Understanding many pathophysiological, psychological, social, and public health issues and creating a differential diagnosis list are core activities of emergency nursing because the exact diagnosis of a patient is unknown.

Emergency nurses work in close collaboration with other disciplines such as medicine with every patient encounter. Respiratory therapy and social services are disciplines that are consulted on a daily basis. In the emergency department, the team approach to every patient is embedded in the care delivery system. All disciplines work together to achieve the same goal: to diagnose the patient's underlying illness and initiate treatment to stabilize the patient's condition. Family-centered care and patient education are also core activities of emergency nursing. Throughout the history of emergency nursing, there is much overlap between the medicine and nursing disciplines (Snyder, Keeling, & Razionale, 2006). For example, emergency nurses are educated and trained to diagnose myocardial ischemia by looking at electrocardiograms and understanding laboratory values. Alternatively, emergency physicians are involved with discharge planning and education of patients.

The patient census can fluctuate wildly throughout the course of a day. In addition, the ED has been described as a place of transition (Chan, 2004). Patients do not usually stay in the ED for the duration of their hospital stay. Rather, they are either discharged to home or admitted to an inpatient unit or to another hospital for specialty care. The focus of ED care is to stabilize the patient's condition and begin treatment with a referral to another service or to the patient's primary care provider for further follow-up.

An important aspect of emergency CNSs' work is to have direct clinical contact with patients who present with complex issues or who are severely ill or injured (Proehl, 2003). These clinical encounters provide opportunities for the emergency CNS to demonstrate, perform, implement, or role model clinical skills of advanced health and social assessment, nursing and medical differential diagnoses, and psychomotor skills. Additional unique issues that have influenced emergency practice includes overcrowding and lack of experienced nurses and physicians (Institute of Medicine [IOM], 2006, p. 622). In addition, the encounters provide an opportunity to assess the knowledge and behavior of clinicians and teach or debrief depending on the situation. Supporting the spheres of influence of nursing and organizations depends on the assessment of clinical practice within the department. Domains of advanced practice nursing in emergency care settings include critical care, urgent care, primary care, behavioral medicine, public health, and social medicine (Chan & Garbez, 2006).

PROBLEM IDENTIFICATION

Providing safe patient care is paramount within hospitals today. Many factors are responsible for the threats to safe patient care. There is a growing concern about the decreasing number of experienced nurses who are aging and getting ready for retirement and an increasing number of novice nurses, as well as high turnover rates of nurses in the workforce (Buerhaus, 2005; IOM Committee on the Work Environment for Nurses and Patient Safety Board on Health Services [IOM Committee], 2004; Norman et al., 2005). Additional factors that may lead to less safe patient care include lack of mentoring and coaching as well as an increased physician workload leading to a decreasing amount of time for collaboration (Buerhaus et al., 2005). Nursing units whose workforce included more experienced registered nurses (i.e., > 5 years of experience) had better quality care as measured by a decrease in medication error and patient fall rates (Blegen, Vaughn, & Goode, 2001). Novice nurses report the need for increased assistance from experienced nurses. Common themes surrounding novice nurses' near-miss or adverse events include an increased need for clinically focused critical thinking, seeking assistance from experienced nurses, knowledge of unit and workflow patters, first-time experiences in situations, time constraints, hand-offs, influence of peer pressure and social norms, losing the big picture, and novice nurses helping other novice nurses (Ebright, Urden, Patterson, & Chalko, 2004). There is an increased workload of staff nurses which leaves little time for mentoring, coaching, and supervision of more novice nurses (IOM Committee, 2004).

Physician inexperience, organizational factors and pressures that inhibit interdisciplinary practice, and communication breakdown are other factors that threaten safe patient care. In order to ensure that process improvement projects are successful, there is a tendency to put pressure on the CNS to implement other parts of the role, by evaluating practices and outcomes and performing audits that take them away from direct patient care. These factors contribute to the need to have CNSs at the bedside providing direct patient care as well as coaching to staff.

With the proliferation of regulatory agency standards and quality initiatives, such as the National Quality Forum and the Institute for Healthcare Improvement (IHI), hospitals struggle to meet all of these mandates for improving care in the hospital setting. CNSs are educated and well-positioned within hospitals to lead the efforts through committee work to comply with these mandates. However, with the increased amount of committee and quality improvement work the CNS engages in, CNSs spend less time in the central activity of all advanced practice nurses—direct clinical practice.

CNS direct clinical practice can be the answer to addressing the issues surrounding patient safety and mentoring less experienced nurses to provide better care. In addition, direct clinical practice can provide the CNS with opportunities to identify staff learning needs and system or process breakdowns. The following exemplar illustrates these concepts and domains of emergency advanced practice nursing and highlights the three spheres of influence of CNS practice.

EXEMPLAR

In my daily practice as the ED CNS, I would round in the department at least twice a day—once in the morning before turning on my computer and beginning to check my e-mails and once in the early afternoon. Often, I would round at 6:30 A.M. to talk with the night shift to ask if there were any unusual incidents or concerns during that time . However, on this particular day, I happened to round in the ED at 8:00 A.M.

The ED was quiet, as there were only three patients. I walked by one of the ED resuscitation rooms and glanced inside. I saw one ventilated patient and three nurses around the patient's bed. As I continued to walk toward the charge nurse desk, I decided to turn around and see what was going on in that room because I thought it was unusual that three very experienced nurses were standing around one patient.

I walked into the room, greeted the nurses, and asked them what was going on with the patient. The primary nurse gave me report. Ms. H was a 14-year-old female who was flown to our hospital from a rural hospital after ingesting a whole bottle of isoniazid in a suicide attempt. Ms. H was paralyzed, sedated, and being mechanically ventilated in the ED awaiting a pediatric intensive care unit (PICU) bed.

Still wondering why there were three nurses at the patient's bedside, I took this opportunity to assess the situation by performing a health and physical assessment and doing some bedside teaching, explaining what I was looking for in each step of the health and physical assessment and paying close attention to the expected normal and potentially abnormal findings in a patient who overdoses on isoniazid. As we were completing the physical exam and reviewing the charting on this patient, the cardiac monitor alarm sounded. The patient's heart rate suddenly went from 80 beats per minute to 180 beats per minute, and the blood pressure was 200/105 mm Hg. The primary nurse informed me that this was the third time this had happened to the patient.

I quickly ran through my differential diagnosis list for probable causes of sudden-onset tachycardia:

1. Seizure secondary to metabolic acidosis
2. Atrial fibrillation/flutter
3. Narrow-complex tachycardias (i.e., multifocal atrial tachycardia, paroxysmal supraventricular tachycardia, AV nodal reentrant tachycardia, ectopic atrial tachycardia, junctional tachycardia)
4. Unstable or stable wide-complex tachycardias (i.e., unknown type, AV reentrant tachycardia, torsades de pointes, or ventricular tachycardia—monomorphic or polymorphic)
5. Thyrotoxicosis
6. Pheochromocytoma
7. Hypoglycemia
8. Hypovolemia/hemorrhage
9. Fever
10. Fear/anxiety
11. Other illicit drug ingestion (e.g., cocaine package rupture, also known as "body packers" or "mules" who traffic packages of cocaine by ingesting them)

As the CNS in a Level II trauma center ED in California, I had to be familiar with the patient demographics and public health issues in my community. For example, in the San Francisco Bay Area, multidrug resistant tuberculosis is on the rise and becoming an epidemic in our communities. Therefore, it was important that I stay informed of the Public Health Department's recommendations for surveillance and treatment of tuberculosis. From my CNS education about advanced pathophysiology, pharmacology, and physical assessment, I recognized that this patient was in metabolic acidosis from the isoniazid overdose.

Symptoms of isoniazid overdose include nausea, vomiting, altered mental status, slurred speech, hallucinations, blurred vision, seizures, and coma. I arrived at the diagnosis that this patient was having a seizure secondary to metabolic acidosis. However, because the patient was being paralyzed and sedated, the patient was not exhibiting the tonic/clonic activity typical of this type of seizure.

I had the nurse draw an arterial blood gas and contact pharmacy to mix more of the antidote, vitamin B_6, as well as a sodium bicarbonate drip. We had the ED physician come in to collaborate with us on our findings. The ED physician agreed with my plan of care.

The arterial blood gas results came back as pH = 6.9, $PaCO_2$ = 17 mm Hg; PaO_2 = 180 mm Hg; HCO_3 = 6 mm Hg; Anion Gap = 30, indicating severe metabolic acidosis with an anion gap. The patient received more vitamin B_6 and lorazepam for her seizures, and she was placed on a sodium bicarbonate drip to correct her severe metabolic acidosis. I made a referral to social services to support the family during this time of crisis. Psychiatry was consulted to follow Ms. H during her hospital stay. Ms. H was then transferred to the PICU and made a full recovery. She was discharged to the care of a local psychiatrist in her home town.

PRACTICE INNOVATION

The CNS in the ED is called upon to effect changes in the three spheres of influence of patient/client, nursing, and organizations, using direct clinical practice skills, education, consultation, research, and change agent skills (NACNS, 2004). To affect patient care and outcomes, the CNSs in EDs must be present in the department. Maintaining a presence in the ED allows the CNS to be visible and to establish or maintain credibility as an expert clinician among the staff. In addition, to affect patient care and outcomes, the CNS must be present in the department to understand the skill level of clinicians, to evaluate current practices of staff, to provide immediate coaching and teaching, to observe the processes of care, to identify opportunities for improvement, and to elicit current issues from the staff. If aspects of clinical care are not well-understood, then planned interventions to address issues or to change processes potentially will not succeed because the CNS does not intimately understand the issues or processes. Additionally, if the staff do not perceive the CNS as being credible, then attempts at process improvement will be seen as extraneous, superfluous, or inappropriate. The goal of this practice innovation is to provide leadership, education, coaching, and mentoring to staff in an effort to ensure quality care is being delivered and to create a culture of excellent care. This goal can be attained through four interventions: direct patient care, bedside teaching, coaching and mentoring of clinicians, and providing evidence-based resources.

To incorporate these four interventions into CNS practice, there are many activities that CNSs in emergency care settings can integrate into their daily routine. First, CNSs can conduct daily rounds in the department across all shifts (i.e., day shift, evening shift, night shift). I would commonly round in the department twice a day—once at 6:30 A.M. at the change of shift to check in with the night staff to determine if there were any issues that occurred during their shift, and once at around 3:00 P.M. Rounding at 6:30 A.M. allowed me to be present when the day shift nurses arrived so they knew I was always available if they needed my assistance. During this time, I would take the opportunity to informally remind the staff nurses of any process improvement (PI) projects the ED was working on and provide rationale for the PI project, answering any of the staff nurses' questions. Rounding with the staff provided the opportunity for the nurses to understand the goals or be educated about the necessity of the PI project. The afternoon rounds provided me with an opportunity to observe and assess nursing practice and care or administrative processes, to assist the department if busy, to assist staff in troubleshooting or managing breakdowns, and to be available to answer questions or provide resources.

Second, my pager was included in all group paging to alert me of any trauma or major medical alert (i.e., patients *in extremis* or in full arrest). When available, I would attend these resuscitations to provide coaching to novice nurses or to experienced nurses in unusual situations, to assist the health care team in incorporating new technology or medications, to assess potential learning needs of the staff, to ensure evidence-based interventions were being included in the care, to acknowledge and reinforce examples of excellent caring interventions, and to debrief and problem solve with staff regarding any issues of concern or breakdown. Participating in the highest acuity patients afforded me the opportunity to be visible in the department and maintain credibility with staff, as well as to practice my skills of advanced health and physical assessment, psychomotor skills in highly stressful situations, and working as a team player in the ED.

Third, I scheduled myself regularly in the department to work 4- or 8-hour shifts across all shifts. These scheduled shifts allowed me to assess and monitor the flow of patients in the ED, to care for patients and maintain clinical competency with patients across all acuity levels and body systems (e.g., obstetric complaints, ear/nose/throat complaints), to be available to staff for any questions they might have, to assess competencies of staff, and to establish credibility with staff in that I could care for all patients who come to the ED. In terms of filling a sick-call shift, I avoided being seen as someone who had nothing else to do but fill in for someone who called in sick or cover for lunches or breaks. In extreme circumstances, I would relieve nurses so that they could take a much needed break or agree to fill an empty slot in the schedule.

Lastly, I realized that I could not be present in the department 24 hours a day, 7 days a week. Therefore, in order to maintain a presence, I developed or participated in the development of educational materials, policies, procedures, and resource guides that were evidence-based. For example, I developed a vasoactive medication binder that listed all the intravenous vasopressor and antiarrhythmic medications and included indications, contraindications, standard concentrations, drip rate charts, adverse side effects, and pediatric through geriatric considerations. Another resource guide was the appropriate assessment and documentation of the neurologic exam in patients with altered level of consciousness due to pathology or medications. At the bottom of each resource I created, I wrote my name and pager number in the event that anyone had a question or concern about the resource.

Empirical indicators to evaluate experience and expertise have been difficult to define (IOM Committee, 2004). Proxy measures of ED quality care include patient flow indicators such as waiting room time, average length of stay, and the number of patients who left without being seen. Clinical performance indicators such as time to 12-lead electrocardiogram, time to antibiotic administration in community acquired pneumonia, and medication error rates are captured for national quality/process improvement initiatives. Patient satisfaction has also been identified as a proxy measure of quality care. However, use caution when including questions about nursing care in patient satisfaction surveys, such as "care and concern shown by nurses" and "courtesy shown to your family and friends"; an incompetent nurse may show a great deal of concern and care for a patient and family yet may not be competent in the technical or social skills required to expertly take care of a patient or family. While these indicators are important in determining whether there are process issues that can be corrected, they do not measure the "near misses" or capture the true expertise of nurses caring for patients in the ED.

Adherence to benchmark standards, facilitation of practice change, creation of clinical resources, implementation of clinical standards, and educational needs assessment potentially averted forces that could have created a sentinel event when I was providing direct clinical care. Additionally, living the clinical practice of a staff and advanced practice nurse, I advocate for or implement processes that support successful changes in practice that are feasible for staff nurses in the ED. Administrators look to the CNS as expert clinicians/practitioners to speak to practice changes that provide safe patient care.

CONCLUSION

Direct patient care is a hidden or often eliminated part of CNS practice in the face of other organizational demands such as The Joint Commission preparation, Magnet Hospital preparation, committee work, and project management. However, direct patient care is an invaluable and core aspect of CNS practice. Because I incorporated these interventions into my practice, I realized that staff were very accepting of changes and improvements I attempted to institute. One nurse said to me that she would incorporate a process change because she knew that I understood the challenges and issues that staff nurses deal with in their daily practice. Without that sense of understanding of the issues of staff nurses, changes to care processes might fail. Competency in the patient/client sphere of influence can take the form of direct care clinician or consulting roles and can maintain the competency of the CNS, identify core issues for the ED, educate nurses to improve nursing and other disciplines' care practices, provide evidence-based rationale for care practices where appropriate, and improve the quality of care for patients.

REFERENCES

Blegen, M. A., Vaughn, T. E., & Goode, C. J. (2001). Nurse experience and education: Effect on quality of care. *Journal of Nursing Administration, 31*(1), 33–39.

Buerhaus, P. I. (2005). Six-part series on the state of the RN workforce in the United States. *Nursing Economics, 23*(2), 55, 58–60.

Buerhaus, P. I., Donelan, K., Ulrich, B. T., Norman, L., Williams, M., & Dittus, R. (2005). Hospital RNs' and CNOs' perceptions of the impact of the nursing shortage on the quality of care. *Nursing Economics, 23*(5), 211, 214–221.

Chan, G. K. (2004). End-of-life models and emergency department care. *Academic Emergency Medicine, 11*(1), 79–86.

Chan, G. K., & Garbez, R. O. (2006). Education of advance practice nurses for emergency care settings: Emphasizing shared competencies and domains. *Advanced Emergency Nursing Journal, 28*(3), 216–225.

Ebright, P. R., Urden, L., Patterson, E., & Chalko, B. (2004). Themes surrounding novice nurse near-miss and adverse-event situations. *Journal of Nursing Administration, 34*(11), 531–538.

Institute of Medicine. (2006). *Hospital based emergency care: At the breaking point.* Washington, DC: National Academies Press.

Institute of Medicine Committee on the Work Environment for Nurses and Patient Safety Board on Health Services. (2004). *Keeping patients safe: Transforming the work environment of nurses.* Washington, DC: National Academies Press.

National Association of Clinical Nurse Specialists. (2004). *Statement on clinical nurse specialist practice and education* (2nd ed.). Harrisburg, PA: Author.

Newberry, L. (Ed.). (2003). *Sheehy's emergency nursing: Principles and practice* (5th ed.). St. Louis: Mosby.

Norman, L. D., Donelan, K., Buerhaus, P. I., Willis, G., Williams, M., Ulrich, B., et al. (2005). The older nurse in the workplace: Does age matter? *Nursing Economics, 23*(6), 279, 282–289.

Proehl, J. A. (2003). The role of the clinical nurse specialist in the emergency department. In V. A. Keough (Ed.), *Advanced practice nursing. Current practice issues in emergency care* (2nd ed.) (pp. 45–46). Des Plaines, IL: Emergency Nurses Association.

Snyder, A., Keeling, A., & Razionale, C. (2006). From "first aid rooms" to advanced practice nursing. A glimpse into the history of emergency nursing. *Advanced Emergency Nursing Journal, 28*(3), 198–209.

Zink, B. J. (2006). *Anyone, anything, anytime: A history of emergency medicine.* Philadelphia: Mosby Elsevier.

Establishing a Private Practice for Diabetes Self-Management

Patricia S. Moore

POPULATION SERVED

Diabetes mellitus is a defined set of metabolic diseases characterized by hyperglycemia (American Diabetes Association [ADA], 2007a). The etiology of diabetes mellitus (diabetes) is multifactorial and includes defects in insulin secretion and/or insulin action. The underlying mechanisms of diabetes are the result of genetic and environmental influences, such as autoimmune process and insulin resistance. Diabetes is classified by the mechanism that influences the onset of the disease. The classification categories include impaired fasting glucose and impaired glucose tolerance, type 1 diabetes, type 2 diabetes, gestational diabetes, and other types of diabetes that result from concurrent diseases, drugs, or chemicals (ADA, 2007a). Diabetes affects children and adults of all ages and ethnicity, with an estimated prevalence rate in the United States of 7%, or 20.8 million people (ADA, 2007c). Type 2 is the predominant form of diabetes accounting for 90%–95% of diagnosed cases. Due to the chronic nature of the disease, multiple complications such as retinopathy, nephropathy, neuropathy, and cardiovascular disease commonly occur in people with diabetes (ADA, 2007a).

Providing health care for the person with diabetes is a complex process that involves a team approach from a variety of disciplines, such as nursing, medicine, dietary, and social work. A plan of care is formulated as an individualized therapeutic alliance among the person with diabetes, his/her family, and the health care team. The person with diabetes and his/her family are encouraged to assume an active role in the management of diabetes by implementing self-management strategies (ADA, 2007b). The role of the diabetes clinical nurse specialist (CNS) is to promote the health of people with diabetes through the diagnosis and treatment of illnesses associated with disease.

In my CNS practice, participation in the care and management of the person with diabetes included the pharmacologic and nonpharmacologic management of the disease as well as the complications that result from the disease. As a member of the health care team, I focused on the delivery of care within the three spheres of influence as described in the National Association of Clinical Nurse Specialists' (NACNS; 2004) *Statement on Clinical Nurse Specialist Practice and Education,* specifically patient/client, nurses/nursing practice, and organization/system.

CNS PRACTICE PROBLEM

The patient population that I have served in my role as a diabetes CNS has primarily been adults with impaired fasting and glucose tolerance, type 1, type 2, and gestational diabetes. My initial CNS practice was based in a university, tertiary health care system as a member of a multidisciplinary team that provided care to preconceptual and pregnant women with diabetes. After approximately 7 years, however, an opportunity to develop a diabetes center in a regional hospital system closer to my home became available.

During the development stages of the diabetes center, a number of visits were arranged to observe a variety of diabetes centers, including hospital-based centers as well as a CNS-owned and operated independent diabetes center. Additionally, a community needs survey was conducted with potential customers of the diabetes center that included physicians, hospital nursing staff, and clients with diabetes and their families. The survey outcomes demonstrated an interest by the respondents to expand the diabetes services outside the traditional setting and into a community setting. The hospital acknowledged the interest and initially sought office space in a free-standing retail location. However, a final decision was made to locate the diabetes center within the main hospital building.

Although the hospital location was convenient, it did not serve the needs of all clients. Over the ensuing two and one-half years, it became evident that a significant percentage of potential clients would not attend a hospital-based diabetes program due to a variety of reasons, including: the expense of the hospital diabetes program; appointment times were not available during the evening and weekend hours; the primary care physician would not refer to a hospital program; the fear of a hospital setting; and inconvenient parking. In addition, my availability to provide individualized CNS care to clients and family members was gradually diminished as my responsibilities were redefined and a greater amount of time was devoted to completion of administrative and committee duties. As a result, I reached the conclusion that establishing a CNS entrepreneurial private practice in a community-based setting would allow me the opportunity to better serve the needs of my clientele.

CNS PRACTICE INNOVATION

My goal was to set up a CNS diabetes private practice in a community-based setting to implement a diabetes self-care management program for clients. Prior to setting up the private practice, it was important to understand the legal and financial aspects of establishing a nursing entrepreneurial business. A literature search was conducted to gather information about establishing a private practice in nursing. The search was expanded to include articles on the development and management of medical and nutrition practices in a community setting. Meetings were arranged with a variety of business advisors, including the director of a business development center, a lawyer with expertise in business development, and an accountant with small business experience. The discussions with each of the experts centered on: (1) the type of business entities that could be legally established for a nursing practice, (2) liability issues, and (3) tax advantages/disadvantages. Each advisor provided pamphlets, books, and Internet site resources for review.

A variety of legal structures were available for the establishment of a private practice, including sole proprietorship, partnership, limited liability company, and S-corporation. The business advisors explained the benefits and liabilities of each structure and how they are regulated by the state and federal agencies. Upon their advice, the practice was established as an S-corporation with the designation as a Professional Corporation. Once the formal name for the corporation was chosen, the legal advisor submitted the application to the state to designate a new corporation. The application included the name of the corporation, the owner, and the primary purpose of the corporation. Upon receiving approval from the state, an application for liability insurance as a self-employed CNS was submitted to the malpractice insurance company.

ESTABLISHING THE NEW OFFICE

Although very few CNSs were in private practice at that time, I was fortunate to meet a mental health CNS in my community who had already established her private practice. After indicating my interest in sharing office space, she agreed to relocate her office to a larger space that would accommodate my practice. Prior to looking at available office space, a conceptual model for the office was developed. The model included the amount of square footage that would be required for two office spaces, a waiting room for clients and families, and storage space considerations.

A variety of office locations were available in the community, however, the selection of the final location was based on the conceptual model and other important factors. These factors included accessibility of the office to persons with disabilities, a centralized location within the community setting, availability of a bus route near the office location, business signage, familiarity of the location to referral sources and potential clients, monthly cost of rent and utilities, and leasing terms. A final location was selected that most closely matched these requirements.

Once a location had been selected, a meeting was arranged with the leasing agent to discuss more specific details that applied to the office rental. These included: office building rules and regulations, rent deposit and monthly charges, average utility costs and hook-up deposits, availability of telephone and cable service, liability issues, and business insurance requirements. A tentative lease was presented for review. The terms were negotiated and adapted to our needs; specifically, the lease allowed us to rent on a year-to-year basis with first option to renew or decline in subsequent years. The percent increase in rent for the second year was established and added to the lease. Once the lease had been signed, the deposit and first month's rent paid, and the business insurance policy purchased, we were allowed access to the office space.

The diabetes office was arranged to enhance the delivery of care to clients and family members. A conference table was added to enhance discussion and education. Education materials were obtained from a variety of diabetes sources, including printed and video materials from the diabetes professional organizations. Additionally, educational materials were developed to support self-management diabetes strategies, such as sick-day rules, glucose monitoring schedules, and nutritional support tools. Office supplies were purchased, including a desk, computer, telephone/fax machine, portable TV/VCR, educational videos, and a filing cabinet with a lock to store patient records.

Office hours were established to meet the needs of clients and families. Daytime, evening, and weekend hours were offered. Appointment times were set to allow for flexibility in scheduling. Two-hour sessions were allowed for new clients that included a 90-minute client and family interaction and 30 minutes for documentation. Return visits were set for 30- to 60-minute client sessions with 15 to 30 minutes between visits for documentation. Clients were provided with return appointment cards that included the office telephone and pager numbers as well as an after-hours number. Clients were scheduled for return visits based on their self-management needs. The return intervals varied from 1 to 4 weeks with the number of sessions determined by the client's progress and ability to master the self-management skills.

MARKETING

In order to establish a collaborative model with physicians, all clients were required to have a physician referral. Therefore, the initial marketing was targeted for the medical community. Appointments were arranged with key physicians to discuss the new diabetes practice. These physicians, who were familiar with my services, had routinely referred clients to me for ongoing diabetes management and self-management education. Pamphlets were developed for distribution to the physicians and office staff that described the goals of the practice, types of clients appropriate for referral, referral methods, location, hours, charges, and contact information. Each practice was provided with referral forms, which were designed as a checklist to indicate the type of services requested, such as diabetes self-management, nutritional counseling, insulin initiation, and self-monitoring of blood glucose. Referral forms were either faxed to the office or given to the client and brought to the initial meeting. These pamphlets and referral forms were also mailed to all primary care and specialty practice physicians. Additional marketing efforts were targeted at nurses in the acute care setting, home care agency, and to the staff of a community free health clinic.

Prior to scheduling the first client, potential customers received an open house invitation to tour the new office location. Invitations were sent to all potential customers as outlined previously as well as business advisors and faculty from the CNS program. Signage listing the name of the new business was placed in strategic locations inside and outside on building marquees. Advertisements announcing the new practice were placed in the community newspaper each week for approximately 3 months, then monthly for another 3 months. Business cards were designed and printed and distributed to all potential customers.

CLIENT VISIT

The initial visit was usually 90 minutes in duration. During this visit, the client's health history was reviewed. The client was interviewed about the duration of diabetes, complications, comorbid diseases and conditions, current pharmacologic regimen, literacy level, and family history. An assessment was conducted with each client to include: (1) knowledge of diabetes; (2) concurrent and potential illness; and (3) culture, age-related factors, and lifestyle behaviors that influenced self-management strategies. Additionally, the client was interviewed about his/her diet plan, exercise routine, and nonpharmacologic treatment strategies. Self-monitored blood glucose and laboratory results were reviewed when available. A physical exam was conducted that included vital signs and neurologic and vascular exams of the lower extremities. Treatment, education, and self-management goals were discussed, and behavioral goals were mutually established with the client and family. Follow-up visits, ranging from 15 to 60 minutes in duration, included a review of the outcomes of self-management strategies, a physical exam, and a review of treatment and education goals.

A variety of nurse sensitive outcomes were used to measure the outcomes of the self-management sessions, including: knowledge; diabetes management; blood glucose control; diet; disease process; health behaviors; health resources; illness care; medication; preconception; pregnancy; treatment regimen; neurological status; nutritional status; risk control: cardiovascular health; sensory function: proprioception; sexual function; symptom control; tissue perfusion: peripheral; vital signs status; and weight control (Moorhead, Johnson, Mass, & Swanson, 2008).

A chart was established for each new patient. The chart contained the following documents: treatment consent form, physician's referral form, laboratory findings, medication sheet, personal and family history, initial visit history and physical summary, and follow-up visit encounter forms. The initial visit summary was dictated and the notes typed up at the end of the day. Eventually, as more clients were referred to the office, a medical transcriptionist was hired to transcribe dictations. All transcribed notes were reviewed and edited for accuracy. Copies of all notes were faxed to the referring physicians. All charts were maintained and kept in a locked filing cabinet.

OBTAINING PROVIDER NUMBERS, DETERMINING CHARGES, AND ESTABLISHING BILLING METHODS

In setting up the practice, a decision was made that it would be advantageous to clients to bill insurance companies for the CNS services. As a result of the previous hospital experience, it was estimated that 30% of the potential clients for the new diabetes office would have insurance coverage through a company insurance plan, 40% would be covered under Medicare, 20% covered by Medicaid (state coverage for the indigent), and 10% would be private pay. An application was completed to obtain provider numbers for Medicare and Medicaid early in the process of setting up the office. A meeting was scheduled with a local third-party insurance agency to provide an overview of my services and to apply as a provider. Additionally, an application was submitted to a large national insurance company that provided coverage in my region.

Charges for the self-management sessions were determined by a variety of methods. The current copy of the physician fee schedule was downloaded from the Internet, charges and reimbursement rates were discussed with my CNS mental health partner, and a voluntary survey was conducted with local providers. A flat rate charge was established for new clients. Charges for returning clients were based on time with increments of 15, 30, 45, and 60 minutes. Clients were advised of the charges in advance of the self-management session, and a handout of billing procedures was made available. A 20% copayment was collected at the time of each visit.

A detailed review of the American Medical Association (2006) *Current Procedural Terminology Coding Manual* was used to determine the evaluation and management codes appropriate for the CNS services. In order to facilitate billing, a superbill was developed that listed the specific code and associated charge. This superbill was used as a reference when billing the insurance company or client.

The Centers for Medicare and Medicaid Services (2007) professional paper claim form (CMS-1500) was completed for each self-management session. Initially, the billing forms were completed by hand and mailed to Medicare, Medicaid, and the appropriate insurance company. As the practice became busier, a billing software program that could function on a desktop computer was

purchased from a medical supply company. Eventually, a billing company was hired to manage the billing process, including completion of the 1500 form, submission to insurance companies, resubmission of bills as necessary, posting of payments, and billing of clients for outstanding balances. The billing company also directly billed private pay clients as well. The billing company handled notices to clients whose bills were in arrears and submitted bills to a collection agency as necessary. This process allowed me to concentrate on the provision of services and provided a degree of separation of the services from the payment issues.

CNS CORE COMPETENCIES RELATED TO PRACTICE INNOVATION

In my role as a diabetes CNS, I designed and implemented an innovative practice solution that provided diabetes self-management services to people with diabetes and their families in a community-based setting. I utilized nurse-sensitive outcomes to evaluate program and client outcomes. As a change agent, I advanced the practice of nursing among other nurses. Hospital staff nurses, home care nurses, and other advanced practice nurses, such as nurse practitioners and nurse midwives, contacted me for questions and routinely referred clients to my office. Additionally, I advanced the practice of nursing within a network of providers. Physicians from a variety of specialties, including obstetrics, family practice and internal medicine, routinely referred clients to my office for advanced practice nursing intervention. I interacted frequently with podiatrists, ophthalmologists, optometrists, and wound specialists to discuss issues and provide referrals.

PRACTICE INNOVATION OUTCOMES

The CNS diabetes practice was a successful endeavor in many ways. The number of client referrals increased over the years. Initially, client referrals were received from the five key physicians who were familiar with my services from the hospital. Eventually, providers from a variety of specialties referred clients to the practice, including obstetrics, family practice, internal medicine, orthopedics, surgery, and podiatry. Additionally, endocrinologists from surrounding communities began to refer clients. Nursing referrals were accepted when the primary care provider agreed to the referral. These referrals were initiated by nurses in the acute care setting, home care, public health, and nurse practitioner providers. The best source for referrals originated from the clients themselves by word of mouth. Clients routinely referred family, friends, and coworkers to the practice. The primary care physicians were usually agreeable to the word of mouth referrals; however, in the rare case when a referral was denied, the client was instructed to contact the regional hospital diabetes center.

Maximum reimbursement for charges was successfully obtained from Medicare and Medicaid, as well as the majority of insurance companies and clients. One large national insurance company that initially declined my request to become a provider eventually recruited me as a preferred provider. Over the years, the practice generated enough money to cover the operating expenses and my salary.

Although the CNS practice was very successful, I discontinued the practice after 8 years due to personal reasons. However, the business and marketing skills that were developed from the practice were invaluable for establishing my future entrepreneurial endeavor, a nurse-owned and operated wellness company.

REFERENCES

American Diabetes Association. (2007a). Diagnosis and classification of diabetes mellitus. *Diabetes Care, 30,* S42–S47.

American Diabetes Association. (2007b). Standards of medical care in diabetes. *Diabetes Care, 30,* S4–S35.

American Diabetes Association. (2007c). *Total prevalence of diabetes & pre-diabetes.* Retrieved October 1, 2007, from http://www.diabetes.org/diabetes-statistics/prevalence.jsp

American Medical Association. (2007). *Current procedural terminology: CPT professional* (2007 ed.). Chicago: Author.

Centers for Medicare & Medicaid Services. (2007). *Professional paper claim form (CMS-1500).* Retrieved October 1, 2007, from http://www.cms.hhs.gov/ElectronicBillingEDITrans/16_1500.asp

Moorhead, S., Johnson, M., Mass, M. L., & Swanson, E. (2008). *Nursing outcomes classification* (4th ed.). St. Louis: Elsevier Mosby Sanders.

National Association of Clinical Nurse Specialists. (2004). *Statement on clinical nurse specialist practice and education* (2nd ed.). Harrisburg, PA: Author.

Improving Outcomes With a Rapid Response Program

Victoria Church

PRACTICE OVERVIEW

As a clinical nurse specialist (CNS) in a Veterans Affairs (VA) hospital, I am one of two CNSs assigned to the medical-surgical wards in our facility. The Portland VA Medical Center (PVAMC) is a Magnet-designated facility that is academically affiliated with the Oregon Health and Sciences University (OHSU). Of our 104 medical-surgical beds, 54 have telemetry monitoring capabilities. An additional 20 beds are designated for inpatient psychiatry. There are 8 operating suites and 22 intensive care beds. Our emergency department (ED) is a Level II center, which is defined as a trauma center that in collaboration with a Level I center provides 24-hour comprehensive care of all essential specialties. The ED is a 19-bed unit that experienced 27,800 visits and 7,867 inpatient hospital discharges in 2006.

The surgical ward population includes general, vascular, orthopedic, neurological, urological, bariatric, thoracic, and/or cardiac surgery patients. Surgical programs also include liver and kidney transplants. The medical ward population includes patients with acute and chronic cardiac, pulmonary, neurological, renal, and metabolic diseases. PVAMC also has an active cardiac and vascular interventional program. Currently, the population of veterans at PVAMC is primarily geriatric with a very high number of co-morbidities. Predominant comorbidities include coronary artery disease (CAD), congestive heart failure (CHF), chronic obstructive pulmonary disease (COPD), and diabetes. These coexisting disease states in a geriatric population mean that high acuity and complex patients present on our four medical-surgical wards. The patient population carries

with it the additional risk of cognitive challenges, especially in light of the presence of post-traumatic stress disorder (PTSD) in many of the veterans. Nationally, the VA patient population is also undergoing change as many younger veterans and an increasing number of female veterans are entering into the system.

As a CNS in this setting, my core goal is to improve patient outcomes. Integral components of my role are: assessing multiple levels of systems; identifying problems at the staff, patient, and system levels; developing and implementing corrective action plans; and evaluating outcomes. I am also available for clinical consultation by all team members and lead educational sessions for staff on a variety of topics related to our patient population and programs. Direct patient care may be performed during my consultative process or during the mentorship of staff in acquiring specific skills.

At PVAMC there is an active CNS committee where the 13 CNSs from across the system work together on projects and network within and outside of our hospital system. As a core member of our CNS team, I assist with coordinating our monthly Nursing Grand Round series. Our CNS group, as a method of integrating evidence into practice, implemented Evidenced Based Fact Sheets within our facility. In addition to serving on the CNS committee, I serve as chair and am a member of multiple committees within the hospital. I also represent the VA nationally by serving as a cochair of the VA Rapid Response System Initiative.

My professional membership in the American Association of Critical Care Nurses (AACN), Sigma Theta Tau, and the Society of Medical Surgical Nurses facilitates my currency on local and national resources.

Membership in online services with organizations such as the Institute for Healthcare Improvement (IHI), the National Database for Nursing Quality Indicators (NDNQI), the National Center for Patient Safety, and the National Guideline Clearing House are essential to staying up to date on research and practice standards.

PROBLEM IDENTIFICATION

Early identification and intervention for patients experiencing clinical deterioration can prevent the patient proceeding to arrest and decrease the mortality associated with cardiopulmonary arrest (Bellomo, 2003; Buist & Bernard, 2002; Kerridge & Saul, 2003). When the system and/or team fail to identify clinical deterioration and the patient arrests, the episode is defined as "failure to rescue" (FTR) (Institute of Healthcare Improvement, 2004). Another definition of FTR is when the staff identifies the patient who is clinically deteriorating, but is unable to obtain timely interventions or resources resulting in the patient arresting. Since 1986, researchers and clinicians have identified cases in which 66% to 84% of patients exhibit signs of clinical deterioration 6 to 8 hours prior to cardiopulmonary arrest (Franklin, 1994; Schein, 1990). In these and subsequent studies the respiratory system has been shown to be the leading body system involved in clinical deterioration among hospitalized patients (Franklin, 1994; Hillman, Bristow, & Chey, 2001; Schein, 1990). In 2004, the IHI, along with the Joint Commission, identified FTR as the number one contributor to hospital deaths. They further identified programs developed for early recognition and intervention of decompensation for hospitalized patients in a medical-surgical environment that could save up to 45 lives per hospital per year. Therefore, the establishment of rapid response programs became one of the primary targets of the 100,000 lives campaign (IHI, 2004).

Shortly after being hired (2003), I recognized a pattern of being called to the bedside at the beginning of the day shift to work with staff on a patient who had become unstable. Frequently, these patients had been deteriorating throughout the night shift but had not been moved to the intensive care unit (ICU). Being familiar with the concept of FTR, it was clear to me that an assessment of the frequency and characteristics of FTR in our veteran population was necessary. A review of the literature and creation of a form that delineated the criteria of FTR aided in the process of patient identification and establishment of a baseline FTR incidence rate. Any patient who had transferred from a medical-surgical unit to the ICU or had experienced code team activation was evaluated against the criteria. A review of 6 months' of data revealed a baseline incidence of 6 to 8 FTR cases a month from a total of 90 medical-surgical beds. In terms of body systems involved in the FTR,

respiratory decompensation was the leading source, followed in turn by cardiac and neurological decompensation. These findings are consistent with national data related to body system involvement in FTR. Chart reviews of the causative factors of the FTR incidences revealed that lack of early recognition of patient decompensation attributed to 40% of the cases, and failure to obtain resources for the decompensating patient attributed to the remaining 60%.

GOALS FOR PRACTICE INNOVATION

It became very clear during the review and participation in FTR cases that the team member pivotal to identifying early signs of decompensation was the bedside nurse on the medical-surgical unit. These registered nurses (RNs) are key to a successful prevention program because they provide direct patient care and 24-hour-a-day surveillance. In addition, early access to clinical resources and early intervention was identified as the second pivotal link essential to impacting FTR. The key players for this link at PVAMC were identified as the primary physician team as well as the medical-surgical and ICU charge nurse and respiratory therapy. Once the model was developed, the outcome goal was identified by improved patient outcomes evidenced by a decrease in cardiac and respiratory arrest as well as a decrease in the incidence of FTR.

INNOVATION SPECIFICS

In the literature, factors that contribute to FTR are grouped into three categories: (1) failure to communicate, (2) failure to assess or plan, and (3) failure to identify cardinal signs of deterioration. Complete assessments of contributing factors at PVAMC could then be grouped into these categories and were prioritized by the nursing staff and leadership. Action plans were established for each item, and a model was selected that identified the medical-surgical RN as the key link in the early identification phase of the model. Success of the program required the involvement of staff from both the medical-surgical wards as well as the ICU in all aspects of assessment, planning, implementation, and evaluation of the project. To paraphrase a method chosen by Peter and William Bridges, known for creating change within organizations, active involvement in the entire process brings far greater success in sustaining change and in creating a true change in culture within the organization (Bridges, 2003; Senge, Kleiner, Ross, Roth, & Smith, 1999).

Focus groups were held with bedside staff, charge nurses, and nursing managers of each medical-surgical unit as well as with the charge nurses and nursing management of the ICU. More then 12 key strategies to reduce FTR were identified and then prioritized. The top five were selected for developing implementation plans to: (1) improve the assessment skills and expand the scope of assessing nursing shifts on the wards; (2) improve communication between the wards and ICU; (3) establish 24/7 clinical resources for ward RNs; (4) establish educational programs related to FTR, resource utilization, communication, and cardinal sign identification; and (5) change the source of ICU bed availability from the nonclinical bed control personnel.

Key strategy number one, implementing a plan to improve assessment skills, included soliciting staff from each medical-surgical ward to review best practice and specialty literature regarding our population of veterans. A total of 55 staff participated in the process and divided into body system groups to identify what should be assessed and documented for each system. I worked with our computer applications personnel to translate this information into a computerized shift assessment note that the group tested and refined. The goal of the template was to standardize the assessment components and documentation as well as provide a charting method that would allow data extraction.

Key strategy number two focused on improving communication between the medical-surgical wards and ICU. An essential component was establishing a system to communicate ICU bed availability to the ward. The charge nurses in ICU agreed on a system whereby the medical and surgical charge nurses would contact the ICU charge nurse directly about any patients experiencing cardinal signs of change. If the patient could not be stabilized on the ward, the information related to bed availability could then be communicated directly with the ward team. Previously, the process was to have the ward team contact a nonclinical individual in bed control to ascertain ICU bed availability.

As the CNS facilitating this project, I had to assess all possible system options or processes that could provide key strategy number three: round the clock access to a clinical resource for the ward staff working with a patient experiencing cardinal signs of decompensation. Without monetary resources to hire additional staff to provide this service, existing options were explored. Ideally, this service is provided by a formalized rapid response team (RRT). The code committee was approached to discuss the development of a RRT and to redefine when the code team could be called.

At the initial presentation, the code committee did not agree with the proposed RRT program or recommended changes. The rationale at that time was that the system had not seen an increase in codes, and FTR was a new term to the committee. Resistance was compounded by the fact that as a new CNS in

the organization and the first of two unit specific CNSs, I did not have established credibility within the organization.

With input from nursing staff and leadership, it was determined that initially the clinical resource for the ward staff would be the ICU charge nurse. The ICU charge nurses agreed that, when called about a medical-surgical patient who was experiencing cardinal signs of deterioration, the ward staff could request a bedside review of the patient by the ICU charge nurse as well as by a respiratory therapist from the ICU. Of note, in our facility at the time of this project, respiratory therapists were located only in the ICU and responded to the wards upon request. When reviewing the literature related to RRT programs, hospitals across the country were using various team groupings. The literature included teams composed of only ICU RNs to those composed of a full complement of ICU personnel, including physicians. It was determined that we would call this a nursing specific RRT or consultative program and have the members of our team include the ICU charge nurse and respiratory therapist.

Key strategy number four, an educational program targeted to the medical-surgical RN, was driven by chart reviews of FTR occurrences. These reviews indicated content needed to focus on definitions and incidences of FTR, cardinal signs for each prominent body system (respiratory, cardiac, and neurological), as well as delineation of resources, team notification, and communication. Part one consisted of in-services for the ward RNs of the previously mentioned content and review of two case scenarios. Reference sheets were developed for the key cardinal signs and resources available to the medical-surgical wards. The ICU charge nurses participated in inservices regarding FTR, resource role, communication, and goals of early identification and treatment. Part two included mock scenarios of a respiratory decompensation patient and was mandatory for all ward RNs and certified nursing assistants (CNAs). The ICU charge nurses were invited to attend a session to become familiar with the content being taught and to reinforce their availability and openness to being a resource.

Once key strategies had been agreed upon, it was a matter of systematically implementing them. All five components were initiated within a 30-day time frame in June 2004.

EVALUATION AND OUTCOMES

Prior to implementation, the medical-surgical and ICU staff chose the end point of success for the rapid response program to be measured by changes in the incidence of FTR. The staff also felt it was important to collect anecdotal feedback from the wards and ICU regarding whether communication was perceived as improving between the ward and ICU when a patient had experienced deterioration.

Three months after implementation, an assessment revealed the incidence of FTR had declined from the baseline of between six to eight a month to only one per month. The one incident per month that remained was consistently that of a patient identified as exhibiting cardinal signs, but for whom timely patient transfer was made impossible by a lack of ICU bed availability. The incidence of FTR continued to remain at one per month for the next 6 months, during which time we began to address ICU throughput, improving shift report and transfer (hand-off) report as well as several other previously identified factors that can contribute to FTR. Of note, the incidence of code team responses decreased by 80% in the medical-surgical wards 3 three months of our initial interventions. To share our successes, I provided a lecture at Nursing Grand Rounds and wrote up our process and results for the hospital executive team. Shortly after the presentation, I was invited to a code committee meeting and asked to join the group. Since that time, we have developed an excellent partnership that has implemented a formalized RRT group to include our senior ICU resident.

Finally, our facility was recently selected at a national VA level as a best practice example for initiation of a successful rapid response program. This selection has led to my participation on a VA wide national panel whose goal is to establish tools and implementation strategies that other VA hospitals could utilize to establish rapid response programs.

REFERENCES

Bellomo, R. (2003). A prospective before-and-after trial of a medical emergency team. *Medical Journal of Australia, 179,* 293.

Bridges, W. (2003). *Managing transitions: Making the most of change* (2nd ed.). Cambridge, MA: Da Capo Press.

Buist, M. D., Moore, G. E., & Bernard, S. A. (2002). Effects of a medical emergency team on reduction of incidence of mortality from unexpected cardiac arrests in hospital: Preliminary study. *British Medical Journal, 324,* 387.

Franklin, C., & Mathew, J. (1994). Developing strategies to prevent in hospital cardiac arrest: Analyzing responses of physicians and nurses in the hours before the event. *Critical Care Medicine, 22*(2), 244.

Hillman, K. M., Bristow, P. J., & Chey, T. (2001). Antecedents to hospital deaths. *Journal of Internal Medicine, 31,* 343.

Institute for Healthcare Improvement. (2004). *Rapid response team how-to guide.* Retrieved January 11, 2009, from http://www.ihi.org/ihi

Kerridge, R. K., & Saul, W. P. (2003). The medical emergency team. Evidence based medicine and ethics. *Medical Journal of Australia, 179*(6), 313.

Schein, R. M. (1990). Clinical antecedents to in-hospital cardiopulmonary arrest. *Chest, 98,* 1388.

Senge, P., Kleiner, A., Roberts, C., Ross, R., Roth, G., & Smith, B. (1999). *The dance of change: The challenges to sustaining momentum in learning organizations.* New York: Broadway Books Publishing.

Specialty Practice Organizations in Nursing

Academy of Medical-Surgical Nurses
East Holly Avenue, Box 56
Pitman, NJ 08071-0056
Phone: 866-877-AMSN
E-mail: AMSN@ajj.com
Web site: http://www.medsurgnurse.org

Specialty:
Medical-surgical

Basic Certification:
Certified Medical-Surgical
Registered Nurse (CMSRN)

Advanced Certification:
None

Certifying Organization:
Medical-Surgical Nursing Certification Board

Academy of Neonatal Nursing
2220 Northpoint Parkway
Santa Rosa, CA 95407-7398
Phone: 707-568-2168
E-mail: None
Web site: http://
www.academyonline.org

Specialty:
Neonatal

Basic Certification:
None

Advanced Certification:
None

Certifying Organization:
N/A

Air and Surface Transport Nurses Association
7995 East Prentice Avenue, Suite 100
Greenwood Village, CO 80111
Phone: 800-897-NFNA (6362)
E-mail: astna@gwami.com
Web site: http://www.astna.org

Specialty:
Emergency

Basic Certification:
Certified Emergency Nurse (CEN)
Certified Flight Registered Nurse (CFRN)
Certified Transport Registered Nurse (CTRN)

Advanced Certification:
None

Certifying Organization:
American Board of Nursing Specialties (ABNS)

American Academy of Ambulatory Care Nursing
East Holly Avenue, Box 56
Pittman, NJ 08071-0056
Phone: 800-262-6877
E-mail: aaacn@ajj.com
Web site: http://www.aaacn.org

Specialty:
Ambulatory

Basic Certification:
Ambulatory Care Nursing
Certification (RN-BC)

Advanced Certification:
None

Certifying Organization:
American Nurses Credentialing Center (ANCC)

American Academy of Nursing
555 East Wells Street, Suite 1100
Milwaukee, WI 53202-3823
Phone: 414-287-0289
E-mail: info@aannet.org
Web site: http://www.aannet.org

Specialty:
General

Basic Certification:
None

Advanced Certification:
None

Certifying Organization:
N/A

American Assembly for Men in Nursing, The
PO Box 130220
Birmingham, AL 35213
Phone: 205-802-7551
E-mail: aamn@aamn.org
Web site: http://www.aamn.org

Specialty:
General

Basic Certification:
None

Advanced Certification:
None

Certifying Organization:
N/A

American Association of Critical-Care Nurses
101 Columbia
Aliso Viejo, CA 92656-4109
Phone: 800-899-2226
E-mail: info@aacn.org
Web site: http://www.aacn.org

Specialty:
Critical care

Basic Certification:
Critical Care Registered Nurse
(CCRN: adult, neonatal, pediatric)
Progressive Care Certified Nurse (PCCN)
Cardiac Medicine Certification (CMC)
Cardiac Surgery Certification (CSC)

Advanced Certification:
Acute/Critical Care Clinical Nurse Specialist (CCNS)
Cardiac Medicine Certification (CMC)
Cardiac Surgery Certification (CSC)

Certifying Organization:
AACN Certification Corporation

American Association of Diabetes Educators
100 W. Monroe Street, Suite 400
Chicago, IL 60603
Phone: 800-338-3633
E-mail: aade@aadenet.org
Web site: http://www.aadenet.org

Specialty:
Diabetes

Basic Certification:
Certified Diabetes Educator (CDE)

Certifying Organization:
National Certification Board for
Diabetes Educators (NCDBE)

Advanced Certification:
Board Certified in Advanced
Diabetes Management (BC-ADM)

Certifying Organization:
American Association of Diabetes
Educators (AADE) and
American Nurses Credentialing Center (ANCC)

American Association of Legal Nurse Consultants
401 N. Michigan Avenue
Chicago, IL 60611
Phone: 877-402-2562
E-mail: info@aalnc.org
Web site: http://www.aalnc.org

Specialty:
Legal

Basic Certification:
Legal Nurse Consultant Certified (LNCC)

Advanced Certification:
None

Certifying Organization:
American Legal Nurse Consultant
Certification Board (ALNCCB)

American Association of Managed Care Nurses
4435 Waterfront Drive, Suite 101
Glen Allen, VA 23060
Phone: 804-747-9698
E-mail: keads@aamcn.org
Web site: http://www.aamcn.org

Specialty:
Managed care

Basic Certification:
None

Advanced Certification:
None

Certifying Organization:
N/A

American Association of Neuroscience Nurses
4700 W. Lake Avenue
Glenview, IL 60025
Phone: 888-557-2266 (U.S. only)
Phone: 847-375-4733
E-mail: info@aann.org
Web site: http://www.aann.org

Specialty:
Neuroscience

Basic Certification:
Certified Neuroscience Registered
Nurse (CNRN)

Advanced Certification:
None

Certifying Organization:
American Board of Neuroscience Nursing (ABNN)

**American Association of
Nurse Attorneys, The**
PO Box 515
Columbus, OH 43216-0515
Phone: 877-538-2262
E-mail: taana@taana.org
Web site: http://www.taana.org

Specialty:
Legal

Basic Certification:
None

Advanced Certification:
None

Certifying Organization:
N/A

**American Association of
Occupational Health Nurses**
2920 Brandywine Road, Suite 100
Atlanta, GA 30341
Phone: 770-455-7757
E-mail: None
Web site: http://www.aaohn.org

Specialty:
Occupational health

Basic Certification:
None

Advanced Certification:
None

Certifying Organization:
N/A

**American Association of Spinal
Cord Injury Nurses**
c/o Paralyzed Veterans of America
801 Eighteenth Street, NW
Washington, DC 20006-3517
Phone: 800-555-9140
E-mail: info@pva.org
Web site: http://www.pva.org/

Specialty:
Neuro

Basic Certification:
None

Advanced Certification:
None

Certifying Organization:
N/A

American Holistic Nurses Association
323 N. San Francisco Street, Suite 201
Flagstaff, AZ 86001
Phone: 800-278-2462
E-mail: info@ahna.org
Web site: http://www.ahna.org

Specialty:
Holism

Basic Certification:
Holistic Nurse—Certified (HN-C)

Advanced Certification:
Advanced Holistic Nurse—Certified (AHN-C)

Certifying Organization:
American Holistic Nurses'
Certification Corporation

**American Nephrology
Nurses' Association**
East Holly Avenue, Box 56
Pittman, NJ 08071-0056
Phone: 888-600-2662
E-mail: anna.webeditor@inurse.com
Web site: http://www.annanurse.org

Specialty:
Renal

Basic Certification:
Certified Nephrology Nurse (CNN)
Certified Dialysis Nurse (CDN)

Advanced Certification:
Certified Nephrology Nurse (CNN)

Certifying Organization:
Nephrology Nursing Certification Commission (NNCC)

**American Nurses Association
American Nurses Credentialing Center
American Nurses Foundation**
8515 Georgia Avenue, Suite 400
Silver Spring, MD 20910-3492
Phone: 800-274-4ANA (4262)
Phone: 1-800-284-CERT (2378)
E-mail: Various, see http://nursingworld.org/
FunctionalMenuCategories/ContactUs.aspx
Web site: http://www.nursingworld.org

Specialty:
Credentialing

Basic Certification:
Registered Nurse-Board Certified (RN-BC):
Ambulatory Care Nursing
Cardiac Rehabilitation Nurse
Cardiac Vascular Nurse
College Health Nurse
Community Health Nurse
Case Management Nurse
Gerontological
High-Risk Perinatal Nurse
Home Health Nurse
Informatics Nurse
Maternal-Child Nurse
Medical-Surgical
Nursing Executive
Nursing Professional Development
Pain Management
Pediatric Nurse

School Nurse
Psychiatric and Mental Health

Advanced Certification for the CNS:
Advanced Practice Registered
Nurse-Board Certified (APRN-BC):
Adult Health
Adult Psychiatric and Mental Health
Child/Adolescent Psychiatric & Mental Health
Diabetes Management
Gerontological Pediatric
Public/Community Health
Advanced Certification for Other:
Diabetes Management—Advanced
Nurse Executive—Advanced
Public Health Nursing—Advanced

Certifying Organization:
American Nurses Credentialing Center (ANCC)

American Nursing Informatics Association
1908 S. El Camino Real, Suite H
San Clemente, CA 92672
Phone: None
E-mail: web@ania.org
Web site: http://www.ania.org

Specialty:
Informatics

Basic Certification:
Certified Professional in Health
Information Technology (CPEHR)
Certified Professional in Electronic
Health Records (CPHIT)

Advanced Certification:
None

Certifying Organization:
Health IT Certification

American Organization of Nurse Executives
1 N. Franklin Street, 32nd Floor
Chicago, IL 60606
Phone: 312-422-2800
E-mail: aone@aha.org
Web site: http://www.aone.org

Specialty:
Administration

Basic Certification:
None

Advanced Certification:
None

Certifying Organization:
N/A

American Psychiatric Nurses Association
1555 Wilson Boulevard, Suite 602
Arlington, VA 22209

Phone: 866-243-2443
E-mail: Various, see http://www.apna.org/i4a/pages/index.cfm?pageid=3291
Web site: http://www.apna.org

Specialty:
Mental Health

Basic Certification:
None

Advanced Certification:
None

Certifying Organization:
N/A

American Society for Pain Management Nursing
PO Box 15473
Lenexa, KS 66285-5473
Phone: 888-34A-SPMN (342-7766)
E-mail: aspmn@goamp.com
Web site: http://www.aspmn.org

Specialty:
Pain management

Basic Certification:
Registered Nurse-Board Certified,
Pain Management (RN-BC)

Advanced Certification:
None

Certifying Organization:
American Nurses Credentialing Center (ANCC)

American Society of PeriAnesthesia Nurses
10 Melrose Avenue, Suite 110
Cherry Hill, NJ 08003-3696
Phone: 877-737-9696
E-mail: aspan@aspan.org
Web site: http://www.aspan.org

Specialty:
Anesthesia

Basic Certification:
Certified Post Anesthesia Nurse (CPAN)
Certified Ambulatory Perianesthesia
Nurse (CAPA)

Advanced Certification:
None

Certifying Organization:
American Board of Nursing
Specialties (ABNS)

Association for Professionals in Infection Control and Epidemiology
1275 K Street, NW, Suite 1000
Washington, DC 20005-4006
Phone: 202-789-1890
E-mail: apicinfo@apic.org
Web site: http://www.apic.org

Specialty:
Infection control

Basic Certification:
Certified in Infection Control (CIC)

Advanced Certification:
None

Certifying Organization:
Certification Board for Infection Control
and Epidemiology (CBIC)

**Association for Radiologic and
Imaging Nursing**
7794 Grow Drive
Pensacola, FL 32514
Phone: 866-486-2762
E-mail: ARIN@dancyamc.com
Web site: http://www.arna.net

Specialty:
Radiology

Basic Certification:
Certified Radiology Nurse (CRN)

Advanced Certification:
None

Certifying Organization:
Radiologic Nursing Certification Board (RNCB)

Association for Vascular Access (AVA)
5526 West 13400 South, Suite 229
Herriman, UT 84096
Phone: 877-924-AVAI (2821)
E-mail: info@avainfo.org
Web site: http://www.avainfo.org

Specialty:
Vascular

Basic Certification:
None

Advanced Certification:
None

Certifying Organization:
N/A

**Association of Nurses in AIDS
Care (ANAC)**
3538 Ridgewood Road
Akron, OH 44333
Phone: 800-260-6780
E-mail: anac@anacnet.org
Web site: http://www.anacnet.org

Specialty:
Medical-surgical

Basic Certification:
AIDS Certified Registered Nurse (ACRN)

Advanced Certification:
Advanced AIDS Certified Registered Nurse (AACRN)

Certifying Organization:
HIV/AIDS Nursing Certification Board (HANCB)

**Association of Pediatric Hematology/
Oncology Nurses (APHON)**
4700 W. Lake Avenue
Glenview, IL 60025-1485
Phone: 847-375-4724
E-mail: info@aphon.org
Web site: http://www.aphon.org

Specialty:
Oncology

Basic Certification:
Certified Pediatric Oncology Nurse (CPON)

Advanced Certification:
None

Certifying Organization:
Oncology Nursing Certification Corporation

**Association of Perioperative
Registered Nurses (AORN)**
2170 S. Parker Road, Suite 300
Denver, CO 80231
Phone: 800-755-2676
E-mail: custsvc@aorn.org
Web site: http://www.aorn.org

Specialty:
Perioperative

Basic Certification:
Certification in Perioperative Nursing (CNOR)
Certified Registered Nurse First Assistant (CRNFA)

Advanced Certification:
Certified Registered Nurse
First Assistant (CRNFA)

Certifying Organization:
Competency & Credentialing Institute (CCI)

Association of Rehabilitation Nurses
4700 W. Lake Avenue
Glenview, IL 60025
Phone: 800-229-7530
E-mail: info@rehabnurse.org
Web site: http://www.rehabnurse.org

Specialty:
Rehabilitation

Basic Certification:
Certified Rehabilitation Registered Nurse (CRRN)

Advanced Certification:
None

Certifying Organization:
Rehabilitation Nursing Certification Board (RNCB)

**Association of Women's Health,
Obstetric and Neonatal Nurses (AWHONN)**
2000 L Street, NW, Suite 740
Washington, DC 20036

Phone: 800-673-8499
E-mail: customerservice@awhonn.org
Web site: http://www.awhonn.org

Specialty:
Women's health

Basic Certification:
None

Advanced Certification:
None

Certifying Organization:
N/A

Case Management Society of America (CMSA)
6301 Ranch Drive
Little Rock, AR 72223
Phone: 501-225-2229
E-mail: cmsa@cmsa.org
Web site: http://cmsa.org

Specialty:
Case management

Basic Certification:
Accredited Case Manager (ACM)
Certified Case Manager (CCM)
Certified Disability Management Specialist (CDMS)
Case Management Administrator Certification (CMAC)
Care Manager Certified (CMC)
Certified Managed Care Nurse (CMCN)
Certified Orthotist (CO)
Certified Occupational Health Nurse (COHN)
Certified Prosthetist (CP)
Certified Prosthetist-Orthotist (CPO)
Certified Professional in Disability Management (CPDM)
Certified Professional in Healthcare Quality (CPHQ)
Certified Professional in Utilization Management (CPUM)
Certified Professional in Utilization Review (CPUR)
Certified Rehabilitation Counselor (CRC)
Certified Rehabilitation Registered Nurse (CRRN)
Certified Social Work Case Manager (CSWCM)
Health Care Quality and Management (HCQM)

Advanced Certification:
Continuity of Care Certification – Advanced (A-CCC) Certified Advanced Social Work Case Manager (CASWCM)

Certifying Organization:
Specific to particular certification; see http://cmsa.org/Individual/Education/Accreditation
Certification/tabid/209/Default.aspx

Dermatology Nurses Association (DNA)
15000 Commerce Parkway, Suite C
Mt. Laurel, NJ 08054
Phone: 800-454-4362
E-mail: DNA@dnanurse.org
Web site: http://www.dnanurse.org

Specialty:
Dermatology

Basic Certification:
Dermatology Nurse Certified (DNC)

Advanced Certification:
None

Certifying Organization:
American Board of Nursing Specialties (ABNS)

Developmental Disabilities Nurses Association (DDNA)
PO Box 536489
Orlando, FL 32853-6489
Phone: 800-888-6733
E-mail: None
Web site: http://www.ddna.org

Specialty:
Disabilities

Basic Certification:
Registered Nurse Certification in Developmental Disability Nursing (CDDN)

Advanced Certification:
None

Certifying Organization:
DDNA Certification Committee

Emergency Nurses Association (ENA)
915 Lee Street
Des Plaines, IL 60016-6569
Phone: 847-460-2630
E-mail: bcen@ena.org
Web site: http://www.ena.org

Specialty:
Emergency

Basic Certification:
Certified Emergency Nurse (CEN)
Certified Flight Registered Nurse (CFRN)
Certified Transport Registered Nurse (CTRN)

Advanced Certification:
None

Certifying Organization:
American Board of Nursing Specialties (ABNS)

Endocrine Nurses Society (ENS)
PO Box 211068
Milwaukee, WI 53211
Phone: 414-421-3679
E-mail: endo.nurses@sbcglobal.net
Web site: http://www.endo-nurses.org

Specialty:
Endocrine

Basic Certification:
None

Advanced Certification:
None

Certifying Organization:
N/A

Hospice and Palliative Nurses Association (HPNA)
One Penn Center West, Suite 229
Pittsburgh, PA 15276-0100
Phone: 412-787-9301
E-mail: hpna@hpna.org
Web site: http://www.hpna.org

Specialty:
Palliative care

Basic Certification:
Certified Hospice and Palliative Nurse (CHPN)
Certified Hospice and Palliative Licensed Nurse (CHPLN)

Advanced Certification:
Advanced Certified Hospice and Palliative Nurse (ACHPN)

Certifying Organization:
National Board for Certification of Hospice and Palliative Nurses (NBCHPN)

Infusion Nurses Society
315 Norwood Park South
Norwood, MA 02062
Phone: 781-440-9408
E-mail: ins@ins1.org
Web site: http://www.ins1.org

Specialty:
General

Basic Certification:
Certified Registered Nurse Infusion (CRNI)

Advanced Certification:
None

Certifying Organization:
Infusion Nurses Certification Corporation (INCC)

National Association of Orthopedic Nurses (NAON)
401 N. Michigan Avenue, Suite 2200
Chicago, IL 60611
Phone: 800-289-NAON (6266)
E-mail: naon@smithbucklin.com
Web site: http://www.orthonurse.org

Specialty:
Orthopedics

Basic Certification:
Orthopedic Nurse Certified (ONC)

Advanced Certification:
Orthopedic Clinical Nurse Specialist Certified (OCNS-C)

Certifying Organization:
Orthopedic Nurses Certification Board (ONCB)

National Gerontological Nursing Association (NGNA)
7794 Grow Drive
Pensacola, FL 32514

Phone: 800-723-0560
E-mail: ngna@dancyamc.com
Web site: http://www.ngna.org

Specialty:
Gerontology

Basic Certification:
See ANCC

Advanced Certification:
See ANCC

Certifying Organization:
American Nurses Credentialing Center (ANCC)

National League for Nursing (NLN)
61 Broadway, 33rd Floor
New York, NY 10006
Phone: 800-669-1656
E-mail: generalinfo@nln.org
Web site: http://www.nln.org

Specialty:
General

Basic Certification:
None

Advanced Certification:
Certified Nurse Educator (CDE)

Certifying Organization:
NLN's Certification Governance Committee

National Nursing Staff Development Organization (NNSDO)
7794 Grow Drive
Pensacola, FL 32514
Phone: 800-489-1995
E-mail: nnsdo@dancyamc.com
Web site: http://www.nnsdo.org

Specialty:
Staff development

Basic Certification:
See ANCC

Advanced Certification:
See ANCC

Certifying Organization:
American Nurses Credentialing Center (ANCC)

Oncology Nursing Society (ONS)
125 Enterprise Drive
RIDC Park West
Pittsburgh, PA 15275-1214
Phone: 866-257-4ONS (4667)
E-mail: customer.service@ons.org
Web site: http://www.ons.org

Specialty:
Oncology

Basic Certification:
Oncology Certified Nurse (OCN)
Certified Pediatric Oncology Nurse (CPON)
Certified Breast Care Nurse (CBCN)

Advanced Certification:
Advanced Oncology Certified Nurse
Practitioner (AOCNP) Advanced Oncology
Certified Clinical Nurse Specialist (AOCNS)

Certifying Organization:
Oncology Nursing Certification Organization

Society of Otorhinolaryngology and Head-Neck Nurses (SOHN)
202 Julia Street
New Smyrna Beach, FL 32168
Phone: 386-428-1695
E-mail: info@sohnnurse.com
Web site: http://www.sohnnurse.com

Specialty:
Ear, nose, throat

Basic Certification:
Certification in Otorhinolaryngology and
Head-Neck Nursing (CORLN)

Advanced Certification:
None

Certifying Organization:
National Certifying Board of Otorhinolaryngology
and Head-Neck Nurses

Society of Pediatric Nurses (SPN)
7794 Grow Drive
Pensacola, FL 32514
Phone: 800-723-2902
E-mail: SPN@dancyamc.com
Web site: http://www.pedsnurses.org

Specialty:
Pediatrics

Basic Certification:
See ANCC

Advanced Certification:
See ANCC

Certifying Organization:
American Nurses Credentialing Center (ANCC)

Society of Urologic Nurses and Associates (SUNA)
East Holly Avenue, Box 56
Pitman, NJ 08071-0056
Phone: 888-827-7862
E-mail: CBUNA@ajj.com
Web site: http://www.suna.org

Specialty:
Genitourinary

Basic Certification:
Certified Urologic Registered Nurse (CURN)
Certified Urologic Associate (CUA)

Advanced Certification:
Certified Urologic Nurse Practitioner (CUNP)
Certified Urologic Clinical Nurse Specialist (CUCNS)
Certified Urologic Physician's Assistant (CUPA)

Certifying Organization:
Certification Board for Urologic Nurses
and Associates (CBUNA)

Society for Vascular Nursing (SVN)
203 Washington Street, PMB 311
Salem, MA 01970
Phone: 888-536-4SVN (4786)
E-mail: svn@administrare.com
Web site: http://www.svnnet.org

Specialty:
Vascular

Basic Certification:
See ANCC

Advanced Certification:
See ANCC

Certifying Organization:
American Nurses Credentialing Center (ANCC)

Wound, Ostomy and Continence Nurses Society (WOCN)
15000 Commerce Parkway, Suite C
Mt. Laurel, NJ 08054
Phone: 888-224-WOCN (9626)
E-mail: info@wocncb.org
Web site: http://www.wocn.org and http://
www.wocncb.org/ (Certification Board)

Specialty:
General

Basic Certification:
Certified Wound, Ostomy and
Continence Nurse (CWOCN)
Certified Wound Care Nurse (CWCN)
Certified Ostomy Care Nurse (COCN)
Certified Wound Ostomy Nurse (CWON)
Certified Foot Care Nurse (CFCN)

Advanced Certification:
Advanced Practice CWOCN (CWOCN-AP)

Certifying Organization:
Wound, Ostomy, and Continence Nursing Certification Board
(WOCNCB)

Index